Modern

Herbal
Medicine

by
Steven Horne, Registered Herbalist (AHG)
and
Thomas Easley, Registered Herbalist (AHG)

The School of Modern Herbal Medicine
dba of Kether-One, Inc

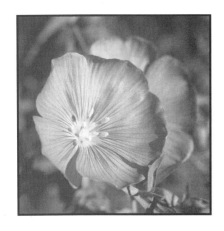
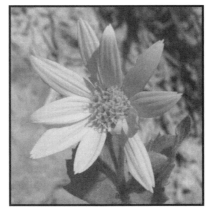
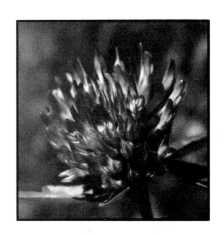

Important Notice

This material is for educational purposes only. It is not intended to replace the services of licensed health care providers. Always obtain competent medical advice for all serious or persistent illness. If you use any of the procedures in this material to treat any disease in yourself or others without the assistance of licensed health care providers, you are doing so at your own risk.

This book is solely the work of the authors and The School of Modern Herbal Medicine and was not authorized by or endorsed by any of the companies whose products are discussed in this book. The authors and publisher are solely responsible for the contents, and have no financial connections to these companies.

Although we have made an effort to make the information contained herein as up-to-date and accurate as possible, there are constant adjustments in company's product lines. New products are added, old products are discontinued and ingredients may change. Please check labels and company websites for possible changes.

Alternative Health/Wellness
ISBN: 978-1-890855-21-5

Published and Distributed by

The School of Modern Herbal Medicine
modernherbalmedicine.com
P.O. Box 911239
St. George, UT 84791
800-416-2887

10 9 8 7 6 5 4 3 2

Table of Contents

Dedication by Thomas Easley

This book, or at least my half of it, is dedicated to my wife Terrie, who put up with me writing nonstop during our first year of marriage. I'd also like to thank my teachers, Rhonda, Phyllis and Steven, for showing me the power that Nature can have in healing. A special thanks goes to all of my family and friends for being mostly-willing test subjects of many horrible tasting concoctions and elixirs. Finally, I'd like to thank the thousands of people who have trusted me to help them find their healing path. Being a small part of their healing process is a sacred trust that I honor and appreciate more than words can describe.

Acknowledgements by Steven Horne

Many people have worked to make this book a reality.
We wish to give special thanks the following people who
contributed their efforts to this book:
Data entry: Kenneth Hepworth, Garret Pittaro,
David Tanner, Amanda Steiner
Editing and proofreading: Leslie Lechner,
Kimberly Balas, Phyllis Light, David Horne
Cover design, layout and programming: David Horne

The photos on the cover are (from left to right): flax flowers, arnica (heart-leafed) and red clover. You can read about these and other herbs in the Key Herbs Section of this book. Flax and arnica photos by Steven Horne; red clover photo is from photos.com.

Introducing Modern Herbal Medicine

Herbal medicine always has been, and always will be, the medicine of the people. For thousands of years human beings have survived on this planet because medicinal plants have been readily available to everyone. In fact, until a few generations ago, most parents and grandparents knew many home remedies and were able to treat common ailments without the aid of medical doctors. Herbal remedies have always been readily and freely available, to anyone who knew how to gather and prepare them.

Today, few people have this knowledge today and most of what people know about herbs is based on marketing hype or shallow information provided by mainstream media. Even those who do have the knowledge of how to pick and prepare their own herbal remedies often find it hard to do so because they live in urban environments, which makes gathering their own herbs difficult. Do-it-yourselfers can purchase bulk herbs to make their own teas, decoctions, tinctures or capsules, but many people just don't have the time to do this because they are busy with families, jobs and other priorities.

This is why the modern herb industry fulfills an important need. It allows people to "harvest" their herbal remedies from their local health food store or other retailer. These commercial herbal products are already packaged in a wide variety of convenient dosage forms, including: tea bags, capsules, tablets, alcohol tinctures, glycerin extracts and topical preparations. The only problem the consumer faces is trying to figure out which herbal remedies are right for them.

Unfortunately, herbal companies and health food store employees are restrained by law from making disease claims about their products, even if these claims are truthful. The only claims that can be made are vague *structure/function* claims, such as "this herb is good for your immune system" or "helps maintain healthy joints."

So, in order to figure out what supplements they need people either have to visit a knowledgeable herbalist or do their own research in third-party literature. Which brings us to the purpose of this book. We designed it to help people figure out which readily-available herbs and herbal formulas may be of benefit to them.

This would be a simple job if herbs had a one-to-one correlation with medical diagnosis. In other words, if we could put together a simple "cookbook" that said, "if you have arthritis take this" and "if you have a headache take that," our task would be a simple one. Unfortunately, herbal medicine can't be reduced to such simple statements.

Working on Root Causes

What most people know about herbal remedies is limited to some very narrow and often misleading information. For instance, they may have heard that ginkgo is for memory, saw palmetto helps with benign prostatic hyperplasia (BPH) and St. John's wort is for depression. These ideas contain an element of truth, but they represent a weak symptomatic approach to using herbs.

Let's take St. John's wort for example. While it can be helpful for depression, most professional herbalists would not consider it the only, or even the best, antidepressant remedy in the plant kingdom. But the problem runs deeper than this. Depression is not really a disease; it is a symptom that can arise from many different root causes. Trying to directly treat depression without identifying why it is there is not what real herbalism is about.

A knowledgeable herbalist (or any other well-trained practitioner) wants to look past the symptom to see its underlying cause. In the case of depression, is it arising from the intestines, the liver, low thyroid or just a person's current life situation? And these are just a few of the possible causes. Depending on the cause, ginkgo, damiana, black cohosh, kava kava or a dozen other remedies might be more appropriate, and more effective, than St. John's wort.

Furthermore, St. John's wort isn't really an anti-depressant, per se, at least not in the way an anti-depressant drug works. Like all herbs it has multiple actions and affects multiple body systems. For starters, it is a nervine that calms anxiety and anxiety-related depression. It also aids repair when nerves have been damaged, is antiviral and is also helpful for healing damaged intestinal mucosa. In short, St. John's wort isn't a "magic bullet" for a particular disease. It is a complex remedy that works on many underlying issues in multiple diseases.

So, this book is designed to help you start thinking like a well-trained herbalist, rather than just applying herbs for symptomatic relief. It provides you with several tools to help you do this.

First, in the *Conditions Section* of this book you'll find descriptions of 471 common health problems. Where possible, we differentiate probable underlying causes of these conditions. This allows you to select potential remedies based on root causes instead of trying to directly treat the condition or its symptoms.

This information is not just information gathered from books. Between them, the authors have 50 years of combined experience in working with clients, as well as connections with other experienced clinical herbalists. So, the insights are based on real-life experience with actual health problems in clients or the clinical experience of other trusted herbalists.

Second, we provide you with a *Therapies Section* containing 33 basic therapies that work on these underlying or root causes. These root causes give rise to multiple disease symptoms. These basic therapies are listed with the various conditions they may help to resolve.

These basic therapies are important, and the first resource a person should turn to in trying to get well. They are important because the body systems do not work in isolation from one another. Thus, you may perceive yourself as having multiple diseases, but these multiple conditions are likely arising from common root causes. As a famous herbalist of the early 1800s, Samuel Thomson, said, "Remove the cause and the effect will cease." So, as you look up various conditions you are working with, you may find that there are common underlying causes. This means these problems are likely interconnected and need to be treated as a whole.

Finally, we also introduce you to the idea of herbal energetics. All traditional systems of herbalism rely on energetic models to help a person select the remedies that are appropriate for them. Most professional modern herbalists use these systems as well. In the beginning of the book we provide you with an easy-to-understand Western energetic model and then give you the energetics of the single remedies throughout this book to help you choose what herb(s) are appropriate for a given situation.

The reliance on energetic systems is not because herbalists are trying to be mystical or obscure. Instead, energetics are helpful metaphors for explaining the broad patterns of illness that herbs are best used to correct. Rather than looking at isolated disease symptoms, we are looking at patterns of symptoms. This approach matches the broad-acting benefits of herbal remedies better than the symptom→disease→treatment system typically used in modern medicine.

Single Herbs versus Herbal Formulas

This brings us to the second major purpose of this book. Most herb books focus primarily on single herbs. If they do discuss formulas, they are the formulas specific to a single herbalist or company.

Ironically, it's harder for a beginner to see results with single herbs than it is with well-crafted herbal formulas. It's the difference between using a rifle and a shot-gun. Using single herbs is like using a rifle. It has a lot of power, but you have to know how to aim it properly to hit the target. Single herbs work best when the person's overall condition matches the overall characteristics of the herb. In other words, they work best when the person has multiple symptoms or issues that closely match the overall pattern of health issues addressed by that herb.

A formula, on the other hand, is like a shotgun. You may not hit the target with as much concentrated force, but your aim doesn't have to be as good. This is because an herbal formula combines many herbs that work on multiple causes of a problem. Returning to the example of St. John's wort and depression, St. John's wort might help a person's depression IF it is the kind of depression that St. John's wort works best on (depression related to anxiety and intestinal problems).

However, if we mix several herbs together that work on several different underlying causes of depression, a person is more likely to get at least some benefit. This is partially because the formula is composed of herbs that address multiple potential root causes of a problem. It is also partly because the synergy of the ingredients often enhances the basic action, and because the multiple ingredients tend to counteract some of the other effects of the single herbs, which also lessens the chance of the remedy throwing the body out of balance in other ways.

To paraphrase Michael Moore, a famous southwestern herbalist, single herbs have subtle and deep actions. Combinations tone down those subtleties to a gray background noise and leave the predominate effects of the herb intact.

The Eclectics, a group of medical doctors who used herbs in the 19th century, emphasized utilizing the subtle effects of the herbs and matching all of a person's problems to one herb in their literature. However, most of the time, in actual practice, they resorted to tried and true formulas.

They, like many practitioners throughout recorded history, recognized that often times disease isn't subtle, it's in your face, and responds best to an herbal formula that addresses several aspects of the disease at the same time.

Traditional Chinese medicine (TCM) also relies heavily on formulas. Basic formulas are used for certain situations, with the ingredients being modified to fit individual needs. One can do a similar thing with commercial herbal formulas by taking a basic blend for a particular problem and also taking one or two more targeted single herbs or nutritional supplements at the same time.

This is why we focus heavily on herbal formulas available in the commercial marketplace. This book contains over 1200 herbal formulas from over 32 different herb companies. It also includes 239 single herbs, which are either available from those companies and/or are key herbs in the formulas. This means that you can readily find all of the herbal remedies discussed in this book at your health food store or online.

To make it easier to understand herbal formulas, we've categorized them into 102 product categories. This allows you to compare formulas with the same basic action or therapeutic purpose. You can easily compare differences in ingredients and dosage forms and look for an alternative to a favorite formula if you can't find it. We've not only explained how each of these categories of formulas can be used, we've also provided you with a list of key herbs to look for in these formulas (and highlighted those key herbs in the ingredient lists).

The goal is to help you to read the label for an herbal formula and have a good idea of what that formula might do based on the key ingredients it contains. Because different companies will often use different common names for the same herb, we've standardized the ingredient names to allow for easier comparison. This means that the name on the label may not exactly match name we use for the herb in the ingredient list, but it's the same plant.

One important note—it's nearly impossible for a book like this to be completely up to date because companies add and drop products regularly. They also change ingredients and product names occasionally. So, always check product labels carefully. If a particular formula has been discontinued, this book provides you with plenty of alternatives.

Will also provide additional information on the modernherbalmedicine.com website. Join our mailing list to be notified when we post more up-to-date information.

Herbs are Safe

A third objective for this book is to make people aware of the wide variety of very safe herbal products that are available in the marketplace. Mainstream media has caused many people to think that herbal medicine is somehow backward, unscientific and even dangerous. This is simply not true. Let's briefly examine the issue of the safety of herbal products.

First, modern herbal medicine is not primitive or unscientific at all. The body of scientific literature concerning herbs and herbal constituents is steadily growing as research on this topic is being carried out around the world. The companies we feature in this book are modern, high-tech companies. Many, if not most of them, have rigorous standards of quality control. Many of them employ qualified scientists, such as chemists and botanists, as well as experienced and well-trained herbalists, to ensure that their products are safe and reliable. You can learn more about each company in the *Companies Section* of the book.

In recent years strict GMPs (good manufacturing practices) have been established by the FDA for herbs and supplements. All major herb companies comply with these standards, which help ensure that the herbal products you purchase are safer than ever.

It is ironic that many people believe pharmaceutical drugs are safe, but herbs are dangerous. The public is led to believe that the FDA doesn't have the authority to remove unsafe products from the marketplace, which is not true. In fact, herbal products are actually held to a higher standard of safety than drugs.

Here's why we can make that claim. All drugs have some level at which they become toxic and therefore involve some measure of risk. Just listen to a TV ad for drugs and you'll hear a list of some of the common side-effects of a medication. This toxicity is considered acceptable because there is a risk/benefit ratio to a drug. If the benefits of the drug are believed to outweigh the risks of taking it, then the drug is considered safe.

In spite of the extensive testing that new drugs undergo, over half of them are removed from the marketplace within ten years due to dangerous side effects. There are also numerous documented cases of people dying from the side effects of prescription drugs each year.

In contrast, regulatory agents do not acknowledge any health benefits to herbal products. Therefore, there is no recognized risk/benefit ratio for herbal products or nutritional supplements. This means that it takes only a few documented cases of potential ill effects from an herb to cause it to be banned from the marketplace.

One example of this was the FDA ban on ephedra. When a number of "ephedra-related" deaths were reported in the media, the FDA banned the herb for sale in the United States. All of the deaths appear to have involved ephedra abuse, that is, taking doses of ephedra that greatly exceeded manufacturer recommendations for extended periods of time. The irony is that the principle active compound in ephedra, ephedrine, is still legal and is found in many over-the-counter medications for colds and weight loss, but herbal products which contain far smaller quantities of ephedrine have been banned.

In pointing this out, we want to make it clear that herbs are not without negative effects. It's just that their potential negative effects are generally far less serious than the potential negative effects of most prescription and non-prescription drugs. There are botanicals remedies that do have a potential for toxicity (and we have covered some of these in this book), but many useful remedies have already been lost due to the fact that regulatory agencies do not accept any risk/benefit associated with these remedies.

The bottom line is that the relative risk of suffering adverse effects from a modern commercially-prepared herbal product are minuscule compared to the risk of suffering adverse reactions to over-the-counter or prescription drugs. In our own experience, and the experience of other professional herbalists we know, adverse reactions to commercial herbal products are rare and when they do occur are usually limited to digestive upset, headaches, rashes or other reactions that people sometimes get from foods. We cover how to deal with these adverse reactions in more detail on page 16.

Herbs are Effective

Finally, we want to discuss the issue of efficacy. Do herbal remedies actually work? The answer is a qualified *yes*. The qualification is this—herbs work, but don't expect them to work like drugs. Allow us to elaborate.

Drugs are isolated chemical compounds and are used to rapidly relieve symptoms. Modern medicine is based on a rather straight-forward paradigm: Measure something in the body such as blood pressure, heart rate, cholesterol levels and so forth; determine that this measurement is out of normal range; then find a chemical compound that will push this measurement back into range.

Under this paradigm, if you have high blood pressure, you take a medication to lower it and you're cured. If you have high cholesterol, you take a medication to lower it and it's considered effective. If you have a pain, you take a drug to suppress it, and the problem is dealt with. If you expect herbs to act in the same way, you'll be disappointed. It's not that herbs can't ease symptoms, it's just that they're not generally as good at doing this as drugs are, and they work primarily by addressing underlying causes, not fixing symptoms.

In contrast to drugs, herbs are complex mixtures of substances with multiple layers of biological activity. Many times we know what some of the so-called "active" constituents are, but each herb contains thousands of chemical compounds (like the foods we eat). These compounds interact with the body in complex ways, acting simultaneously on multiple body systems and functions. They may not provide rapid symptomatic relief, but they can do something which drugs generally don't do—they can move the body back to normal function.

In traditional Chinese medicine, there is a concept of superior and inferior medicine. The medicines that produce rapid symptomatic relief are considered inferior medicines. Superior medicines are slow acting tonics that gradually help to restore the body to health and normal function. In our society, we reverse this. We think that superior medicine is anything that produces a rapid, demonstrable change in symptoms (like Western drugs) and that remedies which slowly act to restore health (like most herbs) are weaker, inferior remedies.

As we'll discuss in the next section, *How to Use This Book*, we believe the Chinese are correct. When you correctly use herbs as tools to restore general health and resolve the underlying causes of disease, you'll generally get good results. If you try to use them for rapid, symptomatic relief, you'll probably be disappointed. This brings us back to the primary reason we wrote this book. A well-designed herbal formula contains many herbs that act on the body in multiple ways to gradually bring the body back to health. Our goal is to help you find the herbal formulas (and single herbs and nutritional supplements) that will help you achieve this goal.

Wishing you the best of health,

Steven Horne and Thomas Easley

How to Use This Book

How to put together an effective health program that addresses the root causes of illness, instead of just treating symptoms

Modern medical care isn't health care; it's disease care. It focuses on disease treatment and symptomatic relief, not on building health. As a result, people have been trained to think in terms of treating specific diseases, or seeking instant relief from annoying symptoms. People carry this attitude with them when they start using herbs and nutritional supplements. They want to use natural products as alternatives to drugs and expect supplements to achieve the same results—rapid symptomatic relief.

Unfortunately, that isn't what natural healing is all about. So, before you look up any health problem or ailment in the *Conditions Section* of this book and try to figure out how to "treat" that ailment naturally, please read this introductory material. It will not only help you get the most out of this book, it will also maximize your chances for success in improving and maintaining your health.

Remove the Cause

The following fictitious story illustrates the basic problem people encounter with modern medical care.

There was once a carpenter who was a little clumsy. He regularly hit his thumb with his hammer. Soon, his thumb became very swollen and inflamed. He went to a doctor who said, "That finger is badly inflamed, let me write you a prescription for an anti-inflammatory."

The man took the medication and noticed that it helped the thumb a little, but because he kept striking it with the hammer, it continued to get worse. The pain was becoming difficult to bear. So the man went to another doctor. This one prescribed a painkiller.

The painkiller really helped take the pain away, but it also made the man's fingers a little numb so that he wound up hitting his thumb more than ever. Soon the thumb was very raw and badly damaged. So, the man sought out a third doctor, a surgeon, who said, "That thumb is badly diseased,

I think we should cut it off before it damages the rest of the body."

Finally, the man went to an herbalist, who took a case history and suggested the man find a different job, since he was obviously too clumsy to be a good carpenter. The carpenter became a salesman and his thumb started to heal without drugs or surgery.

Although the causes of most people's health problems are much more subtle than this, the story illustrates the problem of treating the effect (symptom) without removing the cause. Unfortunately, much of what we encounter in modern medicine is exactly that—treating the symptom without removing the cause. The medical mindset is often oriented towards this symptomatic relief without investigating deeper into what's underneath the symptom.

The first thing one needs to understand if one wants to get consistent, effective results with natural health care is that natural health care isn't about easing symptoms. It's about dealing with root causes. As the herbalist Samuel Thomson, an herbalist who lived in the early 1800s, put so succinctly, "Remove the cause and the effect will cease."

A Holistic Model of Disease

To help people understand how to get to the root causes of disease, we use a model we call The Disease Tree™. The idea for this model came from the writings of Samuel Thomson, who used a systematic approach to treating disease that he summarized in a short poem in his book, *New Guide to Health*. Part of that poem reads:

Let names of all disorders be,
Like to the limbs, joined to the tree,
Work on the root, and that subdue
And all the limbs will bow to you.
The limbs are colic, pleurisy,
Worms and gravel, gout and stone,
Remove the cause and they are gone.

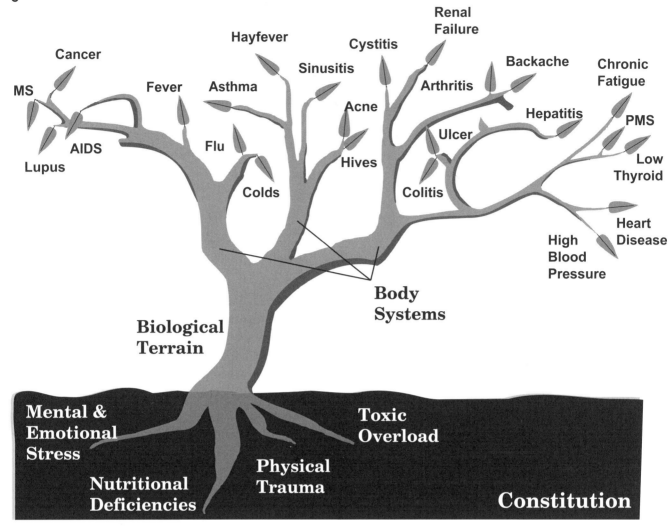

Figure 1—The Disease Tree™

Thomson's poetic metaphor helps us realize that focusing on specific disease symptoms is only attacking the "branches" of disease. Unless we work on the "roots" or underlying causes, the disease will simply get worse or manifest in a new form. Whenever a person takes a drug to relieve a symptom, or has some part of the body cut out, they are not being healed. To be healed is to be made whole, or in other words, to be restored to normal function or balance. Drugs and surgery only remove the branches. The root causes of the problem remain and will grow "suckers"—new diseases that will spring up in place of the old.

Most newcomers to natural health care are still thinking in terms of the symptom→disease→treatment model. They are looking for symptomatic relief. They want the branches of their disease tree to be pruned. Many inexperienced herbalists and natural health consultants try to accommodate this desire by recommending herbs and supplements to replace their medications; however, if the root causes are ignored, the results will be disappointing even if natural substances are used. In order to really correct the problem, a person has to shift his or her focus away from disease symptoms and begin looking at root causes.

Shown in Figure 1, The Disease Tree™ is a model you can use to help clients understand what good health is really all about. Many successful consultants are now using this model to explain what they are doing with their clients. Here is a brief breakdown of the elements in this model.

Soil—Constitution

The first element in the model is the soil, which represents our constitution. This is a person's innate physical and emotional makeup.

We all know that genetics play some role in our health. Heart disease, cancer, diabetes and other chronic ailments tend to run in families. Not all constitutional tendencies are genetically based, since people in the same family often have similar diets, lifestyles and emotional issues, which predisposes them to similar health problems.

Your constitution is what nature and early childhood have given you to work with. A person who has a strong constitution can handle more physical stress than a person with a weaker constitution. In other words, under the same physical conditions, one person may thrive, while another will become ill.

You can't do much about your genetics, but your genetics don't doom you to poor health. New research in the field of epigenetics is showing that the body has mechanisms for regulating genetic expression. Adopting a healthier lifestyle, including better nutrition and mental attitudes, can alter how your genes are utilized in the cells, thus improving your health and preventing you from getting illnesses to which you may be genetically prone.

Roots—Environmental Stress

The roots of disease are the environmental stresses that overwhelm the ability of the physical body to maintain balance. There are four basic root causes of disease, as follows.

1. Physical Trauma. The body can be mechanically damaged. All physical damage, from burns and frostbite to cuts, lacerations and broken bones, causes damage to organs and tissues that can result in disease. In fact, physical trauma, if not addressed appropriately, can lay the foundation for more serious diseases later in life. For example, a damaged joint is more susceptible to developing arthritis than a joint that was never subjected to trauma.

Trauma is something modern medicine is very good at treating, but natural medicine can also help. Nutrition and herbs can help tissues repair themselves more quickly and prevent injured areas from developing into chronic problems later in life.

Although this book is not a manual for trauma care, it does contain some suggestions for dealing with various types of injuries in the *Conditions Section*. The *Therapies Section* contains descriptions of how to do Compresses, Epsom Salt Baths and Poultices, which can help with healing physical trauma.

2. Toxic Overload. Mechanical damage isn't the only way the body can be injured. We can be bitten by a snake, stung by a bee, or encounter a bed of poison ivy, all of which introduce chemical poisons that damage tissues. While these are generally considered forms of physical trauma, the fact that these poisons injure our health shows us that toxins can also be a root cause of disease.

In modern society we are exposed to many potentially toxic chemicals in the form of food additives, pesticides, household cleaning products, cosmetics, heavy metals, solvents and petrochemicals, xenoestrogens, prescription drugs and other chemicals. Since World War II we have developed over 80,000 chemicals that are utilized in modern society.

These toxins are likely the root cause of many modern ailments, including the high rate of cancer, autoimmune diseases and many neurological conditions such as autism and Alzheimer's disease. Reducing exposure to these substances and finding ways to help the body detoxify itself is an important component of treating many modern ailments.

Toxic waste can also come from within the body, which produces waste in the process of metabolism. This waste must be eliminated from the system or it will damage tissues. Adequate intake of water and fiber is essential to ridding the body of these wastes, but most people in modern society are dehydrated and don't get enough fiber. Damage to the eliminative systems can also contribute to a backlog of waste in the tissues. Whatever the reason, when wastes (or toxins) are not properly eliminated tissues are damaged and the roots of disease take hold.

We've listed a variety of therapies that can help deal with the root cause of toxicity in the Therapies Section. Examples include: Colon Cleanse, Drawing Bath, Fast or Juice Fast, Gall Bladder Flush, Heavy Metal Cleanse and Sweat Bath. These detoxification therapies are referred to under health problems they may apply to in the *Conditions Section*.

3. Nutritional Deficiencies. The body needs nutrients in order to function correctly. When essential nutrients are not present in a person's diet the body does not have what it needs to stay healthy. If levels of these nutrients are low, the body may not be able to efficiently resist other environmental stresses.

There are two main reasons most people in modern society are nutritionally deficient. The first is that they consume empty calories in the form of highly processed and refined foods such as refined sugar, high fructose corn syrup, white flour, processed vegetable oils, and canned and prepackaged foods. These foods provide calories, but are low in essential vitamins, minerals and phytonutrients needed to process and utilize those calories for energy and maintain tissue structures.

The solution is to eat more whole, natural foods that are minimally processed and refined, but even then, nutritional deficiencies can occur. Modern agricultural methods deplete the soil of minerals, resulting in produce that has reduced vitamin and mineral content. This is why some supplementation is often a necessity for people living in modern society, even when they eat whole foods.

All chronic illnesses probably involve nutrient deficiencies of one type or another. The bottom line is, a person must eat a healthy diet to avoid or recover from illness. Without a healthy diet, herbs and supplements will not be sufficient to ensure good health.

We've put together several basic therapies for dealing with the problem of nutritional deficiencies in the *Therapies Section* of this book. Examples include: Bone Broth, Gut Healing Diet, Low Glycemic Diet and Mineralization. These basic nutritional therapies are also referred to in the *Conditions Section* where they may be underlying causes of specific health issues.

We've also created a *Nutrients Section* where we cover 60 popular nutritional supplements (from 5-HTP to Zinc) that may address specific nutritional or biochemical imbalances that may be root causes of various ailments. These are also linked to the various health issues in the *Conditions Section*.

4. Mental and Emotional Stress. All of us encounter mental and emotional stress in relationships and life situations. Financial problems, marital problems and other emotional stresses also lay the foundation for disease. This critical root cause is often overlooked in both orthodox and alternative healing circles. People who continue to experience health problems no matter what they do, often have unresolved mental and emotional stress that must be dealt with before healing can occur. Approximately 50% of people's health issues can be related to unresolved mental and emotional stress. All serious chronic and degenerative diseases involve at least some stress component, so this aspect should always be addressed.

We also include therapies that work on the mental and emotional aspect of disease in the *Therapy Section*. Examples include: Affirmation and Visualization, Emotional Healing Work, Flower Essences and Stress Management. All of these are linked to conditions they may help to heal in the *Conditions Section*.

Disease as Disharmony

As these four environmental stressors overwhelm the capacity of a person's constitution to cope with them, the process of disease begins. This concept is expanded in Figure 2. Disease arises from the disharmony that results when our constitution cannot adapt or cope with our environment. The word "dis-ease" suggests this "lack of ease," which develops as these stresses overwhelm the adaptive mechanisms in the body.

This model of disease applies even to trauma. A young person slipping and falling on the ice might experience only a bruise, while an elderly person might fracture their hip. Disease is always a combination of constitutional factors (the internal strength and health of the body) interacting with environmental factors (nutrition, toxins, trauma and stressful circumstances).

Trunk—Biological Terrain

All of the cells of the body live in an internal "ocean" of lymphatic fluid, which is supplied from the blood stream. Just as the health of a plant depends on the health of the soil in which it is grown, so the health of our tissues depends on the composition of these bodily fluids, lymph and blood. An organic farmer knows that if he keeps the soil healthy, the plants he is growing will be healthy and resistant to insect damage and disease.

The fluid medium in which cells live is called the biological terrain and is represented by the trunk of the Disease Tree™. When our biological terrain is healthy, the cells of our body will be healthy—resistant to injury, infections and chronic and degenerative diseases.

All of the root causes of disease previously discussed have an adverse affect on the biological terrain. Just as there is only one trunk to the tree, the biological terrain represents the whole picture of a person's health. By helping to restore balance to the biological terrain, we will restore balance to the entire body.

There are six basic imbalances in biological terrain. Unlike modern reductionist medicine that seeks to isolate tissues and organs and study them independently, the six tissue state imbalances describe broad patterns of imbalance that can influence multiple systems and are fundamentally interconnected.

The six basic imbalances are irritation (heat), depression (cold), stagnation (dampness), atrophy (dryness), constriction (tension) and relaxation (atonic). These six imbalances can occur in combination (such as irritation and constriction or dampness and depression). Once you understand the basic imbalances you will be able to identify the more complex mixtures of imbalance.

The tissue states are uniquely suited to form the framework of using herbs for medicine because, like the tissue states and their description of broad imbalances, herbs also

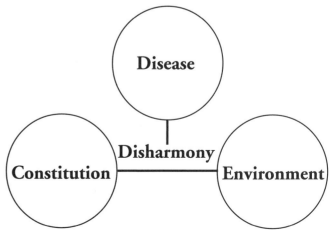

Figure 2—Disease as Disharmony

are broad acting in nature. While there are a few exceptions, most herbs have a multitude of chemical constituents that act on multiple areas of the body and through numerous mechanisms of action. Herbs, and the precise ways they act in the body, are so complicated that we truly understand the mechanisms of action of only a handful of herbs. This isn't a bad thing, because many diseases are very complicated and the current understanding of the exact process of disease is also lacking in many areas.

By moving away from a reductionist model of understanding disease, and seeing disease for what it really is—a breakdown of the interconnected mechanisms maintaining balance in the person's mind, body and spirit—we can more easily recognize the value of herbs and their complex actions.

When thinking about tissue states it is helpful to consider them not as stand-alone issues, but in comparison to other people and other tissue states. It is easy to describe a hot day if you live in an area that has cold days. But the subjective experience of a hot day is quite different for someone living in Hawaii than it is for someone living in Alaska. In a similar manner, the tissue states are easiest to identify if you have observed them in a large number of people.

This type of comparison is easy when you realize that the six tissue states represent three pairs of opposing qualities. To get a better idea of the tissue states, compare two people side by side and look at each set of qualities. Which is more hot, which more cool? Which one is dry, which one moist? Which is more tense, which is more relaxed? This will help you to grasp the concept.

This model of six tissue states was developed by a professional herbalist named Matthew Wood. You can learn more about it by reading *The Practice of Traditional Western Herbalism*. It is also found in his two-volume work *The Earthwise Herbal*. Here is a basic description of these three pairs of opposite qualities.

Energy Production

Irritation and *Depression* have to do with metabolism and energy generation. In irritation energy production is excessive; in depression it is deficient.

Irritation has a strong correlation to oxidation, inflammation and fever, which is why it is often referred to as "heat" in traditional herbalism. Tissues that are irritated are red and warm to the touch. Irritation is often accompanied by sharp pains. A red tongue, a rapid pulse, a ruddy (or reddish) complexion and hyperactivity are also signs of heat or irritation.

Irritation is often caused by chemical, infectious or metabolic irritants. In response to the irritant, the tissues increase their production of energy to throw off the irritant. Irritation (inflammation) is also the mechanism by which cells initiate the healing process. Part of the job of the inflammatory response is to destroy damaged cells and draw immune and stem cells to the area for tissue repair. Acute irritation isn't a bad thing; it's when that irritation becomes chronic that problems arise.

Irritation is treated herbally with cooling and moistening remedies. Directly cooling remedies are often anti-inflammatory and/or antioxidant. Often they are plants with a sour taste (like berries). Indirect cooling remedies or secondary cooling remedies are moistening remedies that typically have a slimy or mildly sweet taste. In our list of the energetic properties of an herb, we refer to remedies that reduce irritation as *cooling*.

Depression is the opposite of irritation. Tissues that are depressed are cool to the touch and pale, which is why it is often referred to in traditional herbalism as "cold." If pain is present it is usually dull and achy. Other signs of tissue depression are hypoactive function, a pale complexion, a pale tongue and a slow pulse rate.

Tissue depression is tricky to treat because it can be mimicked by a false cold, caused by low thyroid function and anemia. Infection in depressed tissues can also give rise to a "false heat." The key to identifying a general state of tissue depression is to look for a general feeling of fatigue, a pale or dark purple tongue and a slow pulse rate.

True tissue depression is treated herbally with warming remedies. These remedies are generally stimulating to circulation and/or metabolism. They are typically aromatic and/or pungent, qualities found in most kitchen spices. We refer to herbs that counteract tissue depression as *warming* in our list of an herb's energetic qualities.

It's important to understand that you aren't going to help balance the body if you treat a hot (irritated) condition with warming herbs, or a cold (depressed) condition with cooling herbs. So, pay attention to the energetics of the condition and select remedies with the correct properties.

Some herbs are neutral or balancing in their effects on energy production. We have labeled these remedies as *neutral* in their energetics.

Minerals and Fluids

Stagnation and *Atrophy* have to do with the balance between the solid (mineral) components of the body and the fluid (water and fat) components in the body. In stagnation, there is too much fluid with insufficient minerals to move it. In atrophy, the mineral content is too high and there is not enough fluid to keep it in solution.

Stagnation can be seen when fluid accumulates in tissues. This can take the form of edema, swollen lymph nodes and sluggish flow of body fluids. In traditional herbalism, stagnation is often called "dampness." Tissues that have stagnation are soft and spongy or hard and swollen to the touch. The tongue will be pale and damp and the pulse feels congested or slippery.

Stagnation was called *torpor* by the Eclectic physicians of the late 1800s and early 1900s. Herbs that removed this stagnation were called alteratives and have also been called blood purifiers. Generally speaking, herbs with a bitter taste fall into this category. Herbs that have this quality are listed as being *drying*.

Atrophy is seen when tissues become hard and brittle. With a loss of good fats and water, tissues become hard and inflexible or brittle. Traditional herbalism often refers to this tissue state as "dryness." Many of the diseases of aging have this quality, such as bone spurs, the formation of arterial plaque, the stiffness of arthritis and the loss of elasticity in the lungs in emphysema. The dry wrinkled skin associated with aging and the brittle bones of osteoporosis are other examples of atrophy. The tongue tends to be dry and withered, and the pulse becomes thin and weak.

Herbs used to treat conditions of atrophy are sometimes called tonics, because they help to revitalize people when they become weak or sickly. Remedies for atrophy include many herbs with a slightly sweet or bland flavor, such as ginseng. Demulcents or mucilaginous herbs (we call them mucilants for short) are also useful for conditions of atrophy. We refer to these herbs as *moistening* in our list of an herb's energetic properties.

Again, it won't be helpful to use drying herbs with atrophy or moistening herbs with stagnation. However, some remedies actually help to balance the solids and liquids within the body. These could also be referred to as neutral, but to avoid confusion we have referred to them as *balancing* in our herbal energetics section.

Tissue Tone

The final pair of opposing imbalances has to do with muscle tension or tone. Muscles act as gates in the body to control the flow of energy and fluids. When muscles tense, flow is reduced or obstructed. Conversely, when tissue is damaged, or muscle tone becomes too relaxed, fluids can drain or leak from tissues. Constriction is the tissue state where muscles are overly tight and relaxation is where muscles are overly relaxed or tissues are damaged and leaking.

Constriction typically happens because muscles get tired from overuse. A muscle expends energy when it contracts, and it rebuilds an energy charge when it relaxes. When muscles fatigue, either due to excessive use or nutritional deficiencies, they spasm. This can not only cause sharp pain and constricted movement, it can also obstruct flow. Examples of conditions involving constriction include some cases of high blood pressure, tension headaches, asthma attacks and a spastic colon.

Conditions involving constriction can periodically relax causing the "dam" to break and excessive flow or secretion to occur. Alternating diarrhea and constipation, alternating fever and chills and migrating pains are examples of this. These are called "wind" disorders in some traditional systems of medicine.

Antispasmodics are the herbal remedies that are helpful for conditions of constriction. These remedies are generally acrid in flavor, although some nervines that are aromatic or slightly bitter also have this quality. We use the term *relaxing* to describe these remedies in our listings of an herb's energetic properties.

Relaxation is when tissues are unable to hold fluids due to damage or loss of muscle tone. Examples of this include diarrhea, leaky gut, excessive mucus production, bleeding, urinary incontinence and excessive sweating.

Herbs containing tannins are used to tighten tissues and stop excessive drainage. These herbs are called astringents and have a slightly bitter and drying taste. We refer to remedies with this property as *constricting* under the herbal energetic listings.

Quick Key to Herbal Energetics

Here, in summary, is how the energetic qualities of herbs balance the biological terrain.

Cooling herbs reduce **irritation** and excess heat.

Warming herbs relieve **depression** and cold.

Neutral herbs are neither warming nor cooling.

Drying herbs treat **stagnation** and water retention.

Moistening herbs restore flexibility and tissue function in **atrophy**.

Balancing herbs help to bring tissues back to normal from either stagnation or atrophy.

Relaxing herbs ease muscle spasms and improve flow of energy and fluids by easing **constriction**.

Constricting herbs stop leakage by toning up tissue **relaxation**.

Nourishing herbs provide nutrients that help the body heal itself and restore normal function.

There is one final energetic property that sort of sits at the center and that is *nourishing*. Herbs that are nourishing in their energetic properties help to build up the body in general by providing nutrition that helps the body function normally.

Branches—Body Systems

The cells of our body need five things to survive—nutrients, water, oxygen, waste removal and a regulated temperature. When biological terrain is in balance, cells will have all of these needs met. In order to maintain this balance, which is called homeostasis, the body contains groups of specialized tissues that regulate the various requirements of homeostasis. These specialized tissues form organs and body systems.

The root causes of disease and the imbalances in biological terrain affect the structure and function of body systems so these systems are less able to perform their proper functions. This is where disease begins to manifest in the body. The major branches and limbs of The Disease Tree™ represent the body systems and tissues that are no longer able to help maintain homeostasis or normal biological terrain.

It is the malfunctioning body systems that eventually give rise to the specific disease symptoms we experience, so a major part of this natural healing model is to determine which body systems are affected. This allows you to use herbs, supplements and natural therapies that support the proper structure and function of these systems. This helps restore balance to the biological terrain, which helps a person recover and maintain health.

Besides having an effect on biological terrain, most herbs also have strong affinity for specific organs and tissues. These herbs become key herbs for certain imbalances within these body systems. This allows us to create categories of products based on their primary herbal ingredients. This categorization of products in the *Herbal Formulas* section is the most unique feature of this book.

Most of these product categories are linked to various systems of the body. Since malfunction of these body systems are involved in various disease states, we can link health problems in the *Conditions Section* to product categories in the *Herbal Formulas* section because these formulas contain key herbs for restoring health to the weakened body systems that are giving rise to the disease.

Here is a list of the body systems and the categories of products in the *Herbal Formulas* section to which they are linked. (Some categories fit in more than one system.)

Circulatory System: Cardiac Tonic, Cardiovascular Stimulant, Cholesterol Balancing, Hypotensive, Iron, Styptic/Hemostatic and Vascular Tonic Formulas.

Digestive System: Antacid, Carminative, Catnip and Fennel, Digestive Bitter Tonic, Digestive Enzyme, Digestive Tonic and Ulcer Healing Formulas.

Glandular System: Adaptogenic, Adrenal Tonic, Blood Sugar Reducing, Hyperthyroid and Hypothyroid Formulas.

Female Reproductive (Glandular) System: Female Aphrodisiac, Female Hormonal Balancing, Menopause Balancing, Menstrual Cramp, Nursing Aid, Phytoestrogen, PMS Relieving, Pre-Delivery, Pregnancy Tonic and Uterine Tonic Formulas.

Male Reproductive (Glandular) System: Male Aphrodisiac, Male Glandular Tonic and Prostate Formulas.

Hepatic System: Blood Purifier, Cholagogue, Cholesterol Balancing, General Detoxifying, Heavy Metal Cleansing, Hepatoprotective and Liver Tonic Formulas.

Immune System: Anti-Inflammatory, Antioxidant, Antibacterial, Anticancer, Antifungal, Antiviral, Cold and Flu, Drawing Salves, Ear Drop, Echinacea Blend, Essiac, Goldenseal & Echinacea, Immune Balancing, Immune Stimulating, Mushroom Blend, Sudorific and Topical Antiseptic Formulas.

Intestinal System: Anti-Diarrhea, Antiparasitic, Fiber Blend, Gentle Laxative, Intestinal Toning and Stimulant Laxative Formulas.

Lymphatic System: Blood Purifier, Echinacea Blend and Lymphatic Drainage Formulas.

Nervous System: Analgesic, Antidepressant, Antispasmodic, Brain and Memory Tonic, Brain Calming, Migraine/Headache, Nerve Tonic, Relaxing Nervine, Sleep and Topical Analgesic Formulas.

Respiratory System: Allergy-Reducing, Bronchialdilator, Cough Remedy, Decongestant, Drying Cough/Lung, Expectorant, Lung and Respiratory Tonic. Moistening Lung/Cough, Quit Smoking and Sinus Decongestant Formulas.

Sensory Systems: Eye Wash and Vision Supporting Formulas.

Structural System: Anti-Itch, Dental Health, Drawing Salves, Joint Healing, Mineral, Poultice. Skin Healing. Tissue Healing, Topical Analgesic, Topical Antiseptic and Topical Vulnerary Formulas.

Urinary System: Diuretic, Kidney Tonic, Lithotriptic and Urinary Infection Fighting Formulas.

The remaining categories, Anti-Alcoholic, Energy-Boosting, Exercise, Superfood and Weight Loss, are not linked to specific body systems. They address specific health issues or needs.

Since herbs work primarily by restoring balance to biological terrain and by strengthening weak body systems, you'll get much better results with them when you start looking beneath the disease symptoms to the underlying imbalances in biological terrain and weakened body systems. As you grasp this concept, you'll become much more effective at selecting appropriate remedies to restore balance to the body.

A more detailed and complete understanding of this approach to biological terrain and body systems is found in some of the courses we offer at modernherbalmedicine.com, particularly the *ABC+D Approach to Natural Healing* and the *Nature's Pharmacy* courses.

Product Categories and Biological Terrain

Besides linking product categories to body systems, it is also worth noting that a few of the product categories also address general biological terrain issues. These include:

Irritation: *Anti-Inflammatory* and *Antioxidant Formulas*

Depression: *Cardiovascular Stimulant* and *Carminative Formulas*

Stagnation: *Blood Purifier* and *Lymphatic Drainage Formulas*

Atrophy: *Female Glandular Tonic* and *Male Glandular Tonic Formulas*

Constriction: *Antispasmodic, Bronchialdilator* and *Relaxing Nervine Formulas*

Relaxation: *Styptic/Hemostatic* and *Vascular Tonic Formulas*

Twigs and Leaves— Specific Disease Symptoms

Finally, we come to the twigs and leaves of the Disease Tree™. These represent the specific diseases and their symptoms. As we have already suggested, most people are only concerned with the treatment of symptoms. Treating symptoms is like pruning the tree. You may be able to eliminate certain branches by suppressing specific symptoms with drugs or by removing diseased tissues with surgery, but these actions do little or nothing to eliminate root causes, bring the biological terrain back into balance, or restore the normal function of body systems. Symptomatic approaches certainly do nothing to strengthen constitution. Treating symptoms (like pain) can be an essential part of a healing program, but the primary goal should be to work on the root of the problem, providing symptomatic relief only to make the person more comfortable or stable during the healing process.

If we focus only on the leaves and twigs (the disease and symptoms), our efforts are misplaced. When a person is obese, diabetic, suffering from depression, high blood pressure, low thyroid and arthritis—things seem very complicated. But this complication only exists when we are looking at the situation from the perspective of disease symptoms. All of these conditions are arising from the same root causes, the same biological terrain and the same imbalanced body systems. The body does not exist in pieces; it exists as a whole, and all of these disease symptoms are simply part of the pattern of the whole.

The body is self-healing when provided with the right tools and environment. So, if we simply remove the environmental stressors that are overcoming the person's natural constitution and support weak body systems while balancing the biological terrain, the body will heal itself to the extent it is able to do so.

With this background, we can now explain how to use this book to help you address the root causes of many health problems, instead of just treating the symptoms.

Putting Your Program Together

When we're sick, we naturally want relief from our illness. This means we have to take a look at our life to discover what may be causing our problems and what we can do to bring the body back to balance. The *Conditions Section* helps you do this.

Conditions Section

When you look up a health problem in the *Conditions Section* you'll find a description of the problem, followed by some suggestions for approaching it using herbs and other natural healing techniques.

Where a particular symptom or problem can have many causes, we've tried to address the most common underlying causes and provide you with information that will help you determine if those causes may apply to the person who has this problem. For each potential cause, we list therapies and remedies that may be helpful. Some conditions list many options as possible remedies because there are many possible root causes.

If you have multiple health problems, look them all up and see if some of the same root causes and therapies show up repeatedly. This is a clue that these may be major underlying factors in your health issues.

Some conditions are serious and potentially life-threatening. In these cases, self-treatment is not wise. Where we encourage you to seek medical attention, *please do so*. Even if you opt to go the natural route for these problems, you should be monitored by modern medical testing to make sure you're on the right track.

You may also want to seek out the help of a qualified herbalist or naturopath for serious health issues. Unfortunately, just because someone calls themselves an herbalist or naturopath, it doesn't mean they are competent. One way to find a competent herbalist is to look for an herbalist who is a Registered Herbalist (RH) with the American Herbalists Guild (AHG). The AHG has a peer-review process to ensure herbalists meet a basic standard of competence. However, many highly qualified herbalists choose not to be members of the AHG. We are creating a database of herbalists online at *herbiverse.com* where you can search for competent herbalists using a variety of search criteria.

Under each condition you will also find the following information.

Related Conditions: These are other health problems that may be associated with or have similar root causes to the condition you are trying to resolve. These may be helpful in better understanding interrelated health problems.

Therapies to Consider: In the preceding pages, we've stressed the importance of working on root causes. The therapies listed under this heading do exactly that. So, before thinking about herbs and supplements, read about the recommended therapies listed under the condition. These therapies will help you address the root causes of that problem and should be your first approach to getting well. We have also indicated which root cause(s) a particular therapy addresses.

Herbal Formulas: These are the categories of herbal formulas that may be helpful for this condition. As previously indicated, these categories of formulas are restoring healthy structure and function to the imbalanced body systems underneath the disease and its symptoms. They also help to balance the biological terrain and may even help with some of the root causes. We've highlighted any formula categories that we feel are particularly helpful for each condition. Look these up in the *Herbal Formulas* section of the book.

Key Herbs: We've also listed single herbs that may be helpful for each condition. We've highlighted our favorite single herbs for each condition. When looking for appropriate herbal formulas, look for ones that contain several of the key herbs recommended for the condition.

Nutrients: In addition to herbal remedies, we've also listed some of the nutritional supplements that may be helpful for each condition. We've highlighted our favorites. Many formulas combine herbs and nutritional supplements, so this can also be a guide to finding the right formula for each condition.

Again, if you are working with multiple health conditions, look all of them up and note the Therapies to Consider, Herbal Formulas, Key Herbs and Nutrients for each. You will probably see some overlap. This will give you clues as to what you can do to balance the entire body and work on multiple conditions at the same time.

Therapies Section

After looking at the condition(s), consult the *Therapies Section* for diet and lifestyle changes that address the underlying causes of the health problems. This is a critical step in the healing process. Generally speaking, herbs and nutrients work best as part of an overall health program. They are called supplements because they are meant to supplement an otherwise healthy diet and lifestyle.

One of the fundamental problems with our modern approach to health care is the idea that we can pop a magic pill (drug, herb or supplement) and that's all we need. In actuality, if we adopt good general health habits, a large portion of health problems would clear up on their own. We realize that there are a lot of conflicting theories about what constitutes a healthy diet and lifestyle. This may be partially due to the fact that we're all a little different biologically and "one size does *not* fit all" when it comes to nutrition. However, what we're recommending are things we have found to be clinically effective.

Herbal Formulas Section

It would be impossible to directly link the 1200+ formulas listed in this book directly to the different conditions. We've solved that problem by dividing the formulas into categories. This section contains 102 product categories, which will help you narrow your search in finding a formula that will work for you.

We've classified these formulas based on their key herbs. Key herbs are herbs with certain major therapeutic actions that may also be very strong remedies for specific body systems. Formulas whose main ingredients fit the key herbs that define that product category were included even if the name of the product on the label didn't exactly match the name of the category.

Many formulas fit into more than one category and some categories are subdivisions of other categories. We've indicated where a category has related product categories, so you can also look for formulas under those related sections. The key herbs that define that category are also listed and these same key herbs are highlighted in the ingredient lists of the actual formulas. This will help you rapidly spot formulas that contain key herbs you are looking for.

Formulas are listed in alphabetical order by product name. Each formula has the following information associated with it.

Company Name: The name of the company that makes the formula appears in italics before the formula name. We've listed all the companies in *Company Appendix*, including contact information and a brief description of the company. We focused primarily on major brands found in most health food stores. There are many smaller companies whose products we had to leave out for the sake of space.

Dosage Form: Each listing also tells what dosage form the product comes in. Dosage forms include capsules, tablets, alcohol tinctures, glycerites, vinegar extracts, bulk powders, liquids, lotions, lozenges, oils, salves and ointments, softgels, sprays, syrups and teas. This allows you to look for appropriate dosage forms for you needs.

Here are some things to consider in selecting dosage forms. Small children can't swallow capsules, so look for dosage forms like alcohol-free extracts, syrups, glycerites or teas. Alcohol extracts can also be used for children, but we recommend avoiding them for children under two. If you do wish to use an alcohol extract for a child under the age of two, pour a small amount of boiling water in a cup and add the extract to the water. Let it stand for about 10 minutes to allow some of the alcohol to evaporate.

Liquid dosage forms often work faster than capsules or tablets because the flavor and aroma of the herb have a direct effect on the body through the nervous system. Many nervines work well as herbal teas, for instance, as the act of making the tea and sipping it helps remind a person to relax. Other remedies, like Digestive Bitters, also don't work well in capsules or tablets.

Many nasty tasting herbs work better in capsules because it's easier to get people to take them regularly. There are even liquid gel capsules available where you can get a liquid form of the herb, but swallow it in a capsule to mask the taste.

There are also topical preparations such as oils, salves and lotions, lozenges that can be sucked on for coughs and sore throats, and even sprays. So, consider which dosage forms will work best for the situation you are addressing.

Ingredients: There is a list of ingredients for each product. Any ingredient that is a key herb for that product category has been highlighted.

Be aware that we standardized the herb names when compiling ingredients for this book. The label may list the same ingredient under a slightly different name. We've tried to include all commonly used names for that herb in parenthesis after the main trade name the plant is sold under. All herbs are listed in the order they appear on the product label. This does not mean that the first ingredient is the main herb in the formula and the last herb is in the least amount. Some companies choose to keep their formulas proprietary and don't list ingredients by percentages.

Non-Herbal Ingredients: We list any non-herbal ingredients separately, since the focus of this book is on herbs. However, sometimes these non-herbal ingredients are an important part of that product category. We chose not to list formulas that were primarily nutritional supplements with herbs added. We list only formulas where herbs form the bulk of the ingredients.

Please note that companies change product names, ingredients and dosage forms on a regular basis. Because of this some discrepancies are expected. Always double-check the actual product labels before purchasing any product.

Key Herbs Section

The formulas in this book contain over 700 single herbs, many of which are very obscure. The 239 singles we selected for the *Key Herbs Section* were chosen because they are key herbs in various product categories or they are important herbs of commerce. In addition to a brief description of some of the basic uses of each herb, we provide the following information for each herb in the *Key Herbs Section*.

Latin Name(s): This is the scientific name or names of the plant being discussed.

Warnings: Here we list any cautions about the use of this herb. We were overly cautious about these warnings, especially regards to pregnancy. That is, we've never personally seen these herbs cause some of these problems, but we wanted to make you aware of any potential problems with that herb. Part of these warnings are contraindications (cases in which a remedy shouldn't be used).

Energetics: This refers to how the herb affects biological terrain as previously discussed. It shows if the herb is warming, cooling or neutral; drying, moistening or balancing; and/or constricting, relaxing or nourishing.

Properties: These are the major actions of the herb upon the body. The definitions for the properties used in this book can be found in *Properties Appendix*.

Key Herbs: We've indicated any product categories in which this single herb is a key ingredient. This helps you see how the herb is used in modern herbalism.

Companies: Finally, we've included a list of companies that sell the herb as a single. This will help you locate a source for the herb if you feel you need it. Some herbs are not sold as singles by any of the companies included in the book, but can be found as ingredients in herbal formulas.

Nutrients Section

The *Nutrients Section* contains information on 60 nutritional supplements which can also be useful for the various conditions in this book. We include a description of each nutrient and appropriate dosages. These nutrients are linked to the conditions for which they may be helpful.

We do not list particular brands or sources for these nutrients. Some of these supplements are offered by the companies in this book, but all of them are readily available in health food stores and online.

Tips for Using Herbs and Supplements

Here are some guidelines for selecting appropriate therapies, herbs and supplements for your health problems, (or the health problems of others).

Don't try to do too many things at once. It can be overwhelming to make too many dietary changes or to take too many supplements. If your plan feels burdensome or overwhelming, pare it down to something you can comfortably handle. Otherwise, you are unlikely to follow through with the program.

This includes limiting the herbs and supplements you pick. There seems to be an almost universal belief in our society that "if a little is good, more is better." This is rarely the case. We find that people who take too many herbs and nutritional supplements generally don't get good results. It's a good idea to start with no more than 2-4 formulas or supplements. If you take too many things it's difficult to tell what's working and what is not.

Monitor your progress. When you put a program together to resolve a health problem, you need to monitor progress. Try keeping a journal or log where you can make notes about changes you observe. For serious health problems we recommend working with a competent health practitioner. (You can search for one at *herbiverse.com*.)

How Quickly Should You See Results?

People have been told that herbs and supplements are slow acting, so they will often take an herbal formula or supplement for a month or more without seeing any results. Herbs and supplements work faster than that!

The perception that herbs and supplements work slowly is due to the difference between healing and symptomatic relief. Drugs generally offer rapid symptomatic relief, but rarely do they actually restore a person's health. Herbs and supplements may not offer rapid symptomatic relief, but they can actually restore a person's health.

Healing takes time. There is no instant relief when it comes to healing a wound or a broken bone. The process takes time. The same is true for healing from chronic or degenerative conditions. It can take months to experience substantial recovery; however, it doesn't take months to start seeing results.

Generally speaking, herbs actually work quite rapidly in terms of speeding the healing process. So, here's a general guide to when you should start seeing results.

- With acute conditions, such as colds, flu and minor injuries, you'll generally see improvement in anywhere from two to eight hours. If you see no improvement after 24 hours, what you're using probably isn't working. In this case, try something else. If the herb or supplement is helpful, you can take it until symptoms are gone and then generally for one to two more days to make sure everything has completely returned to normal.

- With chronic conditions, you will usually notice some improvement in 2-5 days if the herb or supplement is helpful. If you see no improvement after ten days, then the herb or supplement you are taking probably isn't going to work and you can re-evaluate and try something different. If the herb or supplement is helpful, then you can resume taking it and continue until the problem resolves itself. Once the problem is resolved, it is often helpful to continue taking it at a slightly lower dose for an additional 2-4 weeks. You will probably need to take the supplements for at least three to six months (and occasionally a year or two).

- If symptoms recur after discontinuing the product, you can start using the supplement again until symptoms subside. Then you may need to stay on a lower dose for several months to a year.

- With serious degenerative diseases, such as cancer, heart disease and diabetes, it may be hard to detect any subjectively noticeable improvement for a couple of weeks. This is why some type of objective monitoring is necessary to help determine if the program is working. If you see no improvement after four weeks, the program probably isn't working and needs to be re-evaluated.

Don't give up if you don't get it right the first time you try. Even well-trained, experienced practitioners don't always get a program right on the first try. In traditional Chinese medicine (TCM) it has been said that the first prescription is part of the diagnosis. The reason doctors "practice" medicine, is because they do the same thing. If their first prescription doesn't work, they re-evaluate and try something different. There's no harm in doing the same thing yourself, as long as you're using non-toxic herbs and supplements.

Adjusting Dosages

Herbal formulas will be accompanied by a manufacturer's suggested dose. Assume that this dose is meant for an average-sized adult (about 150 lbs.). If you are larger, you may need a slightly higher dose; smaller, you may need a lower dose. If you are sensitive to herbs, you may need to start with a lower dose.

If the herb or supplement is safe for children (and there is no suggested dose for children) adjust the dose by weight. So, for a 50 lb. child, take 1/3 of the suggested adult dose.

For smaller children take 1/4 of the recommended adult dose. For larger children adjust the dose upward.

Dosages with herbs are not as critical as they are with drugs because the potential for adverse reactions is much smaller. In addition, most manufacturer's recommend conservative, safe doses for the general public. In many cases you can safely double (or even triple) the recommended dosage. Still, when trying a new supplement it is a good idea to start with a smaller dose, make sure you tolerate the product well, and then adjust the dose upward if the supplement is having a positive effect but the dose isn't quite strong enough.

Dealing with Negative (Adverse) Reactions

We're all biochemically different and even with relatively safe herbs and supplements people will sometimes react negatively to a product. The most common adverse effects of herbs are digestive upset, nausea, diarrhea and headaches. Skin rashes can also occur. These reactions are not life-threatening. Some herbalists view these as "healing crisis" reactions, signs that the body is detoxifying and urge people to ignore these signs. We disagree.

Even if these signs are symptoms of detoxification, it means you're detoxifying too quickly. If these reactions occur, stop taking the herbs or supplements, drink lots of water and wait a few days. When symptoms have subsided, you can try taking the supplement in a lower dose. If symptoms reappear, stop taking the herb, formula or supplement and don't take it again. Otherwise, you can gradually increase the dose.

Unskilled herbalists sometimes blame all adverse reactions on a detoxification process; however, both herbs and nutritional supplements can have adverse reactions in some people. Examples of adverse reactions include (but are not limited to) increased anxiety, bloating, increased heart rate, increased blood pressure and dizziness. Again, these reactions are not life-threatening, but they are signs that the supplement or herb should be immediately discontinued.

If you go off the herb or supplement for a couple of days, the symptoms generally will stop (unless they are being caused by something other than the herb or supplement). To double-check if the herb or supplement was actually at fault (sometimes these apparent reactions are just co-incidences), you can again try the herb or supplement at a lower dose as described above.

If you have questions about adverse reactions, you may wish to consult with a competent herbalist. (If you don't know a competent herbalist, you can search for one at *herbiverse.com*.) Medical doctors generally know very little about herbs, so they are usually not reliable sources of information on herbs or nutritional supplements.

Conditions Section

A Guide to Herbal Formulas, Single Herbs, Nutritional Supplements and Natural Therapies For Various Health Problems

This section allows you to look up various health problems. It provides you with a brief description of the problem and what natural therapies may be helpful. Where a particular symptom or problem can have many causes, we've tried to address all of the most common underlying causes and provide you with information that will help you determine if those causes may apply to you. For each cause, we list therapies and remedies that may be helpful for that cause. This is why some conditions list so many options as possible remedies.

If you have multiple health problems, look them all up and see if some of the same therapies show up under many of the health problems you have. This is a clue that these may be major underlying factors in your health issues. You may also want to look up related conditions to see if they may also apply to you.

Some conditions are dangerous to engage in self-treatment because of their serious or potentially life-threatening nature. Where we encourage you to seek medical attention, please do so. Even if you opt to go the natural route for these problems, you should be monitored by modern medical testing to make sure you're on the right track.

For each condition we provide you with suggested therapies, herbal formulas, single herbs and nutritional supplements, as appropriate. We've highlighted some of our preferred remedies, but be sure to read the text to help you select the right remedies for the situation you are addressing. Look up suggested therapies in the *Therapies Section*, look up suggested herbal formula categories in the *Herbal Formulas Section*, look up single herbs in the *Key Herbs Section* and look up nutritional supplements in the *Nutrients Section*.

Abrasions

See also *Wounds and Sores*

An abrasion is an injury caused by a scraping away of a portion of skin or mucus membrane. Abrasions can be treated naturally with *Topical Vulnerary Formulas* or topical applications (Poultice or Compress therapy) of the key herbs listed below. If there is a concern about an infection, use a *Topical Antiseptic Formula*. Vitamin E can be applied topically to help prevent scarring.

Therapies: Aromatherapy, Compress, Flower Essences and Poultice

Formulas: Topical Vulnerary and Topical Antiseptic

Key Herbs: Aloe vera, Comfrey, **Calendula**, Goldenseal, Grindelia (Gumweed), Lavender, Plantain and Tea Tree

Key Nutrients: Vitamin E

Abscesses

An abscess is either an open sore, usually surrounded by inflamed tissue, from which there is an oozing of pus, or a cavity formed by a collection of pus-like material in solid tissue as a response to infection or other foreign objects. *Blood Purifier* and *Antibacterial Formulas* can be helpful when taken internally, but an even more effective approach is to use topical remedies.

A *Drawing Salve* or a poultice can be applied to the area directly over the abscess. Another approach is to take a liquid *Blood Purifier* or *Antibacterial Formula* and use it as part of a Compress as described in the *Therapies Section*.

Echinacea is an effective key herb that can be used both internally and externally for abscesses. Other key herbs, used externally, that may be helpful in treating abscesses are, activated charcoal, barberry, chamomile, garlic, pine sap, plantain, propolis, tea tree oil, usnea and yarrow. Also consider irrigating the with a sterile saline solution or herbal tincture. Avoid using comfrey and goldenseal topically because they can heal the abscess from the top, leaving infection beneath the skin. Internally, consider using echinacea, garlic, Oregon grape, usnea, yarrow or an *Antibacterial Formula*.

Therapies: Compress and Poultice

Formulas: Blood Purifier, Antibacterial, Drawing Salve and Poultice

Key Herbs: Echinacea, **Plantain**, Devil's Claw, Garlic, Lobelia, Oregano essential oil, Oregon Grape, Propolis, Tea Tree, Usnea and Yarrow

Key Nutrients: Charcoal (Activated), Vitamin C, Colloidal Silver and Vitamin D

Abuse and Trauma

See also *Mental Illness* and *Anxiety Disorders*

An underlying cause of many people's health problems is unresolved abuse and trauma. They may have experienced it in childhood or later in life. It may have come in the form of physical trauma and abuse or emotional trauma and abuse. For example, accidents, surgery and physical assaults can be traumatizing on a physical level. Abandonment, neglect, ridicule and belittling are emotionally traumatizing. One can also be traumatized through sexual assault.

When we are traumatized, our higher brain shuts down and the amygdala takes over, creating an involuntary fight, flee or freeze response. When we respond to trauma by fight, we get angry and try to fight back against what is hurting or threatening us. Flight involves running away from what is hurting or threatening us. When we perceive ourselves unable to fight or flee (as often happens in childhood abuse) we freeze. In this state, the body remains highly "charged" and ready to fight or flee but doesn't move.

Just as our response to trauma is automatic, so are the responses that allow us to heal from it. When the trauma has passed and we feel safe, we instinctively try to discharge the tension in our bodies, which allows the nervous system to return to normal. Animals in the wild do this automatically and do not remain traumatized.

In human beings, this discharging process may involve one or more of the following:

Anger: shouting, yelling, kicking, punching, stomping one's feet, etc.

Grief: crying, moaning, wailing, sighing, screaming, etc.

Fear and Anxiety: shaking, trembling, breathing rapidly, pacing, ringing one's hands, running, etc.

Laughter: talking about the event or the problem until one starts to find humor in it and begins to laugh.

Once the tension in the body has been discharged, a person is able to reenter the flow of life. Unfortunately, people in our society have been conditioned to interrupt the trauma recovery process. All too often we are told not to get angry, not to be sad, not to be afraid, or not to laugh so loud. This is usually done through criticism or punishment, comforting the person with the intent to make them stop expressing their feelings, or simply showing disapproval for the discharging behavior.

When our attempts to discharge the emotional tension and trauma are repeatedly interrupted, a cycle of trauma is created within us. Every time we encounter situations that remind us of the original traumatic event, the same intense emotions we felt during that event are triggered. We may experience a sense of helplessness, rage, fear, sadness or other intense emotions. Left unresolved, these cycles of trauma can grow stronger over time.

They also contribute to many health problems. These include "mental health" issues such as depression, post traumatic stress disorder, anxiety disorders and feelings of tension and stress as well as physical health problems such as constipation, loss of sex drive, digestive upset, headaches and more.

When a person enters an unresolved trauma cycle, there are two major signs that their trauma is being retriggered. First, the person's thoughts and words become negative and incoherent (don't make sense), and these negative thoughts tend to spiral downwards. Secondly, the person thinks and speaks in absolute terms (everybody does this, nobody does that, this always happens to me and that never happens to me).

Counseling and/or Emotional Healing Work is necessary to help a person discharge the emotional tension from their nervous system, but there are also herbs and supplements that can aid in the person's recovery. *Adaptogen Formulas* are always beneficial, as they help to calm down the production of stress hormones and neurotransmitters. In many cases, the person's adrenal glands are exhausted from chronic stress. In these cases, an *Adrenal Tonic Formula* will be helpful.

When muscles are tense, a *Relaxing Nervine Formula* and magnesium are helpful. Where sleep is disturbed, an herbal *Sleep Formula* may be called for. Cases involving depression will benefit from an *Antidepressant Formula*. B-complex vitamins can help to feed the nerves and reduce anxiety.

Therapies: Affirmation and Visualization, Aromatherapy, Emotional Healing Work, Flower Essences and Healthy Fats

Formulas: Adrenal Tonic, Adaptogen, Relaxing Nervine, Sleep and Antidepressant

Key Herbs: Ashwaganda, Scullcap (Skullcap), Eleuthero (Siberian ginseng), Kava-kava, Passionflower, Pulsatilla, Schisandra (Schizandra) and Self Heal (Heal All) flower essence

Key Nutrients: Vitamin B-Complex, Magnesium and SAM-e

Aches

See *Pain (general remedies for)*

Acid Indigestion (Heartburn, Acid Reflux)

See also *Hiatal Hernia* and *Small Intestinal Bacterial Overgrowth (SIBO)*

Just about everyone has experienced heartburn at least once in their life, but many people suffer from it on a regular basis. Of course, heartburn really has nothing to do with the heart. It's a form of acid indigestion in which acid leaves the stomach and enters the esophagus causing burning and pain.

To understand why people get acid indigestion and conditions related to it, we need to understand the digestive process. When we eat, food passes down the esophagus and into the stomach. There, the stomach secretes hydrochloric acid (an extremely powerful acid) into the food. The acidic environment of the stomach allows pepsin (a stomach enzyme) to break down proteins. The acid also kills harmful microbes in the food (to protect the body from infection) and also helps prepare minerals like calcium, magnesium, copper and zinc for absorption.

Once the digestive process in the stomach is complete, a valve at the bottom of the stomach opens to allow the partially digested food into the small intestines. There, highly alkaline secretions from the pancreas and gallbladder neutralize the acid. The stomach has a mucous lining to help protect it against this acid, but the esophagus and small intestines do not. To hold the acid in the stomach, a muscular valve at the top of the stomach prevents the food from reentering the esophagus. This valve opens to permit belching, then closes again.

The intestines are protected by the valve at the bottom of the stomach, which will not open until there are sufficient alkaline secretions available to neutralize the acid. If this valve doesn't open, food can sit in the stomach long enough that it starts to cause burning pains in the stomach.

Heartburn and GERD

Acid reflux, commonly known as heartburn, occurs when the valve at the top of the stomach allows acid to seep back (reflux) into the esophagus. This acid burns and inflames the esophageal lining. This creates a burning sensation in the center of the chest, which is why it is called heartburn. Acid reflux is the more technical term. One in every four Americans, or about 60 million people, experience heartburn at least once a month and almost 15 million people have heartburn each day.

Although uncomfortable, occasional heartburn is not a serious condition. However, if it happens frequently and persistently, then the repeated burning and inflammation of the esophagus can result in damage to the esophagus that forms scar tissue. This can narrow the passageway and increase the risk of esophageal cancer. This condition is called gastro-esophogeal reflux disease (GERD). GERD is surprisingly common, affecting an estimated 5-7% of the American population.

Medical Treatment

The medical approach to acid reflux and GERD is to give the person anti-acids or acid blockers. While this might be helpful if there is active inflammation that needs a chance to heal, it does not correct the root causes of these problems. Furthermore, long term use of anti-acids and acid blockers weakens the body because proteins and minerals are not digested and absorbed efficiently. The body is also more susceptible to infections.

Natural Therapy for Acid Indigestion

The first thing to understand is that most people's acid indigestion is NOT caused by an excess of stomach acid. Therefore, neutralizing or blocking the acid does not solve the problem. In fact, ironically, most acid indigestion is actually caused by a lack of hydrochloric acid and/or digestive enzymes. This is partially caused by the lack of raw and enzyme-rich foods in our diets and partly due to the fact that acid and enzyme production tends to decline with age.

Furthermore, when food is not thoroughly chewed, it is harder for digestive juices to penetrate the food. Overeating also causes indigestion, as the stomach becomes overburdened with more food than it has digestive secretions to properly break down.

When food is not digested properly due to a lack of enzymes and hydrochloric acid (HCl), overeating or other factors, the undigested food ferments. This typically causes a dull burning pain about an hour after eating. It may also result in a heavy feeling in the stomach after meals, belching, and intestinal gas and bloating.

Dehydration also contributes to acid indigestion. The process of digestion requires a lot of water. If the body is dehydrated it may lack the fluids necessary to make the alkalizing secretions in the gallbladder and pancreas needed to neutralize the stomach acid. This causes the food to remain in the stomach too long, which again results in the heavy, burning feeling in the stomach.

For immediate relief from this type of acid indigestion take something bitter with water. This can be a liquid *Digestive Bitter Tonic Formula* or any bitter herb in liquid or powder form (such as gentian and goldenseal). It is important to actually taste the bitterness as this stimulates digestive secretions. An herbal *Antacid Formula* or a tea made from chamomile, red raspberry leaves, catnip and/or safflowers may also be helpful. Meadowsweet is another useful herb for immediate relief of acid burning and pain.

For severe burning, calcium supplements will be helpful, especially if they contain calcium carbonate. Magnesium glyconate may also be helpful. However, this is a band-aid approach and not a long-term solution as calcium carbonate reduces HCl production, which creates a vicious cycle of continuing indigestion.

For long-term relief start using *Digestive Enzyme Formulas*, digestive enzyme supplements and/or betaine hydrochloric acid (HCl) supplements with meals. It also helps to drink 1-2 glasses of water about 20-30 minutes prior to meals. A *Digestive Bitter Tonic Formula* or a pinch of natural salt with the water may also be helpful as these stimulate HCl production. Many people have also found that taking a little apple cider vinegar with meals to help acidify the stomach also relieves acid indigestion.

If you are a younger person with good digestion and are experiencing acid indigestion without the heavy feeling on the stomach, try slowing down and chewing your food better, drinking more water between meals and eating smaller meals. It can also help follow the Enzyme-Rich Foods therapy, including eating more raw fruits and vegetables and naturally-fermented foods.

If these solutions don't prove helpful keep a food journal and try to figure out if there are any specific foods that trigger acid indigestion. You may have a food sensitivity or allergy. Common foods that cause acid indigestion in some people include onions, peppermint, chocolate, coffee, citrus fruits, tomatoes, garlic and spicy foods.

Natural Therapy for Acid Reflux

The problem that causes acid reflux (heartburn) may also be mechanical. Anything that puts pressure on the valve at the top of the stomach, causing it to open, will allow acid to enter the esophagus, even if acid production isn't excessive. If taking a small amount of apple cider vinegar at the beginning of a meal reduces your acid indigestion, it is NOT due to excess stomach acid.

Some of the mechanical factors that cause this, include intestinal gas and bloating (which is usually due to food sensitivities or allergies or lack of digestive enzymes and HCl), excess body weight, tight fitting clothes, pregnancy and lying down after eating. Stress also tenses the solar plexus area and draws the stomach upward. If you have a lot of gas and bloating after meals, you may also want to try a *Carminative Formula* to help the body expel this gas and relieve the bloating and pressure.

Chronically low HCl allows the migration of bacteria from the large intestines into the small intestines, a condition called Small Intestinal Bacterial Overgrowth (SIBO). The bacterial breakdown of food in the small intestines creates gas and bloating after meals, putting pressure on the diaphragm, occasionally creating enough pressure to force the lower esophageal sphincter open, creating reflux. Many bitter and carminative herbs also have antibacterial properties and are very beneficial.

When a portion of the upper stomach passes through the opening in the diaphragm where the esophagus enters (known as the hiatus), this is called a hiatal hernia. People who have frequent and severe heartburn and/or GERD should use the Hiatal Hernia Correction therapy, which is often necessary for permanent relief. About 80% of the people with GERD have a hiatal hernia.

Healing Tissue Damage from GERD

To heal damage to the esophagus and digestive tract due to acid reflux, soothing mucilaginous remedies are needed. Three of the best are aloe vera juice, licorice and slippery elm, but any *Tissue Healing Formula* will probably be helpful. By sipping small amounts of aloe diluted in water, or sucking on licorice or slippery elm lozenges the burning or inflammation in the esophagus due to the acid reflux can be cooled and soothed. You can also use *Ulcer Healing* or *Tissue Healing Formulas*.

Therapies: Eliminate Allergy-Causing Foods, Gut Healing Diet, Hiatal Hernia Correction, Hydration and Stress Management

Formulas: Antacid, **Digestive Bitter Tonic**, Digestive Enzyme, Ulcer Healing, Tissue Healing, Carminative and Relaxing Nervine

Key Herbs: Aloe vera, Blessed Thistle, Catnip, Chamomile (English and Roman), **Goldenseal**, **Meadowsweet**, Devil's Claw, Gentian, Licorice, Papaya, Pau d' Arco, Red Raspberry, Safflowers, Slippery Elm and Turkey Rhubarb

Key Nutrients: Digestive Enzymes, Calcium, **Betaine Hydrochloric Acid (HCl)** and Magnesium

Acid pH

See *Overacidity*

Acid Reflux

See *Acid Indigestion (Heartburn, Acid Reflux)*

Acne (Pimples, Blackheads)

See also *Hypothyroid* and *Leaky Gut Syndrome*

Acne is an inflammatory condition of the skin. The small glands that excrete oil to lubricate the skin become irritated and inflamed. Microbes get into the pores and as the body fights the infection, the skin pores fill with pus creating pimples.

Medical treatment often involves antibiotics, either topically or internally, to fight the infection. The condition can also be due to hormonal imbalances and may be treated with hormone replacement therapy.

From a natural perspective, acne is seen as a toxic condition of the skin. Fat-soluble irritants are being eliminated through the skin pores and the irritation is creating a breeding ground for microbes.

This is why *Blood Purifier Formulas* have traditionally been used to fight acne. Blood purifiers improve detoxification in the liver and lymphatic drainage. They may also help the kidneys function more efficiently. As waste is eliminated from the system, the irritation diminishes.

Since the irritation is affecting glands that secrete oil, the toxins involved here may result from a problem with the breakdown and utilization of fats in the body. Hydrogenated oils are irritating to the body and should be replaced with healthier fats such as flax seed oil, Omega-3 EPA and olive oil. Cod liver oil supplements may also be helpful.

Both burdock and chickweed (traditional blood purifiers and acne remedies) aid the body in properly metabolizing fats. Fat-soluble vitamins (particularly A, D and E) can also help protect against the oxidation of fats. Oxidation causes fats to become rancid and irritating to the system. This may explain why large doses of vitamin A have helped clear up some cases of acne.

One of the reasons teenagers are so prone to acne is that their hormones are out of balance. Reproductive hormones influence the skin and the metabolism of fats. These breakouts usually occur around the jaw line or chin area. They can also increase eliminative activity in the skin. For this reason, remedies that balance hormones may also be helpful.

For example, chaste tree berries, which regulate reproductive hormones via the pituitary gland, have been beneficial in clearing up teenage acne. A *Female Hormonal Balancing Formula* can be helpful for some girls, but most *Male Glandular Tonic Formulas* would not be suitable for teenage boys. Key glandular herbs that might be helpful include sarsaparilla (which is also a blood purifier) for teenage boys and dong quai (also a blood tonic) for teenage girls.

In some cases, low thyroid can contribute to this problem. The thyroid hormones are needed to properly combust fats in the body. Furthermore, kelp, dulse and other seaweeds found in many Hyopthyroid Formulas are also very nourishing to the skin. If acne is accompanied by a tendency to become cold easily, try supporting the thyroid.

Antibacterial and *Goldenseal & Echinacea Formulas* can be helpful for clearing up the infection part of acne. So can cleansing the skin thoroughly to remove excess oil from the glands and to get rid of unwanted microorganisms. Essential oils found in *Topical Antiseptic Formulas* may be helpful too. However, the problem with internal toxicity and combustion of fats must still be addressed for a long-term solution, so consider working on cleansing the colon, improving liver function and healing the intestinal tract to reduce gut leakage.

Topically, it can be helpful to make a mask out of any fine clay (such as Redmond clay) or red raspberry leaf and apply it to the skin. You can also add a little tea tree oil to the mask, or just place it directly on the blemishes to fight infection.

Therapies: Colon Cleanse, Dietary Fiber, Drawing Bath, Eliminate Allergy-Causing Foods, Gut Healing Diet, Healthy Fats and Low Glycemic Diet

Formulas: Blood Purifier, Female Hormonal Balancing, Hypothyroid, Antibacterial, Goldenseal & Echinacea and **Skin Healing**

Key Herbs: Aloe vera, Blue Flag, Chamomile (English and Roman), Chaparral, Chickweed, **Burdock**, **Red Clover**, Dandelion, Echinacea, Kelp, Lomatium, Milk Thistle, Tea Tree essential oil and Yellow Dock

Key Nutrients: Zinc, Vitamin B-6 (Pyridoxine), MSM, **Vitamin A**, **Vitamin D**, Lipase Enzymes, Lipase Enzymes, Pantothenic Acid (Vitamin B5) and Potassium

Acquired Immune Deficiency Syndrome (AIDS)/HIV

See also *Infection (viral)*

Acquired Immune Deficiency Syndrome, more commonly known as AIDS, is a disease in which the body's immune system is depressed. It is believed to be the result of an infection by the HIV virus, although there are some researchers who dispute this explanation. There are also many drugs that can cause the immune system to be depleted. Malnutrition can also cause immune deficiency.

Late stages of AIDS include severe susceptibility to infections of all kinds and a general weakening of the body. Supporting normal immune function is the key, although preventing secondary infections is also important. *Mushroom Blend Formulas* may have a regulating effect in people with AIDS and depending on the individual case, *Immune Balancing Formulas* or *Immune Stimulating Formulas* may also be helpful.

Swollen lymph nodes and low platelet counts are common in AIDS patients. Red root or a *Lymphatic Drainage Formula* containing red root and echinacea can be helpful here.

Many AIDS patients suffer from systemic yeast infections, so *Antifungal Formulas* are often helpful. Because of its abilities to fight respiratory infections (a common cause of death in people with AIDS) raw garlic can be very helpful.

Because of the seriousness of this condition, professional assistance and medical supervision should be sought when designing a natural program to combat AIDS. Attention should be paid to improving overall diet, lifestyle and basic health, and a professional herbalist (*findanherbalist.com*) or naturopath can help you design a comprehensive program.

Therapies: Affirmation and Visualization, Friendly Flora, Healthy Fats, Mineralization and Stress Management

Formulas: Immune Stimulating, **Immune Balancing**, **Mushroom Blend**, Lymphatic Drainage and Antifungal

Key Herbs: Aloe vera, Barley, **Bitter Melon**, **Garlic**, **Red Root**, Elder, Lomatium, Milk Thistle, Pau d' Arco, Shiitake, St. John's wort and Wild Indigo (Baptista)

Key Nutrients: Co-Q10, N-Acetyl Cysteine, Vitamin B-12, Protease Enzymes, DHEA, **Selenium** and L-Arginine

ADD/ADHD

See *Attention Deficit Disorder (ADD, ADHD)*

Key Nutrients: GABA and Zinc

Addictions (alcohol)

See also *Hypoglycemia* and *Addictions (general remedies for)*

Alcohol is essentially a pure, refined carbohydrate which contributes to hypoglycemia. While a moderate amount of alcohol (such as a glass of wine with a meal) does not seem to cause any serious health problems, excessive alcohol consumption does. Over-consumption of alcohol damages the liver and brain, destroys personal relationships, and is the number one cause of traffic accidents.

As is stressed under *Addictions (general)* alcoholics need to seek outside assistance to obtain the social and emotional support they need to overcome the habit. Good nutrition can help the process. Cravings for alcohol increase with poor nutrition, so following the Low Glycemic Diet and dealing with the problem of hypoglycemia will be helpful.

B-complex vitamins, chromium and licorice root can all help stabilize sugar (glucose) levels in the blood and reduce alcohol cravings. Some research indicates that good fats like evening primrose oil or omega-3 supplements can reduce the craving for alcohol. Alcohol robs the body of large amounts of magnesium, so magnesium supplements may also be helpful. Vitamin C is another nutrient to consider.

To soothe the nerves and resolve headaches when quitting alcohol, use a *Relaxing Nervine Formula*. Kava kava, in moderate doses, can produce a relaxed feeling similar to alcohol, but it leaves the brain clear. However, over consumption of kava can interfere with motor activity like alcohol. People have been convicted for DUI's from over consumption of kava.

In laboratory studies, alcoholic golden hamsters voluntarily and significantly reduced their alcohol consumption when given a water extract of kudzu. In clinical practice, some people have reduced (not stopped) their alcohol consumption. The flowers of kudzu have been used to treat alcohol poisoning (hangover). See *Anti-Alcoholic Formulas*.

The most addictive thing about beer drinking isn't the alcohol. It's an herb used in making the beverage—hops. This herb contains a sedative substance with a mild addictive effect. Hops can be taken to reduce cravings for beer, providing a similar relaxing effect without the negative problems associated with alcohol.

Since the liver works overtime to neutralize alcohol when levels are too high in the blood, the liver itself breaks down after long abuse. The liver can repair itself; all it needs is rest. Milk thistle can be especially helpful for protecting the liver from the effects of alcohol, or in helping the liver to heal. Select a good *Liver Tonic* or *Hepatoprotective Formula* where milk thistle is a major ingredient.

Therapies: Hydration, Low Glycemic Diet and Stress Management

Formulas: Relaxing Nervine, **Anti-Alcoholic**, Hepatoprotective and Liver Tonic

Key Herbs: Chamomile (English and Roman), **Hops**, **Kudzu**, Kava-kava, Licorice, Milk Thistle, Passionflower, Shatavari, Spirulina, St. John's wort and Valerian

Key Nutrients: L-Glutamine, Vitamin B-3 (Niacin), Vitamin B-1 (Thiamine), SAM-e, Magnesium, Vitamin B-Complex, Chromium, Betaine Hydrochloric Acid (HCl) and Potassium

Addictions (coffee, caffeine)

See also *Adrenals (exhaustion, weakness or burnout), Fatigue, Insomnia* and *Addictions (general remedies for)*

Caffeine is a highly addictive drug, yet most adults use it nearly every day and freely offer it in various forms to their children. Caffeine stimulates epinephrine in the nervous system, which temporarily boosts a state of energy and alertness. However, contrary to popular belief, it does not increase energy production in the body. Instead, it tricks the body into using up its energy reserves.

The more a person abuses coffee, tea, cola drinks and "energy" drinks the more depleted their body's energy reserves become. The adrenal glands weaken and fatigue, anxiety, nervousness, insomnia and other nervous symptoms follow. Caffeine constricts arteries, raising blood pressure, and being a diuretic it also tends to be dehydrating. Excessive use can also disrupt sleep patterns, which results in deeper fatigue and more cravings for the stimulus of caffeine to stay alert. In short, caffeine is not the innocent substance many people seem to think it is.

Although research suggests that there are some health benefits to coffee and green tea, because of their antioxidant qualities, it's wise to limit one's intake of these beverages to one or two cups a day. Cola drinks are worse because they also contain loads of sugar and questionable chemicals. The so-called "energy drinks" have the highest caffeine content of all and should be avoided completely

as they have none of the antioxidant benefits of coffee or green tea.

To overcome caffeine addiction one needs to actively support the adrenal glands, reduce one's stress levels and increase energy production. Formulas that support the adrenal glands and can help increase energy while reducing stress include *Adaptogen* and *Adrenal Tonic Formulas*. As an alternative to caffeinated beverages one can also try *Energy-Boosting Formulas*. Be aware however, that some of these natural energy formulas contain herbs with caffeine, such as green tea and guarana. The advantage of these formulas is that they also contain adaptogens and other herbs to help produce a more long-lasting energy boost. Small doses of American or Asian ginseng may also be helpful.

B-complex vitamins and vitamin C can help boost energy naturally by supporting the adrenal function. Vitamin B5 (pantothenic acid) is very helpful if the adrenal glands have become exhausted from excess consumption of caffeine.

The natural way to increase energy is to rest. If you aren't getting enough sleep try using an herbal *Sleep Formula* or look up remedies for insomnia. Also consider reasons why you might be fatigued.

Therapies: Avoid Caffeine, Hydration, Low Glycemic Diet and Stress Management

Formulas: Adrenal Tonic, Adaptogen, **Energy-Boosting** and Sleep

Key Herbs: Ashwaganda, Schisandra (Schizandra), Eleuthero (Siberian ginseng), Ginseng (American), Ginseng (Asian, Korean) and Licorice

Key Nutrients: Vitamin B-Complex, Vitamin C and N-Acetyl Cysteine

Addictions (drugs)

See also *Addictions (general remedies for)*

In discussing drug addiction we're talking about both illegal (meth, rave, crystal, cocaine, etc.) and prescription drugs (such as pain killers, stimulants or barbiturates), which can also be addictive. Of course, professional assistance should be sought with drug addiction, but there are natural remedies that can help too. Specifically, withdrawal from drug addiction requires detoxification and nutritional support for the nervous and glandular system.

Drugs of all kinds place a heavy burden on the detoxification systems of the liver. So, herbs and nutrients that support liver detoxification are probably central to any nutritional program for drug withdrawal. These can include

Hepatoprotective and *Liver Tonic Formulas*, as well as the single herbs milk thistle and schisandra. It is also important to drink lots of pure water to help flush drugs from the system.

Anyone withdrawing from drugs is going to experience mental and emotional stress. Hence, a *Relaxing Nervine Formula* would be another important component to consider in a drug withdrawal program. If the person is suffering from post-traumatic stress disorder or adrenal fatigue, an *Adrenal Tonic Formula* can be very helpful. Omega-3 essential fatty acids and l-glutamine can also be helpful for nervous system support.

Support for the nervous system depends on the type of drugs one is addicted to. If stimulants are the problem, then naturally increase energy with *Energy-Boosting* or *Adaptogen Formulas*. Single herbs like ashwaganda, eleuthero root, schisandra berries, licorice root, ginseng and the B-complex vitamins (especially niacin), along with vitamin C, may also be helpful.

Overcoming an addiction to tranquilizers can be aided by herbs that also provide a relaxing effect, such as *Relaxing Nervine* or *Sleep Formulas*. Single herbs like hops, kava kava, licorice root, lobelia, passion flower, St. John's wort and valerian may be helpful as well. GABA and l-theanine can also be used to ease anxiety.

For addiction to pain killers, try a milder analgesic, such as lobelia, kava kava, passion flower, California poppy, corydalis, valerian, or an herbal *Analgesic Formula*. Licorice root and turmeric can be useful for weaning off corticosteroids. For opiates try California poppy or corydalis. The rule of thumb is to find an herbal remedy with a similar, but milder effect and use it to transition off the drug.

Therapies: Affirmation and Visualization, Healthy Fats, Hydration and Stress Management

Formulas: Hepatoprotective, **Liver Tonic**, Adaptogen, Relaxing Nervine, Sleep, Energy-Boosting, Adrenal Tonic and Analgesic

Key Herbs: California Poppy, Chamomile (English and Roman), Corydalis, **Ashwaganda**, **Blue Vervain**, Hops, Indian Pipe, Kava-kava, Licorice, Lobelia, Milk Thistle, Oat seed (milky), Passionflower, Schisandra (Schizandra), Shatavari, St. John's wort and Valerian

Key Nutrients: L-Glutamine, Vitamin B-3 (Niacin), **GABA**, Vitamin B-Complex and Vitamin C

Addictions (general remedies for)

See also *Addictions (alcohol)*, *Addictions (tobacco smoking or chewing)*, *Addictions (coffee, caffeine)*, *Addictions (drugs)* and *Addictions (sugar and refined carbohydrates)*

When most people think of addiction, they immediately think of serious addictions to substances like drugs and alcohol. In fact, historically addiction has been defined as physical dependence on psychoactive substances such as alcohol, tobacco, opiates and other drugs. However, the definition of addiction has been expanded to include psychological dependency on things such as pornography, sex, food, gambling, computers, the internet, gaming, watching TV, work, exercise, shopping and self-injury. Simply put, when we can't stop a behavior that is damaging to ourselves and others, it is addictive.

The American Society of Addiction Medicine has described addiction as "a primary, chronic disease of brain reward, motivation, memory and related circuitry." Or simply, addiction occurs when there is a compulsive or habitual need to repeat an experience in order to try and feel good. The addiction may be mild or severe, socially acceptable or unacceptable.

Are You Addicted?

Addiction isn't something that's limited to the use of illegal drugs. In fact, many forms of addiction are socially acceptable. The most common addiction is that of caffeine. More than 90% of Americans consume caffeinated beverages daily, and they go through severe withdrawal symptoms if they don't get their daily dose of caffeine. If you have a hard time waking up and getting through the day without a cup of coffee, caffeinated soda or an energy drink, you're probably addicted to caffeine.

Two other commonly used substances in North America that are highly addictive are tobacco and alcohol. But, even if you don't use caffeine, tobacco or alcohol, what about food? Roughly 70% of Americans today are overweight, and many are driven by a need to eat for comfort and pleasure—two classic motivations in addictive behavior. In fact, the addiction to sugar is probably greater than the addiction to caffeine. And, if you don't think sugar is addictive, just try giving it up cold turkey and see what withdrawal symptoms you experience.

Finally, people may seek prescription drugs trying to feel better. If they become addicted to these medications, people have been known to resort to "borrowing" other people's prescriptions, getting multiple prescriptions from different doctors, falsifying prescriptions, or even stealing prescription drugs.

With all the stresses in our modern world, such as economic struggles, threats to security and uncertainty about the future, many people seek to relieve the stress they feel through addictive behaviors. Thus, addiction is very widespread in our culture.

Get Help

With serious addictions, a person needs professional help, because one does not overcome addictions by willpower. It simply doesn't happen. The instinctive drive for pleasure and self-satisfaction is too strong for us to resist. It easily subverts people's best intentions.

That's why the first thing anyone needs to do to overcome an addiction is to seek outside help. One of the reasons for the success of organizations like Alcoholics Anonymous (AA) is that they provide a support system that gives people accountability to a power outside of themselves.

Forming groups of people that meet together to support one another in overcoming addictions to drugs, alcohol or even overeating (weight loss) has proved to be one of the most successful models for helping people become free of addictive behaviors. So first, seek assistance from other people who have overcome the addiction you wish to overcome. Allow yourself to be accountable to outside influences, including spiritual sources, so you are not relying on your own willpower.

Eat Healthy

Secondly, since addictions are motivated by the inner desire we all share to feel good, improving overall health and nutrition will make it much easier to overcome addictions. When our diet contains a proper balance of nutrients, and we are otherwise taking care of the body, it produces the chemicals that make us feel good. This is the healthy way to feel good.

For starters, many addictions are linked to blood sugar problems, so stop eating refined carbohydrates (white sugar, white flour, white rice, corn syrup) and use complex carbohydrates like fresh vegetables, whole fruits and a moderate amount of whole grains instead. Make sure you get adequate intake of protein, especially for breakfast.

It also helps to do an "oil change." Stop using margarine, shortening and refined vegetable oils in favor of organic (preferably grass-fed) butter, olive oil, coconut oil, nuts, seeds and avocados. It may be helpful to supplement your essential fatty acids. Also consider supplementing with vitamin D3, especially during the wintertime.

Heal Emotional Wounds

Thirdly, addictions are often an attempt to escape our fears and run away from emotional pain. Emotional Healing Work can help a person learn to face their fears and find ways to heal their emotional wounds.

Detoxify

Finally, cleansing the body is a great way to begin breaking free of addiction—especially if you are going through withdrawal. Start by getting well hydrated. Drinking a half ounce of water per pound of body weight daily not only flushes toxins from the system, it also tends to create a natural release of neurotransmitters that help us feel good. A *General Detoxifying Formula* can help the body flush the toxins created by the addictive substance out of the system.

Read the entries about specific addictions for ideas on specific supplements that can help a person overcome their addictions.

Therapies: Affirmation and Visualization, Colon Cleanse and Stress Management

Formulas: General Detoxifying and **Adaptogen**

Key Herbs: Barley, Eleuthero (Siberian ginseng), Kava-kava and St. John's wort

Key Nutrients: Omega-3 Essential Fatty Acids, Vitamin B-Complex, Vitamin D and **L-Glutamine**

Addictions (sugar and refined carbohydrates)

See also *Diabetes, Fungal Infections (Yeast Infections, Candida albicans), Hyperinsulinemia (Metabolic Syndrome, Syndrome X), Hypoglycemia* and *Addictions (general remedies for)*

Sugar is a highly addictive substance and the average American consumes between 125 to 175 pounds of refined sugar per year. That's about 1/3 to 1/2 pound per day! Most of this is in the form of table sugar (sucrose) or high fructose corn syrup. Both products are a mixture of glucose and fructose, and both have the same health-destroying effects.

Grains contain a lot of starch, which is broken down into sugar by the digestive tract. Refined grains convert rapidly into simple sugars and have the same problems as refined sugars. Alcohol also rapidly converts to simple sugars and contributes to blood sugar imbalances.

Sugar becomes addictive for several reasons. First, the body needs other nutrients, including B-vitamins, vitamin C and many minerals such as chromium, vanadium and magnesium, to convert sugar into energy. In whole foods these nutrients are present along with the sugar, so the body is able to properly control and regulate sugar metabolism. When we eat refined sugar, however, we wind up still feeling hungry because the body didn't get all the nutrients it needed. This prompts us to eat more.

Sugar also upsets the body's hormonal balance. The pancreas keeps blood sugar levels stable by secreting two hormones, insulin and glucagon. When there is too much sugar in the blood (hyperglycemia), the pancreas secretes insulin to drive this sugar into storage. When the blood sugar level drops too low (hypoglycemia) the pancreas secretes glucagon to bring sugar out of storage.

Insulin depresses glucagon production and glucagon depresses insulin production. This relationship, which is much like a hormonal teeter-totter, is called a hormonal axis.

When large quantities of simple carbohydrates enter the blood stream, the pancreas secretes insulin to try to protect the brain from the excess sugar. This depresses glucagon production, so when the sugar in the blood has been used up, the body has a hard time mobilizing sugar from storage. The result is hypoglycemia, or low blood sugar.

This causes cravings for sugar, which jacks the sugar level up again. This is like a blood sugar roller coaster ride, and your mood goes up and down with it. Blood sugar levels have a powerful impact on the brain, so sugar can contribute to hyperactivity, irritability, depression and nervousness.

These high insulin levels cause fat stores to increase as the body tries to find ways to store the sugar. The hypoglycemic reactions from this can also cause stress on the adrenals, especially when someone is using caffeine to stimulate them. Stress hormones like cortisol are used to try to bring blood sugar levels up again. This contributes to adrenal fatigue.

High insulin levels also depress the production of prostaglandins that control inflammation. As the adrenals become exhausted from excess sugar and caffeine consumption, they also lose their ability to control inflammation. Chronic inflammation sets in, which leads to heart disease, cancer and inflammation in the brain, which contributes to the destruction of brain cells.

You'll never kick the white sugar and carbohydrate habit by trying to avoid all sweets and starchy foods, so forget about it. We need carbohydrates. They give us energy, and we crave sweets because our senses were designed to look for natural foods that contain the carbohydrates we need.

So, instead of just trying to avoid refined sugar and simple carbohydrates, start consciously consuming complex carbohydrates like fresh fruits, vegetables and whole grains in place of products containing refined sugar, white flour and white rice. You can also use more natural sugars in place of refined sugar, such as raw honey, real maple syrup, freeze-dried sugar cane juice and other natural sugars. Because these sugars contain nutrients the body needs they are more satisfying and you'll eat less.

Eating a good breakfast will also help with overcoming sugar addiction because breakfast sets your metabolism for the day. Your blood sugar level is low in the morning because you've been fasting all night. That's why we call the first meal of the day, "break fast."

If you break your fast in the morning by eating simple carbohydrates, such as a pastry, donut, toast or breakfast cereal (even whole grain varieties), you trigger an insulin reaction that starts you on the blood sugar roller coaster ride all day. Conversely, when you break your fast with high protein foods, you stimulate the release of glucagon, which mobilizes stored reserves of sugar and lowers insulin production.

Eating protein for breakfast not only stabilizes your blood sugar level, it also helps you burn fat and lose weight. Eating some good quality fat for breakfast also helps this process. Consider eggs, whole milk yoghurt, organic meats, avocados or breakfast smoothies with protein powder. If you crave carbohydrates and sugar, avoid eating fruit, juice or even whole grain cereal at breakfast until your metabolism stabilizes. Once you don't crave these simple sugars anymore, you can probably have some of these foods for breakfast, too.

See instructions for the Low Glycemic Diet therapy, as this is the ultimate answer to sugar cravings. If you have problems digesting proteins, you may have a hiatal hernia that needs to be corrected.

The final thing you can do to overcome sugar addiction is to use supplements that help balance your blood sugar levels. One of these is licorice root. For adults, the dose is two capsules at breakfast, two at lunch and two more in the mid-afternoon. If you have high blood pressure, however, don't use licorice root.

You can also try *Adaptogen Formulas* as they also tend to balance blood sugar levels. B-complex vitamins and chromium help the body utilize sugar properly and can be very helpful in overcoming sugar addiction. If you are diabetic, use a *Blood Sugar Reducing Formula* to help control blood sugar levels.

Both good fats and fiber help to stabilize blood sugar levels. Good fats reduce sugar cravings and fiber slows the release of sugar into the blood stream resulting in a more stable blood sugar level.

Sugar cravings can be a symptom of chronic yeast infections. Yeast feed on sugar and produce a chemical that makes the brain crave sugar. See Fungal Infections for ideas on dealing with this problem.

Excessive cravings for sweets or food in general can also come from a lack of sweetness (joy) in one's life, which causes one to excessively seek pleasure through food. Learning to find other ways to have joy and pleasure in one's life can be helpful.

Therapies: Dietary Fiber, Healthy Fats, Low Glycemic Diet, Mineralization and Stress Management

Formulas: Adaptogen and Blood Sugar Reducing

Key Herbs: Bee Pollen, **Licorice**, **Spirulina**, Devil's Club and Eleuthero (Siberian ginseng)

Key Nutrients: L-Glutamine, 5-HTP, Chromium and **Vitamin B-Complex**

Addictions (tobacco)

See also *Addictions (general remedies for)*

Nicotine, the addictive substance in tobacco, is one of the most highly addictive substances known. It is an alkaloid that attaches to receptor sites in the sympathetic nervous system, mimicking epinephrine, thus having a similar effect on the body to caffeine and other stimulants. This is why smoking tends to increase the risk of high blood pressure and heart disease.

Lobelia contains lobeline, an alkaloid with a similar structure that attaches to these sites and blocks them. The difference is that lobeline relaxes the nerves, while nicotine stimulates them. Using lobelia can help reduce the craving for nicotine while lessening withdrawal symptoms.

Smokers generally need to build up their depleted nerves and adrenal glands. Smoking also depletes vitamin C levels. B-complex vitamins and vitamin C along with *Relaxing Nervine Formulas* and *Adaptogen Formulas* can be very helpful when people are trying to quit smoking. The single herbs St. John's wort and chamomile have also proven helpful for some people.

Where smoking has damaged the lungs, *General Detoxifying* can help promote healing. Cigarettes contain heavy metals, so consider doing the Colon Cleanse therapy with a *Heavy Metal Cleansing Formula*.

Withdrawal from tobacco products also requires support to the respiratory system. Since tobacco smoke dries the lungs, *Lung and Respiratory Tonic Formulas* can help strengthen and hydrate the lungs and promote healing.

There are a number of companies that sell *Quit Smoking Formulas* you can try. These formulas usually combine herbs for the nerves and lungs into one formula.

Most cigarettes contain heavy metals so you may want to consider doing the Heavy Metal Cleanse therapy or at least taking a *General Detoxifying Formula*. Many people find it easier to quit smoking if they first transition to an additive free tobacco like American Spirit.

Therapies: Affirmation and Visualization, Colon Cleanse, Heavy Metal Cleanse and Stress Management

Formulas: Relaxing Nervine, Adaptogen, General Detoxifying, Heavy Metal Cleansing, **Quit Smoking** and Lung and Respiratory Tonic

Key Herbs: Catnip, Chamomile (English and Roman), **Lobelia**, **St. John's wort**, Oat and Valerian

Key Nutrients: Vitamin C, **Vitamin B-Complex** and **L-Glutamine**

Addison's Disease

See also *Adrenals (exhaustion, weakness or burnout)*

Addison's disease is a severe depletion of the adrenal cortex. It results in extreme weakness, loss of weight, low blood pressure, gastrointestinal disturbances, and brown pigmentation of the skin and mucous membranes. *Adrenal Tonic* and *Adaptogen Formulas* may be helpful for this condition. Even better, an adrenal glandular providing small amounts of hydrocortisone will be very helpful. Prescription cortisol is necessary for most cases of Addison's disease. Other supplements that may be of help include vitamin C, pantothenic acid (vitamin B5), l-theanine and vanadium. See Adrenals (exhaustion, weakness or burnout) for more ideas. Consult with a qualified herbalist (*findanherbalist.com*) or natural healer for assistance.

Therapies: Gut Healing Diet, Low Glycemic Diet and Stress Management

Formulas: Adaptogen and Adrenal Tonic

Key Herbs: Cordyceps, **Licorice**, Eleuthero (Siberian ginseng) and Rhodiola

Key Nutrients: Vitamin C, Pantothenic Acid (Vitamin B5) and SAM-e

Adenitis

See also *Congestion (lymphatic)*

Adenitis is inflammation of a lymph node or gland. *Lymphatic Drainage Formulas*, which improve the flow of lymph are the best choice for this condition. Be sure to drink plenty of water while taking the herbs to help flush the lymphatics. To help fight any infection that may be present, you can also consider Antibacterial, *Echinacea Blend* or *Goldenseal & Echinacea Formulas*. The Drawing Bath or Poultice therapies used with some of the key herbs listed below can also help shrink the lymph node. Physical activity also increases lymphatic flow.

Therapies: Drawing Bath, Exercise, Hydration and Poultice

Formulas: Lymphatic Drainage, Goldenseal & Echinacea, **Echinacea Blend** and Antibacterial

Key Herbs: Cleavers (Bedstraw), **Echinacea**, **Red Clover**, **Wild Indigo (Baptista)**, Garlic, Goldenseal, Lobelia, Myrrh essential oil, Oregon Grape, Rhodiola and Yucca

Key Nutrients: Vitamin C

Adrenals (exhaustion, weakness or burnout)

See also *Addison's Disease*, *Addictions (coffee, caffeine)* and *Stress*

The adrenal glands are part of the endocrine system. They sit just above the kidneys, one on each side. The adrenals are made up of two parts: the outer section is called the adrenal cortex and the central section is called the adrenal medulla.

The adrenal cortex helps in maintaining the balance of salt and water in the body and is involved with metabolizing carbohydrates and regulating blood sugars. It secretes hormones called corticosteroids, which control mineral levels, glucose metabolism and immune responses. One of these corticosteroids is called cortisol and is considered a stress hormone. Cortisol is necessary however for controlling inflammation. The cortex also produces DHEA, progesterone, estrogen and testosterone.

The adrenal medulla is related to the sympathetic nervous system and produces the hormones epinephrine (adrenaline) and norepinephrine (noradrenalin). These hormones speed up metabolism and produce other physiological changes designed to help the body cope with danger (i.e., fight or flee). They may also help in maintaining nervous system control over involuntary functions such as heart rate, respiration and digestion.

The adrenals help the body cope with or adapt to stress. Long-term stress, extreme emotional or physical trauma, excessive use of sugar and caffeine or other stimulants, low thyroid and loss of sleep can weaken the adrenal glands. When the adrenals have been overly stressed for long periods of time they may become exhausted.

Early signs of adrenal exhaustion may be fatigue, continually feeling "stressed out" or "unable to cope," and having reduced resistance to allergies, infection and illnesses. Adrenal stress (both overactivity and exhaustion) creates anxiety, muscle tension, poor digestion, poor elimination, reduced immune response (due to cortisol's immune suppressing effect), high blood pressure, shallow breathing and a difficulty meeting the challenges of life.

Lowered adrenal function causes a deficiency of cortisol, low blood pressure, hypoglycemia, sodium loss, high potassium levels, PMS, heart palpitations and tachycardia, cravings for sweets and carbohydrates, poor memory and concentration, insomnia, nervousness, irritability and mental confusion. When a person feels "burned-out" it is usually a sign of adrenal exhaustion. Typically, the person is tired during the day, but has restless, disturbed sleep. Often they wake up in the middle of the night unable to go back to sleep.

Adrenal exhaustion can also contribute to a broad spectrum of conditions such as angina, asthma, autoimmune disease, cancer, cardiovascular disease, colds, Type II diabetes, depression, headaches, high blood pressure, suppression of the immune system, irritable bowel syndrome (IBS), menstrual irregularities, PMS, rheumatoid arthritis and lupus, ulcerative colitis and ulcers.

A severely underactive adrenal cortex can cause a serious (although relatively rare) condition called Addison's disease. Symptoms of Addison's disease include a deepening of fatigue, loss of appetite, dizziness or fainting, nausea, moodiness, loss of body hair and inability to cope with stress and feeling cold. Discoloration and darkening of the skin and freckles is also common, especially after exposure to the sun.

Adaptogen Formulas and single herbs (such as eleuthero, American and Korean ginseng, rhodiola, suma, schisandra, maca, ashwaganda and astraglus) take stress off of the adrenal glands allowing them to rest and rebuild. *Adrenal Tonic Formulas* will help to strengthen and rebuild the adrenals glands when they are severely depleted. In some cases an adrenal glandular may be needed.

B-complex vitamins (and pantothenic acid in particular) and vitamin C are very helpful for rebuilding the adrenal glands. It is also very important to get extra rest and avoid stimulants, particularly sugar and caffeine, when trying to rebuild the adrenal glands.

Using Stress Management therapy will also help, as will taking some remedies to help the person relax and sleep better. Options include *Relaxing Nervine Formulas*, *Sleep Formulas*, kava kava and blue vervain.

Adrenal fatigue can also lead to chronic inflammation (as in autoimmune disorders) due to a lack of cortisol. Licorice root has a cortisol-sparing effect, and yucca and Devil's claw can also be used to help reduce the inflammation, taking stress off of the adrenal glands.

Therapies: Avoid Caffeine, Eliminate Allergy-Causing Foods, Epsom Salt Bath, Fresh Fruits and Vegetables, Low Glycemic Diet and Stress Management

Formulas: Adaptogen, **Adrenal Tonic**, Sleep and Relaxing Nervine

Key Herbs: Borage, Cordyceps, **Ashwaganda**, **Blue Vervain**, **Eleuthero (Siberian ginseng)**, **Licorice**, Devil's Claw, Ginseng (American), Ginseng (Asian, Korean), Kava-kava, Maca, Reishi (Ganoderma), Rhodiola, Schisandra (Schizandra), Spirulina and Yucca

Key Nutrients: Vitamin B-12, **Pantothenic Acid (Vitamin B5)**, **Magnesium** and **Vitamin C**

Afterbirth Pain

See also *Pain (general remedies for)*

After childbirth there is often discomfort in the abdominal and pelvic regions from the exertion, contractions and stretching that occurred in labor. Baths (particularly sitz baths) using the essential oils of lavender and rose may also be helpful. Using red raspberry or a Pregnancy Formula (where red raspberry is the principle ingredient) during pregnancy helps to prevent this problem by toning the uterine muscles. Consider using *Anti-Inflammatory Formulas* and herbal *Analgesic Formulas* for relief of pain. The mineral magnesium may also be helpful. Clove essential oil or lobelia may be applied topically to ease pain.

Formulas: Anti-Inflammatory, Analgesic and Pregnancy Tonic

Key Herbs: Clove essential oil, **Cramp Bark**, Lavender, Lobelia, Red Raspberry, Valerian and Wild Yam

Key Nutrients: Magnesium, Calcium and Potassium

Age Spots

See also *Free Radical Damage* and *Sunburn*

Also called liver spots or solar lentigo, age spots are pigments on the skin that are usually caused by overexposure to the sun. Age spots are typically treated with methods that cause superficial destruction of the skin which can leave white spots and occasional scars. They may be reduced or eliminated by using antioxidants and nutrients that heal and protect the skin against free radical damage, such as vitamins A, D and E. Cod liver oil is also a good supplement.

Therapies: Fresh Fruits and Vegetables and Healthy Fats

Formulas: Antioxidant and Topical Vulnerary

Key Herbs: Ginkgo, Hawthorn, Pau d' Arco and Rose essential oil

Key Nutrients: Vitamin A, Vitamin D, Vitamin E and Vitamin C

Aging (prevention)

See also *Free Radical Damage*

Many people spend a lot of time and energy saving, investing and planning for retirement. Unfortunately, most of these people will develop chronic and degenerative health problems as they age, which diminish the quality of life they experience in their senior years. It won't do much good to have a fat bank account if they die of a heart attack or cancer, or suffer from crippling arthritis or other conditions that prevent them from enjoying life as they grow older.

When we are planning and preparing for our senior years, we ought to invest some time, effort and money into improving and maintaining our health at the same time. And remember that government health care programs like Medicare and private health insurance policies don't really insure good health. All they cover is the cost of disease care and the use of drugs or surgery to treat symptoms of disease after they develop. This is not the same as investing in creating good health.

An investment in good health isn't all that complex. It doesn't even require that much self-discipline. Self-discipline suggests some type of self-deprivation, but caring for your health is the exact opposite of self-deprivation. Instead, it is self-nurturing.

What it takes to invest in one's health is to form positive health habits. Once you start making these investments and notice how much better you feel, you will want to keep investing because the physical, mental and emotional dividends will become obvious. Here is a checklist of places to invest time, energy and money in your health.

Eat Quality Food

Obviously, good nutrition is the place to start. The basic investment rule here is simple; avoid putting your money into refined and processed foods and purchase whole, natural and organically grown foods instead.

The most important dietary habit you can establish is to eat five to seven 1/2 cup servings of fresh fruits and vegetables every day. It's also important to select whole grain products and natural sugars (such as raw honey, xylitol, organic natural brown sugar, etc.) over their refined and processed counterparts. If you crave sugary snacks and white flour products, you need to eat more healthy fats and protein.

When selecting fats, avoid margarine, shortening and partially hydrogenated vegetable oils. Instead, use olive oil, organic butter and cream from grass-fed cows, coconut oil, avocados, and nuts as good sources of quality fats. Starting your day with a tablespoon of coconut oil will greatly reduce sugar cravings, too.

Food is both the fuel that energizes your body functions and the source of raw materials to produce healthy structures. Eating cheap junk food is no way to save money. It will reduce your energy, weaken your tissues and you'll wind up spending far more in doctor and hospital bills than you saved by eating low quality food.

Drink Water and Breathe Deeply

Two very simple things one can do to insure one's health are to drink plenty of pure water (Hydration therapy) and practice Deep Breathing therapy. For optimal health one needs to drink about 1/2 ounce of water per pound of body weight every day. Practicing any form of deep, abdominal breathing will also greatly benefit one's health. These two practices alone can reduce pain and inflammation throughout the body while increasing energy levels and overall health.

Balance Rest and Exercise

It is very important to stay physically active as one grows older. A rigorous exercise program isn't necessary, but some form of moderate physical activity such as walking, swimming or gentle bouncing on a mini-trampoline is essential to good health. The lymphatic system stagnates when we aren't breathing deeply and moving around. This causes toxins to accumulate in the system and contributes to aging and degenerative disease. A daily stretching routine is also beneficial.

Of course, it's also important to balance activity with rest. As we grow older, it's natural to slow down a little. Taking short naps or otherwise resting when tired is good for our health. It's also important to get a sound night's sleep, something that often becomes a challenge as we get older.

If you're having trouble sleeping, there are numerous herbs and supplements that can help. Try using an herbal

Sleep or *Adaptogen Formula*. *Adrenal Tonic Formulas* can also help when sleep loss is due to chronic stress.

Use Appropriate Supplements

Even if you're eating a healthy diet, you can take out some additional health insurance by selecting a few well-chosen supplements. These can be general supplements designed to support overall nutrition, or specific supplements to address common health concerns associated with aging. Various tonic herbs, like ginseng, ginkgo, cordyceps and he shou wu are used in other cultures to help people stay healthier as they age. Here are a few ideas for some basic herbal formulas and supplements to counteract the aging process.

Antioxidant Formulas can be helpful in counteracting the free radicals associated with the aging process. You can also use individual antioxidants like green tea, ginkgo, alpha lipoic acid and Co-Q10. Fresh or frozen berries are wonderful antioxidants, too.

Brain and Memory Tonic Formulas can help protect the brain and prevent memory loss. Gotu kola and ginkgo are good single herbs to consider for this purpose as they are key herbs in these formulas.

Formulas for supporting the glands can help maintain general health as a person ages. Women can use *Menopause Balancing Formulas* for balancing their hormones and men can use *Male Glandular Tonic Formulas*. Eleuthero, ginseng, gotu kola and he shou wu are single herbs that can help to balance glandular function as one ages.

Elderly people usually have diminished digestive function, so a *Digestive Tonic* or *Digestive Enzyme Formula* can be helpful to improve general nutrition.

These are just some basic suggestions. For help in developing an anti-aging program specifically tailored to your needs, do a little research and/or seek help from a qualified herbalist (*findanherbalist.com*).

Therapies: Deep Breathing, Exercise, Fast or Juice Fast, Fresh Fruits and Vegetables, Healthy Fats, Hydration, Low Glycemic Diet, Mineralization and Stress Management

Formulas: Male Glandular Tonic, Menopause Balancing, Antioxidant, Brain and Memory Tonic, Sleep, Adrenal Tonic, Digestive Tonic and Digestive Enzyme

Key Herbs: Bacopa (Water Hyssop), Barley, Bee Pollen, Cordyceps, Cordyceps, **Eleuthero (Siberian ginseng)**, Ginkgo, Gotu kola, He Shou Wu (Ho Shou Wu, Fo-Ti), Milk Thistle, Rehmannia and Tea (Green or Black)

Key Nutrients: L-Glutamine, Alpha Lipoic Acid, Pantothenic Acid (Vitamin B5), Melatonin, DHEA, Co-Q10, Vitamin E, Zinc, N-Acetyl Cysteine, Selenium and Proanthocyanidins

AIDS

See *Acquired Immune Deficiency Syndrome (AIDS)/HIV*

Alcoholism

See *Addictions (alcohol)*

Alkalosis

See also *Overalkalinity*

This is a serious condition where the body becomes overly alkaline. It should be treated medically.

Allergies (food)

See also *Autoimmune Disorders* and *Leaky Gut Syndrome*

Allergies are an adverse reaction in the immune system to a substance that most people would consider harmless. Symptoms of food allergies are many and varied, but may include gastrointestinal disturbances (inflammatory bowel disorders and leaky gut syndrome), respiratory and lymphatic congestion (excess mucus, swollen lymph nodes), rashes, fatigue, headaches, autoimmune disorders, and even emotional disturbances. There is research and clinical experience that suggests food allergies may be a factor in hyperactivity, restlessness, irritability, anxiety and depression.

This is because food allergies can actually produce a profound alteration in the brain function. These are known as cerebral allergies. In fact, in some rare cases extremely aggressive or psychotic behavior may appear after eating certain foods.

In children, frequent earaches are often a sign of dairy or wheat allergies. In adults, arthritis, migraines, glaucoma, colitis and eczema are often connected with food allergies. In short, many common health problems may trace back to food allergies.

Understanding Food Allergies

Why do people have these negative reactions to what should be nourishing foods? The medical explanation is that the immune system is "out of whack" and is recognizing a substance (such as a protein molecule) as something "foreign or bad" when it really isn't. Consequently, there is an immune system response whenever foods containing that particular substance are eaten.

Improper functioning of the immune system may be brought about by an overload of toxic irritants. Our immune systems may be unnecessarily burdened for many reasons, such as: all forms of environmental pollution, repeated vaccinations and immunizations, malnutrition, and destruction of the healthy bacteria in the intestines due to overuse of antibiotics, Non Steroidal Anti-inflammatories (NSAIDs) and steroids (especially birth control pills).

Many natural healers believe that part of the problem in food allergies may be poor digestion, especially poor protein metabolism. The essential basis of the immune system is the ability of the body to sense the difference between self and what is not self. Somehow, bodies are able to tell the difference between a protein manufactured by our own bodies and a protein manufactured by another living thing. This is why someone who receives an organ transplant must be given immune depressing drugs. Otherwise, the body will recognize that the transplanted organ does not belong to the body and will destroy it.

As a result, we have an immune system response (or in other words an allergic reaction) to various foreign protein structures. The purpose of protein digestion is to break all the proteins we eat down into free amino acids (the basic building blocks of protein). We then assimilate the free amino acids and recombine them to make our own proteins. One can readily see that if digestion of proteins is incomplete, undigested protein fragments would trigger the immune system to produce antibodies because these protein fragments are actually foreign invaders.

Food Allergies and Gut Health

Thus, food allergies may be closely related disturbances of the gastrointestinal tract resulting in poor digestion and improved assimilation. So, food allergies may begin as a food intolerance or sensitivity that occurs when the body lacks certain enzymes needed for digestion. For example, many people lack the enzyme necessary to digest the lactose (milk sugar) in dairy foods. Thus, dairy foods cause these people to develop symptoms of indigestion, such as gas, bloating and intestinal distress. However, since there is no antibody (immune) response, lactose intolerance is not considered a food allergy.

People who are allergic to milk are allergic to the proteins in milk, which trigger an antibody response. The body cannot break down the A-1 Beta Casein in dairy products, especially after a heating process like pasteurization. This causes bloating, excess mucus and allergy responses that can be labeled as lactose intolerance. Many do not have this reaction with low temp processed A-2 Beta Casein dairy.

The same problem occurs with gluten in grains like wheat, rye, barley and spelt. Other common food allergies/intolerances include grains in general (corn, oats, etc.) legumes (peas, beans, peanuts, etc.), broccoli, cabbage, mushrooms, oranges, eggs, and some wines.

There is some evidence to back up the theory that food allergies signal a lack of enzymes in the body. Enzyme deficiency is caused by the fact that we eat so many cooked and processed foods and so few raw, sprouted or fermented foods.

Another reason why certain enzymes might be depleted is simply over-consumption of a particular food. Any "good" thing becomes a "bad" thing when it is out of balance. Most Americans are heavy consumers of wheat, corn, dairy, oranges and other common "allergic" foods. In his studies, one physician found that most sufferers of allergies had diets that consisted of thirty foods or less, which they ate all the time. In fact, it is said that if people eat the same food consistently, they could easily develop an allergy to that food since their immune systems are constantly exposed to it. Hence, a food allergy may be the body's way of saying, "I've had enough of this, give me something else."

Overworked Liver

Another major cause of food allergies may be an over-burdened liver. The liver is responsible for filtering all of the blood from the intestines before it is released into the rest of the body. All foods contain small amounts of irritating substances that the liver must filter out and destroy. Add to these naturally occurring irritants all of the man-made chemicals (food additives, pesticide residues, water pollutants, etc.) which the liver must also filter out and one can readily see how the liver can be very overworked.

The liver performs its tasks by means of thousands of enzyme reactions. Each of these enzyme reactions requires the presence of certain minerals that act as chemical "spark plugs" to trigger that reaction. So enzymes come into the picture again.

With our diets of processed, mineral-deficient foods, it is easy to see how the liver could fail to keep the blood free of irritants from the digestive tract. Once these irritants and chemicals get past the liver, it falls on the immune system response to eliminate them. So, this is another key factor in understanding the mechanism of food allergies.

Natural Therapy

To combat food allergies start by eliminating the foods that cause the allergic reaction for a while to allow your digestive system and immune system to heal and rebalance. For help identifying what foods to avoid, see the Eliminate-Allergy Causing Foods therapy. There are also allergy tests you can obtain from your health professional.

As suggested above, the most important supplements to help with food allergies are enzymes, so take digestive enzyme supplements or *Digestive Enzyme Formulas*. Since the liver may also need support, consider a *General Detoxifying* or a *Liver Tonic Formula* as part of your program. *Digestive Bitter Tonic Formulas* work on both the stomach and the liver to improve digestion.

Many food allergies involve Leaky Gut Syndrome, so improving the health of the intestinal tract is also helpful. Start with the Colon Cleanse therapy and then use probiotics (or fermented foods) and antioxidants to reduce intestinal irritation and improve gut health. *Intestinal Toning* and *Mushroom Blend Formulas* can help to desensitize the immune system to foods. See Leaky Gut for more suggestions.

Homeopathics may also help to desensitize a person's allergies. The homeopathic provides the energy signature of the allergen without actually providing the substance, which can adjust the body's immune system to better tolerate the food.

When a person suffers from allergic responses to raw, unprocessed foods like strawberries, pineapple or papaya, it may not be that the person's body is so toxic or out of balance that it can't handle this healthy food. By taking very tiny amounts of the food and gradually increasing them, the person's body may be able to gradually discharge the irritant and the food will no longer cause a reaction. This also works for many so-called "allergic" reactions to herbs, too.

Therapies: Colon Cleanse, Eliminate Allergy-Causing Foods, Fresh Fruits and Vegetables, Friendly Flora, Gut Healing Diet, Hiatal Hernia Correction and Hydration

Formulas: Digestive Enzyme, General Detoxifying, Liver Tonic, Intestinal Toning, Mushroom Blend and **Digestive Bitter Tonic**

Key Herbs: Aloe vera, Burdock, **Black Walnut, Cats Claw (Uña de Gato, Gambier)**, Devil's Claw, Ginger, Nettle (Stinging), Osha and Plantain

Key Nutrients: Protease Enzymes, Lactase Enzymes, **Digestive Enzymes**, Probiotics and **Betaine Hydrochloric Acid (HCl)**

Allergies (respiratory)

See also *Adrenals (exhaustion, weakness or burnout), Allergies (food), Congestion (lymphatic), Fungal Infections (Yeast Infections, Candida albicans) and Leaky Gut Syndrome*

As nature awakes each spring and plants begin to bud and bloom, flowers release their pollen and millions of Americans are suddenly miserable. Most people call this condition hayfever, but technically it is allergic rhinitis, and pollen isn't the only thing that causes it. Rhinitis is an inflammatory condition that affects the sensitive membranes of the nasal and sinus passages, the eyes and the throat. In allergic rhinitis, the inflammation is caused by allergic reactions. However, rhinitis can have other causes besides allergies.

Respiratory allergies like allergic rhinitis are caused by an overly sensitive immune response reacting to environmental substances. In the case of an allergic reaction, the immune system overproduces immunoglobulin E (IgE) antibodies. When antibodies attach to an allergen, it causes your body to release histamine. This causes inflammation and the symptoms associated with rhinitis and respiratory allergies, which can include congestion, sinus discharge, sneezing, watery eyes, itchy eyes, sinus pain and/or pressure, coughing and/or sore throat. It may even upset the digestive tract, causing bloating, gas, loss of appetite and abdominal discomfort.

Seasonal allergic rhinitis, which occurs during specific seasons of the year, is always caused by pollen. Tree and grass pollens, as well as pollen from flowers like ragweed, plantain and dandelion, are common culprits. However, when the rhinitis symptoms occur year-round, the allergic reactions are usually caused by indoor irritants such as dust, dust mites, pet dander, feathers and mold. The non-allergic rhinitis can be caused by household cleaning agents, cosmetics, perfumes and other chemicals.

Most of the medical treatments available for these conditions only treat the symptoms, but never actually cure the underlying problem. Fortunately, there are natural ways to relieve respiratory allergies and create more permanent relief.

It's pretty obvious that the place to start in getting relief from rhinitis is to remove the source of the respiratory irritants, whenever possible. For example, get rid of toxic household cleaning products and chemicals and, if air pollution is a serious problem, purchase an air filtration system. Even if it's pollen you're allergic to, reducing the amount of irritants your sensitive membranes have to deal with will go a long way to easing your problems.

You can also gain relief from rhinitis by dealing with a number of underlying health issues that are often contributing to the problem. These include all of the following:

Food Allergies

Allergic reactions to foods in the intestinal tract will hypersensitize the immune system and make you more susceptible to respiratory allergies. Common food allergies that may be contributing to rhinitis include wheat, corn, dairy, citrus, eggs, peanut butter, shellfish and soy. Food additives, dyes and preservatives in processed foods may also be a contributing factor.

There are signs that indicate food allergies may be a contributing factor. If a person experiences any of the following after eating a food, they probably have an allergic reaction to it, such as: dark circles under the eyes, redness of the ears, face or eyes, a glassy look, an increased pulse rate, bloating, fatigue or mood changes. If a person craves certain foods excessively, they may be allergic to them.

If you suspect food allergies may be contributing to your respiratory allergies, eliminate all suspected allergy-producing foods or do a short fast for two or three days. If symptoms improve, then food allergies are probably an underlying factor. Reintroduce suspected foods one at a time and watch for symptoms or reaction. See Allergies (food) for more information.

Dehydration

A little known contributing factor to respiratory allergies is dehydration. Normally mucus traps irritating particles and allows them to be swept off the surface of the membranes. Tears wash away irritants from the eyes. When a person is dehydrated, their mucus membranes and eyes can be dry. This allows irritants to sit on the membranes. In response, the body creates an inflammatory reaction, driven by histamine, to flush the irritants from the nose, eyes and throat.

Staying well hydrated by drinking lots of water can greatly reduce allergic reactions. It also helps to take a little natural salt with the water as mucus and tears are salty. Allergic reactions can often be calmed down rapidly by drinking water and taking a pinch of salt.

Intestinal Inflammation and Leaky Gut Syndrome

Inflammation in the colon tends to congest the lymphatic system and trigger inflammation in the respiratory tract. If you're eating a standard American diet and have allergies, cleansing the colon will probably help relieve respiratory allergy symptoms. Take a *Fiber Blend Formula*, along with a good *General Detoxifying Formula*. Also take digestive enzyme supplements. An enzyme from pineapple called bromelain is especially helpful if you have allergies.

Since allergies are an inflammatory response, *Anti-Inflammatory Formulas* may be useful, too. Vitamin C is a great antioxidant and anti-inflammatory remedy with the added benefit that it helps break down histamine. MSM and Co-Q10 are other anti-inflammatory remedies that may calm down allergic reactions.

It takes about three to four weeks before you'll start seeing significant results, but this cleaning out the colon and restoring intestinal health with probiotics, enzymes and *Mushroom Blend Formulas* has helped many people obtain permanent relief from respiratory allergies. See Leaky Gut Syndrome for more information on how to heal the intestinal membranes.

Liver Problems and Toxicity

The liver is the primary organ of internal detoxification and when it is overburdened with toxins, people become more susceptible to allergies. A number of toxins have been shown to contribute to allergies, including mercury, sodium benzoate, atazine yellow, MSG, aspirin and a number of other drugs. The liver also breaks down excess histamine, so if liver function is sluggish histamine will not be eliminated efficiently from the body.

If you get stuffy, bloated feelings in your abdomen, especially under the right rib cage and feel very groggy and sluggish in the mornings, you may need to support your liver. Irritability, headaches and difficulty getting to sleep are also indications your liver may be overwhelmed with toxins.

Cleansing the colon will also help the liver clear toxins better, but in addition, consider adding a more specific remedy to aid liver detoxification. Good choices include *Blood Purifier* and *Hepatoprotective Formulas*.

Inhibited Lymphatic Drainage

The lymphatic system drains fluid away from inflamed areas, so if you have poor lymphatic drainage, this may contribute to your problems with rhinitis. If you can feel swollen lymph nodes or tenderness in your neck, then poor lymphatic drainage may be a factor in your stuffed up head. Try using a *Lymphatic Drainage Formula*, drinking more water and mild exercise, like walking, to improve lymph flow.

Adrenal Insufficiency

The adrenal medulla regulates histamine reactions and inflammation in the body. So, reduced function of the adrenals may contribute to excessive allergic responses. If you feel tired, or under a lot of stress, this may be a factor

in your allergies. In this case *Adrenal Tonic Formulas* may be helpful. Vitamin B5 is also helpful for overcoming adrenal insufficiency.

Specific Nutritional Deficiencies

Nutritional deficiencies may play a role in respiratory allergies. The over sensitivity of the immune system may be due to a lack of essential nutrients needed to regulate the immune response. For instance, vitamin C and bioflavonoids (especially quercitin) have been shown to reduce histamine reactions. Deficiencies of calcium and magnesium have also been linked with respiratory allergies. Many Americans are particularly low in magnesium.

Omega-3 essential fatty acids help produce compounds which mediate inflammation and reduce inflammatory reactions. Other nutrients that may be beneficial to allergy sufferers include vitamin A, selenium, zinc, pantothenic acid and *Antioxidant Formulas*.

Homeopathic Remedies

Homeopathy addresses the hypersensitive reaction of the allergen. By giving diluted doses of remedies that can cause allergy-like symptoms, homeopathic remedies can desensitize the immune system so that it no longer overreacts. Look for an appropriate homeopathic remedy made from the substances that trigger your allergies. Sometimes you can find locally-made homeopathic remedies from the pollen of local species known to cause allergic reactions.

Many people with pollen allergies have been able to achieve an effect similar to that of homeopathic remedies by taking locally gathered bee pollen internally actually helps diminish allergic reactions to pollen. Locally-grown honey which has not been filtered can also be helpful. Start by taking a very small amount (just a few grains) and gradually work up to several capsules a day.

Symptomatic Relief

There are herbs that desensitize mast cells and calm down allergic reactions. These include blessed thistle, burdock, nettles, eyebright, goldenrod and ambrosia. Taking these remedies throughout the allergy season won't solve the underlying causes of the allergies, but they can reduce reactions and symptoms. Many of these herbs are found in *Allergy-Reducing Formulas*. So, try using one of these formulas or one or more of the aforementioned herbs to provide symptomatic relief. Large amounts of water, taken with a little natural salt and large doses of vitamin C, will also offer symptomatic relief.

Symptomatic relief can also be had through using herbs that help to decongest respiratory passages and dry up excessive secretions. Yerba Santa, horseradish, marshmallow and mullein are all good choices for decongesting the airways. So, a *Decongestant Formula* may be helpful. Bitter orange and Mormon Tea can dry out excessive secretions, although this is not the best approach for long-term relief (see Dehydration above).

Balancing the function of the immune system will also help alleviate symptoms. *Mushroom Blend* or *Immune Balancing Formulas* help to stabilize immune reactions (reducing excessive immune reactions while enhancing normal ones).

Therapies: Colon Cleanse, Eliminate Allergy-Causing Foods, Eliminate Gluten, Fresh Fruits and Vegetables, Friendly Flora, Gut Healing Diet, Healthy Fats, Hiatal Hernia Correction and Hydration

Formulas: Anti-Inflammatory, **Allergy-Reducing**, Fiber Blend, General Detoxifying, Blood Purifier, Hepatoprotective, Lymphatic Drainage, Adrenal Tonic, Antioxidant, Mushroom Blend, Decongestant and Immune Balancing

Key Herbs: Bee Pollen, Blessed Thistle, Burdock, Butterbur Root, Cherry (Wild), **Eyebright**, **Goldenrod**, **Nettle (Stinging)**, Devil's Claw, Holy Basil, Horseradish, Licorice, Lomatium, Maitake, Mangosteen, Marshmallow, Mullein, Triphala and Yerba Santa

Key Nutrients: Vitamin C, Omega-3 Essential Fatty Acids, MSM, Co-Q10, Vitamin A, Selenium, Zinc, Bromelain, Fiber, Digestive Enzymes, Potassium and **Quercitin**

Alzheimer's Disease

See also *Free Radical Damage, Heavy Metal Poisoning, Memory and Brain Function* and *Dementia*

Alzheimer's is a degenerative disease of the central nervous system characterized by mental deterioration. Neurons in the brain that produce a neurotransmitter called acetylcholine are destroyed by free radical damage.

High levels of aluminum have been found in the brains of some, but not all, Alzheimer's patients. Although many experts feel that aluminum doesn't cause Alzheimer's disease, Charles Walters in *Minerals for the Genetic Code* indicates that aluminum absorbed into the body readily travels to the brain where it deactivates phosphorus (a mineral needed for ATP production, the molecule that powers cellular activity). Aluminum also depletes boron and silica.

So, while Alzheimer's isn't conclusively linked to aluminum toxicity it is easy to avoid and may offer some benefit. Avoid aluminum cookware and aluminum foil, especially when preparing acidic food like tomatoes. Also avoid antiperspirant deodorants that contain aluminum compounds and baking powder with aluminum. Aluminum is also used in processed American cheese, certain food dyes, cosmetics, coated aspirin, certain brands of antacids and many vaccines.

A *Heavy Metal Cleansing Formula* is an option, although these formulas are more likely to help remove mercury (which also damages brain function) than aluminum. N-Acetyl-Cysteine is also useful for heavy metal detoxification.

Recent research into Alzheimer's shows that at least some cases are caused by elevated insulin levels and oxidative damage causing faulty glucose metabolism in the brain. Moderately high insulin levels are associated with increased levels of inflammatory markers and beta-amyloid in cerebrospinal fluid, suggesting a causal link between hyperinsulinemia and Alzheimer's disease. Therefore, eliminating refined starches and sugar from the diet is the best prevention. According to Maciej Gasior in the *Journal of Behavioral Pharmacology*, Ketogenic diets with added medium chain triglycerides seem to provide "symptomatic and disease-modifying activity in a broad range of neurodegenerative disorders" including Alzheimer's. Consult a qualified practitioner before starting a Ketogenic diet.

Researchers agree that free radical damage is at work in Alzheimer's. The brain is mostly fat (50% by dry weight) and needs adequate amounts of antioxidants (especially fat soluble vitamins like A, D, E and K) to protect it from damage. *Antioxidant Formulas* and antioxidant herbs and nutrients like green tea, rosemary, alpha lipoic acid and Co-Q10 may be of benefit in both preventing and slowing the progression of Alzheimer's.

Ginkgo, gotu kola, rosemary and other key herbs found in *Brain and Memory Tonic Formulas* may be helpful in enhancing cognitive function in Alzheimer's patients. They are unlikely to affect an actual cure, but herbalists have found them to be of benefit. A specific form of magnesium, magnesium threonate, can also be helpful.

One of the most hopeful remedies for helping improve brain function in Alzheimer's is the use of good fats. Eating coconut oil every day has proven beneficial for some. Also consider omega-3 essential fatty acids, especially DHA.

To protect the brain, minimize exposure to alcohol, tobacco and environmental toxins. Eat generous servings of fresh fruits and vegetables every day and stay mentally active. These general tips help to protect against memory loss due to aging, which includes reducing the risk of Alzheimer's. For more tips see Memory and Brain Function.

Therapies: Fresh Fruits and Vegetables, Healthy Fats and Heavy Metal Cleanse

Formulas: Brain and Memory Tonic, Antioxidant and Heavy Metal Cleansing

Key Herbs: Bacopa (Water Hyssop), **Ginkgo**, **Rosemary**, Gotu kola and Tea (Green or Black)

Key Nutrients: Alpha Lipoic Acid, **N-Acetyl Cysteine**, Vitamin B-3 (Niacin), **Vitamin B-12**, SAM-e, MSM, DHEA, Co-Q10, Omega-3 Essential Fatty Acids, DHA, Magnesium, L-Glutamine and Potassium

Amenorrhea

Amenorrhea is a lack of periods or menstrual flow. When periods are scant, infrequent, or absent it is important to try to identify the cause. The most common causes are extreme diets (especially diets low in fats and protein), excessive exercise, stress, general poor health, thyroid imbalances, and medications. Seek appropriate professional assistance in identifying the cause, but you can also try some basic remedies for balancing hormones, such as: Female Hormonal Balancing, General Glandular Tonic and *Hypothyroid Formulas*.

Herbs that were traditionally used to bring on "delayed menstruation" were called emmenagogues. Some of these herbs are actually abortifacients, meaning they were used to abort the fetus and restart menstruation in early pregnancy. Blue cohosh is one of these herbs and should be avoided if there is a possibility one is pregnant as it can be very harmful to the fetus.

Therapies: Healthy Fats, Mineralization and Stress Management

Formulas: Hyperthyroid and Female Hormonal Balancing

Key Herbs: Cinnamon, **Blue Cohosh**, **Dong Quai**, False Unicorn (Helonias), Ginger, Motherwort, Myrrh, Peony and Rhodiola

Key Nutrients: Omega-3 Essential Fatty Acids and Vitamin B-Complex

Amyotrophic Lateral Sclerosis

See *Lou Gehrig's Disease (Amyotrophic Lateral Sclerosis)*

Anal Fistula or Fissure

See also *Hemorrhoids*

An anal fistula is an abnormal passageway in the anal area. It is also known as an anal fissure. To heal an anal fistula, it is important to keep the stool soft. Take a *Fiber Blend Formula* and a *Gentle Laxative Formula* along with plenty of water to keep the bowels moving without strain. Apply astringent herbs like white oak bark or stone root (collinsonia) topically mixed with *Topical Vulnerary Formula* (salve) and *Topical Antiseptic Formulas* can be applied to help close the fissure, fight infection and promote healing. You can also take these astringents internally.

Therapies: Dietary Fiber and Hydration

Formulas: Vascular Tonic, Fiber Blend, Gentle Laxative, Topical Vulnerary and Topical Antiseptic

Key Herbs: Butchers Broom, Calendula, **Collinsonia (Stoneroot)**, Horse Chestnut, Horsetail, Plantain, White Oak and Witch Hazel

Key Nutrients: Magnesium, Bioflavonoids and Fiber

Anemia

Anemia indicates that there is a deficiency in red blood cells, hemoglobin (the component in red blood cells that carries oxygen) or in total blood volume. This results in fatigue, reduced resistance to illness and other symptoms. Iron alone is not necessarily the solution, since there are many other nutrients necessary for the utilization of iron and the production of hemoglobin.

In working with your doctor, it is important to get all levels of iron measured and not just serum iron. Check transferrin, total iron binding capacity (TIBC) ferritn, hemoglobin and hematocrit. The whole picture needs to be evaluated.

A nutrient dense diet should be combined with supplements to correct deficiency. Unless you are losing blood or have malabsorption, you should be able to get plenty of folate from green vegetables. The best food sources of iron are beef liver, beef, and eggs. If you have to supplement with iron be sure to take it with foods containing vitamin C.

To supply the body with iron take a chelated iron supplement or, better yet, an herbal *Iron Formula*. Herbs like nettles, yellow dock, dong quai and alfalfa can be very helpful for building up anemic blood. A tea made of equal parts nettle leaf, alfalfa herb and red raspberry has been used in pregnancy as a tonic and is very helpful at preventing anemia during pregnancy.

Vitamin B-12 supplementation if often necessary with SIBO and always necessary with pernicious anemia. A good way to supplement this is to take 5,000 mcg. of methyl B12 (methylcobalamin) sublingually daily. In severe cases B-12 injections may be needed. If you do have anemia it is best to work with a competent practitioner to figure out the cause.

Although it does not contain iron, chlorophyll may be helpful in building up iron poor blood Supplements that help the utilization of iron in the body include vitamin C, l-glutamine, vitamin B-12, folate (not folic acid), vitamin B-6 and zinc. Red meat from organic, exclusively grass-fed animals is also a good blood-building tonic for anemia.

Megaloblastic anemia is caused by a defect in red cell DNA synthesis and is most often due to vitamin B12 and folate deficiency. In a recent broad study covering people with varied diets and ages, an average of 60% of Americans had sub-optimal B12 levels, with 20% being severely deficient. B12 deficiency can not only directly result in anemia, it can cause low stomach acid and indirectly contribute to anemia. When taking vitamin B-12, make sure the form is methylcobalamin, not cyanocobalamin). B-12 shots may also be needed.

The absorption of iron also requires hydrochloric acid in the stomach, so a *Digestive Bitter Tonic Formula* may be helpful in stimulating the absorption of iron. You may even need to try a betaine hydrochloric acid (HCl) supplement.

Therapies: Gut Healing Diet and Mineralization

Formulas: Iron, Digestive Bitter Tonic and Pregnancy Tonic

Key Herbs: Alfalfa, Angelica, Beet Root, Blue Vervain, Burdock, Chickweed, **Nettle (Stinging)**, **Yellow Dock**, Dong Quai, Gentian and Marshmallow

Key Nutrients: Chlorophyll, L-Glutamine, Iron, Vitamin B-6 (Pyridoxine), **Vitamin B-12**, Zinc, Vitamin C, **Betaine Hydrochloric Acid (HCl)**, Folate (Folic Acid, Vitamin B9) and Vitamin B-2 (Riboflavin)

Aneurysm

An aneurysm is a blood-filled dilation of a blood vessel wall as a result of a blood vessel disease or weakness. Appropriate medical attention should be sought for this condition as it is life-threatening. Herbs like yarrow and capsicum can be administered during transport for medical care. *Vascular Tonic* and *Cardiovascular Stimulant Formulas* may assist in recovery, as can bioflavonoids from berries like blueberries. Hawthorn solid extract will also be helpful.

Formulas: Cardiovascular Stimulant and Vascular Tonic

Key Herbs: Butchers Broom, Capsicum (Cayenne), **Horse Chestnut**, **Yarrow**, Hawthorn and Rose hips

Key Nutrients: Magnesium and Bioflavonoids

Anger (excessive)

See also *Irritability*

While not commonly thought of as a "mood" disorder like depression or anxiety, excessive anger is harmful both to our health and our relationships. In Traditional Chinese Medicine (TCM), excess anger is thought to damage the liver and gallbladder. The liver/gallbladder connection to anger is also found in traditional Western medicine and culture, as shown in the expression, "that really galls me," (gall being another word for bile).

When people are thinking about adopting better health habits they usually try to improve their diet, exercise, get a good night's sleep and perhaps take a few herbs or supplements. Some people also work on changing their attitude to be more positive. Few people work on their emotions or even consider the role that emotions play in their health problems.

This is a shame, because traditional healing systems all over the world have recognized that our emotional state has a huge impact on our health and is also an important clue as to what organs in the body may need help.

Modern Western medicine recognizes that angry people are at much higher risk for cardiovascular problems. Again, our language intuitively recognizes this when we talk about angry and controlling people as being "hard-hearted." Anger and aggression also inhibit elimination, hence the phrase "pissed off," suggesting that anger turns "off" our ability to urinate. Constantly being angry and controlling makes us constipated or "tight assed." Phrases like "venting one's spleen," suggest that anger also affects the digestive organs.

As if the damage to our physical health isn't bad enough, anger also destroys relationships. Constantly venting anger destroys love in marriages, ruins parent-child relationships, and adversely affects other personal and business relationships.

Clearly, we need to learn how to manage anger to preserve both our health and the health of our relationships. Let's begin by understanding two important facts about anger.

Facing and Understanding Anger

First of all, let's make it clear that anger is not a "bad" or "negative" emotion, per se. Anger is the emotion that allows us to protect and defend ourselves. It only becomes a destructive influence in our lives when we aren't able to express it constructively. Most people only know two ways of dealing with anger. They either "vent" their anger by attacking and belittling others, or they "suppress" their anger and let other people have their way to avoid a fight. Both of these approaches are unhealthy.

The second thing we need to understand is that the relationship between anger and our physical health goes both ways. Anger can damage our health, but health problems can make us more prone to being angry and irritable. Just like depression can have physical causes, so can being easily angered.

Because of this, we're going to explore learning how to manage anger from both directions, emotionally and physically. If you have problems with anger, work on it from both directions for best results.

There are three primary health issues that can make us feel irritable (easily angered). They are liver toxicity, blood sugar problems and stress. We'll look at each of these issues and then talk a little bit about managing anger.

Clean Up Your Liver

TCM associates the element of "wood" with the liver and gallbladder. The element of wood represents our ability to grow, expand and live. When this ability to flow is disrupted, we feel irritable and anger. To understand this, just imagine that you are driving down the freeway and are running a little late. You are anxious to get to your destination when suddenly you run into a huge traffic jam that grinds traffic to a halt.

If you're normal, this block in your "flow" probably makes you feel frustrated at the least and angry at the worst. This inhibition of flow is something similar to the concept of "constricted liver chi (energy)." When our liver is congested and toxic, we tend to feel defensive and irritable. This is why excessive anger is associated with an imbalance in the wood element in Chinese medicine.

This is why taking a good liver cleansing formula, such as a *Blood Purifier*, *Cholagogue* or *Liver Tonic Formula* can help cool down irritable feelings. The Chinese herb bupleurum root can be particularly helpful because it is said to remove feelings of anger and sadness from the liver.

In detoxifying the body to reduce anger, you may also want to consider working with the kidneys. The kidneys help to flush toxins processed by the liver, so if your kidneys can't keep up with the toxic load you may also feel angry and irritable because your ability to piss is "off." If you're angry and you're having problems with your kidneys or bladder, use a *Diuretic Formula*.

Balance that Blood Sugar

Refined carbohydrates cause rapid increases in blood sugar, which over-stimulates the brain. If you're a careful observer, you will notice how a relaxed and calm child can suddenly become a "little monster" after eating a bunch of sugary foods. The same thing happens to adults, who can become agitated and aggressive after consuming lots of sugar and caffeine.

When blood sugar levels rise dramatically, they also tend to fall dramatically, sort of like a blood sugar roller coaster ride. So, later, when the blood sugar drops, one may feel shaky, agitated, defensive or withdrawn. Barbara Reed, a juvenile parole officer in upstate New York, found that delinquent teenagers often had serious blood sugar issues. When fed a diet designed to control hypoglycemia (low blood sugar) these kids never got in trouble with the law again. This diet consisted of fresh fruits, vegetables, whole grains and meat with no sugar, alcohol and caffeine.

Other studies have shown that criminals in prisons become less violent when put on a similar diet to balance blood sugar. Clearly, regulating blood sugar helps regulate our mood so we can face the problems of life with a calmer, clearer head.

To regulate blood sugar, start the day with a good breakfast that includes some form of high quality protein and fat. Choose low glycemic carbohydrates such as fresh fruits and vegetables, rather than refined sugar or white flour. Licorice root can help reduce cravings for sugar and a *Hypoglycemic Formula* and/or a B-complex vitamin supplement with vitamin C can also help keep blood sugar levels more stable. Spirulina and bee pollen are other single remedies that may help here.

Adaptogens Help You Stay Calm

Stress is the natural response of our adrenal glands to danger. The adrenal hormones that pump through the body when we experience stress make our heart beat faster, raise our blood pressure, tense our muscles and otherwise prime the body for action. This is called the "fight or flight" response because it is preparing us to flee the danger or fight it off.

One of the effects of this response is that the flow of blood to our higher brain (cortex) diminishes leaving our "animal instincts" in charge. Since we are primed to "fight" one of the reactions we might have is to lash out in anger to "protect" ourselves. Unfortunately, lashing out in anger often makes the situation worse, rather than better, so we need to find a way to calm the production of stress hormones.

This is where adaptogens come to the rescue. Adaptogens reduce the output of stress hormones, which can help us think more clearly, feel calmer and less stressed and deal with problems without flying off the handle. A good *Adaptogen Formula* will help reduce your stress hormones, which can ease feelings of anger, irritability and anxiety.

Since adaptogens also help to balance blood sugar, they provide a double benefit for reducing our tendency to anger and irritability. Add to this the facts that adaptogens can make us more productive and efficient, increase stamina and energy, decrease our risk of getting sick and help us live longer.

Anger Management

To understand how to use anger constructively, we need to understand a concept called personal boundaries. Our personal boundary separates the things we are in control of from the things we are not. We are responsible (that is, able to respond) to the things inside our personal boundaries, but we are not responsible for what is outside of them, or what we have no control over. This means that we are only responsible for our own thoughts, feelings and choices (actions), as nothing else is in our control.

Problems with anger involve problems with personal boundaries. We are either trying to control something that is not in our control, or allowing others to control something inside our personal boundary. When we try to control something not in our control, we "vent" our anger, using it to threaten, attack, belittle and manipulate others. When we "vent" anger, we are trying to solve our problem by controlling other people.

This is impossible, of course, and it is not a positive way to use anger. It is a sign that we have a poor understanding of our personal boundaries and lack responsibility for ourselves. Venting anger pushes other people away, creating feelings of loneliness and isolation that can lead to heart disease, increased stress and other health problems.

Another choice we have would be to suppress our anger. This often means we "cave in" to unreasonable demands and expectations of others, allowing them to control us. This is also not healthy. It weakens our immune system and eventually leads to frustration and resentment that can destroy relationships. This is a sign that we are not taking control of our own life, which is also a sign of holes in our personal boundaries.

These two ways of dealing with anger are the only two options most people are aware of (it is either control or be controlled). However, there is a third option. We can *assert* our right to control our own life, and *affirm* the right of others to control theirs. This means that we embrace our personal boundaries, we aren't trying to attack others, and we aren't allowing others to push us around. We are standing up for, or asserting, ourselves. This is the constructive way to deal with anger.

A good anger management course or book can help you learn to be assertive without being controlling, but here are a few basic tips. First, when you are feeling angry, train yourself to pause and take a few deep breaths. This is particularly important if you are prone to vent your anger (that is to attack other people, trying to belittle or control them). Before speaking or acting in anger, first try to understand the real source of your frustration.

If you are trying to control someone else's behavior, take a look at why you feel you have the right to demand that they change for your benefit. Ask yourself, "How do I feel my personal well-being is being threatened?" Then ask, "What could I do about this that doesn't involve trying to attack or control someone else?"

We can communicate that something bothers us without having to make the other person's actions wrong. We can just state that we like or dislike certain things. We can also decide what our course of action is going to be to resolve a problem. In other words, how could we change our own behavior in a way that would make us feel better about something that is causing us to feel angry?

All of this does not come easy at first, but it is worth the effort. If you need help, get some counseling, read some books, or take an anger management class.

Therapies: Aromatherapy, Deep Breathing, Emotional Healing Work, Exercise, Gall Bladder Flush, Hydration, Low Glycemic Diet and Stress Management

Formulas: Cholagogue, Blood Purifier, Relaxing Nervine, **Adaptogen**, Liver Tonic, Diuretic and Hypoglycemic

Key Herbs: Agrimony, Bee Pollen, Blue Vervain, Chamomile (English and Roman), **Bupleurum**, Dandelion root, Lavender, Licorice, Linden flowers, Rose petals, Shatavari, Spirulina and Suma

Key Nutrients: Vitamin B-Complex, Vitamin C, Chromium, SAM-e, Pantothenic Acid (Vitamin B5), L-Glutamine and N-Acetyl Cysteine

Angina

See also *Cardiovascular Disease (Heart Disease), Gall Bladder (sluggish or removed), Gas and Bloating* and *Anxiety Disorders*

Angina is chest pain that can range from mild to severe and is caused by lack of blood flow to the heart muscle. Anxiety, gallbladder problems or digestive problems like severe abdominal bloating, atypical acid reflux and esophageal spasms can cause a similar type of pain. Seek appropriate medical attention for a proper diagnosis and then select appropriate remedies based on the cause.

In true angina, due to constriction of blood vessels in the heart, magnesium supplements, Co-Q10, l-arginine (5 grams daily) and *Antispasmodic* Remedies can ease blood flow to the heart.

If the problem is related to the gallbladder, *Cholagogue Formulas* and the Gall Bladder Flush therapy may be helpful.

Where there is no arterial blockage and stress and anxiety are the primary factors, *Adaptogen* and *Relaxing Nervine Formulas* should be helpful. Also consider B-complex vitamins and magnesium.

Therapies: Fresh Fruits and Vegetables, Gall Bladder Flush, Healthy Fats, Hiatal Hernia Correction and Stress Management

Formulas: Cardiac Tonic, Cholagogue, Relaxing Nervine, **Antispasmodic** and Adaptogen

Key Herbs: Arjuna, Arnica, Black Cohosh, **Cramp Bark**, **Khella**, Ginkgo, Hawthorn, Lily of the Valley, Lobelia and Motherwort

Key Nutrients: L-Carnitine, Bromelain, Magnesium, Folate (Folic Acid, Vitamin B9), **Co-Q10**, **L-Arginine** and Vitamin E

Anorexia

See also *Appetite (deficient)* and *Anxiety Disorders*

Anorexia nervosa is a eating disorder characterized by severe food restriction. It occurs most commonly among teenage women and includes an irrational fear of weight gain and distorted body image. Seek appropriate medical attention when dealing with this condition.

To stimulate appetite take bitter herbs such as gentian or goldenseal, or a *Digestive Bitter Tonic Formula*. It is absolutely essential that you taste these herbs as it is the bitter taste that has the effect. Use a liquid product or open the capsules and put the powders directly into the mouth. *Carminative Formulas* may also stimulate appetite when taken

as teas prior to mealtime. Teas with chamomile or alfalfa and peppermint as a primary ingredients would be good choices.

Digestive Enzyme or *Digestive Tonic Formulas* may improve digestion and utilization of nutrients to support healthy weight gain. Dehydration can cause a loss of appetite because it takes water to digest food.

Adaptogen and *Nerve Tonic Formulas* may help to balance nervous and glandular function while doing the Emotional Healing Work that is typically necessary with this condition. It may also be necessary to support the heart with *Cardiac Tonic Formulas* and to stabilize blood sugar levels with the Low Glycemic Diet therapy.

Therapies: Affirmation and Visualization, Healthy Fats, Hydration, Low Glycemic Diet, Mineralization and Stress Management

Formulas: Digestive Bitter Tonic, Carminative, Digestive Tonic, Digestive Enzyme, Adaptogen and Cardiac Tonic

Key Herbs: Alfalfa, Angelica, Bee Pollen, Blessed Thistle, Borage, Cardamom, Catnip, Chamomile (English and Roman), Cinnamon, **Gentian**, **Goldenseal**, Licorice, Peppermint, Sage, Saw Palmetto and St. John's wort

Key Nutrients: Probiotics, **Digestive Enzymes**, Vitamin B-Complex and Colloidal Minerals

Antibiotics (alternatives to)

See also *Infection (bacterial)*

There is no question about it. Antibiotics are one of the wonders of modern medicine and they have saved countless lives through their appropriate use.

Unfortunately, these valuable drugs are also commonly prescribed for conditions where they have little or no effect. For starters, antibiotics only work on bacterial infections, so they are worthless on viral or fungal infections. This means that there is absolutely no reason to take an antibiotic for the common cold or flu. Antibiotics are also ineffective in many, if not most, cases of sore throats, sinus infections, bronchitis, respiratory congestion and earaches (otitis media).

In spite of these facts, many people run to their doctor and practically insist on getting a prescription for an antibiotic for these types of health problems. What these people don't realize is that using antibiotics in this inappropriate manner will actually harm their health in the long run.

This is partly because antibiotics kill friendly bacteria in the intestinal tract. When these friendly bacteria are destroyed, yeast and infectious bacteria proliferate causing intestinal inflammation, Leaky Gut Syndrome and a weakened immune system. This makes the person even more susceptible to future infections.

An even more serious problem created by antibiotic overuse is the development of antibiotic resistant bacteria, sometimes called "superbugs." Here's how this happens: Antibiotics never kill all the bacteria and the few that survive are the ones that are most resistant to the drug. Over time, the process of natural selection gradually creates strains of bacteria which can't be killed by that particular antibiotic.

Antibiotic resistance can develop very quickly. For instance, penicillin became widely used after World War II, and it only took four years for microbes to start becoming resistant to penicillin. This is why new antibiotics have to be introduced regularly, but it's becoming a losing battle. Antibiotic resistance is now a worldwide problem, especially in hospitals and medical clinics. It has made diseases such as tuberculosis, gonorrhea and childhood ear infections more difficult to treat than they were a few decades ago.

Prescribing antibiotics for colds and other viral infections and feeding livestock antibiotics for "prevention" has hastened the development of antibiotic resistance, which is why we need to put a halt to this abuse of antibiotics, especially when there are natural ways to treat most infections. There are many natural remedies that are not only effective against bacterial infections, they also work on viral and fungal infections. More importantly, bacteria do not seem to develop resistance to natural substances.

Some of the best single herbs to use in fighting bacterial infections are garlic, echinacea, thyme, usnea, wild indigo, and cryptolepsis. These are some of the key herbs in *Antibacterial Formulas*. You can also consider *Goldenseal & Echinacea Formulas* or just *Echinacea Blend Formulas*, as these are very popular remedies for fighting bacterial infections.

Topically, tea tree oil is a great infection-fighting remedy. It is one of the key herbs in *Topical Antiseptic Formulas*, which, along with tinctures of single antiseptic herbs, can be applied directly to wounds.

Formulas: Antibacterial, Echinacea Blend, **Goldenseal & Echinacea** and Topical Antiseptic

Key Herbs: Echinacea, Garlic, Goldenseal, Myrrh, Oregano, Oregon Grape, Tea Tree, Thuja, Thyme, Usnea and Wild Indigo (Baptista)

Key Nutrients: Vitamin C, Zinc and Colloidal Silver

Antibiotics (side effects of)

See also *Fungal Infections (Yeast Infections, Candida albicans)*

Antibiotics are antibacterial agents. They have no effect against viral conditions for which they are frequently prescribed. Unfortunately, antibiotics also destroy beneficial bacteria in the gastrointestinal and female reproductive tracts. This allows yeast and occasionally pathogenic bacteria to multiply out of balance with other organisms in the gut. Yeast produce a toxin that weakens the immune system. Long-term use of antibiotics results in reduced immunity.

After completing a round of antibiotics it is important to take probiotics and eat cultured vegetables in order to replace the friendly bacteria that have been destroyed. There are many species of friendly bacteria or Lactobacillus besides the commonly recommended Lactobacillus acidophilus.

It may also be helpful to take *Antifungal Formulas* following antibiotic therapy to knock down yeast. See Fungal Infections for more information.

Therapies: Friendly Flora

Formulas: Antifungal

Key Herbs: Barberry, Black Walnut, Garlic, Oregano, Pau d' Arco and Tea Tree

Key Nutrients: Probiotics and Pantothenic Acid (Vitamin B5)

Anxiety Disorders

See also *Adrenals (exhaustion, weakness or burnout), Insomnia* and *Stress*

If you've ever had to speak or perform in front of a large group of people, you've probably felt a little anxiety. Most people do. In fact, it's perfectly normal to feel anxious when facing difficult, dangerous or even challenging situations. People often feel anxious about financial difficulties, health problems, talking to a boss about a raise, job interviews and big decisions like buying a house or car.

When a person experiences mild to severe apprehension or uneasiness over a present or impending event, with symptoms such as a cold sweat, heart palpitations, trembling, faintness, a sense of pressure in the chest over the heart area, and/or dry mouth, he or she is experiencing anxiety.

Anxiety is a complex combination of feeling apprehension, dread, fear, nervousness and worry, in anticipation of problems or misfortune. So, when facing unknown or "scary" situations, it's perfectly normal to experience the sensation of "butterflies" or "knots" in your stomach that signal a touch of anxiety. However, for a large number of people, anxiety is something far more serious and persistent.

When anxiety is severe enough to interfere with family relations, socializing and work, it can be debilitating. It can manifest as shortness of breath, rapid heartbeat or heart palpitations, muscle tension, trembling, insomnia, irritability, chest pain, cold sweats, feeling faint and general feelings of stress. These symptoms are bad enough, but to make matters worse, anxiety contributes to the development of other health problems, including heart disease, high blood pressure, cancer, diabetes, and pain-related disorders such as arthritis and fibromyalgia. There is also a high correlation between anxiety and addiction to alcohol, smoking and drug use.

Clinicians recognize about 12 relatively distinct subtypes of anxiety disorder, but the major ones are: panic disorder (panic attacks), phobias, obsessive-compulsive disorder, post-traumatic stress disorder and generalized anxiety disorder. These anxiety-related problems have reached epidemic proportions in the United States. According to the Surgeon General, 16 percent of adults ages 18 to 24 experience one subtype of an anxiety disorder that lasts at least a year. That's a lot of anxiety!

The large majority of those suffering with these disorders are holding full-time jobs, many at executive and managerial levels, and are experiencing a relatively high degree of workplace stress. Most are just masking the symptoms of their problem by taking some sort of medication, such as tranquilizers, antidepressants or sleeping pills. Others are "self-medicating" through alcohol, cigarettes and drugs. There are better ways of dealing with anxiety, however.

For starters, we need to realize that anxiety is not a "bad" thing. It is a natural reaction to real or perceived dangers. The perception of possible danger triggers the release of hormones and neurotransmitters that prime the body and mind for action. These physiological changes can help us push beyond our normal limits and may actually help us perform better.

For instance, coming back to the example of giving a speech or performing in front of a group, the perceived "danger" of humiliating oneself in front of a large group of people creates a release of hormones that actually prime the person to perform better. So, the key is not to eliminate anxiety, but to keep our anxiety at manageable levels so we can perform well in the tasks before us, and not be paralyzed from action by excessive anxiety.

It can also be thyroid related as well. This can be due to high T3 uptake or low TSH. Dominant parasympathetic types are prone to anxiety as well.

Fortunately, there are many simple, natural therapies that can regulate the production of stress-related hormones and ease anxiety-related problems. These natural approaches don't just temporarily relieve the symptoms, either. They can actually resolve anxiety problems and help a person get rid of that crippling anxiety for good. Natural remedies can be very effective in reducing anxiety and helping a person heal from anxiety disorders. Here are five strategies one can employ to reduce anxiety.

Reduce Stress Hormones with Adaptogenic Herbs

Anxiety is part of the normal reaction we have to difficult or challenging circumstances. It is a reaction of the nerves and glands that primes the body for action. When one is suffering from anxiety-related disorders, the chemical messengers (hormones, neurotransmitters and prostaglandins) involved in this process are chronically out of balance.

Fortunately, there is a class of herbal remedies that have been shown to help balance and modulate these messenger chemicals. These remedies are called adaptogens, and are of major benefit to anyone suffering from anxiety or any other stress-related health problem.

Adaptogens reduce the output of stress-related hormones from the pituitary and adrenal glands. They reduce both fatigue and insomnia, while improving memory and cognitive function. Many adaptogens enhance immunity, reduce cholesterol and high blood pressure and balance blood sugar. So, adaptogens not only relieve anxiety, they reduce the health problems associated with it.

There are many adaptogenic herbs and formulas, so your only challenge may be in deciding which one is the best for you. Consider one of the *Adaptogen Formulas* or the single herbs eleuthero, schizandra, ashwaganda or suma. If you feel completely burned out and unable to cope, try an *Adrenal Tonic Formula*.

Make Time for Rest and Relaxation

Since anxiety is created by the release of stress-related hormones and neurotransmitters, it is obvious that reducing stress is important to reducing anxiety. But stress is a part of life, so we all have to deal with it everyday. In fact, trying to avoid stress is downright stressful!

The truth is, one doesn't have to try to avoid stress to reduce the effects of stress in one's life. It turns out that a pleasurable experience causes the release of hormones and neurotransmitters that counteract the effects of stress. And, a pleasurable experience creates more positive benefits than a stressful experience causes harm. So, instead of reducing stress, we should be deliberately creating pleasure and enjoyment in our lives.

It's likely that a major part of the reason anxiety-related disorders are epidemic in our society is because we are just too busy. We are constantly on the go, and take very little time for pleasure and recreation. Making sure to *plan* time for doing enjoyable things is very important to our emotional and physical health.

Many people feel they are too busy for this. Well, the truth is, that the busier you are, the more important it is for you to make time for rest and relaxation. If a woodcutter doesn't take time to sharpen his saw or ax, he will find himself working harder and harder while becoming less and less productive. Rest and relaxation is "saw-sharpening" time—it makes you more productive the rest of the time. If you are busy, you can't afford to *not* take time for rest and relaxation.

Watching TV doesn't count. Generally speaking, TV is designed to be stimulating, not relaxing. Instead, look for activities that feel pleasurable to the body, such as a warm bath, a soak in a hot tub, a massage, listening to relaxing music or taking a walk in nature. Moderate exercise is helpful, but strenuous exercise and extreme sports may aggravate the anxiety.

Find things that make you laugh and awaken a childlike delight in life. Slow down when you eat and really enjoy the flavor of the food. Remember that anything that brings a sensation of bodily pleasure counteracts the effects of stress and reduces anxiety.

Get a Good Night's Sleep

One surefire way to increase anxiety is to get short-changed on sleep. Unfortunately, a large percentage of Americans have trouble sleeping or simply do not get enough sleep.

If you have trouble getting to sleep there are several remedies you can try. What works for you will depend on the specific problems inhibiting your sleep. Sometimes, just taking something that helps relax the nervous system shortly before bedtime is enough. See Insomnia for suggestions on how to get a better night's sleep.

Relax Tense Muscles

People who suffer from anxiety usually have a lot of tension in their muscles. Anything that helps to stretch muscles and get them to relax will reduce feelings of stress and anxiety. Good choices include stretching exercises, yoga, tai chi or massage therapy.

You can also use supplements to help muscles relax. Lobelia, blue vervain and kava kava are great antispasmodic herbs that can relax muscles and reduce anxiety. For long-term use, take more magnesium. Most people are deficient and magnesium helps muscles relax.

Calm the Mind and Nerves

Most of us have a constant flow of verbal "monkey chatter" going on in our minds. In some people, these thoughts can become so obsessive that they lead to constant states of worry, fear, anxiety and obsession. Learning to calm the mind through prayer and meditation can be very helpful. In many cases, counseling may be needed to help a person learn to "step back" from these negative thoughts and replace them with more positive ones.

One way of calming the mind is to center one's attention more on directly experiencing the world around us. While breathing slowly and deeply, look around you and notice colors, sounds, textures and smells. Touch things and feel their texture. Coming to your "senses" in this manner counteracts the effects of stress and reduces anxiety. And guess what? It doesn't cost anything!

Herbs and herbal formulas can help with this process. Good sedative herbs that can calm anxiety include bacopa, blue vervain, chamomile, hops, mimosa, motherwort, passion flower, St. John's wort and valerian. Choose a *Relaxing Nervine* or *Brain Calming Formula*. If you have obsessive thoughts, passion flower and GABA can help reduce anxiety by easing the mental chatter.

It's also a good idea to avoid nicotine, caffeine and other stimulants and stay well hydrated. Taking B-complex vitamins, particularly B6, and eliminating refined sugar from the diet by adopting the Low Glycemic Diet therapy will also be helpful.

These techniques, along with basic good health practices, can help you recover from anxiety disorders. If the problem is severe, be sure to seek appropriate professional help.

Therapies: Affirmation and Visualization, Aromatherapy, Deep Breathing, Emotional Healing Work, Exercise, Healthy Fats, Hiatal Hernia Correction, Hydration, Low Glycemic Diet, Mineralization and Stress Management

Formulas: Adaptogen, Brain Calming, Antispasmodic, Relaxing Nervine, Sleep and **Adrenal Tonic**

Key Herbs: Bacopa (Water Hyssop), Bugleweed, California Poppy, Chamomile (English and Roman), **Ashwaganda**, **Blue Vervain**, **Eleuthero (Siberian ginseng)**, **Kava-kava**, **Mimosa (Albizia, Silk Tree)**, Holy Basil, Hops, Lavender, Lemon Balm, Lobelia, Motherwort, Oat seed (milky), Passionflower,

Rhodiola, Schisandra (Schizandra), Shatavari, St. John's wort and Valerian

Key Nutrients: Vitamin B-Complex, Omega-3 Essential Fatty Acids, **GABA**, **Magnesium**, Pantothenic Acid (Vitamin B5), Vitamin B-6 (Pyridoxine) and Zinc

Anxiety or Panic Attack

See also *Anxiety Disorders*

An anxiety or panic attack is an acute form of anxiety that causes rapid, shallow breathing, paralyzing fear and can even cause a person to experience tetany, where the muscles cramp so strongly that movement is impaired. These acute attacks of anxiety can be relieved naturally using a three-step process. Each step is helpful by itself, but when all three are combined the effect is powerful and rapid.

1. Breathe Slowly and Deeply

When someone is having a panic attack, have them concentrate on their breathing. Coach them to take slower, deeper breaths and to exhale more completely. It helps if the person experiencing the panic attack starts counting the time of their inhalation and exhalation and seeks to lengthen it. Breathe in—one, two, three, four... Breathe out—one, two, three, four. This immediately starts reducing the anxiety.

2. Take Bach Rescue Remedy

Take 5-10 drops of the Bach Flower Rescue Remedy (or an equivalent like FES Five Flower Remedy or Nature's Sunshine's Distress Remedy) under the tongue. Rescue remedy helps reduce emotional shock and trauma and should be in everyone's first aid kit.

3. Take Antispasmodic Herbs

Administer 1-5 drops lobelia or pulsatilla and/or 10-15 drops kava kava (tinctures or extracts) every 2-3 minutes, until the person experiencing the attack starts to relax. Lobelia is a good choice, because it slows breathing and calms the heart rate. It also relaxes muscle cramps and spasms. If liquids are not available, empty the powder from the capsules directly onto the tongue and follow it with a drink of water.

Therapies: Aromatherapy, Avoid Caffeine, Deep Breathing, Hydration, Low Glycemic Diet and Stress Management

Formulas: Relaxing Nervine and **Antispasmodic**

Key Herbs: Blue Vervain, **Kava-kava**, **Lobelia**, **Pulsatilla**, Eleuthero (Siberian ginseng), Hops,

Lavender, Linden, Motherwort, Passionflower, St. John's wort and Valerian

Key Nutrients: Magnesium and **GABA**

Apathy

See also *Adrenals (exhaustion, weakness or burnout)*, *Depression* and *Anxiety Disorders*

Apathy is an "I don't care" attitude that may have its roots in wounds to the self-esteem or a lack of energy or drive. Severe apathy will probably require counseling or Emotional Healing Work, but consider herbal remedies for depression, anxiety and adrenal exhaustion. Low thyroid may also be a factor.

Therapies: Aromatherapy

Formulas: Adaptogen, Adrenal Tonic, **Antidepressant** and Hypothyroid

Key Herbs: Mimosa (Albizia, Silk Tree), **Rose petals**, Oat seed (milky), Peppermint and Rosemary essential oil

Key Nutrients: Vitamin B-Complex, Vitamin C and SAM-e

Appendicitis

Inflammation of the appendix is called appendicitis. It is characterized by inflammation (heat, swelling and pain) in the lower abdomen, just inside the right hip. This is a serious condition because the appendix can rupture resulting in a life-threatening infection of the abdominal cavity. For this reason, stimulant laxatives and enemas should be avoided when having an acute episode of appendicitis.

In his book *Food is Your Best Medicine*, Dr. Henry Bieler speaks of treating appendicitis without surgery by putting the patient on a diet of clear liquids (no solid food) and giving doses of antibiotics. It is possible that similar results could be achieved with large doses of an *Antibacterial Formula*. Five hundred milligrams of vitamin C every 2-4 hours would also be helpful.

In an emergency situation where surgery isn't an option, antibiotics are often successful for treating uncomplicated appendicitis. However according to the British Medical Journal, about 20% of the time the appendicitis reoccurred within a year.

Due to the seriousness of this condition, however, we recommend that appropriate medical attention be sought before undertaking any course of treatment and that a natural approach only be tried under medical supervision.

Formulas: Antibacterial, Echinacea Blend and **Goldenseal & Echinacea**

Key Herbs: Goldenseal, Echinacea, Garlic, Wild Indigo (Baptista) and Wild Yam

Key Nutrients: Vitamin C

Appetite (deficient)

See also *Anorexia* and *Wasting*

A deficient appetite is a lack of desire for food. A loss of appetite is often due to illness, nervous or glandular system problems, stress, or a congested digestive tract and liver. A short-term loss of appetite when sick is normal and is nothing to worry about. However, a long term loss of appetite can result in loss of weight and health.

The appetite can be stimulated by taking *Digestive Bitter Tonic* or *Digestive Tonic Formula* in liquid form about 20 minutes prior to eating. *Carminative Formulas* that are teas will also be helpful if taken prior to or with meals. Emotional Healing Work may be needed. If these approaches don't work, seek appropriate assistance.

Therapies: Colon Cleanse and Hydration

Formulas: Carminative, **Digestive Bitter Tonic**, Digestive Tonic and Relaxing Nervine

Key Herbs: Alfalfa, Astragalus, Blessed Thistle, Chamomile (English and Roman), Codonopsis, **Artichoke**, **Gentian**, Dandelion, Devil's Claw, Fringe Tree, Goldenseal, Horehound, Licorice, Myrrh and Oregon Grape

Key Nutrients: 5-HTP, Vitamin C, Zinc and Copper

Appetite (excessive)

See also *Weight Loss (aids for)*

When a person craves food beyond what is nutritionally necessary to sustain life, health and optimum body weight, there may be a need for substances that curb appetite. Often the problem is related to eating too many "empty calories," or foods that have a very low content of vitamins, minerals and other micronutrients such as refined sugar and white flour. By supplying the body with micronutrients, the body will crave less food because its nutritional requirements are satisfied. There may also be hormonal or nervous system imbalances.

Supplements that help to curb appetite in this manner include mineral rich supplements like alfalfa, spirulina, barley juice powder, essential fatty acids, and flax seed oil. Coconut oil is also helpful.

Excessive appetite can also be a sign of hormonal imbalances. Serotonin helps control both mood and appetite, so an *Antidepressant Formula* or 5-HTP can sometimes help.

A number of herbalists have designed *Weight Loss Formulas*, which may be helpful in stimulating fat burning and reducing appetite. However, be cautious about using any Weight loss Aid containing caffeine. The Low Glycemic Diet and Hydration therapies will also help.

Therapies: Dietary Fiber, Exercise, Fast or Juice Fast, Healthy Fats, Hydration, Low Glycemic Diet, Mineralization and Stress Management

Formulas: Antidepressant and Weight Loss

Key Herbs: Barley, Black Walnut, Chickweed, **Hoodia**, Psyllium and Spirulina

Key Nutrients: 5-HTP, Omega-3 Essential Fatty Acids, Colloidal Minerals, Iodine and L-Glutamine

Arrhythmia (Irregular Heartbeat)

Arrhythmia is a medical term referring to an irregular heartbeat. This can be very serious and should be examined and monitored medically. In many cases drugs may be needed to stabilize the condition. It is sometime congenital (inherited) and in this case cannot be effectively eliminated. Arrhythmias can be difficult to treat with herbs and nutrition, but there are natural therapies that sometimes prove helpful. One of the first things to look at is the possibility of a hiatal hernia. The stomach protruding into the diaphragm can stress the heart and when this is mechanically corrected it takes the stress off of the heart.

Arrhythmias can also be a sign of mineral deficiencies. Magnesium, in particular is often lacking in people's diets and may be helpful. Sometimes calcium, potassium or trace mineral deficiencies may also play a role. If the person is under a lot of stress, *Adaptogen Formulas* may help to regulate the cardiac rhythm. It is also wise to avoid stimulants like caffeine, tobacco and alcohol. Even peppermint oil can be a problem for some.

Herbally, arrhythmias will sometimes respond to *Cardiac Tonic* or *Relaxing Nervine Formulas*, especially ones containing motherwort, passion flower, lobelia or valerian. However, some of the best herbs for arrhythmia are toxic botanicals available only from a professional herbalist or naturopath. These include lily of the valley and mistletoe. If you decide to try any of these stronger botanicals, do so under the supervision of an herbalist familiar with their contraindications (*findanherbalist.com*).

Therapies: Hiatal Hernia Correction, Hydration and Mineralization

Formulas: Cardiac Tonic, Relaxing Nervine and Adaptogen

Key Herbs: Black Cohosh, **Arjuna**, **Motherwort**, Eleuthero (Siberian ginseng), Hawthorn, Horehound, Khella, Lily of the Valley, Lobelia, Night Blooming Cereus (Cactus), Passionflower and Rhodiola

Key Nutrients: Magnesium, Pantothenic Acid (Vitamin B5) and Calcium

Arteriosclerosis (Hardening of the Arteries, Atherosclerosis)

See also *Cardiovascular Disease (Heart Disease)*, *Cholesterol (high)* and *Free Radical Damage*

Arteriosclerosis or hardening of the arteries, occurs when there is damage to the lining of the blood vessels in the body through poor diet, infection and/or free radical damage. There is a thickening of interior vessel walls, usually by fatty or mineral deposits that reduce the opening size and obstruct blood flow.

Restricted blood flow prevents tissues from getting oxygen and nutrients, which prevents wounds from healing, causes coldness in the extremities and affects memory and cognitive function. When a blood clot forms in the circulatory system it may get lodged in the heart, causing cardiac arrest, or in the brain, causing a stroke.

Although most people believe that high cholesterol causes arteriosclerosis, there is research to suggest that cholesterol itself has little to do with the problem. It is mostly due to free radical damage caused by a lack of antioxidant nutrients, an elevation of stress hormones, excess carbohydrate consumption and general poor nutrition. It may also occur in response to infection.

To reduce your risk of arteriosclerois use healthy fats and increase your antioxidant nutrients. If you have gum infections, you need to get them under control as there is a link between gum infections and arterial infections and hardening of the arteries. Co-Q10 is a nutrient that helps both the gums and the arteries.

If you have already developed arteriosclerosis try doing Heavy Metal Detoxification. See related conditions, especially Cardiovascular Disease, for more information.

Therapies: Fresh Fruits and Vegetables, Healthy Fats, Heavy Metal Cleanse, Low Glycemic Diet and Stress Management

Formulas: Cardiac Tonic and Antioxidant

Key Herbs: Capsicum (Cayenne), **Arjuna**, **Hawthorn**, Garlic, Ginkgo, Guggul, Kelp, Khella, Olive, Periwinkle (Lesser), Reishi (Ganoderma), Rose and Tea (Green or Black)

Key Nutrients: Vitamin B-3 (Niacin), **Omega-3 Essential Fatty Acids**, L-Arginine, Folate (Folic Acid, Vitamin B9), Chromium, Vitamin E, Zinc, **Co-Q10**, Vitamin D, Vitamin C and Digestive Enzymes

Arthritis

See also *Rheumatoid Arthritis (Rheumatism)*

The word arthritis means quite simply "inflammation of a joint," but there are many different kinds of arthritis and many different causes. So, when dealing with this disturbingly common disease (more than 20 million Americans are thought to suffer from it) it is necessary to look at its underlying causes and deal with them to achieve any kind of real results.

Most people are familiar with the two most common forms of arthritis, osteoarthritis and rheumatoid arthritis. Osteoarthritis affects more than 15 million Americans and occurs most frequently in older people. In osteoarthritis, the cartilage that coats the ends of the bones in our joints begins to break down, starting a vicious cycle of damage, reduced function and health, leading to more damage. It is not a systemic disease but the result of damage from local wear and tear, trauma, surgery or infection to a specific joint. It can also result from the effects of other diseases.

Symptoms of osteoarthritis include:

Pain in the affected joint(s) after repeated use, especially later in the day.

Swelling, pain and stiffness after long periods of inactivity, like sleep, that subside with movement and activity.

Continuous pain, even at rest, with advanced osteoarthritis.

In contrast, rheumatoid arthritis is much more rare, occurring in less than one percent of the population. Unlike osteoarthritis, rheumatoid arthritis is an autoimmune disease, meaning the tissues that surround and cushion the joints are attacked by the body's own immune system. This happens throughout the whole body, not just in joints that have been subjected to wear and tear. It usually occurs between the ages of 25 and 50, but it can develop at any age, and generally strikes women three times as often as men.

Symptoms of rheumatoid arthritis include:

Swollen, warm, painful joints, especially after long periods of inactivity.

Fatigue and occasional fever.

Symmetrical pattern of inflammation if one wrist is involved, the other will be also.

The small joints of the body (hands, fingers, feet, toes, wrists, elbows and ankles) are usually affected first.

As the disease progresses, the joints often will become deformed and may freeze in one position, making it difficult to move them.

Other Forms of Arthritis

In addition to these most common forms of arthritis, there are some other recognized forms.

Allergic arthritis, as the name implies, is triggered by an allergic reaction. This type of arthritis has actually been produced in the laboratory by injecting research subjects with allergenic substances. The connection between allergies and arthritis is easier to understand if we consider that both of these conditions are caused by inflammation in the body, and that the inflammation itself can become chronic when an individual is repeatedly exposed to allergenic substances over time.

Gonorrheal arthritis is inflammation of the joints resulting from gonorrheal infection.

Gouty arthritis was the most widely known variety until the 20th century. Caused by an elevation of uric acid in the blood, it also causes joint inflammation and usually affects one joint at a time.

Hemophilic arthritis results from bleeding into a joint in someone who has hemophilia. This often results in joint stiffness and inflammation.

Menopausal arthritis can occur because of hormonal imbalances experienced during menopause.

Tuberculous arthritis is joint inflammation found in people infected by tuberculosis where the infection has spread into the joints.

Understanding Arthritis

What all these forms of arthritis have in common is that the joints have been subjected to some kind of stress: mechanical, biochemical or infectious. The stress leads to irritation of the tissues that causes inflammation. The irritation and inflammation lead to physical and chemical changes that send the joint(s) into a downward spiral of breakdown, then toxification, which creates more irritation, more inflammation, and further breakdown.

In advanced cases of arthritis, irreversible deformation and degeneration may have occurred. But even in these situations, the foundation for healing lies in breaking the vicious cycle by reducing the inflammation and removing the sources of irritation that have caused or resulted from the tissue damage. Once this is done, then nutrition can be used to aid the body's ability to heal itself.

One of the misperceptions people have about bones is they associate them with the bleached-white and dried-out bones from creatures which have died. Living bones aren't static, dead objects, they are composed of living tissue. This makes them capable of growth, change and repair. In fact, if joints weren't alive they couldn't become inflamed in the first place. Recognizing that bones and joints are living tissue helps us realize that they are capable of self-repair, if we remove the sources of irritation and supply them with the tools they need to repair themselves.

Think of an engine that hasn't had its oil changed in a long time. As it gets dirtier and dirtier, it will start to function less and less effectively until it finally stops working. To extend the analogy, an engine that has been stressed by contaminants or poor quality fuel or by being driven at excessive speeds or under excessive loads will eventually malfunction.

Joints are meant to endure a certain amount of wear and tear, but when toxins and inflammation are present, it creates more friction in the joints (just like the dirty oil in the car). Furthermore, when nutrients needed for joint health aren't there then repairs can't be made, which makes the joint more easily damaged and inflamed.

Healing Arthritis

There are three things that need to be done to help arthritis to heal. First we need to identify and remove sources of stress, whether they are mechanical, biochemical or infectious. Secondly, we need to reduce inflammation and tissue toxicity, which is like changing the dirty oil in the engine and replacing it with fresh oil. Lastly, we need to supply nutrients necessary for joint health to aid the body in effecting repairs.

1. Remove Sources of Irritation

In osteoarthritis, reducing mechanical stress to the joints is an important key. This mechanical stress is often the result of repetitive habits of movement and posture that were not properly balanced. Correcting structural alignment through stretching, yoga, massage, or other forms of bodywork will help to take mechanical stress off joints and allow better blood flow and alignment. If excess weight is putting stress on joints, then obviously losing weight is going to help. Mild exercise that doesn't put stress on the joints will improve blood and lymph flow to bring healing energy to the joints. Self-massage will also improve blood and lymph flow.

Where there is an infectious cause, obviously the infection will need to be dealt with using whatever remedies are appropriate to that type of infection. Where the cause of stress is biochemical, as in rheumatoid, allergic or gouty arthritis, improving the diet is a crucial step. Here are some things to consider.

Wheat, dairy (A-1 Beta Casein), corn, GMO's and chemicals in our food have been implicated in triggering arthritis through what is called chemical onset inflammation. Nightshade vegetables like eggplant, tomatoes, potatoes and green peppers should be eliminated, as they have also been implicated in joint inflammation. Coffee and tobacco have also been linked to increased risk of arthritis and should be avoided. Citrus fruits may cause problems in some people, too.

Gentle fasting, fruit and vegetable juice diets and mild food diets can all help to strengthen the body's ability to naturally reduce inflammation, while helping to clear toxins from the system. Inflammation can be combated nutritionally by cooking with herbs like ginger and turmeric, which have been shown to have anti-inflammatory properties. Oily fish such as salmon, are excellent sources of omega-3 fatty acids, which also combat inflammation.

2. Reduce Inflammation

Since arthritis is an inflammatory condition, remedies that reduce inflammatory reactions are an obvious place to start. So, consider *Anti-Inflammatory Formulas*.

Herbs containing salicylates have been used for thousands of years to ease arthritic pain. Salicylates, the forerunners of modern aspirin, reduce joint swelling and inflammation and ease pain. The most famous of these salycilate-bearing herbs is white willow bark, which has been used since the time of Hippocrates for arthritis. Other plants containing salicylates include black cohosh, meadowsweet and wintergreen. So, another category of remedies to consider is herbal *Analgesic Formulas* that utilize these natural anti-inflammatory and pain-reducing agents. They can be used as an effective natural replacement for NSAIDs, without the side-effects. It goes without saying that short-term pain relief also needs to be accompanied by working on the underlying causes of the pain.

If massage relieves pain, then massage around sore joints several times a day using a *Topical Analgesic Formula*. Besides easing pain, this keeps fluid out of the tissue spaces and allows more oxygen and nutrients to reach the tissues better for more effective healing. The use of massage for reducing inflammation and easing pain is discussed in detail in The School of Modern Herbal Medicine's *Fundamentals of Natural Healing* course.

Certain plant seed oils containing the fatty acid GLA (gamma-linolenic acid) can help alleviate the pain and discomfort of arthritis. Found in evening primrose, borage, black currant, and flax seed oils, GLA is important because the body converts it to compounds with strong anti-inflammatory and immune regulating effects. Omega 3 essential fatty acids are also highly beneficial.

Joint Healing Formulas are formulas designed by herbalists to ease pain and promote healing in arthritic joints. These formulas typically rely on anti-inflammatory herbs (like boswellia, white willow, Devil's claw, turmeric and yucca), tissue healing and mineralizing herbs (like alfalfa) and detoxifying herbs (like burdock and sarsaparilla), providing a multi-action relief.

3. Provide Nutrition to the Joints

Even in osteoarthritis, where the original stress is mechanical, nutrition plays a critical role. Healthy joints need good nutrition. When joints have the nutrients they need, they have a greater capacity to resist damage or to heal from damage when it occurs. So, appropriate supplements should be considered with all forms of arthritis.

Minerals are extremely critical to aiding joint repair. Silica adds resiliency to joints so they are less susceptible to damage. It is found in herbs like horsetail and dulse.

Calcium is important for joints, but taking calcium supplements doesn't help unless you are taking the right forms of calcium and other elements are present for assimilation and utilization, including vitamin D, silica, boron and magnesium. Many people actually do better with formulas of mineral-rich herbs that contain silica, calcium and other nutrients to aid tissue repair. So, also consider herbal *Mineral* and *Tissue Healing Formulas*.

There are some very popular nutrients sold to aid joint health, which can be combined with herbs to enhance their effectiveness. These include MSM, glucosamine and chondroitin.

MSM (MethylSulfonylMethane) is a sulfur compound. Sulfur, the eighth most abundant element in the human body, has a long history as a healing agent. For centuries, mankind has soaked in sulfur-rich mineral hot springs to help heal a variety of ailments. MSM supplies biologically active sulfur. It helps with liver detoxification and studies show it helps ease arthritis pain in many individuals. Most people don't see results because they under-dose. Try 3000 mg, twice daily.

Glucosamine is an amino sugar normally found in the human body and is the base material for making mucous membranes, ligaments, tendons and synovial fluid in the joints. It helps joints to heal and can help them become more fluid and well lubricated.

Chondroitin is a long chain of repeating sugars found naturally in the joints and connective tissues. It helps to produce new cartilage and protects existing cartilage. Chondroitin helps by interfering with enzymes that destroy cartilage molecules and enzymes that prevent nutrients from reaching the cartilage.

Collagen is another major supportive tissue in the human body. Cartilage, ligaments and tendons are primarily made of collagen. Collagen supplements can be useful in preventing damaged cartilage from hardening and in promoting healing.

A great way to get the nutrients needed for healthy joints and bones is to make homemade stock. This is done by simmering bones, meat scraps and vegetables in water for a long time. Directions for making stock can be found in the *Therapies Section* under Bone Broth.

Looking closely at the causes and effects of arthritis shows both the complexity and the simplicity that underlie its symptoms—complexity in just how many factors there are to consider and simplicity because all the factors and symptoms ultimately boil down to some very straightforward concepts. If we remove the stresses causing the disease, detoxify the body and build up the structural system with good nutrition arthritis can not only be relieved, it can actually be cured in many cases.

Therapies: Affirmation and Visualization, Bone Broth, Colon Cleanse, Compress, Drawing Bath, Eliminate Allergy-Causing Foods, Fast or Juice Fast, Fresh Fruits and Vegetables, Healthy Fats, Hiatal Hernia Correction, Hydration and Mineralization

Formulas: Anti-Inflammatory, Analgesic, **Joint Healing**, Mineral, Tissue Healing and **Topical Analgesic**

Key Herbs: Alfalfa, Aloe vera, Boneset, Borage, Boswellia, Burdock, Camphor, Capsicum (Cayenne), Cats Claw (Uña de Gato, Gambier), Celery, **Devil's Claw**, **Solomon's Seal**, **Turmeric**, **Willow**, **Yucca**, Dandelion, Horsetail, Hydrangea, Jamaican Dogwood, Licorice, Meadowsweet, Nettle (Stinging), Nopal (Prickly Pear), Prickly Ash, Reishi (Ganoderma), Safflowers, Sarsaparilla, Stillingia, Valerian and Yerba Santa

Key Nutrients: Chondroitin, Colloidal Minerals, Vitamin D, **Omega-3 Essential Fatty Acids**, **MSM**, Magnesium, **Glucosamine**, DHA, Copper, Selenium, Silicon, Magnesium, Betaine Hydrochloric Acid (HCl), Pantothenic Acid (Vitamin B5), Potassium and SAM-e

Asthma

See also *Adrenals (exhaustion, weakness or burnout), Allergies (food), Allergies (respiratory), Congestion (bronchial), Congestion (lymphatic), Hiatal Hernia and Leaky Gut Syndrome*

Helplessness. Panic. Fear. These are the feelings invoked by an asthma attack, both for the sufferer and for parents or other loved ones. During an asthma attack the muscles surrounding the bronchial passages in the lungs constrict. This interferes with the outflow of stale air and causes a feeling of suffocation in the victim. Typical symptoms of asthma include a feeling of tightness in the chest and difficulty breathing often coupled with wheezing and coughing.

Asthma is on the rise, affecting about seventeen million Americans (five million children and twelve million adults). The dramatic increase in asthma appears to be linked to the increase in air pollution and other lung irritants, including chemicals in food such as pesticides, preservatives, sugar in refined foods, and GMO's. For instance, in Mexico City, the most heavily air-polluted city in the world, as high as 50% of the children may have asthma. The majority of these cases are ages 4 and under.

This respiratory disorder is often unpredictable; and this is what makes it so intimidating. Those who suffer from it experience bouts of breathlessness which can come on suddenly during periods of stress, anxiety, exercise, low blood sugar, laughing, changes in temperature, extremes of dryness or dampness or exposure to allergens such as dust, animal dander, smoke, mold or food additives. Asthma attacks can last from minutes to hours and can come daily or annually.

Everyone's lungs will react to irritants by the process of inflammation, swelling, mucus production and coughing. Yet, for the person with asthma these reactions appear to be exaggerated or hyperactive. Swelling and inflammation in the lung tissue triggers spastic reactions in the lungs, which further constrict airways. As air is trapped in the lungs, excess carbon dioxide builds up in the blood creating the suffocating feeling.

Asthma is commonly treated with antihistamines (substances which reduce allergic reactions), anti-inflammatories (substances that reduce swelling and inflammation) and bronchial dilators (substances that relax the bronchial passages, allowing air to escape). These therapies are effective for symptomatic relief and can ease attacks and even save lives. However, they do not help to relieve any of the underlying causes of this disease.

If more than symptomatic relief is to be obtained, one has to investigate what may be causing the irritation in the lungs and removing it. Here are some of the underlying causes to consider and work on.

Food and Respiratory Allergies

Most individuals who experience asthma notice that it is prompted by substances such as pollen, dander, smoke, cold air or excessive exercise. Along with dust, mites, molds and pet dander that tend to cause an onset of allergies or asthma, diet has also become a part of the picture.

Dairy products and grains with gluten have come to be known as contributing factors. Most asthma sufferers notice tremendous relief once these allergens have been eliminated.

A number of herbs and nutrients can be helpful in reducing allergic reactions. Try *Allergy-Reducing Formulas* for a start and look for more information under Allergies (respiratory) and Allergies (food).

Excess Estrogen

Adult asthma tends to be most prevalent in women. Many physicians believe this to be hormonally related. With the rising number of asthma cases, this could be due to the influence of xenoestrogens (estrogen-like chemicals such as pesticides and plastics) present in our environment. Women who are estrogen dominant (with estrogen too high relative to progesterone) display signs of asthma more often than those who are more hormonally balanced.

The balancer for estrogen is progesterone, which can be applied topically in a progesterone cream. This has helped to ease symptoms in some women. Synthetic progestins, conversely, have shown no such benefit. Herbs that could be of help here include false unicorn (helonias root) and chaste tree. So, a *Female Hormonal Balancing Formula* with these herbs as principle ingredients could also be helpful.

Stress and Adrenal Fatigue

Epinephrine (adrenaline) acts as a bronchial dilator. Forms of it can be injected or are used in bronchial inhalers in order to halt asthma attacks. Epinephrine is both an adrenal hormone and a sympathetic neurotransmitter.

Corticosteroid drugs are also used to treat asthma. These drugs are mimics of another adrenal hormone, cortisol, which reduces inflammation in the body.

This suggests a connection between stress and adrenal fatigue in asthma cases. People who have been involved in any type of organized athletics are bound to have met individuals with exercise-induced asthma. These individuals, as well as others under chronic stress, generally have exhausted their adrenals and are lacking the naturally produced steroids and epinephrine necessary to prevent these attacks.

So, rebuilding the adrenals is often critical to overcoming asthma. The difficulty in this is that the drugs usually used to treat asthma contribute to adrenal fatigue. The best approach, therefore, is to start rebuilding the adrenals while slowly backing off the medications.

A number of nutrients can help to rebuild the adrenals. The combination of B-complex and vitamin C has a rebuilding effect on the adrenals, especially when combined with adaptogens. Consider an anti-stress vitamin supplement (with B-complex and C) and an *Adaptogen Formula*. In particular, pantothenic acid is very important for adrenal function and can also help to rebuild exhausted adrenal glands. In severe cases an *Adrenal Tonic Formula* or perhaps even an adrenal glandular (from a naturopath, chiropractor or holistically-minded MD) will be helpful.

Licorice root helps preserve cortisol levels (the adrenal hormone that reduces inflammation) and can help to rebuild exhausted adrenals. Licorice is also anti-inflammatory. This herb can be taken regularly by most asthmatic children to reduce frequency and severity of attacks.

When rebuilding the adrenals, it is very important to avoid refined sugar, and foods and beverages containing caffeine, as these substances tax the adrenals. See *Adrenals (exhaustion, weakness or burnout)* for more information.

Digestive Problems

Many asthmatics have a hiatal hernia, which inhibits free movement of the diaphragm and contributes to poor digestion of proteins, which causes mucus congestion. Food allergies, leaky gut and lymphatic congestion are all common in asthmatics.

If present, start by using the Hiatal Hernia Correction therapy. Taking *Digestive Enzyme Formulas*, *Digestive Bitter Tonic Formulas* and or digestive enzyme supplements can help reduce allergic reactions to foods that contribute to asthma.

Cleansing the liver and colon also has tremendous benefits for healing the lungs. So consider doing the Colon Cleanse therapy.

Congestion

Mucus buildup in the lungs may be a contributing factor in asthma. This can occur partly because the epinephrine-based inhalers used to stop asthma attacks have a drying action that tends to dry out mucus secretions in the lungs. Yerba santa, grindelia, mullein and plantain are particularly good remedies for loosening this mucus in the lungs, so look for *Decongestant* or *Expectorant Formulas* where these herbs are key ingredients.

Lymphatic drainage may also be poor in people with asthma, so another class of remedy to consider is *Lymphatic Drainage Formulas*. See *Congestion (lymphatic)* and *Congestion (bronchial)*.

Natural Bronchial Dilators

To stop asthma attacks it is necessary to dilate the bronchial passages to let in more air. Lobelia is a very effective bronchial dilator and antispasmodic that can be used as a natural alternative to inhalers. It has a long history of successful use in easing asthma attacks. A tincture or extract of lobelia can be administered in doses of 3-20 drops at one to two minute intervals starting at the beginning of the attack until it subsides. Lobelia can also be rubbed onto the chest to relieve feelings of tightness and to relieve coughing.

Occasionally, taking lobelia internally will cause a person to vomit. However, the attack nearly always subsides as soon as the person expels the contents of the stomach (which interestingly enough often contains a large quantity of mucus).

Another herb that can help to stop asthma attacks is black cohosh. Although not commonly used for this purpose by modern herbalists, eclectic physicians at the turn of the century used both lobelia and black cohosh for asthma. Both of these herb are key ingredients in *Bronchialdilator* and *Antispasmodic Formulas*, both of which can be used to help prevent and stop asthma attacks. *Bronchialdilator Formulas* often combine these antispasmodic remedies with herbs to relieve congestion and inflammation.

Asthma is a serious condition, yet one that can be dealt with effectively by natural means. It will, however, take some determination, study and a commitment to a generally healthier lifestyle.

Therapies: Avoid Xenoestrogens, Colon Cleanse, Colon Hydrotherapy, Eliminate Allergy-Causing Foods, Fast or Juice Fast, Fresh Fruits and Vegetables, Healthy Fats, Hiatal Hernia Correction, Hydration and Stress Management

Formulas: Allergy-Reducing, Female Hormonal Balancing, Adaptogen, Adrenal Tonic, Digestive Enzyme, Decongestant, Expectorant, **Bronchialdilator**, **Antispasmodic** and Digestive Bitter Tonic

Key Herbs: Astragalus, Bloodroot, Blue Vervain, Butterbur Root, Cherry (Wild), Coleus, Coltsfoot, Cordyceps, **Khella**, **Lobelia**, **Skunk Cabbage**, **Yerba Santa**, Elecampane, Eucalyptus, Fenugreek, Garlic, Grindelia (Gumweed), Holy Basil, Hyssop, Jamaican Dogwood, Licorice, Lomatium, Mangosteen, Marshmallow, Mullein, Oregano, Pleurisy Root, Sage and Thyme

Key Nutrients: Pantothenic Acid (Vitamin B5), MSM, **Magnesium**, Co-Q10, Vitamin B-Complex, N-Acetyl Cysteine, Betaine Hydrochloric Acid (HCl) and Quercitin

Atherosclerosis

See *Arteriosclerosis (Atherosclerosis, Hardening of the Arteries)*

Key Nutrients: Chromium

Athlete's Foot

See also *Fungal Infections (Yeast Infections, Candida albicans)*

Athlete's foot is a fungal infection of the foot most often between the toes and on the soles of the feet. Symptoms include pain, burning and itching. The problem in treating athlete's foot is that it exists inside the skin where it is difficult to reach via the circulatory system and also difficult to completely eradicate topically. Therefore, the best approach is to use *Antifungal Formulas* both topically and internally. When there is a topical fungal infection like this, it is wise to treat for yeast internally as well, so see *Fungal Infections* for more information.

Therapies: Friendly Flora and Low Glycemic Diet

Formulas: Antifungal and Topical Antiseptic

Key Herbs: Calendula, **Black Walnut**, **Tea Tree**, Garlic, Myrrh, Oregano, Pau d' Arco, Thuja and Usnea

Key Nutrients: Zinc

Athletic Performance or Exercise (aids to)

A number of herbalists have formulated products specifically for aiding athletes and/or people engaged in exercise. These are listed under *Exercise Formulas*. However, there are other classes of formulas that can aid exercise and promote improved athletic performance.

For example, there is a lot of research showing that adaptogens like eleuthero root or cordyceps can improve athletic performance. So, consider using an *Adaptogen Formula* as part of your training or exercise regime.

Energy-Boosting and *Cardiovascular Stimulant Formulas* may also be helpful in exercise programs.

When muscles are sore from exercise, try taking safflower along with drinking lots of water to ease muscle soreness. You can also massage sore muscles using *Topical Analgesic Formulas.*

Therapies: Affirmation and Visualization, Hydration, Low Glycemic Diet and Mineralization

Formulas: Exercise, Energy-Boosting, **Adaptogen**, Cardiovascular Stimulant and Topical Analgesic

Key Herbs: Cordyceps, **Eleuthero (Siberian ginseng)**, Ginseng (American), Ginseng (Asian, Korean), Rhodiola, Safflowers, Schisandra (Schizandra) and Spirulina

Key Nutrients: Colloidal Minerals, Selenium and N-Acetyl Cysteine

Attention Deficit Disorder (ADD, ADHD)

See also *Heavy Metal Poisoning, Hypoglycemia* and *Leaky Gut Syndrome*

ADD (Attention Deficient Disorder) and ADHD (Attention-Deficit Hyperactive Disorder) are characterized by inappropriate inattention, impulsivity and hyperactivity. There is a tendency to haphazard, poorly organized activity. In true ADHD, there is often a weakness of the sympathetic nervous system and a corresponding overactivity of the parasympathetic nervous system. This is why a child suffering from ADHD is calmed down by the use of small doses of a stimulant like Ritalin (which is an epinephrine mimic). Ritalin is in the same class of drugs as all speed or uppers like cocaine, so this does not seem like a very wise way to deal with the problem.

It was once thought that Ritalin changed the faulty brain chemistry in children with ADD/ADHD. New research shows that it has the same action on the brain in children with or without ADD/ADHD. Research also shows that the benefits of Ritalin and other stimulants are short lived, with a return of behavioral problems within 5 years.

Before selecting remedies to try, determine whether the child is truly ADHD or is just stressed and anxious. This is easy to tell by looking at their pupils. Enlarged pupils signal an excess of sympathetic nervous system activity, which means that they are simply stressed and anxious. In this case, *Relaxing Nervine Formulas* will calm them down. Chamomile and lavender are good single herbs for young children suffering from this problem. B-complex vitamins and vitamin C may also be helpful.

If the pupils are small and contracted, then there is an excess of parasympathetic nervous system activity, which means the child actually has ADHD. When this is the case, relaxing herbs like lavender can actually make the child more agitated, while stimulants like caffeine will have a calming effect. If your child has small pupils, look for *Energy-Boosting Formulas* that contain a source of caffeine, like green tea or guarana. Since the adrenals are often insufficient, *Adrenal Tonic Formulas* may also help. Iodine supplements have also helped children with ADHD.

Essential fatty acids are absolutely essential to brain function since the brain structure is mostly composed of fat. Children's brains need a lot of good fats, particular fats with omega-3 essential fatty acids and DHA.

Protein is also very important, both for balancing blood sugar and creating neurotransmitters. The amino acid l-tyrosine is very important because it is the precursor to epinephrine and norepinephrine. One of its richest sources is in red meat. Feeding children with ADHD a hearty breakfast that includes eggs and red meat often helps them become more focused. Simple carbohydrates (such as sugar sweetened cereals) should not be eaten for breakfast.

Heavy metal poisoning, particularly with lead or mercury, can be another root problem in these learning disabilities. These metals may have been introduced into the nervous system through vaccines or environmental pollution. Consider using a *Heavy Metal Cleansing Formula.*

There are specific neurotransmitters that calm down excess nervous system reactions. *Brain Calming Formulas* are herbal formulas designed to help calm down brain activity, making them potentially helpful in many cases of ADHD. The nutritional supplement GABA may also help to calm down the brain.

Hypoglycemia and leaky gut syndrome may also play a role in ADD. Licorice root may be helpful in both. See Hypoglycemia for more tips on balancing blood sugar and Leaky Gut Syndrome for information on how to heal the intestinal tract. The Low Glycemic Diet therapy is important in balancing blood sugar.

Don't substitute artificial sweeteners for sugar. Food additives, including aspartame, can be linked with hyperactivity and other behavioral disorders. Artificial colorings have also been linked with ADHD.

For more information and suggestions read the article *Back to School Shouldn't Mean Back to Ritalin* at *modernherbalmedicine.com.*

Therapies: Friendly Flora, Healthy Fats, Low Glycemic Diet and Stress Management

Formulas: Relaxing Nervine, Energy-Boosting, Adrenal Tonic, Heavy Metal Cleansing and **Brain Calming**

Key Herbs: Bacopa (Water Hyssop), Bee Pollen, Chamomile (English and Roman), **Ashwaganda**, **Jujube**, **Lemon Balm**, **Schisandra (Schizandra)**, Lavender, Licorice, Spirulina, Tea (Green or Black) and Wood Betony

Key Nutrients: Magnesium, Probiotics, Vitamin B-Complex, Vitamin C, **GABA**, Omega-3 Essential Fatty Acids, **DHA**, **L-Glutamine**, Pantothenic Acid (Vitamin B5) and Iron

Autism (Autism Spectrum Disorder)

See also *Heavy Metal Poisoning* and *Vaccines (detoxification from)*

Autism is a mental condition of self-centered subjective mental activity (daydreams, fantasies, delusions, hallucinations, etc.) often accompanied by a marked withdrawal from reality.

Two theories link autism and vaccines. The first theory suggests that the MMR (Mumps-Measles-Rubella) vaccine may cause intestinal problems leading to the development of autism. The second theory suggests that a mercury-based preservative called thimerosal, used in some vaccines, could be connected to autism. The medical community has soundly refuted these theories, but a very passionate group of parents and researchers continue to disagree, based on anecdotal evidence.

There is some evidence that autism is linked to problems in the immune system. Autistic individuals often have other physical issues related to immune deficiency. Some researchers say they have developed effective treatments based on boosting the immune system.

There is also evidence that allergies to certain foods could contribute to autistic symptoms. Most people who hold to this theory feel that gluten (a wheat product) and casein (dairy) are the most significant culprits

Finally, research also suggests several genetic factors. Autistic children have differences in the shape and structure of their brain.

Because of the complexity and seriousness of this condition, professional assistance and support should be sought. The following may be helpful in getting started.

First, improve the diet in general so children are getting the nutrients they need. For starters, avoid refined carbohydrates (simple sugars and starches) and using more fresh fruits and vegetables. Make sure the child is getting high quality fats and proteins. Use the Eliminate Aller-gy-Causing Foods therapy. Dairy products and grains are often major contributing factors to this condition. The Specific Carbohydrate Diet and the GAPS diet have been successful for many children.

Heal the intestinal tract, as intestinal inflammation is often a major issue. See the information under Leaky Gut Syndrome.

Immune overactivity, specifically antibodies to certain brain proteins have been found in several small studies. Many children with ASD also have other autoimmune disorders including celiac and eczema. A general approach of balancing the immune system through diet, nutritional supplements and herbs has been helpful in many children. Astragalus, codonopsis and medicinal mushrooms have a balancing action on the immune system and should play a role in natural ASD treatment.

Gently supporting the body's own detoxification pathways by increasing the nutrient density in the diet and supplementing with NAC, glutathione creams, Co-Q10, B-complex vitamins, methyl B12, and methyl folate can be very beneficial.

Some specific nutritional deficiencies that are common with autism include B12, folate, vitamin C, vitamin A and vitamin D.

For more information see Thomas Easley's class *Working with Autism* available at *modernherbalmedicine.com*.

Therapies: Fresh Fruits and Vegetables, Friendly Flora, Healthy Fats and Heavy Metal Cleanse

Formulas: Heavy Metal Cleansing, General Detoxifying and Brain and Memory Tonic

Key Herbs: Black Walnut, **Lemon Balm**, Linden flowers, Mimosa (Albizia and Silk Tree)

Key Nutrients: Vitamin B-6 (Pyridoxine), Protease Enzymes, **Magnesium**, **Vitamin B-Complex**, DHA, **Omega-3 Essential Fatty Acids** and **L-Glutamine**

Autoimmune Disorders

See also *Fibromyalgia Syndrome (FMS), Hyperthyroid (Grave's Disease), Hashimoto's Disease (Thyroiditis), Lou Gehrig's Disease (Amyotrophic Lateral Sclerosis), Lupus, Multiple Sclerosis (MS), Myasthenia Gravis* and *Rheumatoid Arthritis (Rheumatism)*

The immune system's job is beautifully orchestrated to determine what is self and what is not self and to get rid of anything that is not self by destroying or eliminating that not-self substance. But sometimes things go awry and the immune system becomes confused enough to begin to attack the body's own tissues. This is what causes autoimmune disorders. In essence, the immune system goes renegade.

Think of the renegade immune system as an army that has received confusing messages on who and where the enemy is. Acting on this critical misinformation, the commanding officers order an attack on what they think is the enemy, while in reality they are attacking their own troops and destroying them with "friendly fire."

Like the confused commanding officers, instead of being the protector of health, the confused immune system has become the destroyer of health. These attacks are directed at different tissues, systems and parts of the body in different people, creating symptom clusters that have been named as various diseases.

Before our modern society started experimenting with our health and environment, immune disorders were relatively uncommon. In the last few decades, the incidences of immune disorders have risen at alarming rates. In order to turn the tide and stop the onslaught, we need to understand what we are doing to ourselves and to our environment that may be major contributors to these increases in autoimmune disorders. We also need to know what we can do to prevent further health damage and how to recapture our health through diet, life style changes, and natural health supplements.

There are many possible causes of autoimmune disorders. Here are the major ones and what to do about them.

Viruses

Certain viruses are known to trigger immune problems. A good example is Epstein-Barr virus which is often at the root of many fatigue and pain related autoimmune disorders. *Antiviral Formulas* may be helpful as long as they are not immune stimulants.

Vaccinations

Immunizations bypass our body's first line of immune defense, the skin and mucus membranes. This can confuse the body's immune system and may cause the viral material in the vaccine to get mixed in with the body's own DNA. The body then associates some of its own tissues with disease organisms. The polio vaccine is particularly suspect in multiple sclerosis. Vaccines have been loosely associated with type I diabetes and autism. They may also be involved in multiple sclerosis (MS).

While we are not 100% anti-vaccines, we believe there is still much we do not know about the long term effects of vaccines. If you choose to vaccinate, consider a slower vaccination schedule and only vaccinate if healthy.

Mercury Fillings

One of the most toxic of all substances on earth is the liquid metal mercury. Among other things, it damages our immune system. Just touching it is extremely dangerous, and yet we mix it with silver and put it in our mouths where it stays for the rest of our lives, leaching tiny amounts into our bodies. Consider having a properly trained dentist remove the mercury/silver fillings and replace them with composite fillings, then do the Heavy Metal Cleanse therapy.

Air Pollution

If the air we breathe is loaded with toxins and chemicals, it will negatively affect the immune system. If you live where the air has been damaged by pollutants, use filters and ionizers in your home and make sure you take frequent trips to places with clean air. We have to do everything we can to protect our air. Plant trees and other greenery and have an active voice in environmental issues.

Water Pollution

Our bodies are made of nearly 70% water, and we need to constantly replenish our water supply. When we put bad water and chemically loaded liquids into our bodies, we suffer immediate loss of energy. Some of the most dangerous viruses are waterborne, as are chemicals and toxins, so filter and purify your water.

Chemicals in Food

Commercially grown and processed foods typically contain numerous chemicals. These chemicals also contribute to immune problems. Non-organic foods are grown with artificial chemical fertilizers and toxic chemical pesticides in dead soil. This greatly reduces the nutritional value of the foods, as well as being questionably safe for human consumption. Non-organic meats are raised with steroids, antibiotics, and hormones. These are passed through to us when we eat them. So, wherever possible, insist on certified organic foods.

Avoid eating highly processed foods, refined sugars (including corn syrup), fried foods, prepackaged foods, artificial dyes, flavorings and additives. Avoid pesticides by eating organically grown foods and washing produce carefully. Also avoid GMOs. Hydrogenated fats are a major problem for people with autoimmune problems because they directly contribute to inflammation.

Other Negative Environmental Influences

Many cleaning fluids are made of highly toxic chemicals. Toxic paint fumes, formaldehyde in new carpets, chemicals in particle board, and the electromagnetic frequencies from high tension electrical wires that scramble our energy can be invisible enemies. Microwave ovens and cell phones are also suspect in our quest to find and eliminate factors that can be negatively affecting our immune systems. Some medications can also negatively affect the immune system.

Aids to Balanced Immunity

The key to overcoming and healing autoimmune disorders lies in calming down the immune system response, detoxifying the body gently, and building health from within. Natural therapy for autoimmune disorders includes undoing the damage we have done to our bodies and our environment. Massage, accupressure, acupuncture, chiropractic treatment, spas, gentle exercise, regular stress-breaks, calm and quiet, and rest are valuable possibilities. The only way to recover from autoimmune disorders is to pamper and take care of yourself.

Stress

Avoid or reduce stress wherever possible. Stress can push one's health to the breaking point and exacerbates autoimmune problems. Practice meditation, prayer, yoga or tai chi, take walks, do gentle stretching, garden, journal, enjoy life, take a nice bath or listen to quiet music. Nearly everyone with an autoimmune disorder has exhausted adrenals. The adrenals make cortisol that helps regulate the immune system by dampening excessive inflammation. *Adrenal Tonic* and *Adaptogen Formulas* can be helpful for reducing stress and helping the adrenals balance cortisol to control inflammation.

Inflammation

Autoimmune disorders involve chronic, low grade inflammation. *Antioxidant* and *Anti-Inflammatory Formulas* can be very helpful. Licorice root, yucca and wild yam all have a cortisol-like anti-inflammatory action and can be used as alternatives to the corticosteroid drugs often used to treat these conditions.

Emotional Factors

Find the attitude or feeling that may be presenting itself as a health condition in your life. For instance, Multiple Sclerosis (MS) eats at the nervous system, so try to identify unresolved feelings that may be eating at your nerves. If the inner body is attacking itself in any way because of self-guilt, shame, anger, etc., then self-care and self-love, the antithesis of the attack, can be a powerful tool for turning the autoimmune condition around.

Exercise

Exercise has to be the right kind for the autoimmune profile. It's very important not to overdo on exercise and stress the body! Hard aerobics and intense team sports are out.

What is needed most is oxygen in the system and staying flexible. Yoga, tai chi and other flowing martial arts and dance disciplines, hiking, walking, swimming, light bicycle riding and other enjoyable activities that stretch the body and gently oxygenate the blood are appropriate choices. Keep the exercise regime on the gentle side, but be regular about it.

Diet

Consume fatty, cold water fish at least four times a week. Organic grass fed beef has a much better fat profile than chicken or pork and can be consumed regularly. Cut out any laboratory made fats and avoid fried foods. Hydrogenated oils are very aggravating to autoimmune conditions. Use olive oil, coconut oil, flax seed oil and other good fats. Essential fatty acid supplements are often helpful for autoimmune disorders. Stay off of sugars and sweets by following the Low Glycemic Diet therapy.

Make sure your diet is two-thirds fresh veggies and fruits, organic when possible. Watch out for grains and legumes, especially dairy, corn and wheat/gluten allergies. Many people with autoimmune disorders also need to eliminate eggs and foods in the nightshade family. Screen for other food allergies, too. This eliminates foods that are most likely to cause an immune reaction.

People with autoimmune diseases generally require extra enzymes, especially protease enzymes, to break down protein better. Their lack of the ability to digest proteins may be due to low stomach acid from a hiatal hernia, B12 deficiency, not relaxing while eating or the consumption of food allergens.

When a person's small intestines are inflamed, they can lose structural tone, a condition known as leaky gut. Inflammation of the Small Intestine allows partially digested proteins to cross the intestinal membranes into the blood stream. These proteins trigger immune reactions, which may also trigger the immune system to go after body tissues with a similar protein structure.

Enzymes, fiber, cultured vegetables and probiotics are all helpful for restoring intestinal health. See Leaky Gut Syndrome for ideas on how to heal this underlying problem in autoimmune diseases.

Balancing the Immune System

Avoid herbs and supplements that stimulate the immune system, such as *Immune Stimulating*, *Echinacea Blend* and *Goldenseal & Echinacea Formulas*. Caffeine containing foods and beverages may also overstimulate the immune system. Avoid ylang ylang, geranium and thyme essential oils, as they are too stimulating to a hyperactive immune system.

What is needed in autoimmune disorders is remedies that balance the immune system. *Immune Balancing*, *Mushroom Blend* and *Adaptogen Formulas* may all have this effect. *Mushroom Blend Formulas* can also be helpful in healing the gastrointestinal tract.

Other Supplements

The autoimmune disorder profile includes digestive weakness and malabsorption, so digestive bitters or enzyme supplementation is essential. Consider taking *Digestive Enzyme* or *Digestive Bitter Tonic Formulas*. Extra doses of protease enzyme supplements may also be helpful.

As mentioned under inflammation, essential fatty acids can be very helpful for reducing pain and inflammation. Consider taking a relatively high dose of omega-3 with EPA and DHA for a short period of time. Try to get 10,000 mg of combined EPA/DHA for 5 days. Then back down to a maintenance dose of 2,000 mg of combined EPA/DHA. You should also try to eliminate polyunsaturated vegetable oils as much as possible.

Gentle detoxification may be helpful. Other helpful supplements can be found under the headings for specific autoimmune disorders.

Therapies: Affirmation and Visualization, Bone Broth, Dietary Fiber, Eliminate Gluten, Fresh Fruits and Vegetables, Friendly Flora, Gut Healing Diet, Healthy Fats, Heavy Metal Cleanse, Hiatal Hernia Correction, Hydration, Low Glycemic Diet and Stress Management

Formulas: Adrenal Tonic, Adaptogen, Anti-Inflammatory, Digestive Enzyme, Antioxidant, **Immune Balancing**, **Mushroom Blend**, Digestive Tonic, Blood Purifier, General Detoxifying and Heavy Metal Cleansing

Key Herbs: Aloe vera, Ashwaganda, Cordyceps, **Astragalus**, **Codonopsis**, **Licorice**, **Maitake**, He Shou Wu (Ho Shou Wu, Fo-Ti), Rehmannia, Solomon's Seal and Yucca

Key Nutrients: Vitamin D, Protease Enzymes, Omega-3 Essential Fatty Acids, Digestive Enzymes, **Betaine Hydrochloric Acid (HCl)**, Potassium, **Bromelain** and DHEA

Backache (Back Pain, Lumbago)

See also *Disks (bulging or slipped)*

Pain in the back can be caused by many things, but it often ties to poor kidney function. It can also be due to mechanical stress on the back from poor posture, heavy lifting and other factors. Interestingly, 50% of people with chronic low back pain have no structural damage and 50% of people with herniated disk have no back pain. This leads many in the natural world to correlate stress and systemic inflammation as primary factors in low back pain.

For immediate relief, try applying equal parts lobelia and capsicum tinctures or an *Antispasmodic Formula* in tincture form to the back, especially around the area of pain. Massage that in, then follow it with a *Topical Analgesic Formula*. This will help muscles to relax, realigning the spine and helping vertebrae to move into place. It will also help ease the pain. It may also be helpful to take an herbal *Analgesic Formula* or an *Anti-Inflammatory Formula* internally.

Strengthening the kidneys in their ability to flush waste using a *Kidney Tonic Formula* and drinking more pure water is often helpful. Consuming more fresh fruits and vegetables and less grain will also help. Herbal *Mineral Formulas* can provide nutrients that can strengthen the spine and aid healing.

Check the alignment of your hips by standing in front of a mirror and placing your fingers on the hip bones on both sides of your body. Notice if they are level. If they are not (that is, if one hip is higher than the other), this could be causing your back pain. It can also cause neck and shoulder pain because the pelvis is the foundation for the spine. If the pelvis is out of alignment, then the whole spine will be stressed all the way to the neck.

If your pelvis is out of alignment, chiropractic adjustments, along with structural tonics like Solomon's seal or herbal *Mineral Formulas*, will be helpful. You can also vigorously rub the front of your pelvis, the sides of your legs and your back from your kidney area (the small of your back) to the bottom of your buttocks. This will often help to align the pelvis temporarily.

To help realign the pelvis, stand on one foot. Put all your weight on the leg where the hip is higher. You can even walk favoring that side. This compresses the high side and stretches the low side, creating better alignment.

Your back can also be stressed because you don't have good posture front to back. Many people sit, walk and stand leaning forward. This places constant stress on the back muscles which are forced to hold the weight of the body up against gravity. Practice standing, sitting and walking with your back straight. Stretch your back backwards as well. This eases tension in the muscles. Also consider stretching exercises, yoga or massage therapy.

Therapies: Compress, Hydration, Mineralization and Poultice

Formulas: Antispasmodic, **Topical Analgesic**, Analgesic, Anti-Inflammatory, **Kidney Tonic** and Mineral

Key Herbs: Arnica, Blue Vervain, Buchu, Cramp Bark, **Corydalis**, **Jamaican Dogwood**, Devil's Claw, Kavakava, Lobelia, Mullein root, Scullcap (Skullcap), Stillingia and Wood Betony

Key Nutrients: Magnesium, Bromelain, Digestive Enzymes, **MSM** and Glucosamine

Bacterial Infection

See *Infection (bacterial)*

Bad Breath

See *Halitosis (Bad Breath)*

Therapies: Colon Cleanse

Baldness

See *Hair (loss or thinning)*

Bedwetting

See also *Incontinence (urinary)*

When a child loses bladder control while sleeping and wets the bed, it can be caused by the same problems that cause some adults to wake up during the night to use the bathroom. One of these is adrenal fatigue, because the adrenals help to regulate fluid balance in the body. This can be a sign of stress or blood sugar problems.

Severe stress inhibits urinary function, which may resume when a person is resting at night. Blood sugar problems can cause the adrenals to respond at night waking an adult up or causing a child to wet the bed. *Adrenal Tonic Formulas* or licorice root can be helpful when this is the case. So can a protein snack before bedtime (such as a couple of ounces of peanut butter, cottage cheese or beef jerky). Don't feed children high sugar foods in the evening.

Believe it or not, dehydration is another cause of bedwetting. Drinking more water during the day, and less in the evening, will often help. Taking a mild *Diuretic Formula* during the day (but not in the evening) may also be helpful.

Mineral deficiencies may also play a role in bedwetting, so herbal *Mineral Formulas* might help. The mineral magnesium can be especially helpful.

Children who wet the bed may have fears that affect the adrenals and kidneys. These fears may need to be addressed for the problem to stop.

If the problem is a lack of tone in the sphincter of the bladder then uva ursi, sumach berry or another astringent herb might be helpful. See Incontinence (urinary).

Therapies: Hydration and Low Glycemic Diet

Formulas: Diuretic, Adrenal Tonic and Mineral

Key Herbs: Cranberry, **Cornsilk**, **Uva ursi**, Eleuthero (Siberian ginseng), Hydrangea, Licorice, Marshmallow, Parsley, Red Raspberry, St. John's wort and White Oak

Key Nutrients: Magnesium, Chromium and Pantothenic Acid (Vitamin B5)

Belching

See also *Gas and Bloating*, *Hiatal Hernia* and *Small Intestinal Bacterial Overgrowth (SIBO)*

Belching, gas bubbles from the stomach expelled through the esophagus and mouth, usually signals a problem with poor digestion. *Digestive Enzyme* and *Digestive Bitter Tonic Formulas* may be helpful.

This is particularly true when a person belches and a foul, rotten egg odor and taste accompany the belch. This is a sign that proteins are not being properly broken down in the stomach. In fact, they are decaying. A lack of hydrochloric acid and digestive enzymes often cause this problem, although a hiatal hernia and small intestinal bacterial overgrowth are also possible factors.

If there is a lot of intestinal gas, too, a *Carminative Formula* may be helpful. See *Gas and Bloating*.

Therapies: Hiatal Hernia Correction

Formulas: Digestive Enzyme, Digestive Bitter Tonic, **Carminative** and Catnip & Fennel

Key Herbs: Catnip, Clove, Coptis (Chinese Goldenthread), **Fennel**, **Peppermint**, Papaya and St. John's wort

Key Nutrients: Protease Enzymes, **Digestive Enzymes** and Charcoal (Activated)

Bell's Palsy

See also *Neuralgia and Neuritis*

Paralysis of the facial nerve producing distortion on one side of the face is called Bell's Palsy. This is a form of neuralgia. There are several conditions that can cause facial paralysis, including Lymes disease, stroke and a brain tumor. In Bell's Palsy, however, the cause is unknown. It is thought to be caused by inflammation of the facial nerve, possibly by latent viral infections or an autoimmune response. It can also be caused by an injury or other irritation to the nerves.

Since it is an inflammatory condition, *Anti-Inflammatory Formulas* can be helpful. Essential fatty acids can also be helpful for controlling inflammation and acting as a food for repairing nerves.

Wood betony and blue vervain are good single remedies for this problem. B-complex vitamins, magnesium and calcium can also be helpful.

Therapies: Healthy Fats

Formulas: Antiviral and Anti-Inflammatory

Key Herbs: Alfalfa, **St. John's wort**, **Wood Betony**, Horsetail and Prickly Ash

Key Nutrients: Omega-3 Essential Fatty Acids, N-Acetyl Cysteine, **Vitamin B-Complex**, **Magnesium** and Calcium

Benign Prostate Hyperplasia (BPH)

See also *Prostatitis*

This is a nonmalignant, abnormal growth of the prostate tissue. The severity is measured in stages I-IV (mild-serious), which refers to the size of the growth (walnut-sized to grapefruit-sized) and the impact this enlargement has on one's quality of life. The enlargement of prostate tissue can cause partial or complete obstruction of the urethra leading to urinary hesitancy, painful urination, frequent urination and increased risk of urinary tract infections. Having BPH can elevate the PSA test but fortunately BPH doesn't lead to an increased risk of cancer.

There are several theories as to the cause of BPH. Some research suggest that an excess of a special form of testosterone called dihydrotestosterone (DHT) is to blame, while other research indicates that elevated estrogens and venous stagnation is the cause.

A popular key herb in the treatment of BPH is Saw Palmetto. In several clinical trials Saw Palmetto has been shown to be at least as effective in treating BPH as the most common prescription drug Proscar. Saw Palmetto works not only to inhibit DHT, one of the possible causes of BPH, but it also seems to balance estrogen and testosterone.

Other key herbs for prostate problems are described under *Prostate Formulas*. Men who have been diagnosed with BPH will find these formulas helpful in preventing prostate enlargement or reducing an already enlarged prostate. Some *Male Glandular Tonic Formulas* may also be helpful.

A key nutrient for preventing prostate problems is the mineral zinc. Zinc has been found to be a potent inhibitor of 5a-reductase, the enzyme that converts testosterone to DHT. A reasonable dose of zinc for inhibiting BPH would be 50 mg daily with an added 2 mg of copper.

Excess estrogens, or an imbalance of estrogens and androgens have been implicated in BPH. Estrogen production naturally increases as fat stores increase. Exercise is very beneficial in BPH partially due to the decrease of estrogens that occur with exercise and weight loss. Xenoestrogens are also a major factor in BPH. Reduce or eliminate dairy products and minimize exposure to pesticides, soft plastics and other sources of xenoestrogens. Cruciferous vegetables contain sulfur compounds that can help the liver to help break down excess estrogens. *Liver Tonic* and *Hepatoprotective Formulas* may also be helpful in purging estrogens from the body.

Avoid grapefruit as this inhibits estrogen breakdown. Beer should also be avoided, as the hops in beer is also estrogenic.

Recent research has focused on venous stagnation as a cause of BPH. Enlargement of the prostate is associated with a sedentary lifestyle and is more common in men with desk jobs and those who sit for long periods of time like truck drivers. Regular physical activity and pelvic floor exercises (kegel exercises) can be helpful in stimulating pelvic circulation. Sitz baths also are beneficial for BPH. Many of the most successful herbal formulas for BPH combine herbs like saw palmetto with circulatory remedies like collinsonia.

Therapies: Avoid Xenoestrogens, Colon Cleanse, Exercise and Healthy Fats

Formulas: Prostate, Male Glandular Tonic, Hepatoprotective and Liver Tonic

Key Herbs: Cramp Bark, **Collinsonia (Stoneroot)**, **Nettle (Stinging) root**, **White Sage**, Damiana, Eleuthero (Siberian ginseng), False Unicorn (Helonias), Pumpkin Seed, Pygeum Bark and Saw Palmetto

Key Nutrients: Indole-3 Carbinol (DIM), Omega-3 Essential Fatty Acids, DHEA, **Zinc** and Indole-3 Carbinol (DIM)

Bipolar Mood Disorder (Manic Depressive Disorder)

See also *Depression*

Bipolar mood disorder, formerly known as manic depressive disorder, is a psychological condition where a person has dramatic swings between depression and mania. In the depressed phase the person may sleep a lot, have very little motivation, feel discouraged, anxious, sad or irritable and have thoughts of suicide. During the manic phase the person may have grandiose thoughts, insomnia, poor judgment, increased sex drive, and feel like they can do anything. The exact cause of Bipolar mood disorder is not known, although it does seem to run in families, whether from genetic or learned lifestyle habits is not clear.

Providing general nutritional support for the nervous system is helpful with bipolar disorder. The amino acid l-tyrosine may be helpful in balancing dopamine, a neurotransmitter that may be involved. Eating red meat (ideally from organically raised, grass-fed animals) for breakfast, or taking a protein supplement for breakfast can be helpful in supplying the amino acids, especially tyrosine, necessary to regulate neurotransmitters. L-tyrosine can also be taken as a supplement.

Other nutritional supplements that may be helpful include: l-taurine, coenzymated B-complex vitamins and Omega 3 essential fatty acids. Lithium is used to treat this disorder medically. Lithium is one of the trace elements found in colloidal mineral supplements and is available commercially as a single mineral. Use caution when supplementing with lithium.

Herbally, *Antidepressant Formulas* can be helpful during depressive phases and *Nerve Tonic Formulas* may be helpful during manic phases. Supporting the liver with *Liver Tonic Formulas* may also help to balance out nervous system responses because the liver breaks down excess neurotransmitters.

This disorder may involve environmental sensitivities and food allergies. Avoid food additives and chemicals and screen for food allergies. Heavy metals can be involved, so *Heavy Metal Cleansing Formulas* could be helpful.

Emotional Healing Work is often needed because this problem is frequently triggered by abuse in early childhood. Healing the emotional scars from the abuse helps to stabilize the person's nervous system and mood.

Bipolar mood disorder is a serious disease. Find a qualified practitioner to help you explore natural therapies safely.

Therapies: Affirmation and Visualization, Colon Cleanse, Emotional Healing Work, Healthy Fats, Heavy Metal Cleanse, Low Glycemic Diet, Mineralization and Stress Management

Formulas: Antidepressant, Liver Tonic and Heavy Metal Cleansing

Key Herbs: Ashwaganda, Damiana, Eleuthero (Siberian ginseng), Holy Basil, Linden flowers and Sage

Key Nutrients: Colloidal Minerals, **Vitamin B-Complex**, Omega-3 Essential Fatty Acids and DHA

Birth Control (countering side effects)

See also *Fungal Infections (Yeast Infections, Candida albicans)* and *Leaky Gut Syndrome*

Birth control pills contain hormones which can disrupt the body's normal hormonal balance. They may also contribute to yeast overgrowth and the development of intestinal inflammation and leaky gut syndrome.

Formulas: Female Hormonal Balancing

Key Herbs: Chastetree (Vitex) and Milk Thistle

Key Nutrients: Vitamin B-6 (Pyridoxine), Magnesium and L-Glutamine

Birth Control (natural)

Wild yam has been promoted as a natural birth control agent, but the evidence suggests that this isn't effective. A much more effective way to practice natural birth control is to chart a woman's menstrual cycle.

On a normal 28 day menstrual cycle, a woman is fertile about 14 days after the beginning of her period, and this period of fertility lasts from 5-7 days. Generally speaking there is little risk of pregnancy if unprotected intercourse is limited to 7 days after menstrual flow ceases and the 7 days prior to the beginning of the period.

Another natural approach to birth control is natural lambskin condoms. These do not interfere with pleasure as much as latex condoms. They are effective at preventing conception, but not sexually transmitted diseases, so they should only be used in a monogamous relationship.

Birth Defects (prevention)

See also *Pregnancy (herbs and supplements for)* and *Pregnancy (herbs and supplements to avoid during)*

When a woman is pregnant, she needs extra nutrition to ensure she has adequate nutrients for her developing child. Many birth defects are caused by nutritional deficiencies and toxins. Women planning to get pregnant might benefit from doing a cleanse before getting pregnant. They should also minimize their exposure to tobacco, alcohol, drugs (including over-the-counter and prescription medications), food additives and chemicals of all kinds. Many women have found that they have fewer problems with pregnancy and healthier children if they do a high nutrient diet for three months before trying to conceive. Focusing on vibrantly colored, locally grown vegetables, grass fed or pastured meats, wild caught fish and seasonal fruits, while avoiding packaged and processed foods, helps supply essential nutrients to mothers.

A good prenatal vitamin and mineral supplement (with extra folate) is helpful. Adequate intake of minerals, essential fatty acids and protein is also important. Herbally, *Pregnancy Tonic Formulas* can also be used to ensure a healthier pregnancy.

Therapies: Fresh Fruits and Vegetables, Healthy Fats, Mineralization and Stress Management

Formulas: Pregnancy Tonic

Key Herbs: Alfalfa, **Red Raspberry**, Kelp and Nettle (Stinging)

Key Nutrients: Folate (Folic Acid, Vitamin B9), Colloidal Minerals and **Omega-3 Essential Fatty Acids**

Bites and Stings

There are many herbs that can be applied topically to help heal bites and stings from ants, chiggers, mosquitos and other insects. These natural remedies reduce swelling and inflammation, relieve itching and ease pain, often very rapidly. Single herbs that are helpful for bites and stings include black cohosh, echinacea, lobelia, white oak bark and yarrow. These herbs should be applied topically by either crushing fresh plants, moistening dried powders for the Poultice therapy, or using tinctures and extracts in the Compress therapy.

Commercial herb preparations that may be helpful for bites and stings include *Topical Vulnerary* and *Topical Analgesic Formulas*. These should be kept in an herbal first aid kit so they are readily available when needed.

For poisonous spider bites a poultice of fresh plantain or activated charcoal is often helpful. These should be changed every hour. *Drawing Salve Formulas* may also be helpful. High doses of vitamin C, about 1,000 milligrams, can be taken internally every two hours to aid recovery. Medical assistance should be sought in treating poisonous spider bites.

Bites from poisonous snakes have been eased by the use of poultices of herbs like plantain, echinacea and black cohosh. However, these treatments should be used en route to the emergency room for medical treatment.

For allergic reactions to bee stings *Allergy-Reducing Formulas* may be used in conjunction with topical applications, but again medical assistance should be sought immediately.

Therapies: Aromatherapy, Compress and Poultice

Formulas: Poultice, **Topical Vulnerary**, Allergy-Reducing, Echinacea Blend, Antispasmodic and Drawing Salve

Key Herbs: Aloe vera, Bayberry, Blackberry, Calendula, **Black Cohosh**, **Grindelia (Gumweed)**, **Plantain**, **White Oak**, Echinacea, Hyssop, Lemon Balm, Lobelia, Pennyroyal, Yarrow and Yerba Santa

Key Nutrients: Charcoal (Activated) and Vitamin C

Blackheads

See *Acne (Pimples, Blackheads)*

Bladder (irritable)

See also *Urethritis*, *Urination (burning or painful)*, *Urinary Tract Infections* and *Urination (frequent)*

With an irritable bladder there is a constant urge to urinate, even when there is only a small amount of urine in the bladder. This can be due to dehydration (lack of water) or inflammation of the bladder.

Most people who have this problem drink less water trying to avoid having to urinate so frequently, but this is the wrong approach as it concentrates irritating compounds excreted from the kidneys even more, causing greater irritation. Drinking more water dilutes the toxins and helps the body flush them more effectively.

Herbs that soothe the urinary passages, like cornsilk, pippsessiwa, marshmallow or kava kava, will be helpful. Look for *Kidney Tonic Formulas* that contain these ingredients. You should also consider the possibility of a urinary tract infection. Use *Urinary Infection Fighting Formulas* internally.

Cautions: Uva ursi and juniper are both warming herbs that can irritate the bladder in some people. Do not use these herbs if you are experiencing burning or painful urination. For many people the alcohol in tinctures can be irritating. If you are sensitive to alcohol use a tea, a glycerite, or an encapsulated herb.

Emotionally, an irritable bladder may be a symptom of unresolved angry feelings, in other words, being pissed off. Dealing with whatever is making you angry will ease the irritation.

Therapies: Hydration and Stress Management

Formulas: Urinary Infection Fighting and Kidney Tonic

Key Herbs: Buchu, Cleavers (Bedstraw), **Cornsilk**, **Marshmallow**, **Pipsissewa**, False Unicorn (Helonias), Goldenseal, Kava-kava and Uva ursi

Key Nutrients: MSM

Bladder (ulcerated)

See also *Bladder (irritable)*

When bladder tissues become damaged through continuous inflammation, they may become chronically inflamed and sore. Ulcers may develop in the bladder just as they can in the stomach or intestines.

Single herbal remedies that may be helpful here include goldenseal, cornsilk and marshmallow. If there is blood in the urine consider adding horsetail. Look for *Diuretic, Kidney Tonic* or *Urinary Infection Fighting Formulas* where these herbs are key ingredients.

You should also consider using *Anti-Inflammatory Formulas* to reduce tissue irritation. *Tissue Healing* and *Goldenseal & Echinacea Formulas* may also be helpful.

Therapies: Fresh Fruits and Vegetables and Healthy Fats

Formulas: Urinary Infection Fighting, Tissue Healing, Goldenseal & Echinacea, Kidney Tonic, Anti-Inflammatory and Diuretic

Key Herbs: Cornsilk, **Goldenseal**, Horsetail, Hydrangea and Marshmallow

Key Nutrients: MSM

Bladder Infection

See also *Urinary Tract Infections*

The bladder can easily become infected, especially in women, from bacteria in the feces. This is especially true when the microflora of the intestinal tract has been upset due to the use of antibiotics, birth control pills and other medications. An imbalance in the pH of the body will also make one more prone to bladder infections. Invasion of the bladder by bacteria can result in pain, itching, burning urination, and frequent urgency to void.

To prevent bladder infections, unsweetened cranberry juice is helpful. Also look for *Urinary Infection Fighting Formulas* where cranberry is a major ingredient.

When there is an active infection, use *Urinary Infection Fighting, Antibacterial* or *Goldenseal & Echinacea Formulas*.

Cautions: An untreated or poorly treated bladder infection can lead to a kidney infection, a serious condition. Home test kits that check urine for leukocytes and nitrites are available in any pharmacy. If after several days of using herbal urinary antiseptics you still test positive for a UTI, please go to a doctor for antibiotics.

Therapies: Friendly Flora and Hydration

Formulas: Urinary Infection Fighting, Antibacterial and Goldenseal & Echinacea

Key Herbs: Cranberry, **Goldenseal**, **Juniper Berry**, **Pipsissewa**, **Uva ursi** and Olive leaf

Key Nutrients: Vitamin C

Bleeding (external)

See also *Cuts* and *Nose Bleeds*

To stop bleeding, styptic herbs should be applied directly into the bleeding wound. Two of the best styptics are yarrow and capsicum. You can also use a commercial *Styptic/Hemostatic Formula* both internally and topically. Just about any astringent herb, such as bayberry rootbark, white oak bark, lady's mantle or cranesbill, will also be helpful. For arterial bleeding, pressure should be applied as instructed in any good first aid manual. For any serious bleeding or blood loss, seek appropriate medical attention.

Therapies: Poultice

Formulas: Styptic/Hemostatic

Key Herbs: Bayberry, Calendula, Capsicum (Cayenne), **Erigeron (Fleabane)**, **Tienchi Ginseng**, **Yarrow**, Lady's Mantle and White Oak

Key Nutrients: Vitamin C

Bleeding (internal)

See also *Bleeding (external)*, *Blood in Stool* and *Blood in Urine*

To stop internal bleeding, homeostatic herbs, such as those found in *Styptic/Hemostatic Formulas*, are used. These herbs should be taken internally at frequent intervals (anywhere from every few minutes to every couple of hours, depending on the situation). Vitamin C with citrus bioflavonoids is helpful for strengthening blood vessels and preventing easy bleeding. Horsetail is very helpful for strengthening mucus membranes in the kidneys and lungs for minor bleeding in these organs. For serious bleeding, especially internally, seek appropriate medical attention.

Formulas: Styptic/Hemostatic

Key Herbs: Agrimony, Bayberry, Black Haw, Butchers Broom, Capsicum (Cayenne), Coptis (Chinese Goldenthread), **Tienchi Ginseng**, **Yarrow**, Erigeron (Fleabane), Goldenseal, Horse Chestnut, Horsetail, Lady's Mantle, Periwinkle (Lesser) and White Oak

Key Nutrients: Vitamin C and Bioflavonoids

Bleeding Gums

See *Gingivitis (Bleeding Gums, Gum Disease, Pyorrhea)*

Blisters

Blisters are formed by an irritation that causes a bump filled with lymphatic fluid on the skin. *Poultice* or *Topical Vulnerary Formulas* can be applied directly to blisters to promote healing. When blisters pop, a *Topical Antiseptic Formula* can use used to prevent infection and promote healing.

Therapies: Compress and Poultice

Formulas: Topical Vulnerary, Poultice and Topical Antiseptic

Key Herbs: Aloe vera, **Calendula**, **Comfrey**, Goldenseal, Tea Tree and Yarrow

Bloating

See *Gas and Bloating*

Blood Clots (prevention of)

See also *Thrombosis*

Blood contains a protein called fibrinogen, which helps to form blood clots when we cut ourselves, an important defense mechanism that protects us from bleeding to death. Unfortunately, this same substance can cause our death when a blood clot forms inside the circulatory system and lodges in our heart or brain, resulting in a heart attack or stroke.

When a person's blood is too thick with fibrin, doctors prescribe blood thinners. There are some natural options, however, to prevent the formation of blood clots in the circulatory system. One of these options is vitamin E, which acts as an antioxidant and helps to thin the blood naturally.

Butcher's broom is an herb most commonly used to treat varicose veins. However, it also appears to inhibit clot formation in blood vessels without thinning the blood, especially when taken with vitamin E.

Many herbs for the cardiovascular system have mild blood thinning properties, including alfalfa and ginkgo. Generally speaking, *Cardiovascular Stimulant* and *Vascular Tonic Formulas* can help to reduce the risk of blood clot formation. Other formulas used for this purpose include *Blood Purifier* and *Antioxidant Formulas*.

Therapies: Fresh Fruits and Vegetables, Healthy Fats and Hydration

Formulas: Vascular Tonic, Cardiovascular Stimulant, Blood Purifier and Antioxidant

Key Herbs: Capsicum (Cayenne), **Butchers Broom**, **Ginkgo** and Garlic

Key Nutrients: Omega-3 Essential Fatty Acids, **Vitamin E** and Bromelain

Blood in Stool

See also *Inflammatory Bowel Disorders (Colitis, IBS)*

Blood in the stool can be a sign of severe intestinal inflammation or other injuries in the colon or rectum. It can also be a sign of cancer or other serious problems. Appropriate medical diagnosis should be sought to determine the exact nature of the problem before determining what remedies to use.

To help stop bleeding, use *Styptic/Hemostatic Formulas*. To soothe intestinal inflammation and reduce irritation, consider *Intestinal Toning* and *Fiber Blend Formulas*.

Therapies: Fresh Fruits and Vegetables, Friendly Flora and Mineralization

Formulas: Styptic/Hemostatic, Intestinal Toning, Anti-Diarrhea and Fiber Blend

Key Herbs: Aloe vera, Capsicum (Cayenne), Coptis (Chinese Goldenthread), **Bayberry**, **Yarrow** and White Oak

Key Nutrients: MSM

Blood in Urine

See also *Bleeding (internal)*

Blood in the urine can be caused by severe irritation and inflammation in the kidneys or bladder. It can also be caused by tumors or other serious problems. Appropriate medical diagnosis should be sought to determine the exact nature of the problem before determining what remedies to use.

Horsetail is a very good herb for blood in the urine and can be used alone or with a *Kidney Tonic Formula*. *Styptic/Hemostatic Formulas* can also be used to control the bleeding.

Therapies: Fresh Fruits and Vegetables

Formulas: Styptic/Hemostatic and Kidney Tonic

Key Herbs: Bayberry, Coptis (Chinese Goldenthread), **Horsetail**, Marshmallow, Tienchi Ginseng and Uva ursi

Key Nutrients: Vitamin C and Bioflavonoids

Blood Poisoning (Sepsis)

See also *Infection (bacterial)*

Blood poisoning involves an invasion of the bloodstream by microorganisms. This is usually accompanied by chills, fever and weakness, which may result in secondary abscess in other organs. Seek appropriate professional assistance for this serious problem.

Application of a *Topical Antiseptic Formula* to injuries and wounds can help prevent blood poisoning and may be helpful when it actually develops. You can also use the Poultice or Compress therapy with a mixture of two or three of any of the key herbs listed below.

An herb traditionally used internally to treat blood poisoning is echinacea, which means that *Echinacea Blend*, *Goldenseal & Echinacea*, and *Antibacterial Formulas* containing echinacea are good remedies to consider. *Blood Purifier Formulas* could be taken along with the infection-fighting remedies to speed recovery.

Therapies: Compress, Hydration and Poultice

Formulas: Antibacterial, Echinacea Blend, Goldenseal & Echinacea, Topical Antiseptic and Blood Purifier

Key Herbs: Echinacea, Wild Indigo (Baptista), Garlic, Isatis, Lobelia, Red Clover, Thuja and Usnea

Key Nutrients: MSM, Charcoal (Activated) and Vitamin C

Blood Pressure (high)

See *Hypertension*

Blood Pressure (low)

See *Hypotension*

Bloodshot Eyes

See also *Eyes (red or itching)*

Blood shot eyes are eyes with many red blood vessels showing in the whites of the eyes. This may be caused by fatigue, stress or irritation. An herbal *Eye Wash Formula* can be used topically to reduce irritation to the eyes in the form of a wash or a compress. A simple tip is to dip a tea bag (chamomile or green tea work great) into hot water for a second or two just to get the herbs damp. Let the bag cool until it is safe to put on the skin. Close your eyes and lay the warm tea bag over your closed eyelid for an instant compress. *Vision Supporting Formulas* usually contain herbs that can reduce eye irritation and inflammation when taken internally, too. If stress is an issue, look for a *Relaxing Nervine Formula*.

Therapies: Compress, Fresh Fruits and Vegetables, Hydration and Stress Management

Formulas: Eye Wash, Vision Supporting and Relaxing Nervine

Key Herbs: Chamomile (English and Roman), Eyebright, Goldenseal and Tea (Green or Black)

Key Nutrients: Vitamin C

Body Building

See also *Exercise*

Herbal formulas can be a useful adjunct to body building. For starters consider herbal *Exercise Formula*. These formulas contain herbs that may assist the body in energy production and recovery after a workout. Adaptogens have been shown to improve athletic performance, so *Adaptogen* and *Adrenal Tonic Formulas* that contain adaptogens may also be helpful for body builders. When you overexert yourself, a tea made of safflowers helps to reduce acid buildup in the muscles and ease muscle aches.

Therapies: Affirmation and Visualization, Avoid Xenoestrogens, Hydration and Mineralization

Formulas: Exercise, Adaptogen and Adrenal Tonic

Key Herbs: Cordyceps, Eleuthero (Siberian ginseng), Ginseng (American), Ginseng (Asian, Korean) and Safflowers

Key Nutrients: MSM

Body Odor

When there is an excessively offensive odor associated with sweat, it is an indication of a need for cleansing the body. Doing the Colon Cleanse therapy will often reduce body odor, so *Blood Purifier* and *General Detoxifying Formulas* can be helpful here. Also consider *Digestive Enzyme Formulas* to enhance digestion of nutrients. Liquid chlorophyll is a natural deodorizer when taken internally.

Therapies: Colon Cleanse and Hydration

Formulas: Blood Purifier, General Detoxifying and Digestive Enzyme

Key Herbs: Parsley, Pau d' Arco and Sage

Key Nutrients: Chlorophyll, Vitamin B-Complex, Vitamin B-12 and Zinc

Boils

A boil is an infection of a skin gland resulting in localized swelling and inflammation, having a hard central core often filled with pus and/or watery fluid. Boils are best treated by using remedies that cleanse the blood and help drain the lymphatics. Topically, echinacea is one of the best remedies. *Blood Purifier Formulas* can be used internally.

Therapies: Poultice

Formulas: Blood Purifier, Lymphatic Drainage, General Detoxifying and Poultice

Key Herbs: Black Walnut, Burdock, Chickweed, **Echinacea**, **Tea Tree**, Poke Root, Red Clover and Wild Indigo (Baptista)

Bone Spur

See *Calcium Deposits (Calcification)*

BPH

See *Benign Prostate Hyperplasia (BPH)* and *Prostatitis*

Brain Fog

See *Confusion*

Breast (infection)

See *Mastitis*

Breast Lumps

See also *Cancer (natural therapy for)* and *Cystic Breast Disease*

If you have a lump in your breast be sure to obtain an appropriate medical diagnosis to find out if you are dealing with benign breast lumps or breast cancer. If the lumps are

cancerous, see Cancer (natural therapy for). If the lumps are benign, then the following information may be useful.

Start by eliminating caffeine as this is a major cause of breast lumps. Since lumps are usually a sign of too much estrogen stimulation, also consider using *Phytoestrogen Formulas* and the therapy Avoid Xenoestrogens.

Female Hormonal Balancing Formulas can also help to regulate the balance between estrogen and progesterone in the body, particularly if chaste tree berries are a principle ingredient. Progesterone creams may also help to reduce excess estrogen stimulation to breast tissue.

Herbal formulas that help the liver and lymphatics to function better may also be helpful for eliminating benign breast lumps. Generally speaking, *Blood Purifier* and *General Detoxifying Formulas* will be helpful. Use these along with a good *Lymphatic Drainage Formula*. The oil of poke root can be massaged topically into the breasts to further increase lymphatic drainage. One can also use the Castor Oil Pack therapy.

Therapies: Avoid Xenoestrogens, Castor Oil Pack, Colon Cleanse and Fresh Fruits and Vegetables

Formulas: Blood Purifier, General Detoxifying, Female Hormonal Balancing, Phytoestrogen and Lymphatic Drainage

Key Herbs: Chastetree (Vitex), False Unicorn (Helonias) and Poke Root oil

Key Nutrients: Vitamin E and **Indole-3 Carbinol (DIM)**

Breast Milk (dry up)

See *Nursing*

Breast Milk (increase or enrich)

See *Nursing*

Breasts (enhance size)

Certain phytoestrogens in plants appear to encourage breast development. Saw palmetto, in particular, has been reported helpful for this purpose, but the effect is temporary and only lasts while taking the herb. Breast size enhancement with herbs is not a claim any legitimate herbalist is likely to make.

Key Herbs: Saw Palmetto

Breasts
(swelling and tenderness)

See also *PMS Type H*

Tenderness or pain in the breast tissue may be due to lymphatic congestion. Hormonal imbalances may also cause breast swelling and tenderness.

Lymphatic Drainage Formulas, which improve the flow of lymph, are often helpful when used with plenty of water. *Diuretic Formulas* can also be used if the swelling occurs in other tissues of the body.

Poultices with herbs like mullein and slippery elm have also eased this problem. You can use a *Poultice Formula* directly on the breasts.

When associated with PMS this problem may be due to elevated aldosterone. Vitamin B6, magnesium, vitamin E, omega-3 fatty acids, evening primrose oil and the essential oils of frankincense and lemon are all remedies that may help.

Hormonal balancers such as black cohosh and dong quai may also help ease breast swelling when hormones are involved. Consider using a *Female Hormonal Balancing Formula*.

Therapies: Avoid Xenoestrogens, Compress, Healthy Fats, Hydration and Poultice

Formulas: Lymphatic Drainage, Diuretic, Female Hormonal Balancing and **Poultice**

Key Herbs: Black Cohosh, Calendula, Cleavers (Bedstraw), **Chastetree (Vitex)**, **Mullein**, Dong Quai, Eleuthero (Siberian ginseng), Parsley, Poke Root, Red Clover and Violet

Key Nutrients: Vitamin B-6 (Pyridoxine), Omega-3 Essential Fatty Acids, Magnesium and Vitamin E

Broken Bones

Herbal remedies can speed the healing of broken bones. In particular, consider using herbal *Mineral* and *Tissue Healing Formulas*. In cases where it is possible to apply a poultice topically, you can use a *Poultice Formula*. You can also apply a compress. (See Poultice and Compress in the *Therapies Section*.)

In addition to herbal remedies, a good mineral supplement with calcium, magnesium and phosphorus will be helpful. Vitamins D3 and K2 are also helpful for speeding the healing of broken bones.

Therapies: Bone Broth, Compress, Mineralization and Poultice

Formulas: Mineral, Tissue Healing and Poultice

Key Herbs: Comfrey, **Mullein**, Horsetail, Mimosa (Albizia, Silk Tree) and Solomon's Seal

Key Nutrients: Vitamin D, Calcium, Colloidal Minerals, Magnesium, Vitamin C, **Vitamin K**, MSM and Silicon

Bronchitis

See also *Congestion (bronchial)*

Bronchitis is an inflammation of the small tubes of the lungs, usually as a result of a respiratory infection. If the inflammation is due to an infection, *Antibacterial* or *Antiviral Formulas* should be helpful. Generally speaking, *Expectorant* and *Decongestant Formulas* are also needed to remove congestion and aid healing.

Since this is an inflammatory condition, an *Anti-Inflammatory Formula* may also be used in conjunction with expectorants and decongestants to speed recovery, as will drinking plenty of fluids.

Therapies: Fresh Fruits and Vegetables and Hydration

Formulas: Bronchialdilator, **Decongestant**, Expectorant, Anti-Inflammatory, Antibacterial and Antiviral

Key Herbs: Astragalus, Black Cohosh, Bloodroot, Blue Vervain, Butterbur Root, Camphor, Cherry (Wild), Cinnamon, Clove, Coleus, **Echinacea**, **Horehound**, **Licorice**, **Marshmallow**, **Osha**, Elecampane, Eucalyptus, Garlic, Goldenseal, Grindelia (Gumweed), Horseradish, Hyssop, Irish moss, Khella, Lobelia, Lomatium, Mullein, Myrrh, Oregano, Pine (White), Plantain, Reishi (Ganoderma), Skunk Cabbage, Thyme, Usnea and Yerba Santa

Key Nutrients: N-Acetyl Cysteine, MSM, **Vitamin A** and Vitamin D

Bruises

Bruises are caused by an injury to the tissues where stagnation sets in causing the area to turn a purplish black color. When a bruise has already formed apply a *Topical Vulnerary* or a *Topical Analgesic Formula* to speed healing. In particular, look for formulas that contain arnica, Solomon's seal or yarrow.

If a person bruises easily, this is a sign of fragile capillaries and poor circulation. *Cardiovascular Stimulant Formulas* can be taken internally along with rose hips and/or vitamin C with bioflavonoids to correct this problem. herbal *Mineral Formulas* may also strengthen blood vessels to reduce easy bruising.

Therapies: Aromatherapy and Fresh Fruits and Vegetables

Conditions

Formulas: Topical Vulnerary, Topical Analgesic, Cardiovascular Stimulant, **Vascular Tonic** and Mineral

Key Herbs: Bilberry (Blueberry, Huckleberry), Butchers Broom, Comfrey, **Arnica**, **Yarrow**, Horse Chestnut, Horsetail, Lomatium, Rose hips, Tienchi Ginseng, Witch Hazel and Yerba Santa

Key Nutrients: Vitamin C, Bioflavonoids and **MSM**

Bulimia

See also *Anorexia* and *Anxiety Disorders*

Bulimia is a disorder characterized by binge eating followed by self-induced vomiting and the use of laxatives, fasting or diuretics to prevent weight gain. Herbs and supplements may help with appetite or nerves, but this disorder is psychologically based and requires counseling and Emotional Healing Work. Seek appropriate professional assistance.

As an adjunct to professional assistance you can use *Digestive Bitter Tonic Formulas* to stimulate appetite and *Digestive Enzyme Formulas* or digestive enzyme supplements to improve digestion. *Adaptogen* and *Nerve Tonic Formulas* may help with the stress factor in this disorder. Avoid cleansing programs and herbal laxatives.

Therapies: Affirmation and Visualization, Healthy Fats, Low Glycemic Diet, Mineralization and Stress Management

Formulas: Digestive Bitter Tonic, **Adaptogen** and Digestive Enzyme

Key Herbs: Bee Pollen, **Ashwaganda**, Eleuthero (Siberian ginseng), Gentian and Spirulina

Key Nutrients: Digestive Enzymes

Bunions

A localized swelling at a joint in the foot caused by an inflammation of the bursa is called a bunion. *Anti-Inflammatory Formulas* can be used internally to reduce inflammation and pain while *Topical Vulnerary Formulas* can be applied to inflamed areas to promote healing. A *Poultice Formula* could also be applied topically.

Therapies: Compress and Poultice

Formulas: Topical Vulnerary, Poultice and Anti-Inflammatory

Key Herbs: Arnica, Burdock, **Solomon's Seal** and St. John's wort

Key Nutrients: MSM

Burning Feet or Hands

See also *Anemia, Circulation (poor), Diabetes, Hyperinsulinemia (Metabolic Syndrome, Syndrome X)* and *Inflammation*

Burning hands and feet are caused by an abnormal nervous system signal or by a lack of circulation. This causes a tingling sensation in the extremities.

To help the nerves to function better, methyl B12, folate, B-complex vitamins and *Nerve Tonic Formulas* may be helpful. herbal *Mineral Formulas* may provide additional healing and relief.

Where the problem is circulatory in nature as in peripheral artery disease, *Cardiovascular Stimulant Formulas* may be helpful. Many people find contrast therapy helpful in cases of poor circulation. Simply fill two small tubs, one with water as hot as you can stand, the other with ice water. Soak your feet for 3 minutes in hot and then 30 seconds in cold. Repeat this rotation several times every night.

This problem may be due to complications of poor circulation caused by diabetes. In this case *Blood Sugar Reducing Formulas* may be helpful. See Diabetes and Hyperinsulinemia (Syndrome X) for more information.

Because inflammation is involved, an *Anti-Inflammatory Formula* and omega-3 essential fatty acids may also be helpful in reducing the burning sensations.

Tingling or burning in the feet is also commonly caused by anemia from a B12 or folate deficiency. In alcoholics or those with severe malabsorption, thiamine deficiency can cause burning feet.

Therapies: Fresh Fruits and Vegetables, Healthy Fats, Hydration and Low Glycemic Diet

Formulas: Blood Sugar Reducing, Anti-Inflammatory and Mineral

Key Herbs: Capsicum (Cayenne), **Schisandra (Schizandra)**, Ginger, Prickly Ash and St. John's wort

Key Nutrients: Vitamin B-Complex, Omega-3 Essential Fatty Acids, Chromium, **Vitamin B-12**, **Folate (Folic Acid and Vitamin B9)**

Burnout

See *Adrenals (exhaustion, weakness or burnout)*

Burns and Scalds

See also *Sunburn*

Burns and scalds can be very painful. Minor burns (1st degree) involve normal symptoms of inflammation—redness, pain and swelling. More severe burns (2nd degree) can result in blisters and the most severe burns (3rd degree) can have permanent skin damage that prevents skin regeneration and can threaten life due to infection or fluid loss if the area is extensive. The remedies here are primarily for 1st and 2nd degree burns. Third degree burns, especially if over a large area of the body, should be treated medically.

Effective topical remedies for burns include: aloe vera gel, tea tree essential oil, lavender essential oil, real vanilla extract, raw honey and plantain leaf. Many of these remedies are readily available in most kitchens. Running the burned area under cold water to cool the heat, or using ice water to soak the burned area is very helpful for pain. Remedies can be applied by using the Compress or Poultice therapy. Vitamin E can be applied once the pain is gone from the burn to prevent scarring and speed tissue repair. Zinc and vitamin C, taken internally, help to speed the healing of burns. An herbal *Analgesic Formula* may be helpful for pain.

Therapies: Aromatherapy, Compress and Poultice

Formulas: Topical Vulnerary and Analgesic

Key Herbs: Aloe vera, **Lavender**, Lomatium, Marshmallow, Plantain, Slippery Elm and Tea Tree essential oil

Key Nutrients: Vitamin C, Zinc and **MSM**

Bursitis

See also *Arthritis*

Bursitis is an inflammation of the connective tissue capsule of joints resulting in pain and inflammation. It is treated naturally in a similar manner to arthritis, but some of the more specific remedies that can be helpful for it are listed here.

Therapies: Eliminate Allergy-Causing Foods, Healthy Fats and Hydration

Formulas: Anti-Inflammatory, Joint Healing and Topical Analgesic

Key Herbs: Boswellia, Burdock, Cats Claw (Uña de Gato, Gambier), Chaparral, **Solomon's Seal**, Devil's Claw, Licorice, Pleurisy Root, Turmeric and Willow

Key Nutrients: Magnesium and **MSM**

Calcium Deficiency

See *Osteoporosis*

Calcium Deposits (Calcification)

See also *Kidney Stones*

In the presence of mineral imbalances and a vitamin K2 deficiency, calcium can come out of solution and form kidney stones, hardened tissue or bone spurs. Calcium deposits often signal a lack of magnesium or other nutrients used in conjunction with calcium. Herbs that have lithotriptic properties can help bring calcium back into solution in the body. These include hydrangea, gravel root and lemon juice.

Use these herbs as singles or select a *Lithotriptic Formula* and take it along with lots of purified water. Since lemon juice is also lithotriptic, adding freshly-squeezed lemon to the water will enhance the effectiveness.

If you have been taking calcium supplements, discontinue their use and take 500-1,000 milligrams of magnesium each day. If you feel you still need a calcium supplement try using an herbal *Mineral Formula*. Remedies that reduce inflammation may also be helpful when bone spurs are involved.

Formulas: Lithotriptic, Mineral and Anti-Inflammatory

Key Herbs: Hydrangea, Gravel root and Lemon

Key Nutrients: Omega-3 Essential Fatty Acids and **Magnesium**

Cancer (natural therapy for)

See also *Leukemia* and *Lymphoma*

Anyone who has ever had cancer, or had a loved one with cancer, knows the feelings of fear, anxiety, worry and often hopelessness that this very serious illness can bring. This is understandable considering cancer is the second leading cause of death in civilized nations. Furthermore, conventional treatments such as chemotherapy, radiation and surgery are often dangerous in and of themselves. So, it's little wonder that cancer generally causes intense emotional distress in everyone involved. However, one should always believe that there is hope, even when orthodox medicine offers none. As long as the body has life, there is hope.

Of course, the subject of cancer is far too involved to adequately address in this book. We can acquaint you with some important information about cancer from a natural healing perspective and give you some ideas about options you may not be familiar with. However, we strongly encourage you to seek professional help when dealing with cancer. You need competent health care professionals helping you with your program and monitoring your progress, but you should also do some study on your own and learn about things you can do for yourself.

Cancer is a disease involving cells that have undergone a genetic mutation so they are no longer responsive to messages from the body that regulate cell metabolism and growth. Some of these mutations are believed to be the result of free radical damage that causes the cells to develop an anaerobic metabolism and turn cancerous. Other mutations seem to be genetic, or caused by cellular injuries from infection or chemicals. Normal cells have an aerobic metabolism, which means they produce energy by means of oxygen and oxidation. Anaerobic cells produce energy without oxygen via a process of fermentation.

This is important to know because if the body is highly oxygenated, the environment for cancer does not exist. In fact, in 1931, Dr. Otto Warburg won a Nobel Prize for proving that whenever any cell is denied 60% of its oxygen requirements, it can become cancerous. So, conditions that deprive cells of oxygen (such as chronic inflammation, buildup of toxins or problems with red blood cells or circulation) increase the risk of cancer. Cancer creates a low oxygen, acidic environment to encourage its growth.

Another important thing you should know is that cancer cells are forming in the body on a regular basis. Very likely, you have a few inside you right now. Don't worry, the immune system normally recognizes these deviant cells and destroys them.

Therefore, in order for you to develop cancer, two factors must exist. First, your body has to have a toxic, low oxygen environment that encourages the development of anaerobic cancer cells, and second, your immune system must be weakened so that it is not able to recognize and destroy these cells.

So, while killing cancer cells (the goal of conventional cancer therapy) is an important part of treating cancer, it does not fix the underlying problems that created the cancer in the first place. This is the weakness of the standard medical approach to cancer. An effective protocol for cancer should do more than just destroy cancer cells; it should try to restore a normal, healthy environment in the body and rebuild the immune system.

Even if one chooses to use orthodox cancer therapies, they would be wise to consider doing natural therapy both to restore the body's state of health and prevent the cancer from reoccurring. Here are the basic principles of natural cancer therapy.

Principle Number One: Increase Oxygen Levels

Cancer cells are anaerobic. They get their energy by metabolizing nutrients, notably sugars and carbohydrates, without oxygen via a fermentative process. Cancer cells cannot survive in a high oxygen environment, so keeping the body well oxygenated inhibits cancer. Do this by getting plenty of fresh air and exercise. Breathe deeply. If you smoke, quit.

Liquid chlorophyll is a great way to enhance oxygen transport. It helps the blood carry more oxygen to the tissues, and research has shown that it reduces the risk of cancer. The natural way to get more chlorophyll is to consume dark green, leafy vegetables, wheat grass, barley grass and other green plant foods.

If you have problems with the lungs, *Lung and Respiratory Tonic Formulas*, particularly those containing astragalus or cordyceps can also be helpful. Both of these herbs enhance lung function and boost the immune system.

Principle Number Two: Increase Nutrient Intake From High Quality Foods.

Eat large quantities of fresh, preferably organic, fruits and vegetables every day. This is well-recognized as one of the best ways of decreasing your risk of cancer, but unfortunately, its benefit in helping people recover from cancer is often ignored. Fresh fruits and vegetables not only have vitamins, minerals and phytonutrients that are anti-cancerous, they also strengthen immunity, aid detoxification and provide antioxidants.

A lack of hydrochloric acid leads to excess lactic acid in the body and poor digestion and absorption of nutrients, which sets the stage for cancer. *Digestive Bitter Tonic Formulas* can be taken before meals to stimulate appetite and increase hydrochloric acid production. You may also want to use an enzyme supplement that contains Betaine HCl.

Principle Number Three: Strengthen the Immune System

The body normally and regularly produces cancer cells due to free radical damage, environmental factors or other causes. A healthy immune system recognizes and destroys these defective cells. When the immune system is unable to recognize these deviant cells or is too weak to destroy them, the disease we call cancer develops.

There are many reasons why the immune system becomes weakened. Poor nutritional intake is a major factor. The loss or destruction of friendly bacteria in the intestinal tract is another. Excessive sugar consumption causes chronic inflammation that distresses the immune system.

Improving nutritional intake, especially eating those 7-9 servings of fruits and vegetables daily, will help the immune system, as will eliminating chemical-laden processed foods. Reducing intake of sugar, white flour and other simple carbohydrates will also help.

Immune Stimulating and *Mushroom Blend Formulas* are the principle immune-boosting remedies that are helpful with natural cancer therapy. There is a lot of research supporting the use of medicinal mushrooms in helping the body fight cancer. These formulas can be used in conjunction with medical cancer therapy as well.

Fu Zheng therapy is a combination of herbs from China that strengthen the immune system and help with the side effects of chemotherapy. It has been found to substantially decrease the immune suppression associated with chemotherapy and it increases survival time. Fu Zheng therapy uses a combination of astragalus, ligustrum, ginseng, codonopsis, atractylodes and reishi (ganoderma).

Principle Number Four: Detoxify

The human body is bombarded with toxins, heavy metals, chlorine and thousands of chemicals that we breathe in, consume in our diet, or absorb through our skin. These all cause free radicals in the body and contribute to the environment of cancer. Avoiding these toxins is part of both cancer prevention and holistic cancer therapy. In particular, avoid or eliminate refined and processed foods (especially foods raised with pesticides, antibiotics or steroids), toxic cleaning products (such as laundry detergents, skin care items, fluoridated toothpaste, etc.) and chlorinated and fluoridated water. Also, avoid microwaved or irradiated foods and protect yourself from electrical equipment (electromagnetic pollution may be a major causal factor in cancer).

It is also helpful to assist the body in detoxifying from these substances using *Blood Purifier* and *General Detoxifying Formulas*. Blood purifiers like burdock, red clover and sheep sorrel are used in all traditional herbal remedies for cancer, including Essiac Tea, Jason Winters Tea and the Hoxsey Formula. Variations of these traditional cancer formulas can be found under the heading *Anticancer Formulas*.

It is important to note that cleansing is often overstressed in natural cancer therapy. It is also essential to build the body with good nutrition and to address stress and other mental and emotional factors.

Principle Number Five: Use Antioxidants

Our need for oxygen exceeds the demand for any nutrient, even water, because we need oxygen for normal energy production in the cells. However, oxygen can also produce free radicals that can damage normal cells and cause cancer. Antioxidant nutrients protect the body from this free radical damage, thereby reducing cancer risk. Antioxidants can also be used in a treatment program for cancer because they help protect the body from harmful side effects of radiation and chemotherapy. So adding an *Antioxidant Formula* can be helpful for cancer recovery whether a person is using a natural approach or a medical approach.

Some antioxidants to consider here include green tea extract, mangosteen and turmeric. Green tea contains polyphenols called catechins, powerful antioxidants that protect cells from cancer and kill cancer cells. One of these catechins is epigallocatechin gallate (EGCG), which was shown in several lab studies to kill cancer cells without harming healthy tissue.

Mangosteen contains xanthones, powerful antioxidants that have been shown in numerous studies to inhibit cancer cells and aid in tumor reduction. These compounds cause apoptosis (preprogrammed cell death) in cancer cells. Xanthones exert cytotoxic (cancer cell killing) effects against human hepatocellular carcinoma cells, and have been shown to inhibit the growth of human leukemia HL60 cells. Xanthones have also been shown to be effective against human breast cancer SKBR3 cells.

Turmeric, a spice commonly used in Indian food, also has powerful anticancer and antioxidant properties. In one study, curcumin (an active constituent in turmeric) induced apoptosis in cancer cells without cytotoxic effects on healthy cells. In an animal study, curcumin inhibited the growth of cancer cells in the stomach, liver and colon as well as oral cancers.

Principle Number Six: Kill Cancer Cells

For those diagnosed with cancer, it is important to kill the cancerous cells. The problem is that chemotherapy and radiation also cause damage to healthy cells. Killing cancer cells also produces toxins that the body must eliminate.

There are some natural compounds that can help kill cancer cells, too. Two of these remedies are graviola (*Annona muricata*) and the American paw paw tree (*Asimina triloba*). These plants contain compounds called acetogenins that have been shown in scientific studies to cause apoptosis in cancer cells by inhibiting their energy production. Unfortunately, the acetogenins that are anti-cancerous also cause nausea, so getting an effective dose is sometimes challenging.

Other possible cancer-destroying remedies discussed in the *Key Herbs Section* include mistletoe, Venus fly trap, bloodroot, chaparral and poke root. Many of these plants are toxic and should only be used under the guidance of a skilled professional herbalist. You will probably need to locate a professional herbalist to even obtain most of them (*findanherbalist.com*).

Principle Number Seven: Increase Joy and Pleasure

One German study shows the commonality that all cancer patients experienced a trauma and an unresolved psychological issue shortly before the cancer developed. Stress is a big component of cancer because psychological stress creates physical stress that dramatically reduces immune function.

Reducing stress should be a stress free task. That's why the goal here is not to reduce stress, but rather to deliberately seek out joy and pleasure. A pleasurable, happy experience has a more positive effect on the immune system and healing than a stressful experience.

So, seek out pleasurable experiences. Find things that make you laugh. Spend time with family, friends or pets. Take a walk in the fresh air and sunshine. Surround yourself with pleasing colors, smells and sounds. Listen to your favorite music; get up and dance. Listen to calming, meditative music. Take a hot bath in Epsom salts and lavender oil. Treat yourself to a massage, take a mini-vacation or go to a spa for the day.

You can also reduce stress by taking *Adaptogen* and *Relaxing Nervine Formulas*. B-complex vitamins and vitamin C will also help reduce feelings of stress. They will also help with detoxification and have antioxidant properties.

Cancer is a difficult disease to work with, but many people have successfully recovered from cancer using both natural therapies and conventional therapies or a combination of the two. Seek out professional assistance in designing the holistic program that's right for you. Remember, there is hope!

Therapies: Affirmation and Visualization, Avoid Xenoestrogens, Colon Cleanse, Colon Hydrotherapy, Deep Breathing, Emotional Healing Work, Epsom Salt Bath, Fresh Fruits and Vegetables, Heavy Metal Cleanse, Hiatal Hernia Correction, Hydration and Stress Management

Formulas: Anticancer, Blood Purifier, **Mushroom Blend**, Immune Stimulating, General Detoxifying, Antioxidant, Digestive Enzyme, Drawing Salve, Lung and Respiratory Tonic, Digestive Enzyme, Adaptogen, Relaxing Nervine and **Essiac**

Key Herbs: Aloe vera, Astragalus, Barberry, Bitter Melon, Bloodroot, Boswellia, Codonopsis, Cordyceps, **Burdock**, **Cats Claw (Uña de Gato, Gambier)**, **Chaparral**, **Paw Paw**, **Reishi (Ganoderma)**, **Turmeric**, **Venus Fly Trap**, Echinacea, Eleuthero (Siberian ginseng), Garlic, Ginseng (American), Ginseng (Asian, Korean), Maitake, Pau d' Arco, Poke Root, Red Clover, Sheep Sorrel, Shiitake, Sweet Annie (Ching-Hao), Tea (Green or Black) and Yellow Dock

Key Nutrients: Indole-3 Carbinol (DIM), N-Acetyl Cysteine, **Protease Enzymes**, Probiotics, Folate (Folic Acid, Vitamin B9), **Digestive Enzymes**, Chlorophyll, Vitamin B-Complex and Potassium

Cancer (prevention)

See also *Cancer (natural therapy for)* and *Cancer Treatment (reducing side effects)*

Anyone who has ever had cancer, or had a loved one with cancer, knows the feelings of fear, anxiety, worry and often hopelessness that this very serious illness can bring. This is understandable considering cancer is the second leading cause of death in civilized nations. Furthermore, while death rates from heart disease have been declining over the past decade, death rates from cancer have been increasing. According to recent statistics, heart disease and cancer deaths are close to equal and it is likely that cancer will become the leading cause of death within the next five years.

Cancer is already the leading cause of death during middle age (45-75), while heart disease is the leading cause of death in old age (after 75). In people between the ages of 35 and 45–and beyond age 75–cancer is the second leading cause of death. In other words, if you're interested in a long and healthy life, you should be interested in preventing cancer.

Cancer is largely a disease of modern civilization. Environmental toxins and electromagnetic pollution are major factors in the development of cancer. There is also a big emotional component, as the typical cancer patient is usually neglecting their own care while taking care of others.

Most experts agree that increasing one's intake of antioxidants and other nutrients by eating 5-9 one-half cup servings of fresh fruits and vegetables (ideally organic or at least washed to remove chemical residues) is the best way to prevent cancer. A number of specific nutrients also have cancer inhibiting properties, including vitamins A, C and D, zinc, selenium and chlorophyll.

Eating organic food, using natural personal care and household cleaning products, and otherwise avoiding chemicals will help reduce one's risk of cancer. It is also helpful to minimize exposure to electromagnetic fields. For example, use a headset when talking on a cell phone, avoid using microwave ovens, and take periodic breaks when working on computers or around electronic equipment. Avoid living near high power electric lines or electrical substations. There are devices called diodes that reportedly help to reduce electromagnetic interference in the body. This is controversial, but there are people using them (including some of the authors) who have noticed they have more energy and feel better when using them.

Since it is impossible to avoid all toxins, doing some periodic cleansing and eating lots of fresh fruits and vegetables to obtain adequate amounts of antioxidants are also important keys to cancer prevention. If you are exposed to chemicals on a regular basis in your job, you should probably consider using an *Antioxidant Formula* and a *Hepatoprotective Formula* on a regular basis.

To reduce the risk of estrogen-dependent cancers like breast, uterine and prostate cancer it is also important to follow the program Avoid Xenoestrogens in the *Therapies Section*. Foods rich in phytoestrogens like beans, green leafy vegetables and whole grains as well as *Phytoestrogen Formulas* may also be helpful.

Keeping the immune system healthy is also important to avoiding cancer. Consider taking *Mushroom Blend Formulas* to tonify the immune system. *Immune Stimulating Formulas* may also be helpful if you have a weak immune system (that is, you catch contagious diseases easily).

As for the stress component, there is research that suggests that major stresses in life can trigger tumor growth. People with cancer are often taking care of others, while neglecting to take care of themselves. Since stress can weaken the immune system, Stress Management therapy is a major part of preventing cancer and many other diseases. The bad news is that none of us can avoid stress. The good news is that we don't have to. We simply have to make time for pleasure and recreation. Pleasurable experiences do more good for the body than stressful experiences do harm.

Therapies: Avoid Xenoestrogens, Colon Cleanse, Deep Breathing, Dietary Fiber, Fresh Fruits and Vegetables, Healthy Fats, Heavy Metal Cleanse and Stress Management

Formulas: Antioxidant, Phytoestrogen, Immune Stimulating, **Mushroom Blend** and **Hepatoprotective**

Key Herbs: Astragalus, Burdock, Cordyceps, **Milk Thistle**, **Reishi (Ganoderma)**, **Turmeric**, Maitake, Red Clover and Shiitake

Key Nutrients: Indole-3 Carbinol (DIM), **Vitamin D**, **Vitamin C**, **Vitamin A**, Omega-3 Essential Fatty Acids, Lycopene, Chlorophyll, Bromelain, **Zinc**, **Selenium**, Fiber, **Iodine**, Lutein and Proanthocyanidins

Cancer Treatment (reducing side effects)

See also *Cancer (natural therapy for)*, *Chemical Poisoning* and *Radiation Sickness*

Surgery, chemotherapy and radiation all have one goal—to remove or destroy cancer cells, but, they don't do anything to deal with the underlying causes of the disease. The pioneer herbalist, Samuel Thomson, once said that the same thing that will prevent a disease will cure it. So, even if you're receiving medical treatment for cancer, it makes sense to adopt a diet and lifestyle that would have helped to prevent it in the first place. So, first read the section on Cancer (prevention) and Cancer (natural therapy for) and then read this section for tips on handling specific side effects of orthodox cancer therapy.

Reducing Side Effects of Radiation and Chemotherapy

Radiation causes free radical damage and can actually turn healthy cells cancerous. Chemotherapy generally targets fast growing cells, which means it tends to damage healthy cells that are also fast growing. These include the cells lining the digestive tract and white blood or immune cells.

Antioxidants can help protect healthy cells from both radiation and chemotherapy. Organically grown fresh fruits and vegetables should be used freely and may be supplemented with *Antioxidant Formulas* and individual antioxidants. Particularly helpful is an intracellular antioxidant called glutathione. n-acetyl cysteine and alpha lipoic acid can enhance glutathione production, thus protecting healthy cells from damage. High doses of vitamin C can also be helpful.

Adaptogens are also helpful for improving the body's ability to resist chemicals and radiation. They also enhance the function of the immune system. Eleuthero, rhodiola or schisandra would all be options. You can also use one of the many *Adaptogen Formulas*. These are also helpful for rebuilding health and energy between treatments.

Digestive Upset

Chemotherapy and radiation can disrupt the function of the gastrointestinal tract by damaging the fast growing cells that line the digestive membranes and by killing off friendly bacteria in the gut. This can result in nausea, vomiting, diarrhea or constipation, weight loss, and loss of appetite.

Probiotics can be taken to replace friendly gut flora and support normal immune functions. Slippery elm and aloe vera juice can be taken to reduce gastrointestinal irritation and ease diarrhea. If diarrhea is severe, an astringent like bayberry root bark or blackberry root may also be helpful. Activated charcoal can also be used to gently detoxify the gastrointestinal tract and reduce irritation from chemotherapy and radiation treatments.

Where nausea and vomiting are a problem, try using some ginger (especially in the form of ginger tea or an all natural ginger beer) to settle the stomach. Peppermint or chamomile tea, or a drop of peppermint essential oil in a cup of warm water, can be sipped slowly to ease nausea, too. Eat small, but frequent meals to avoid stressing the digestive tract.

If appetite is poor, take a *Digestive Bitter Tonic Formula* prior to meals. Also consider *Digestive Enzyme Formulas* or digestive enzyme supplements to help the body break down food. Taken between meals, these same enzymes will help the body fight the cancer.

Immune Suppression

Mainstream cancer treatments tend to depress immune function, and since the immune system tends to be deficient in people with cancer in the first place, it is very important to build immune function. *Mushroom Blend* and *Immune Stimulating Formulas* can be helpful for raising white blood cell counts and helping the body rebuild between chemotherapy sessions. General Glandular Tonic Formulas may also help rebuild the body between sessions.

Antibiotics are often used to prevent infection in cancer patients. Both antibiotics and chemotherapy disrupt friendly gut bacteria, which can lead to yeast infections. *Antifungal Formulas* may be helpful along with probiotics to restore gut flora and immune health.

Supporting Detoxification

Toxins are part of the reason people get cancer in the first place and fighting cancer results in an increase of toxins, partly due to the drugs and partly to the die-off of cancer cells. Most traditional *Anticancer Formulas* are based on herbs that act as blood purifiers or alteratives, meaning they have a gentle detoxifying action. It is very helpful to do detoxification therapy to help the body get rid of this waste. It can be helpful to alternate cleansing and building during therapy, too.

Start by drinking plenty of water (one-half ounce or more per pound of body weight daily). *Fiber Blend* and *General Detoxifying Formulas* are helpful, along with regular enemas or colonics. This can also help to ease pain in cancer.

A number of nutrients can support this detoxification, particularly in the liver. This helps the body break down chemotherapy agents faster to avoid damage to healthy tissues. These include B-complex vitamins, magnesium and MSM.

Cancer die-off sometimes causes lymphatic congestion and swelling. This can be eased by using *Lymphatic Drainage Formulas* and drinking lots of water. *Vascular Tonic Formulas* containing butcher's broom and horse chestnut can also be helpful if there is lymphedema.

Additional Tips

Pain can be a problem in cancer. Remedies that relax tension and/or relief pain like kava kava, lobelia, corydalis, California poppy or a good herbal *Analgesic Formula* may be helpful. A good nervine for this purpose is medicinal marijuana, which is legal for medical use in 13 states but illegal in the rest.

Eating a very clean diet with lots of fresh, raw, organic produce and drinking lots of water also eases pain. Echinacea is also helpful for easing pain in cancer, while boosting the immune system and aiding detoxification.

Overcoming Drug Resistance

A standardized extract of paw paw has anticancer activity of its own, but it also has the ability to inhibit a pumping mechanism in the membranes of cancer cells that enables them to purge toxic drugs and become drug resistant. Cancer patients who have a relapse after a few years often have drug resistant cancer cells. Paw paw can be used to restore the effectiveness of chemotherapy.

Since cancer is a very serious disease, we recommend you work closely with skilled professionals to develop a treatment plan that is right for you.

Therapies: Affirmation and Visualization, Dietary Fiber, Epsom Salt Bath, Fresh Fruits and Vegetables, Friendly Flora and Healthy Fats

Formulas: Antioxidant, **Mushroom Blend**, **Intestinal Toning**, Fiber Blend, **Immune Stimulating**, Antioxidant, Digestive Bitter Tonic, Digestive Enzyme, Adaptogen, Lymphatic Drainage, **Anticancer**, Antifungal, **Essiac** and General Detoxifying

Key Herbs: Ashwaganda, Astragalus, Bayberry, Blackberry root, Butchers Broom, Cats Claw (Uña de Gato, Gambier), Chamomile (English and Roman), Codonopsis, Corydalis, **Aloe vera juice**, **Eleuthero (Siberian ginseng)**, **Reishi (Ganoderma)**, **Slippery Elm**, Echinacea, Ginger, Horse Chestnut, Kavakava, Maitake, Mangosteen, Pau d' Arco, Paw Paw standardized extract, Peppermint, Poke Root, Red

Raspberry, Rhodiola, Schisandra (Schizandra) and Shiitake

Key Nutrients: Co-Q10, Vitamin C, Vitamin E, Alpha Lipoic Acid, N-Acetyl Cysteine, Probiotics, Charcoal (Activated), Vitamin B-Complex, Magnesium, MSM, **Vitamin D** and Digestive Enzymes

Candida Albicans or Candidiasis

See *Fungal Infections (Yeast Infections, Candida albicans)*

Canker Sores (Mouth Ulcers, Stomatitis)

A small painful ulcer usually in the mouth is called a canker sore. It has a grayish-white base surrounded by a red inflamed area.

Goldenseal, taken internally and applied topically, is very effective at healing canker sores. A drop of a *Topical Analgesic Formula*, made with essential oils, can be applied topically to the sore to rapidly relieve the pain and promote healing. L-lysine is an amino acid that helps prevent canker sores. Since this can be viral-related, *Antiviral Formulas* may also help. In several small studies, supplementing with vitamin B12 has decreased canker sore occurrence by 75%.

Formulas: Topical Analgesic, Antiviral and Goldenseal & Echinacea

Key Herbs: Black Walnut, Blackberry, **Goldenseal**, **Propolis**, Echinacea, Myrrh, Prickly Ash, Tea Tree and White Oak

Key Nutrients: L-Lysine, Vitamin B-Complex and Vitamin B-12

Capillary Weakness

See also *Bruises* and *Spider Veins*

Capillaries are the smallest of blood vessels that allow the passage of nutrients and oxygen from the bloodstream to the cells of the body. Some are so small that red blood cells must pass through them in single file. Nutritional deficiencies can cause these thin walls to become fragile and prone to rupture causing bleeding and bruising. *Vascular Tonic* and *Antioxidant Formulas* can help to strengthen capillaries. Rose hips and vitamin C are also helpful.

Therapies: Fresh Fruits and Vegetables and Healthy Fats

Formulas: Vascular Tonic and Antioxidant

Key Herbs: Bilberry (Blueberry, Huckleberry), **Butchers Broom**, **Rose hips**, Hawthorn, Horse Chestnut, Lemon and Yarrow

Key Nutrients: Vitamin C, Omega-3 Essential Fatty Acids and **Bioflavonoids**

Carbuncles

A carbuncle is a deep-seated infection of the skin, usually arising from several hair follicles that are close together. Because it is a bacterial infection, *Antibacterial* or *Echinacea Blend Formulas* taken internally are generally helpful. Also consider applying a *Topical Antiseptic Formula* directly to the afflicted area.

Therapies: Compress and Poultice

Formulas: Topical Antiseptic, Antibacterial and Echinacea Blend

Key Herbs: Coptis (Chinese Goldenthread), **Tea Tree**, Echinacea and Poke Root

Cardiac Arrest (Heart Attack)

See also *Cardiovascular Disease (Heart Disease)*

A cardiac arrest or heart attack is caused by an acute episode of insufficient blood supply to the heart muscle often resulting in damage to the heart and possibly even death. This lack of blood supply to the heart may be triggered by a blood clot or a muscle spasm constricting already partially blocked blood vessels. Prompt medical treatment is essential.

When a person is having a heart attack, capsicum and lobelia extracts or powders placed under the tongue can help support the heart and may save the person's life. Massive doses of vitamin E (400 IU every 10-20 minutes) can also be helpful. These remedies should be administered while awaiting an ambulance or en route to the emergency room.

After a heart attack, high doses of Co-Q10 (100 milligrams or more) will aid repair of the damage. Other supplements that may aid recovery from a heart attack include *Cardiac Tonic* and *Cardiovascular Stimulant Formulas*. Magnesium supplements are also helpful with recovery.

Therapies: Affirmation and Visualization and Stress Management

Formulas: Cardiac Tonic and Cardiovascular Stimulant

Key Herbs: Capsicum (Cayenne), **Hawthorn** and **Lobelia**

Key Nutrients: Magnesium, Co-Q10, Vitamin E and Potassium

Cardiovascular Disease (Heart Disease)

See also *Arteriosclerosis (Atherosclerosis, Hardening of the Arteries), Blood Clots (prevention of), Hypertension, Cholesterol (high), Hypothyroid and Anger (excessive)*

Cardiovascular disease is still the leading cause of death in Western civilization. One out of two people die from it. It makes sense, then, to do what we can to reduce our risk of becoming one of the "one in two" statistics. Unfortunately, much of the information in the popular media about reducing one's risk of heart disease is based on outdated research.

For instance, most people believe that high cholesterol causes heart disease and that the lower your cholesterol level, the less risk you have of dying of heart disease. This simply isn't true. More recent research shows that chronic inflammation (not cholesterol) is the major cause of heart disease and that having your cholesterol get too low is more dangerous to your health than having high cholesterol.

Most people also believe that fats cause heart disease and that low fat diets will prevent heart disease. This is partially true because the wrong kinds of fats (such as margarine and partially hydrogenated vegetable oils) do contribute to the development of heart disease. However, it's also true that good fats (such as olive oil, omega-3 essential fatty acids and the medium chain saturated fats found in organic butter from grass fed cows) actually protect your heart and reduce your risk of heart disease. Foods marketed as fat free or low fat often contain high amounts of refined sugars that actually increase inflammation and heart disease risk, which means they are not good for heart health.

Eating refined carbohydrates is far worse for your heart than eating fats. This is because sugar, white flour and other empty calorie foods spike insulin levels. High insulin levels are a bigger risk factor for heart disease than high cholesterol or high triglycerides. If this information comes as a surprise to you, it's time to update your knowledge a little.

Evaluating Your Risk of Heart Disease

Most people feel that heart disease strikes without warning, but the truth is that there are many subtle clues that demonstrate the heart needs help long before a person has a heart attack. Besides high blood pressure and high cholesterol, here are some things to consider.

Gum Disease: There is a high correlation between inflammation of the gums and the risk of dying of a heart attack. If your gums are inflamed, so are your arteries.

Varicose Veins and Hemorrhoids: These problems are reflections of sluggish circulation and poor blood vessel tone.

Weakness: Fatigue and shortness of breath, feeling no desire for physical activity, getting winded with minor exertion, and feelings of pressure or pain in your chest are early warning signs that your heart may need some help.

Facial Clues: a red, bulbous tip on the nose, spider veins in the nose, and a vertical crease in the left earlobe are all early warning signs that your heart may need help. A bright red tip and pointed tongue is also an indicator of heart stress.

Iridology: If you know an iridologist or are familiar with iridology, markings in the heart area of the iris, having a spleen heart transversal and/or having a lipemic diathesis (lipid ring) are all indicators of a genetic tendency to heart disease.

Blood Tests: Besides cholesterol and triglycerides, consider tests for homocysteine, fibrinogen, C-reactive protein, hemoglobin A1C, fasting insulin, fasting blood glucose, Lp(a) and ferritin (iron). These tests can be more revealing of heart disease risk. If you are concerned about your heart and circulation, consider getting these blood tests done and working with a good practitioner to interpret the results.

If you show signs of needing help with your heart, take action now. Waiting until you have a heart attack or stroke is too late. Here are some steps to take.

Step One: Reduce Inflammation and Free Radical Damage

Oxidative stress and the inflammation that accompanies it is what allows cholesterol and minerals to stick to our arteries, forming arterial plaque. This lessens blood flow to the heart, brain and other parts of the body, increasing the risk of heart attack, stroke and other arterial blockages.

That's why the single most important thing you can do to reduce your risk of heart disease is to obtain adequate amounts of antioxidant and anti-inflammatory nutrients. If you're one of the millions of Americans who aren't eating enough fresh fruits and vegetables, start now! Get the extra antioxidants you need either from foods like blueberries, blackberries and raspberries, or from supplements. This is one of the best things you can do to reduce your risk of heart disease, cancer, dementia and other degenerative diseases associated with aging. You can also consider using *Antioxidant Formulas* to supply your body with antioxidants.

When it comes to protecting your heart, one of the best antioxidants is Co-Q10. It reduces blood pressure, aids recovery from heart attacks, keeps LDL cholesterol from oxidizing and improves energy production in the heart muscle. Statin drugs deplete Q-10, so this supplement should always be taken by people using statin drugs to lower cholesterol.

If your cholesterol level is high (over 250 mg/dl.), then you can help to lower it naturally by using *Cholesterol Balancing Formulas* along with *Fiber Blend Formulas*. This helps the liver get rid of excess cholesterol and bind it in the intestines. Elevated cholesterol is often due to a sluggish thyroid. Unfortunately most medical doctors don't run the correct test nor prescribe the correct treatment for low thyroid. See Hypothyroid for more information.

Step Two: Get an Oil Change

For a long time we've heard the dogma preached that high fat diets contribute to heart disease, and that margarine and vegetable oils are healthier for us than butter, coconut oil or animal fats. In response to this propaganda many people have adopted low fat diets, avoiding eggs, whole milk and red meat in an effort to stay healthier. Unfortunately, this hasn't reduced deaths from heart disease.

The fact is that fatty acids are the preferred fuel of the heart. In other words, the heart needs fats to be healthy, but not just any kind of fats; it needs good fats.

Margarine, shortening, processed vegetable oils and most deep-fat-fried foods are examples of bad fats. These fats have been molecularly altered and do contribute to chronic inflammation, heart disease and other health problems. The natural fats found in high quality foods actually have the opposite effect. So, if you want a healthy heart, keep it well-oiled with the right kinds of fats. Don't eliminate them from your diet, just make an oil change and change the kinds of fats you eat.

What has blown the whole high fat equals heart disease myth is the discovery of cultures (such as Mediterranean and Eskimo) that have both high fat diets and low incidence of heart disease. Part of the secret is an essential fatty acid called omega-3, which is in short supply in most Western diets. Taking omega-3 fatty acids actually reduces the risk of heart disease.

Besides omega-3 supplements, use other good fats. Butter from organically raised, grass-fed cows is a very healthy fat. So is organic, virgin coconut oil. The medium chain saturated fats in these oils are the preferred fuel of the heart and are also important for your immune system.

Step Three: If You Smoke, Quit

Tobacco smoke contains almost 5,000 different chemicals, many of which damage and inflame the artery walls, starting a cascade of damage-inflammation-plaque buildup which ultimately leads to atherosclerosis, or a narrowing of artery walls. In addition, nicotine constricts blood vessels, increasing blood pressure and forcing the heart to work harder. And the carbon monoxide in cigarette smoke replaces some of the oxygen in the bloodstream, meaning your heart has to work harder just to get the same amount of oxygen to the heart and other tissues.

The good news is that people who quit smoking start to get significant benefits immediately. Their risk of heart disease drops dramatically within one year of quitting.

Step Four: Get Physically Active

Regular exercise has almost the opposite effect of smoking: it increases blood flow to the heart and strengthens the heart so that it pumps more blood with less effort. It also controls weight and reduces fat—a big gain if you consider that one pound of fatty tissue contains *one mile* of capillaries that the heart has to pump blood through. Exercise also can reduce your chances of developing other conditions that may put strain on your heart, such as high blood pressure and diabetes. And finally, exercise can reduce stress, which is generally considered a contributor to high blood pressure.

Step Five: Control Your Temper

Anger damages the heart. It is well documented that angry people are more prone to heart disease. If you have a problem with your temper, learn how to manage your anger and develop closer relationships. Having loving relationships reduces your risk of heart disease.

If you are prone to anger and stress consider using *Adaptogen Formulas* to reduce stress hormones. Look up some of the tips for managing stress in the Introduction of this book. If you have a serious problem, take a stress management or anger management class, learn meditation or develop other ways of learning to keep your "cool." See Anger (excessive) for more suggestions.

In general, the heart is highly responsive to emotions, so Emotional Healing Work can be very helpful for preventing and healing from cardiovascular disease. For more information, read the article *Let's Stop Attacking our Hearts* at *modernherbalmedicine.com*.

Step Six: Use Appropriate Supplements to Support Heart Health.

There are numerous herbs and nutritional supplements that can help to both prevent and reverse heart disease. We can't cover them all, but here are a few of the most important ones (besides Co-Q10 and omega-3 which we've already discussed).

L-carnitine for Heart Energy: This important amino acid, found primarily in red meat, transports fatty acids to be metabolized for energy in the mitochondria. It improves energy production and oxygen utilization in the heart and can be very helpful for improving heart health.

Magnesium to Prevent Spasms: About half of all Americans are deficient in magnesium, a critical mineral for heart health. Magnesium helps the heart and blood vessels to relax properly, which reduces stress on the heart, helps protect the heart against spasms and helps lower blood pressure. Magnesium is also essential for energy production in the heart.

Cardiac Tonic Formulas: These are formulas built around hawthorn berries and other key herbs for strengthening the heart. They may also enhance peripheral circulation, although formulas aimed more specifically at general circulation are classified as *Cardiovascular Stimulant Formulas* in this book. These are very safe remedies that elderly people at risk for heart disease could take every day.

Hypotensive Formulas: If your blood pressure is high, consider using a *Hypotensive Formula* and take other steps to keep your blood pressure under control such as taking l-arginine. L-arginine helps synthesize nitric oxide, which dilates the blood vessels to reduce blood pressure. Taking 5 grams a day can not only lower blood pressure, it may even help with erectile dysfunction in some men. See Blood Pressure (high) for more information.

Brain and Memory Tonic Formulas: These formulas generally contain ginkgo, an herb that enhances peripheral circulation and improves blood flow to the brain. It also helps prevent blood clots from forming in the cardiovascular system.

Don't be one of the statistics. Alter your lifestyle and start using some of the many supplements that can keep your heart healthy.

Therapies: Affirmation and Visualization, Deep Breathing, Exercise, Fresh Fruits and Vegetables, Healthy Fats, Hydration, Low Glycemic Diet and Stress Management

Formulas: Cardiac Tonic, **Cardiovascular Stimulant**, Hypotensive, Cholesterol Balancing, Antioxidant, Adaptogen and Brain and Memory Tonic

Key Herbs: Açaí, Capsicum (Cayenne), **Arjuna**, **Hawthorn**, **Prickly Ash**, Ginkgo, Ginseng (American), Ginseng (Asian, Korean), Holy Basil, Kelp, Mangosteen, Night Blooming Cereus (Cactus) and Tribulus

Key Nutrients: Alpha Lipoic Acid, **Omega-3 Essential Fatty Acids**, **Magnesium**, L-Arginine, Co-Q10, Chromium, Vitamin E, Vitamin C, Selenium, Folate (Folic Acid, Vitamin B9), Lycopene and Potassium

Carpal Tunnel Syndrome

Carpal tunnel syndrome is a narrowing of the bony passage in the wrist that constricts blood vessels and nerves passing to and from the hand, causing pain and disturbances of sensation in the hand. Repetitive movements such as constant typing cause carpal tunnel syndrome.

Vitamin B-6 has helped many people with carpal tunnel syndrome. Anti-inflammatory Formulas may also be helpful along with massage and stretching exercises that keep the wrists flexible. Chiropractors and other body workers can also make adjustments to the wrists to aid in healing. *Topical Analgesic* or herbal *Analgesic Formulas* may provide temporary relief from pain, and *Joint Healing Formulas* may help tissues to heal.

Therapies: Fresh Fruits and Vegetables

Formulas: Topical Analgesic, Anti-Inflammatory, Analgesic and Joint Healing

Key Herbs: Boswellia and **Solomon's Seal**

Key Nutrients: Vitamin B-6 (Pyridoxine), MSM, Vitamin B-Complex, Magnesium and Vitamin B-2 (Riboflavin)

Cartilage Damage

See also *Arthritis*

Cartilage is a spongy material that cushions the ends of bones at the joints. Nutritional deficiencies may prevent its proper production, or immune disorders may cause enzymes to destroy healthy cartilage. Cartilage may also be torn during injuries such as those that occur in sports. Cartilage generally heals slower than bone since it relies on passive fluid movement for nutrients rather than blood vessels.

Glucosamine and collagen supplements can be helpful for repairing cartilage. Herbal remedies that may also be helpful include herbal Mineral, *Joint Healing* and *Tissue Healing Formulas*.

Therapies: Fresh Fruits and Vegetables, Mineralization and Poultice

Formulas: Mineral, **Joint Healing** and Tissue Healing

Key Herbs: Boswellia, Cats Claw (Uña de Gato, Gambier), **Solomon's Seal** and Turmeric

Key Nutrients: SAM-e, **MSM** and Glucosamine

Cataracts

See also *Free Radical Damage*

Any clouding of the lens in the eye is called a cataract. Cataracts usually develop from age-associated free radical damage but they may also be caused by injury. Symptoms include hazy vision, glare, trouble focusing, rapid eye fatigue and double vision. Worldwide, cataracts are the number one cause of blindness in the elderly. Cigarette smoking greatly increases the risk of cataracts.

Hydration therapy, a healthy liver and a diet high in antioxidants (fruits and vegetables) reduce cataract risk. Because cataracts are due to free radical damage from the sun, wearing sunglasses in bright light can also be helpful.

If you are concerned about developing cataracts, you can reduce your risk by increasing your intake of antioxidants and omega-3 essential fatty acids. *Antioxidant* and *Vision Supporting Formulas* may also be beneficial in preventing cataracts and other vision problems. *Vision Supporting Formulas* contain antioxidants more specifically beneficial to the eyes.

In Chinese medicine there is a connection between eye and liver health. Both the eyes and the liver require large quantities of antioxidants. A formula to support liver health, such as a *Hepatoprotective Formula* may also be helpful for preventing cataracts.

Large doses of vitamin C may be helpful for cataracts. Some people have reported benefits from using herbal *Eye Wash Formulas* or n-acetyl cysteine eye drops, but this does not seem to be a very dependable approach to reversing cataracts. Surgery will probably be necessary in most cases after cataracts have formed.

Therapies: Fresh Fruits and Vegetables and Healthy Fats

Formulas: Antioxidant, **Vision Supporting**, **Eye Wash**, Heavy Metal Cleansing and Hepatoprotective

Key Herbs: Chickweed, Eyebright, Ginseng (American), Ginseng (Asian, Korean) and Spirulina

Key Nutrients: L-Carnitine, **Zeaxanthin**, Vitamin C, Vitamin B-3 (Niacin), Vitamin B-2 (Riboflavin), Vitamin B-1 (Thiamine), Vitamin A, Quercitin, MSM, N-Acetyl Cysteine, **Lutein**, Folate (Folic Acid, Vitamin B9), Vitamin E and Zinc

Cavities

See *Tooth Decay (prevention)*

Celiac Disease

See also *Inflammatory Bowel Disorders (Colitis, IBS)*

Celiac disease is an inflammatory condition of the colon, a chronic condition that causes breakdown of the intestines due to a gluten allergy. Gluten is a protein found in wheat and other grains such as oats, barley and rye. This disease requires avoiding gluten foods, but some supplements can help as well.

For starters, using some soothing mucilaginous herbs can remove irritation, reduce inflammation and encourage tissue healing.

Digestive Enzyme Formulas or digestive enzyme supplements can aid in the breakdown of foods and further reduce intestinal irritation. Taking probiotics will also improve general intestinal health.

Fiber Blend Formulas can soothe irritated intestinal tissue and promote healing, but it is best to stick with soft, mucilaginous fibers and start very slowly, taking small amounts and gradually increasing them as they can be tolerated.

Ulcer Healing Formulas may also help to reduce inflammation and speed healing of tissues. *Intestinal Toning* and *Gentle Laxative Formulas* containing triphala may also be of benefit. Vitamin B12 and magnesium supplements may also be of benefit for people suffering from Celiac disease.

Therapies: Eliminate Allergy-Causing Foods, Eliminate Gluten, Fresh Fruits and Vegetables, Friendly Flora and Gut Healing Diet

Formulas: Fiber Blend, **Gentle Laxative**, Digestive Enzyme, Ulcer Healing and **Intestinal Toning**

Key Herbs: Chamomile (English and Roman), **Aloe vera**, **Marshmallow**, **Slippery Elm**, Plantain and Yarrow

Key Nutrients: Vitamin B-12, **Probiotics**, **Magnesium**, **Betaine Hydrochloric Acid (HCl)** and Lipase Enzymes

Cellulite

See also *Weight Loss (aids for)*

Cellulite is made of fatty deposits trapped by collagen that give the skin a dimpled, orange peel look. It tends to develop on the thighs, hips and buttocks of women.

It is a myth to think that certain remedies are going to specifically target cellulite. However, some herbs that help the body metabolize fats and release toxins, such as chickweed and burdock, will help to burn cellulite and excess fats in general. See more information under *Weight Loss.*

Therapies: Healthy Fats and Low Glycemic Diet

Formulas: Blood Purifier, Cholagogue and Weight Loss

Key Herbs: Burdock and Chickweed

Key Nutrients: L-Carnitine and Omega-3 Essential Fatty Acids

Cervical Dysplasia

Cervical dysplasia occurs when abnormal squamous cells develop on the surface of the cervix. It results from a chronic infection of HPV and is associated not only with viral HPV infection but also nutrient deficiencies and oral birth control. There are three stages of cervical dysplasia, each having a high risk for potentially developing into cervical cancer. For many, the body's immune system will resolve the dysplasia on its own. Supporting the body's immune system with *Immune Stimulating Formulas* and herbal *Antiviral Formulas* can help remedy one of the causes of cervical dysplasia.

The lining of the cervix is comprised of very fast growing cells. These cells have a much larger requirement for folate than normal cells. Many people have reversed their cervical dysplasia by supplementing with high doses (10 mg daily) of natural folic acid and 5MTHF. For higher grades of dysplasia an experienced herbalist (*findanherbalist.com*) can guide you through the use of echinacea and/or vitamin A suppositories, both of which are effective treatments.

Formulas: Antiviral and Immune Stimulating

Key Herbs: Echinacea, Elder berry, Isatis and Wild Indigo (Baptista)

Key Nutrients: Folate (Folic Acid, Vitamin B9) and Indole-3 Carbinol (DIM)

Chemical Poisoning

See also *Heavy Metal Poisoning*

In the modern world we are exposed to thousands of chemicals on a regular basis—many of which are toxic. These chemicals come from many sources. Pesticides, herbicides and fungicides are used on our crops. Antibiotics and hormones are routinely fed to animals. Artificial colorings, flavoring agents, preservatives and other food additives are also added to processed foods. In fact, the average person eats two to three pounds of chemical food additives each year.

We are also exposed to chemicals in household cleaning products and personal care products. Chemicals are found in building materials, paint, solvents, carpets, fabrics, and our water and air due to pollution.

Reducing our exposure to these chemicals is one of the key things we can do to improve overall health. For starters, buy organic food as much as possible and wash commercial produce in a natural soap like Dr. Bronner's Supermild Baby Soap to remove pesticide residues. Use natural cleaning and personal care products and drink purified water.

Of course, we can't eliminate all exposure to these chemicals in our modern world, so we need to assist the body in removing them. For example, many people work at jobs that expose them to chemicals on a daily basis, such as carpet cleaners, dry cleaners, painters, auto mechanics and beauticians. The liver bears the primary burden of having to process all of these chemicals.

If one has to work around chemicals, it's a good idea to take *Hepatoprotective Formulas* to help the liver process these chemicals. Antioxidants, as found in fresh fruits and vegetables, and herbal *Antioxidant Formulas*, are also important for helping the liver deal with chemicals. Nutritional supplements like N-acetyl-cystine, alpha lipoic acid, and SAM-e are all helpful for liver detoxification.

A periodic cleanse using a *General Detoxifying* or *Blood Purifier Formulas* with a *Fiber Blend Formula* is helpful for eliminating chemicals from the system. Periodically doing the Fast or Juice Fast therapy is also helpful.

For acute chemical poisoning it is best to consult a poison control center for advice. Activated charcoal can be taken to absorb many kinds of poisons after they have been ingested, but ask the poison control center for specific instructions. Acute cases of chemical poisoning should be treated medically, with herbal and nutritional therapies used for backup support.

Therapies: Colon Cleanse, Dietary Fiber, Drawing Bath, Fast or Juice Fast, Fresh Fruits and Vegetables, Friendly Flora, Healthy Fats, Heavy Metal Cleanse and Hydration

Formulas: Fiber Blend, Blood Purifier, **Hepatoprotective**, General Detoxifying and Antioxidant

Key Herbs: Milk Thistle, Red Clover, Reishi (Ganoderma), Rhodiola and Schisandra (Schizandra)

Key Nutrients: N-Acetyl Cysteine, Probiotics, Omega-3 Essential Fatty Acids, **Charcoal (Activated)** and Alpha Lipoic Acid

Chest Pain

See also *Acid Indigestion (Heartburn, Acid Reflux), Angina, Gall Bladder (sluggish or removed), Pain (general remedies for)* and *Pleurisy*

Chest pain can have several causes, including a gallbladder attack, heartburn or acid reflux, inflammation in the pleura, muscle tension, or angina. Get a proper diagnosis and see appropriate related conditions.

Chicken Pox

See also *Itching* and *Shingles*

Chicken pox is an acute, contagious infection of the *Varicella zoster* virus. The immune response to this infection creates a low-grade fever and oozing, itching sores almost anywhere on the surface of the body. They may even occur on mucous membrane surfaces such as the throat. If sores are scratched or picked they can leave scars.

Chicken pox is aided naturally by enhancing the immune system's ability to expel the virus from the body. This is accomplished by taking frequent doses (every 2-4 hours) of alterative or blood purifying herbs such as burdock, goldenseal, Oregon grape, safflowers or yellow dock along with plenty of water. Look for a *Blood Purifier Formula* with these herbs as principle ingredients.

Sudorific Formulas can be used to help reduce fever and inflammation. Aspirin is not recommended because it suppresses the body's ability to eliminate the virus, which causes problems with shingles later in life.

Remedies used to ease topical itching may be helpful as well. These include using the Drawing Bath or Compress therapies with herbs like burdock, comfrey, goldenseal, chickweed or Oregon grape. Check out *Anti-Itch* and *Topical Vulnerary Formulas* to ease itching and promote healing of the pox.

Antiviral Formulas may also be helpful for chicken pox. Safflowers, St. John's wort, lemon balm and lomatium are some of the single herbs that may be helpful for chicken pox.

Therapies: Compress, Drawing Bath and Hydration

Formulas: Antiviral, Blood Purifier, **Anti-Itch** and Topical Vulnerary

Key Herbs: Burdock, Chickweed, **Oregon Grape, St. John's wort, Yellow Dock**, Goldenseal, Lemon Balm, Lobelia, Lomatium, Olive, Poke Root and Safflowers

Key Nutrients: Vitamin E

Childbirth

See *Labor and Delivery* and *Pregnancy (herbs and supplements for)*

Chills

Chills are usually associated with an increased internal body temperature during a fever but can also be present in severe blood loss or shock. Mild, chronic feelings of cold, especially in the extremities, is usually caused by poor circulation or hormonal imbalances, particularly low thyroid. The hypothalamus regulates the body temperature and opens and closes the vents or pores in the skin to help regulate the body temperature.

Cardiovascular Stimulant Formulas can help when a person is experiencing chills because they usually contain capsicum, a circulatory stimulant. *Adaptogen Formulas* may also help with chills.

Formulas: Cardiovascular Stimulant and Adaptogen

Key Herbs: Capsicum (Cayenne), Cinnamon, **Eleuthero (Siberian ginseng)**, Garlic and Licorice

Cholera

See also *Diarrhea*

Cholera is an acute infection caused by the bacterium *Vibrio cholerae*. It generally causes diarrhea and dehydration. Since it is a bacterial condition, use *Antibacterial* or *Goldenseal & Echinacea Formulas*. In severe cases, however, it may be best to seek medical treatment and get an antibiotic. The big issue with cholera is severe dehydration. Staying hydrated will allow the infection to run its course without serious complications in most cases. You can use commercial rehydration salts or make you own. To make your own rehydration drink remember the 8-8-8 rule: 8 oz of boiled water or fruit juice, 1/8 tsp salt and 8 tsp of sugar mixed together. You can also help the diarrhea by taking *Anti-Diarrhea* and *Fiber Blend Formulas*. Activated charcoal is also a good diarrhea remedy.

Formulas: Antibacterial, Goldenseal & Echinacea, Fiber Blend and Anti-Diarrhea

Key Herbs: Goldenseal, Garlic, Marshmallow and Slippery Elm

Key Nutrients: Charcoal (Activated)

Cholesterol (high)

See also *Cholesterol (low)* and *Hypothyroid*

High cholesterol is not really a disease. It is a symptom of metabolic imbalance, not a root cause of any health problem. The lab ranges for cholesterol have been artificially reduced due to pressure from the pharmaceutical industry in order to sell more highly profitable statin drugs. Normal cholesterol ranges should probably be 175 to 275, with the optimal range between 200 and 250.

Cholesterol below 175 is too low and can cause serious health risks, including infertility, depression, increased risk of cancer and a higher tendency to death from a heart attack.

Cholesterol plays a very important role in the body. The primary use of cholesterol (60-80%) is to make bile for the digestion of fats. Cholesterol is also used to make adrenal and reproductive hormones and to sequester toxins in the body.

The following can help to lower cholesterol when it is too high.

Fiber in the diet helps to reduce cholesterol levels for a couple of reasons. First, it binds toxins in the gut. Second, it binds to cholesterol being released in the bile to prevent it from being reabsorbed. So, if you want to lower your cholesterol naturally, start by increasing fiber in your diet or taking a good *Fiber Blend Formula* and drinking lots of water.

Cholagogue herbs, like milk thistle, fringetree, yellow dock and barberry, promote the flow of bile, which eliminates excess cholesterol from the liver. When there is adequate fiber in the intestinal tract to bind this cholesterol it can't be reabsorbed. So using a *Cholagogue Formula* with a *Fiber Blend Formula* is a very good strategy for reducing cholesterol.

Cholesterol levels can also be lowered by consuming adequate quantities of high quality fats. Eating a lot of olive oil will actually help to lower cholesterol because more bile has to be produced to break down the fats. Again, this strategy works best if you are taking plenty of fiber and drinking lots of water. Essential fatty acids in flax seed oil and omega-3 supplements will also help lower cholesterol.

There are a number of herbs and nutrients that help to maintain normal cholesterol levels. These include red yeast rice, ho shu wu, niacin, lecithin, garlic and guggul. Use one of the *Cholesterol Balancing Formulas* that contains these herbs. These formulas usually include chologogue herbs as well.

Low thyroid may be a cause of high cholesterol. In this case, consider using *Hypothyroid Formula*. If your thyroid is really low, you may need a thyroid glandular or even thyroid medication to bring cholesterol into normal range.

Anyone on statin drugs should also be taking Co-Q10, as statin drugs deplete levels of this important antioxidant nutrient. Co-Q10 should be taken when using red yeast rice, as well.

Therapies: Colon Cleanse, Dietary Fiber, Fresh Fruits and Vegetables, Gall Bladder Flush, Healthy Fats and Hydration

Formulas: Cholesterol Balancing, **Fiber Blend**, Cholagogue and Hypothyroid

Key Herbs: Barberry, **Artichoke**, **Guggul**, **He Shou Wu (Ho Shou Wu, Fo-Ti)**, Fringe Tree, Garlic, Maitake, Milk Thistle, Myrrh, Reishi (Ganoderma), Turmeric and Yellow Dock

Key Nutrients: Vitamin B-3 (Niacin), **Omega-3 Essential Fatty Acids**, DHA, Chromium, Charcoal (Activated), **Fiber**, Proanthocyanidins and Sodium Alginate (Algin)

Cholesterol (low)

See also *Adrenals (exhaustion, weakness or burnout)*, *Fat Metabolism (poor)*, *Gall Bladder (sluggish or removed)* and *Grave's Disease*

A cholesterol level below 175 should be considered low. Low cholesterol increases one's risk of death from cardiovascular diseases and cancer. In fact, the lower the cholesterol, the higher the risk of cancer. Low cholesterol also interferes with glandular function, especially the adrenal and reproductive hormones. It may be a cause of infertility and depression. Low cholesterol is also linked with increased risk of suicide.

There are many possible causes of low cholesterol, which include: taking statin drugs, low thyroid, lack of bile flow or production, low fat diets, low protein diets, poor fat or protein metabolism and adrenal fatigue. Remedies will depend on the cause, so talk to a holistically-minded practitioner who understands this problem to help you determine an appropriate approach.

If low thyroid is the cause, see *Hypothyroid*. It may be helpful to take iodine supplements or a *Hypothyroid Formula*. It may also be helpful to get a prescription for a thyroid glandular or thyroid medication.

A *Cholagogue Formula* may be helpful in increasing bile production to improve digestion of fats. *Digestive Bit-*

ter Tonic or *Digestive Enzyme Formulas* may be needed if digestion is poor. Supplementation with lipase enzymes and bile salts in particular will aid digestion and metabolism of fats.

Many people are not eating enough good fats because they have been led to believe that all fats are "bad." If a person is on a low fat diet, they need to add good fats back into the diet in the form of olive oil, coconut oil, butter from grass-fed cows, avocados, nuts and/or deep ocean fish.

Cholesterol is a lipoprotein, meaning it is a combination of fat and protein, so low protein diets and/or problems with protein metabolism may also contribute to low cholesterol. If this is the case increase intake of protein foods and/or take protease enzyme supplements and hydrochloric acid supplements to aid protein metabolism.

Adrenal fatigue may be another factor in low cholesterol. If stress and exhaustion are problems consider using an *Adrenal Tonic* to improve glandular function.

Therapies: Healthy Fats

Formulas: Adrenal Tonic, Hypothyroid, Cholagogue, Digestive Bitter Tonic and Digestive Enzyme

Key Herbs: Black Walnut, Chickweed, Kelp and Oregon Grape

Key Nutrients: Vitamin B-12, SAM-e, Omega-3 Essential Fatty Acids, Vitamin B-Complex, Lipase Enzymes, Betaine Hydrochloric Acid (HCl), Protease Enzymes and **Iodine**

Chronic Fatigue Syndrome (CFS)

See *Epstein Barr Virus*

Key Nutrients: Magnesium

Chronic Obstructive Pulmonary Disorder (COPD)

See also *Allergies (respiratory)*, *Asthma*, *Bronchitis* and *Hiatal Hernia*

Chronic obstructive pulmonary disease (COPD) is a slow-developing disorder that causes chronic obstruction in the lungs, making breathing difficult. There are two main forms of this disease, chronic bronchitis and emphysema. Symptoms include cough with mucus, shortness of breath, fatigue, frequent respiratory infections and wheezing.

Medical treatment for this disorder is to use inhalers, like those used in asthma, to open airways. Corticosteroid drugs and antibiotics are often used during flare-ups, and oxygen therapy may be used in severe cases.

It is important to avoid smoking and breathing very cold air. Reducing air pollution by getting an in-house air filtration system may be helpful. It is also important to eat plenty of fresh fruits and vegetables for their inflammation-reducing antioxidants.

There are several categories of herbal remedies that may be helpful here. *Lung and Respiratory Tonic Formulas*, which contain herbs like astragalus, licorice and mullein, can be used to strengthen the lung tissue and reduce risk of infection. Anti-inflammatory formulas can be used to reduce tissue swelling and make breathing easier. *Bronchialdilator Formulas* or lobelia will help to open airways and make breathing easier. Finally, *Adaptogen Formulas* can reduce stress and improve general health.

Using the Eliminate Allergy-Causing Foods therapy is often helpful with chronic lung conditions. There is a big connection between the health of the mucus membranes of the digestive tract and the mucus membranes of the lungs. So, digestive enzymes, probiotics, fiber and other supplements that improve gastrointestinal health will often help respiratory conditions clear up as well.

Most people with asthma or COPD have a hiatal hernia. Correcting this will greatly improve lung function and breathing capacity. See Hiatal Hernia in the *Therapies Section*.

Therapies: Colon Cleanse, Dietary Fiber, Eliminate Allergy-Causing Foods, Fast or Juice Fast, Fresh Fruits and Vegetables, Friendly Flora, Healthy Fats, Hiatal Hernia Correction and Hydration

Formulas: Bronchialdilator, **Lung and Respiratory Tonic**, Adaptogen and Anti-Inflammatory

Key Herbs: Astragalus, Cherry (Wild), Cordyceps, **Licorice**, **Lobelia**, **Mullein**, Eucalyptus, Khella, Reishi (Ganoderma) and Thyme

Key Nutrients: Magnesium, Omega-3 Essential Fatty Acids, Digestive Enzymes, Probiotics and **N-Acetyl Cysteine**

Circulation (poor)

See also *Anemia*, *Cardiovascular Disease (Heart Disease)* and *Hypothyroid*

Poor circulation is characterized by a variety of symptoms. It may result in cold hands and feet, fatigue, loss of memory, wounds or sores that won't heal in the extremities, loss of eyesight, swelling in the legs and tingling sensations in the arms, hands, legs and feet. Poor circulation can be related to dehydration, lack of physical activity and nutritional deficiencies. *Cardiovascular Stimulant Formulas* or single herbs like capsicum, garlic, prickly ash or ginkgo help to stimulate good circulation. Capsicum, in particular, tends to normalize blood flow throughout the body.

Therapies: Exercise and Hydration

Formulas: Cardiovascular Stimulant

Key Herbs: Capsicum (Cayenne), Cinnamon, **Ginger**, **Prickly Ash**, Dong Quai, Garlic, Ginkgo and Hawthorn

Key Nutrients: Omega-3 Essential Fatty Acids, Vitamin E and Vitamin B-3 (Niacin)

Cirrhosis of the Liver

See also *Hepatitis*

Cirrhosis is an end stage liver disease associated with functional failure of liver tissues and eventual liver failure. The liver tissue becomes scarred from viral infections, alcohol abuse, reactions to drugs and exposure to environmental toxins. This disease usually results in the need for a liver transplant. The best natural remedy is to go on a completely mild food diet (nothing but fresh fruits and vegetables, preferably in juice form) to give the liver a rest. Juices made from greens (chard, celery, etc.) are extremely beneficial. Salads are also beneficial. Of course, all alcohol, drugs and chemicals must be avoided. Also avoid all spicy food and heavy fats and oils.

Liver Tonic Formulas can be used to support the health of liver tissue. SAM-e and milk thistle are two specific supplements that are useful for cirrhosis of the liver. Helichrysum essential oil and/or use the Castor Oil Pack therapy over the liver area to help break up scar tissue and promote healing. Licorice root, MSM and dandelion are also potentially useful supplements here. Seek appropriate medical assistance with this very severe disease.

Therapies: Castor Oil Pack, Fresh Fruits and Vegetables, Gut Healing Diet and Hydration

Formulas: Liver Tonic

Key Herbs: Dandelion, **Milk Thistle**, Goldenseal, Licorice, Schisandra (Schizandra) and Yellow Dock

Key Nutrients: SAM-e, MSM, N-Acetyl Cysteine and Vitamin B-Complex

Cold Hands and Feet

See also *Circulation (poor)*, *Hiatal Hernia*, *Hypothyroid* and *Stress*

Mild, chronic feelings of cold, especially in the extremities, can be a symptom of several different health problems. Seek appropriate assistance to determine the cause before embarking on a course of therapy. Here are a few of the more common causes of cold hands and feet.

Low thyroid is a common cause and taking remedies like *Hypothyroid Formulas* to boost the metabolism often resolves the problem. In some cases thyroid medication may be needed. See *Hypothyroid.*

Another common cause is poor circulation to the extremities. Try taking a *Cardiovascular Stimulant Formula* or otherwise taking steps to improve circulation. Exercise will be helpful in these cases. See Circulation (poor).

Cold hands and feet may also be a symptom of a lowered immune response. If the person is tired and catches colds and flu easily, then try *Immune Stimulating Formulas.*

Chronic stress can cause a constriction of peripheral blood vessels, leading to cold extremities. If stress, anxiety or insomnia are present use *Relaxing Nervine* and *Adaptogen Formulas*. See Stress.

Poor digestion may also be a factor. People with a hiatal hernia are often pale and cold. *Digestive Tonic Formulas* may be helpful in these cases. See Hiatal Hernia.

Therapies: Exercise and Hiatal Hernia Correction

Formulas: Hypothyroid, **Cardiovascular Stimulant**, Immune Stimulating, Digestive Tonic, Relaxing Nervine, Adaptogen and Relaxing Nervine

Key Herbs: Blue Vervain, **Capsicum (Cayenne)**, **Ginger**, Garlic, Ginkgo, Hawthorn, Prickly Ash and Scullcap (Skullcap)

Key Nutrients: Vitamin B-3 (Niacin) and Omega-3 Essential Fatty Acids

Cold Sores (Fever Blisters)

See also *Herpes*

A cold sore is an infection of the *Herpes simplex* virus that causes a painful, oozing group of blisters usually located around the lips. They turn into a scabby sore. Cold sores are also known as fever blisters.

Black walnut, goldenseal, olive leaf and St. John's wort are all potential remedies for cold sores. Look for an *Antiviral Formula* that contains some of these remedies. You can also look for a *Topical Vulnerary Formula* that contains some of these ingredients. Some people find supplementation with l-lysine helpful. L-arginine is contraindicated with this condition. Since outbreaks are often stress-related, Stress Management therapy may be helpful in reducing the frequency of outbreaks.

Therapies: Friendly Flora and Stress Management

Formulas: Antiviral and Topical Vulnerary

Key Herbs: Black Walnut, Garlic, Lemon Balm, Olive, Peppermint, St. John's wort and Tea Tree essential oil

Key Nutrients: L-Lysine, Probiotics, Omega-3 Essential Fatty Acids, Chlorophyll, Vitamin B-Complex and Zinc

Colds (prevention)

See also *Congestion (general)*, *Fever*, *Flu (Influenza)* and *Cough (general)*

Maintaining a strong immune system can help prevent colds. *Immune Stimulating Formulas* containing echinacea, astragalus and medicinal mushrooms like reshi (ganoderma) and shitake can all be used to boost the body's immune response in people with weak immune systems. *Echinacea Blend Formulas* and *Mushroom Blend Formulas* are also helpful for boosting immune responses. For people with weak respiratory systems, *Lung and Respiratory Tonic Formulas* can be used, especially during the winter months, to prevent colds. Deficiencies of vitamins A and D are associated with an increased risk of colds. Of course, attention to basic hygiene and sanitation also helps prevent colds, but it is not necessary to disinfect everything. Basic cleanliness is sufficient.

Therapies: Colon Cleanse, Eliminate Allergy-Causing Foods, Friendly Flora and Stress Management

Formulas: Immune Stimulating, Mushroom Blend, Lung and Respiratory Tonic and Echinacea Blend

Key Herbs: Astragalus, **Echinacea**, Elder, Eleuthero (Siberian ginseng), Garlic and Reishi (Ganoderma)

Key Nutrients: Probiotics, **Vitamin C**, **Zinc**, **Vitamin D** and **Vitamin A**

Colds (remedies for)

See also *Infection (viral)* and *Cough (general)*

Colds are a group of acute, contagious infections characterized by malaise, fever, chills (thus the name) and respiratory congestion. The goal in working with colds should be to help the body eliminate the toxins it is trying to expel from the body.

Although echinacea or *Goldenseal & Echinacea Formulas* are commonly used for colds, these are not the most effective cold remedies, especially during the early stages of a cold. They are more helpful in the later stages of a cold when there is thick, discolored mucus.

During the early stages of a cold, when mucus is thin and clear or pale white, one of the best remedies for a cold is to use aromatic or pungent (spicy) herbs and take it every hour or two with plenty of fluids. Examples of aromatics that are helpful for colds include yarrow, peppermint, chamomile and catnip. These work best when taken as hot teas. Pungent herbs include capsicum, ginger, garlic and horseradish. These are often easier to take as capsules or extracts and should also be taken with warm or hot liquids.

Many *Cardiovascular Stimulant Formulas* contain a lot of aromatics and can be taken in doses every hour or two with plenty of fluids to help get rid of colds quickly. You can try this same strategy with any of the *Cold and Flu* or *Sudorific Formulas*.

Taking an enema to clear the colon and/or doing the Sweat Bath therapy to stimulate perspiration is highly effective for getting rid of colds. Taking aromatic and pungent herbs every 2-4 hours after these procedures usually clears colds in less than 24 hours.

Topical Analgesic Formulas can often be rubbed on the chest or throat to help get rid of colds. By breathing these aromatic vapors it helps to open airways and clear congestion.

When there is congestion in the sinuses during a cold take a *Sinus Decongestant Formula*, again with plenty of water. If the congestion is in the lungs, you can use a *Decongestant Formula* to break it up or an *Expectorant Formula* to help the body cough out the mucus. You can also consider using an herbal *Cough Remedy Formula*.

When you have a cold, stop eating. The famous saying "feed a cold, starve a fever" means "if you feed a cold, you'll have to starve a fever." If you are hungry when you have a cold, drink some fresh fruit or vegetable juices or a little soup or broth. Avoid grains, animal proteins, nuts, beans and other heavier foods when sick.

Other potential options for natural cold treatments include *Antiviral* and *Immune Stimulating Formulas*. You will probably need to experiment a little to find which remedies work best for you, but it is possible to dramatically reduce the recovery time with colds using natural remedies.

Therapies: Colon Hydrotherapy, Fast or Juice Fast, Hydration and Sweat Bath

Formulas: Antiviral, **Cold and Flu**, Echinacea Blend, Goldenseal & Echinacea, Immune Stimulating, Cough Remedy, Decongestant, Sinus Decongestant, Expectorant, Cardiovascular Stimulant, Lymphatic Drainage, Topical Analgesic and **Sudorific**

Key Herbs: Astragalus, Blue Vervain, Capsicum (Cayenne), Catnip, Chamomile (English and Roman), Cinnamon, Clove, Coltsfoot, **Andrographis**, **Boneset**, **Osha**, **Yarrow**, Devil's Club, Echinacea, Garlic, Ginger, Holy Basil, Horseradish, Hyssop, Lemon, Lobelia, Pennyroyal, Peppermint, Rosemary, Thyme and Usnea

Key Nutrients: Zinc, **Vitamin A**, Vitamin D and Vitamin C

Colic

See also *Fungal Infections (Yeast Infections, Candida albicans)* and *Gas and Bloating*

Colic involves acute abdominal pain, characterized by cramping and gas. It is common in infants, but adults can also have this problem.

The combination of catnip and fennel is a tried-and-true remedy for colic. There are several *Catnip & Fennel Formulas* in the commercial marketplace that can be used for colic in infants, young children and even adults.

Yeast infections in infants can also cause colic. Use a little lavender and tea tree essential oil topically over the abdomen to help with the yeast infections. Dilute these essential oils in olive oil before applying. You can also use 2-3 drops of a liquid *Antifungal Formula* twice daily. Giving the child probiotics, especially bifidophilus, will also help. Probiotics can be administered orally by mixing with food or rectally in an enema.

For colic in adults, *Antispasmodic* and *Carminative Formulas* can be helpful. If the problem is frequent also consider using *Digestive Enzyme* and/or *Digestive Bitter Tonic Formulas* to improve digestive function.

Therapies: Friendly Flora

Formulas: Catnip & Fennel, Antifungal, Antispasmodic, **Carminative**, Digestive Bitter Tonic and Digestive Enzyme

Key Herbs: Chamomile (English and Roman), **Anise**, **Catnip**, **Fennel**, Lavender, Lemon Balm, Lobelia, Peppermint, Safflowers, Tea Tree, Thyme and Wild Yam

Key Nutrients: Digestive Enzymes

Colitis

See also *Inflammatory Bowel Disorders (Colitis, IBS)*

Colitis is inflammation of the colon and small intestine. To reduce inflammation use *Anti-Inflammatory Formulas* and *Fiber Blend Formulas. Digestive Enzyme Formulas* are helpful for improving digestive function. Colitis is an Inflammatory Bowel Disorder, so see that heading for more detailed information on this condition.

Therapies: Dietary Fiber, Fast or Juice Fast, Fresh Fruits and Vegetables, Friendly Flora, Healthy Fats and Stress Management

Formulas: Fiber Blend, Digestive Enzyme, Anti-Inflammatory and **Intestinal Toning**

Key Herbs: Cats Claw (Uña de Gato, Gambier), Chamomile (English and Roman), Coptis (Chinese Goldenthread), **Aloe vera**, **Marshmallow**, **Plantain**, Licorice and Slippery Elm

Key Nutrients: L-Glutamine, Omega-3 Essential Fatty Acids, Probiotics, Betaine Hydrochloric Acid (HCl) and DHA

Colon (atonic)

See also *Constipation (adults)* and *Diverticulitis (Diverticuli)*

An atonic colon is one that has lost muscular tone and balloons, lacking sufficient peristaltic strength to push material forward. This is the less common form of constipation and results in very slow, but regular, bowel eliminations. *Stimulant Laxative* and *Fiber Blend Formulas* are the primary remedies for an atonic colon, but *Intestinal Toning* and *Tissue Healing Formulas* may also help.

Therapies: Friendly Flora and Mineralization

Formulas: Stimulant Laxative, Fiber Blend, Tissue Healing, Intestinal Toning and Digestive Bitter Tonic

Key Herbs: Black Walnut, Buckthorn, Cascara Sagrada, **Butternut bark**, **Turkey Rhubarb**, Psyllium, Senna Leaves and White Oak

Key Nutrients: Digestive Enzymes, Fiber, Vitamin C and **Probiotics**

Colon (spastic)

See also *Irritable Bowel Syndrome (IBS)* and *Stress*

A spastic colon is caused by muscle spasms in the colon that inhibit peristalsis. It is characterized by irregular bowel movements and constipation that is aggravated by stress. Most adults and children who are constipated have a spastic bowel condition. Stimulant laxatives can actually aggravate a spastic bowel condition. What is needed are *Gentle Laxative Formulas*, *Antispasmodic Formulas*, and *Relaxing Nervine Formulas*. The more modern term for a spastic bowel is Irritable Bowel Syndrome (IBS). See more under that heading.

Therapies: Eliminate Allergy-Causing Foods and Stress Management

Formulas: Gentle Laxative, Antispasmodic and Relaxing Nervine

Key Herbs: Chamomile (English and Roman), **Catnip**, Lobelia, Marshmallow, Valerian and Wild Yam

Key Nutrients: Magnesium

Concentration (poor)

See also *Adrenals (exhaustion, weakness or burnout)*, *Attention Deficit Disorder (ADD, ADHD)*, *Circulation (poor)* and *Memory and Brain Function*

Poor concentration is often due to a lack of circulation to the brain or imbalances in glandular function. Where circulation is the issue, *Cardiovascular Stimulant Formulas* may be helpful. *Adrenal Tonic* or *Adaptogen Formulas* often help improve concentration when the problem is due to chronic stress. As a person ages, *Brain and Memory Tonic Formulas* may also be helpful for keeping the mind clear and focused. When the problem is associated with ADD, *Brain Calming Formulas* may be the answer. See related conditions for more information.

Therapies: Deep Breathing, Healthy Fats and Low Glycemic Diet

Formulas: Brain Calming, **Brain and Memory Tonic**, Adaptogen, Adrenal Tonic and Cardiovascular Stimulant

Key Herbs: Bee Pollen, Blessed Thistle, **Bacopa (Water Hyssop)**, **Gotu kola**, **Rosemary**, Ginkgo and Peppermint

Key Nutrients: GABA, Omega-3 Essential Fatty Acids, Magnesium, Vitamin B-Complex and **DHA**

Concussions

See also *Injuries*

A concussion is an injury to the soft tissue of the brain. It usually results from being shaken violently or receiving a blow to the head. Seek medical assistance. As an aid to healing, take St. John's wort internally and apply a *Topical Vulnerary Formula*. It may also be helpful to supplement one's diet with essential fatty acids.

Therapies: Fresh Fruits and Vegetables and Healthy Fats

Formulas: Topical Vulnerary

Key Herbs: Yarrow and St. John's wort

Key Nutrients: Digestive Enzymes, DHA and Omega-3 Essential Fatty Acids

Confusion

See also *Adrenals (exhaustion, weakness or burnout)* and *Hypoglycemia*

This is often a sign of low blood sugar or adrenal exhaustion. When a person feels confused when they haven't eaten in a few hours, it is probably hypoglycemia or low blood sugar. Avoiding refined sugar and simple carbohydrates and using licorice root to stabilize blood sugar levels can be helpful. When the problem is due to chronic stress, consider using *Adaptogen* or *Adrenal Tonic Formulas*. *Brain and Memory Tonic Formulas* may also be helpful for mental confusion.

Therapies: Deep Breathing, Hydration, Low Glycemic Diet and Stress Management

Formulas: Adaptogen, **Brain and Memory Tonic** and Adrenal Tonic

Key Herbs: Bacopa (Water Hyssop), **Licorice**, **Peppermint**, **Rosemary**, Eleuthero (Siberian ginseng), Ginkgo, Gotu kola and Thyme

Key Nutrients: MSM, Magnesium, Omega-3 Essential Fatty Acids and Potassium

Congestion (bronchial)

See also *Bronchitis* and *Chronic Obstructive Pulmonary Disorder (COPD)*

When the bronchial passages are inflamed, swollen, congested with mucus or constricted due to stress, a person will have a difficult time breathing. When inflammation is the cause, the condition is known as bronchitis. When chronic mucus congestion is the cause, it is classified as COPD (chronic obstructive pulmonary disorder).

When inflammation is the culprit, an *Anti-Inflammatory Formula* will probably be helpful. If the inflammation is accompanied by infection, then an *Antiviral* or *Antibacterial Formula* will help, depending on the nature of the infection.

Decongestant Formulas can be helpful for breaking up congestion and loosening mucus, and *Expectorant Formulas* will help to get rid of excess mucus.

To relax bronchial constriction, use an *Antispasmodic Formula* or a *Bronchialdilator Formula*. As a single herb, lobelia works extremely well as a bronchial dilator.

Therapies: Colon Cleanse, Hydration and Stress Management

Formulas: Decongestant, Antispasmodic, **Bronchialdilator**, Allergy-Reducing, Anti-Inflammatory, Antibacterial, Antiviral and Expectorant

Key Herbs: Cherry (Wild), Cordyceps, **Anise**, **Camphor**, **Mullein**, Grindelia (Gumweed), Khella, Licorice, Lobelia and Yerba Santa

Key Nutrients: Pantothenic Acid (Vitamin B5), MSM and **N-Acetyl Cysteine**

Congestion (general)

See also *Congestion (bronchial)*, *Congestion (lungs)*, *Congestion (lymphatic)*, *Congestion (sinus)* and *Chronic Obstructive Pulmonary Disorder (COPD)*

Excessive mucous collected in the nasal and/or lung passages causes congestion, which can interfere with breathing. The lymphatics can also become congested, resulting in swollen lymph nodes, earaches, sore throats and frequent respiratory infections.

Decongestant and *Expectorant Formulas* can be used to break up and expel mucus from the body. It is important to understand that expectorant and decongestant remedies won't necessarily dry up the sinuses. Since they promote breakup of congestion and the expulsion of mucus, they may cause a temporary increase in drainage as the lungs and sinuses clear out irritants. This is normal. Just keep drinking plenty of water. It may also help to use the Colon Hydrotherapy and/or the Sweat Bath therapy.

The long-term solution to congestion involves normalizing the intestinal tract, as there is a strong connection between the mucus membranes of the digestive system and the respiratory system. Enzymes will help the body break down food better, which will result in less congestion. A colon cleaning program using a *General Detoxifying* and a *Fiber Blend Formula* may also be helpful.

See other headings for dealing with specific types of congestion, such as sinus and lymphatic congestion.

Therapies: Colon Hydrotherapy, Dietary Fiber, Fast or Juice Fast, Friendly Flora, Hydration and Sweat Bath

Formulas: Decongestant, Lymphatic Drainage, General Detoxifying, Expectorant and Fiber Blend

Key Herbs: Blue Vervain, Capsicum (Cayenne), **Red Clover**, **Yerba Santa**, Fenugreek, Garlic, Lobelia, Marshmallow, Mullein, Orange Peel, Rosemary and Thyme

Key Nutrients: Alpha Lipoic Acid, Protease Enzymes, N-Acetyl Cysteine and Vitamin C

Congestion (lungs)

See also *Congestion (general)*, *Cough (damp)*, *Pneumonia* and *Cough (general)*

When the lungs are congested it can be very difficult to breath. *Decongestant* and *Expectorant Formulas* can be used to break up and help the lungs expel excess mucus. Remedies for a damp cough will also be helpful. Be sure to drink plenty of water to thin the mucus secretions.

When the problem is associated with infection, it can also help to use the Colon Hydrotherapy or Sweat Bath therapies.

Antibacterial Formulas can be helpful if there is an infection in the lungs and, unlike antibiotics, will also be helpful if the infection is viral. Garlic, in particular, is good at fighting both bacterial and viral infections in the lungs and is also helpful in expelling excess fluid and mucus. When the lungs are easily congested and weak, a *Lung and Respiratory Tonic* should be helpful.

Therapies: Aromatherapy, Colon Hydrotherapy, Eliminate Allergy-Causing Foods, Hydration and Sweat Bath

Formulas: Decongestant, General Detoxifying, Antibacterial, **Expectorant** and Lung and Respiratory Tonic

Key Herbs: Elecampane, **Garlic**, **Horehound**, Horseradish, Lomatium, Mullein, Platycodon (Balloon Flower) and Pleurisy Root

Key Nutrients: Bromelain and Pantothenic Acid (Vitamin B5)

Congestion (lymphatic)

See also *Lymph Nodes or Glands (swollen)* and *Hodgkin Lymphoma (Hodgkin's Disease)*

We have all experienced the frustration of a clogged drain. We understand that stagnant water isn't healthy, so we do whatever is necessary to unclog that drain and prevent wastewater from standing around polluting the internal environment of our home.

Most people aren't aware that the body has a drainage system. It's called the lymphatic system, and it works hand in hand with the circulatory system to keep the various tissues and organs alive and healthy. It's the lymphatic system's job to make certain the fluid around the cells in the body doesn't become stagnant. Sometimes, however, the lymphatic system becomes congested, and like a clogged or sluggish drain, an unhealthy stagnation of fluids occurs. Without the lymphatic drainage working properly, the tissues in the body become like a clogged kitchen sink, a trash-laden back alley or a stagnant swamp, none of which can be considered healthy conditions.

Lymphatic congestion contributes to swollen lymph nodes, earaches, sore throats, chronic sinus and respiratory congestion, tonsillitis, appendicitis, breast swelling, lumps and tumors, lymphatic cancers and other health problems. Here are some ways to clear lymphatic congestion.

First, Deep Breathing therapy, combined with muscular movements, is the key to pumping our lymph and keeping it moving. Exercise, for example, increases lymph flow as much as five to fifteen times. One of the best forms of lymphatic exercise is gentle bouncing on a mini trampoline. If a person is unable to stand on the mini trampoline, he or she can still obtain benefit by sitting in a chair next to the trampoline with his or her feet on the trampoline. Another person stands on the trampoline and gently bounces up and down. This passively moves the lymphatics as the seated person's legs move up and down. If you don't own a mini trampoline, don't worry. Just walking and breathing deeply will greatly enhance lymphatic circulation, as will any other form of moderate exercise.

The second key to reducing lymphatic sluggishness is to drink an adequate amount of water. Even moderate dehydration will contribute to poor lymphatic drainage.

Dietary therapy may also be helpful. Certain foods seem to clog up the lymphatic system more than others. For many people, dairy products are major culprits. Wheat and other gluten-bearing grains are another lymphatic congestant for many people. However, any food that creates allergic reactions for a person may contribute to lymphatic stagnation. Avoiding these foods is the third key.

The fourth key is using herbs that improve lymphatic function such as those found in *Lymphatic Drainage Formulas*. *Echinacea Blend Formulas* are also very good at promoting better lymph drainage. Some *Blood Purifier Formulas* will also improve lymph flow, particularly if they contain herbs like echinacea, red clover, mullein and lobelia.

Finally, cleansing the colon is helpful for improving lymph flow. Try using *General Detoxifying* and *Fiber Blend Formulas* to improve bowel function.

Therapies: Aromatherapy, Colon Cleanse, Deep Breathing, Dietary Fiber, Exercise and Hydration

Formulas: Lymphatic Drainage, General Detoxifying, Fiber Blend, Blood Purifier and Echinacea Blend

Key Herbs: Cleavers (Bedstraw), **Echinacea**, **Red Clover**, **Red Root**, Garlic, Lobelia, Mullein and Ocotillo

Key Nutrients: Digestive Enzymes

Congestion (sinus)

See also *Allergies (respiratory)*, *Leaky Gut Syndrome*, *Polyps*, *Headache (sinus)* and *Sinus Infection*

When sinuses are congested, the first and most obvious remedy to try is a *Sinus Decongestant Formula*. *Decongestant Formulas* are also helpful.

However, when sinus problems are chronic, it is usually a sign of poor diet and chronic problems with digestion and the gastrointestinal tract. Start by following the Eliminate Allergy-Causing Foods therapy. Then improve digestive function with *Digestive Bitter Tonic* or *Digestive Enzyme Formulas*.

Cleansing the colon will also help. Use *General Detoxifying* and *Fiber Blend Formulas* to improve elimination and bind toxins in the colon. In some cases, leaky gut syndrome may be a factor and *Intestinal Toning Formulas* may be helpful.

Using a neti pot to wash the sinuses with salt water can help to cleanse the sinuses. If infection is present, *Goldenseal & Echinacea Formulas* may be helpful. These can be taken internally, or used as teas or highly diluted extracts in a neti pot for washing our the sinuses.

Therapies: Aromatherapy, Colon Cleanse, Colon Hydrotherapy, Dietary Fiber, Eliminate Allergy-Causing Foods and Hydration

Formulas: Sinus Decongestant, Decongestant, Fiber Blend, Intestinal Toning, Digestive Bitter Tonic, Digestive Enzyme, General Detoxifying and Goldenseal & Echinacea

Key Herbs: Bayberry, Brigham Tea, Burdock, **Fenugreek**, **Horseradish**, **Thyme**, Lomatium, Nettle (Stinging) and Triphala

Key Nutrients: Digestive Enzymes, Pantothenic Acid (Vitamin B5) and Bromelain

Congestive Heart Failure

See also *Cardiovascular Disease (Heart Disease)*

Congestive heart failure is a decline in the function of the heart due to damage of the heart muscle, normally from ischemic heart disease. Hawthorn may be helpful, but many of the best botanical remedies for congestive heart failure are toxic botanicals like lily of the valley and arnica that require the assistance of a professional herbalist (*findanherbalist.com*). Appropriate medical assistance should be sought for this condition. *Cardiac Tonic* and *Diuretic Formulas* may be helpful along with appropriate medical treatment. Nutritional supplements that may be helpful include Co-Q10, magnesium, l-arginine and l-carnitine.

Therapies: Fresh Fruits and Vegetables and Healthy Fats

Formulas: Diuretic and **Cardiac Tonic**

Key Herbs: Arnica, Astragalus, Coleus, **Arjuna**, **Hawthorn**, **Lily of the Valley**, Khella, Night Blooming Cereus (Cactus) and Pleurisy Root

Key Nutrients: Co-Q10, **L-Carnitine**, **L-Arginine**, **Vitamin B-1 (Thiamine)**, **Magnesium** and **Omega-3 Essential Fatty Acids**

Conjunctivitis (Pink Eye)

See also *Stye*

Conjunctivitis is an inflammation of the lining of the eye that causes redness in the whites. It may be due to allergic reactions or infections such as pink eye—a contagious viral condition. A closely related condition is a stye, which is a staph infection in the eyelid that causes swelling of the eyelid.

These conditions may be treated naturally using an herbal *Eye Wash Formula* or a tea of any of the following herbs: chamomile, eyebright or goldenseal. A cotton ball can be soaked with the tea from the *Eye Wash Formula* or single herbs listed above and applied over the closed eye as a compress. You can also use a piece of clean, soft cloth soaked in the tea. The cotton ball or cloth should be warm, not hot, and should be allowed to rest over the closed eyelid for about 15 minutes.

Another way to do this is to quickly dunk a tea bag of chamomile tea into hot water just long enough to moisten it and then apply the tea bag over the closed eyelid. Again, it should be warm, not hot, and left in place for about 15 minutes.

A liquid extract of *Goldenseal & Echinacea* or an *Antiviral Formula* can be used topically over the closed eyelid as a compress. These can also be rubbed around the closed eye, but avoid putting them directly into the eye. They can be taken internally, too. If the condition is bacterial, use an *Antibacterial Formula*.

Another remedy that helps is to poke a pin hole into a gel capsule of vitamin A (or vitamin A and D) and rub this around the closed eyelid and eye socket, but again, not directly into the eyeball. A solution of colloidal silver can be dropped directly into the eye as a natural eye drop.

Therapies: Compress

Formulas: **Eye Wash**, Antibacterial, Antiviral and **Goldenseal & Echinacea**

Key Herbs: Barberry, Calendula, **Chamomile (English and Roman)**, **Goldenseal** and Eyebright

Key Nutrients: **Vitamin A** and Vitamin D

Constipation (adults)

See also *Fungal Infections (Yeast Infections, Candida albicans), Gall Bladder (sluggish or removed), Inflammatory Bowel Disorders (Colitis, IBS), Parasites (general)* and *Colon (spastic)*

Constipation is a lack of normal bowel movements. Many people are slightly constipated and don't know it.

Ideally, the stool should move two to three times a day, depending on the number of meals consumed, and should be soft and easy to pass. It should come out in long "banana-like" pieces. Hard, round balls that are difficult to pass are a sign of dehydration and a form of constipation.

A slow colon transit time could also be considered constipation. Colon transit time is the time it takes for food materials to move through the length of the entire gastrointestinal tract. A great way to check colon transit time is to eat red beets or take liquid chlorophyll and see how long it takes to pass the red or green color of these substances in the stool.

It should take less than 24 hours for this material to show up in the stool and it should be cleared from the system in less than 36 hours. The average colon transit time of most people is 48-72 hours, which is too long and a sign of constipation.

Dehydration is the main cause of constipation in adults. So, start by drinking plenty of pure water.

Lack of sufficient dietary fiber is the second main cause of constipation. Increasing fibrous foods in the diet (like vegetables, fruits, beans and whole grains) helps keep the colon healthy. You can also take a *Fiber Blend Formula* once or twice daily. Always drink plenty of water when taking fiber.

Temporary constipation can be relieved by the use of *Stimulant Laxative Formulas*. These formulas contain herbs like cascara sagrada and senna, which contain anthraquinone glycosides that hold moisture in the stool and decrease colon transit time.

These herbs are fine for an occasional cleanse, but should not be used regularly as they tend to deplete the tone of the bowel. They also cause the colon to become stained, which can alarm doctors who give colonoscopies. There is no evidence this harms the bowel, but it is still not the best approach to long-term bowel health.

Long-term constipation is often due to intestinal inflammation and disruption of the friendly microbes living in the intestines. Probiotics and enzyme supplements are very important to long-term bowel health in these cases. *Anti-Inflammatory* and *Intestinal Toning Formulas* will also be helpful with long term-constipation.

Gentle Laxative Formulas containing three fruits used in Ayurvedic medicine to tone the bowel (collectively known as triphala) are a good tonic for long-term bowel problems. They reduce intestinal inflammation, tone the bowel and have a gentle laxative action.

Magnesium supplements work well with *Gentle Laxative Formulas* for promoting long-term bowel health. About 70% of North Americans do not get enough magnesium. Magnesium hydroxide, combined with vitamin C, is also a good laxative for long-term use.

Constipation can also be stress related. If the bowel is spastic (tense), *Antispasmodic Formulas* can have a mild laxative action. See Colon (spastic) for more detailed information.

The bile from the liver also has a laxative action, so *Cholagogue Formulas* may also be helpful for some cases of constipation. *General Detoxifying Formulas* combine cholagogue and liver cleansing action with small amounts of stimulant laxatives. They are good for "cleansing" the colon when used with *Fiber Blend Formulas* and plenty of water.

In some cases yeast infections or parasites may be an underlying problem. So, *Antiparasitic* and *Antifungal Formulas* may also be helpful.

Therapies: Colon Cleanse, Colon Hydrotherapy, Dietary Fiber, Fast or Juice Fast, Fresh Fruits and Vegetables, Friendly Flora, Gall Bladder Flush, Gut Healing Diet, Hiatal Hernia Correction and Hydration

Formulas: Fiber Blend, Gentle Laxative, **Stimulant Laxative**, Antifungal, Antispasmodic, Anti-Inflammatory, Cholagogue, General Detoxifying, Intestinal Toning and Antiparasitic

Key Herbs: Aloe vera, Buckthorn, **Butternut bark**, **Cascara Sagrada**, **Turkey Rhubarb**, Culver's root, Flax Seed, Milk Thistle, Peppermint, Psyllium, Senna Leaves, Triphala and Yellow Dock

Key Nutrients: Probiotics, Magnesium, Chlorophyll, Digestive Enzymes and Fiber

Constipation (children)

Children, like adults, can suffer from constipation and sluggish colon transit time. It is not wise, however, to use Stimulant Laxatives with children in most cases, except for very mild laxative herbs like yellow dock. However, *Gentle Laxative Formulas* are suitable for use with children.

A little prune juice or fresh apple juice is often enough to overcome constipation in children. Children with constipation may also be magnesium deficient or need essential fatty acids for intestinal health. Flax seeds and slippery elm make good bulk laxatives with children.

Like adults, children may need enzymes and probiotics for bowel health. Papaya is a good source of enzymes for children, and cultured dairy products like yoghurt and kiefer can supply probiotics. (Just make sure they aren't loaded with refined sugar, which feeds yeast overgrowth.)

Children are often constipated due to stress. So, if a child seems stressed, use a liquid *Relaxing Nervine Formula* and extra water or fresh fruit and vegetable juices to help their colon move normally.

Therapies: Colon Hydrotherapy, Friendly Flora, Healthy Fats and Hydration

Formulas: Gentle Laxative and Relaxing Nervine

Key Herbs: Flax Seed, Licorice, Papaya, Slippery Elm, Triphala and Yellow Dock

Key Nutrients: Magnesium, Digestive Enzymes and **Probiotics**

Contagious Diseases

See also *Chicken Pox, Colds (remedies for), Flu (Influenza), Infection (bacterial), Infection (viral), Measles* and *Mumps*

Contagious diseases are caused by infectious organisms like viruses and bacteria. Most people subscribe to the "germ theory," which says that these microbes are the direct and immediate cause of illness. However, there is another theory of contagious disease, known as the biological terrain theory, which says that the organism has to be weakened in order to be susceptible to contagious diseases.

The biological terrain theory is validated by the fact that everyone exposed to a germ does not get sick. The health of a person's body determines their natural resistance, so by paying appropriate attention to good health (eating a healthy diet, getting adequate rest and exercise, drinking pure water and other good health practices) one can largely avoid contagious diseases. These same practices speed recovery from contagious diseases.

As more and more people have started to use herbal remedies, they have tended to use them in the context of modern medical theory. This doesn't always yield the best results. That is, many herbs that have been historically used to fight infection aren't nearly as powerful at killing germs as modern drugs. However, in clinical experience, they still work, partially because they also help to boost the immune system and otherwise alter the body's biological terrain.

Immune Stimulating, Mushroom Blend or *Echinacea Blend Formulas* can be taken when contagious diseases are "going around" to boost the immune system. These remedies put the immune system on "red alert" so that it is better prepared to fight off an infection when the body is exposed to it. When coupled with basic hygiene and sanitation, this can help to protect a person from "catching" most contagious diseases.

Affirmation and Visualization and Stress Management therapies help to keep the immune system strong as well. Keeping a good balance of friendly microbes (probiotics) in the intestinal tract also helps to both prevent and fight contagious diseases.

If a person does "catch" a contagious disease, there are many categories of remedies to select from in combating these ailments, including *Antiviral, Antibacterial, Cold and Flu, Echinacea Blend* and *Goldenseal & Echinacea Formulas*. These remedies work best when taken about every two hours with plenty of water and rest. It also helps to avoid eating heavy food and sticking primarily to a diet of fresh fruit and vegetable juices, broth and clear soups.

You can also look up specific contagious diseases for more specific recommendations.

Therapies: Affirmation and Visualization, Colon Hydrotherapy, Friendly Flora and Stress Management

Formulas: Immune Stimulating, Echinacea Blend, Goldenseal & Echinacea, Antiviral, Antibacterial, Cold and Flu, Lung and Respiratory Tonic, Urinary Infection Fighting and **Mushroom Blend**

Key Herbs: Echinacea, Garlic, Goldenseal, Lobelia, Olive and Reishi (Ganoderma)

Key Nutrients: Probiotics and Digestive Enzymes

Convalescence

After a prolonged illness, the body is often in a debilitated state and needs special nutritional support to aid in rebuilding and recovering good health. This period of recovery from debility is called convalescence.

Adaptogen Formulas are good basic remedies for convalescence. Where there has been a lot of stress associated with the illness, a *Nerve Tonic Formula* would also be a good idea. After a bout with intestinal infection, diarrhea, flu, nausea and vomiting, etc., a *Digestive Tonic Formula* may be helpful. After a bout with a long-term contagious disease or cancer, it may also be helpful to tonify the immune system using a *Mushroom Blend Formula*.

Therapies: Fresh Fruits and Vegetables and Healthy Fats

Formulas: Adaptogen, Digestive Tonic, **Mushroom Blend** and **Superfood**

Key Herbs: Alfalfa, Aloe vera, Barley, Bee Pollen, Blue Vervain, Borage, **Ashwaganda, Astragalus, Codonopsis**, Irish moss, Slippery Elm, Tea (Green or Black) and Turmeric

Key Nutrients: Digestive Enzymes, Omega-3 Essential Fatty Acids and Co-Q10

Convulsions

See also *Epilepsy*

Convulsions are abnormal, violent and involuntary contractions or a series of contractions of the muscles. Nervines and Antispasmodics like blue vervain, kava kava, lobelia, scullcap and passion flower should be helpful. Look for *Antispasmodic* or *Relaxing Nervine Formulas* with these herbs as major ingredients.

Therapies: Fresh Fruits and Vegetables and Healthy Fats

Formulas: Antispasmodic and Relaxing Nervine

Key Herbs: Aloe vera, Blue Vervain, Catnip, **Lobelia, Scullcap (Skullcap)**, Kava-kava and Passionflower

Key Nutrients: Omega-3 Essential Fatty Acids, **Vitamin B-Complex**, Potassium and Magnesium

Copper Toxicity

Copper is an important nutrient, but can be toxic when there is too much of it in the system. Zinc and copper are antagonists, so increasing zinc intake should help to flush excess copper from the system. Pumpkin seeds are naturally high in zinc. MSM is a supplement that helps the liver flush excess copper. A *Heavy Metal Cleansing Formula* may also help.

Therapies: Heavy Metal Cleanse

Formulas: Heavy Metal Cleansing

Key Nutrients: Zinc, Potassium and MSM

Corns

Corns are a lesion of the skin formed between two toes as a result of pressure between them. The surface of the skin is macerated and yellowish in color. Remedies that can be applied topically for relief include vitamin E, chamomile, aloe vera and tea tree oil. A *Topical Vulnerary Formula* should also help.

Therapies: Compress and Poultice

Formulas: Topical Vulnerary

Key Herbs: Celandine, Chamomile (English and Roman), **Tea Tree** and Garlic

Key Nutrients: Vitamin E

Cough (damp)

See also *Congestion (lungs)*, *Pneumonia* and *Cough (general)*

A damp cough is a cough that produces a lot of phlegm. There is excess mucus production and fluid in the lungs. Remedies that help to tone mucus membranes and reduce excess secretions are helpful for damp coughs. These include bayberry, pine (white), wild cherry, eucalyptus, thyme, osha and yerba santa. Use *Cough Remedy Formulas* with these herbs as major ingredients or remedies listed under Cough Remedies (Drying).

Therapies: Colon Hydrotherapy, Eliminate Allergy-Causing Foods and Sweat Bath

Formulas: Drying Cough/Lung and Cough Remedy

Key Herbs: Bayberry, **Cherry (Wild)**, **Osha**, **Pine (White)**, **Yerba Santa**, Elder, Eucalyptus, Garlic,

Horehound, Horseradish, Hyssop, Platycodon (Balloon Flower), Rosemary and Thyme

Key Nutrients: Vitamin D and Vitamin C

Cough (dry)

See also *Cough (general)*

When a cough is unproductive (dry and hacking) so that there is little mucus production, the lungs are dehydrated. Moistening expectorants and decongestants, like astragalus, licorice, mullein, marshmallow and slippery elm are needed. Choose *Cough Remedy Formulas* that contain these herbs as major ingredients or formulas listed under Cough Remedies (Moistening).

Therapies: Hydration

Formulas: Cough Remedy and **Moistening Lung/ Cough**

Key Herbs: Aloe vera, Astragalus, Bloodroot, Coltsfoot, Comfrey, Cordyceps, **Licorice**, **Marshmallow**, **Mullein**, Fenugreek, Grindelia (Gumweed), Irish moss, Lycium (Wolfberry, Gogi), Plantain, Pleurisy Root and Schisandra (Schizandra)

Key Nutrients: Pantothenic Acid (Vitamin B5)

Cough (general)

See also *Cough (damp)*, *Cough (dry)* and *Cough (spastic)*

Under normal conditions, the lungs and sinuses secrete a thin, protective layer of mucus that traps dust and other particles in the air. Thin, hair-like projections called cilia sweep this mucus to the back of the throat (from the sinuses) or to the top of the throat (from the lungs). When the mucus gets trapped in the lungs and the cilia are unable to move it out of the lungs, this creates an involuntary, explosive expulsion of air from the lung in an attempt to expel the mucus and irritants from the lungs.

All over-the-counter cough medicines contain cough suppressants that suppress the cough reflex. This does not help the body eliminate the irritants. Decongestants help thin the mucus so that it can move more freely, and expectorants stimulate the cilia to move it out of the system.

Remedies that primarily contain decongestant herbs are listed under *Decongestant Formulas* and remedies that primarily contain expectorant herbs are listed under *Expectorant Formulas*. However, there is a lot of crossover in these formulas as most *Decongestant Formulas* are also expectorant and vice-versa. There are also herbal formulas designed specifically for coughs listed under Cough Formulas. These formulas are typically both decongestants and expectorants.

Always take these formulas with plenty of water. Also look at the specific types of coughs listed in this book for more specific cough remedies.

Therapies: Eliminate Allergy-Causing Foods and Hydration

Formulas: Cough Remedy, Decongestant, **Expectorant**, Drying Cough/Lung and Moistening Lung/Cough

Key Herbs: Horehound, Thyme, Yerba Santa, Elecampane, Garlic, Horseradish, Lobelia, Oregano and Rosemary

Key Nutrients: Vitamin C

Cough (spastic)

See also *Croup* and *Pertussis (Whooping Cough)*

A spastic cough is one in which there is muscle constriction in the bronchials. This can come as a result of muscle exhaustion after an extended period of coughing. Coughs that have a whooping sound or constricted quality to them need remedies with an antispasmodic action. Pertussis and Croup are diseases that typically have spastic coughs as part of their symptomology.

Bronchialdilator and *Antispasmodic Formulas* can be used along with *Expectorant, Decongestant* and *Cough Remedy Formulas* for spastic coughs. These formulas can also be used to calm coughs when excessive coughing is leading to exhaustion.

Therapies: Stress Management

Formulas: Bronchialdilator, Antispasmodic and Adrenal Tonic

Key Herbs: Black Cohosh, Blue Vervain, **Khella, Lobelia, Skunk Cabbage**, Jamaican Dogwood, Rosemary and Thyme

Key Nutrients: Pantothenic Acid (Vitamin B5) and Vitamin C

Cradle Cap

Cradle cap is a skin condition affecting the scalp of babies. It is characterized by large oily, yellow flaking from the baby's scalp. It is a form of dermatitis and is related to eczema. It may involve yeast infections. Often babies who have this are severely deficient in essential fatty acids, most likely due to a deficiency in the mother's diet during pregnancy. Vitamin E and aloe vera gel make good topical applications for cradle cap.

Therapies: Healthy Fats

Formulas: Antifungal

Key Herbs: Aloe vera, Black Walnut, Calendula, **Tea Tree essential oil**, Pau d' Arco and Violet

Key Nutrients: Probiotics, **Omega-3 Essential Fatty Acids**, Vitamin E and Colloidal Silver

Cramps (leg)

See also *Cramps and Spasms (general)*

Cramps in the legs are usually a sign of magnesium and/or potassium deficiencies. Stress can be a contributing factor. In addition to supplementation with magnesium and potassium, *Antispasmodic* or *Nerve Tonic Formulas* may be helpful. In some cases, B-complex vitamins may also help.

Therapies: Mineralization and Stress Management

Formulas: Antispasmodic

Key Herbs: Cramp Bark, Hops, Kava-kava and Valerian

Key Nutrients: Potassium, Magnesium, Vitamin B-6 (Pyridoxine) and Vitamin B-Complex

Cramps (menstrual)

See also *Cramps and Spasms (general), Dysmenorrhea (Painful Menstruation)* and *PMS (general)*

Menstrual cramps often signal a lack of magnesium and/or vitamin B-6 in the diet. These are also general nutrients for PMS symptoms. There are specific *Menstrual Cramp Formulas* that may help to bring relief. *Antispasmodic Formulas* may also help to ease menstrual cramps. See *Cramps and Spasms (general)* for more ideas on dealing with cramps.

Therapies: Healthy Fats, Mineralization and Stress Management

Formulas: Antispasmodic and **Menstrual Cramp**

Key Herbs: Angelica, Black Haw, Blue Cohosh, Butterbur Root, Chastetree (Vitex), **Black Cohosh, Cramp Bark, Khella, Wild Yam**, Dong Quai, Motherwort, Muira Puama, Pennyroyal and Thyme

Key Nutrients: Potassium, **Magnesium**, DHEA, Omega-3 Essential Fatty Acids and Vitamin E

Cramps and Spasms (general)

See also *Tension*

A cramp is a painful, involuntary spasmodic contraction of a muscle. A spasm is an involuntary and abnormal contraction of a muscle that can be extremely painful. Cramps can also be signs of magnesium and potassium deficiencies.

Antispasmodic herbs, such as lobelia, black cohosh and kava kava, will help to relax cramps and muscle spasms when taken internally and applied topically. These are key herbs in *Antispasmodic Formulas*.

Muscles expend energy to contract and must regenerate energy in order to relax again. A muscle that cramps is low in energy. Because of this, *Nerve Tonic Formulas* may also be helpful for problems with cramps and spasms. Stretching exercises help to rebuild energy charges in muscles and promote relaxation of cramps, as does Deep Breathing therapy.

Therapies: Affirmation and Visualization, Aromatherapy, Compress, Deep Breathing, Epsom Salt Bath, Mineralization and Stress Management

Formulas: Antispasmodic

Key Herbs: Black Cohosh, Black Haw, **Cramp Bark**, **Lobelia**, **Scullcap (Skullcap)**, Hops, Jamaican Dogwood, Kava-kava, Skunk Cabbage, Valerian, Wild Yam and Wood Betony

Key Nutrients: Potassium, Pantothenic Acid (Vitamin B5) and **Magnesium**

Crohn's Disease

See also *Inflammatory Bowel Disorders (Colitis, IBS)*

Crohn's disease is an inflammatory condition of the small intestine and colon. It is a severe form of colitis that causes fistulas to form in the colon. There is atrophy and ulceration of the intestines. Symptoms include diarrhea, cramping, loss of appetite, loss of weight and intestinal abscesses and scarring.

Remedies to reduce inflammation, absorb irritants and restore normal intestinal flora are needed. *Intestinal Toning* and *Ulcer Healing Formulas* are good choices for Crohn's disease. *Tissue Healing Formulas* may also be helpful. In particular, look for formulas containing herbs like slippery elm, wild yam, cat's claw (una d'gato), licorice root and aloe vera.

Fiber Blend Formulas, particularly those containing softer fibers like gums, pectins and mucilages and *Gentle Laxative Formulas* may also be helpful for Crohn's disease. Probiotics and enzyme supplements are essential to general gastrointestinal health in inflammatory diseases like Crohn's.

This is a serious condition and requires competent medical assistance. See Inflammatory Bowel Disorders for more ideas on how to deal with Chron's disease.

Therapies: Dietary Fiber, Fast or Juice Fast, Fresh Fruits and Vegetables, Friendly Flora, Gut Healing Diet, Healthy Fats and Stress Management

Formulas: Fiber Blend, **Intestinal Toning**, Ulcer Healing, Tissue Healing and Gentle Laxative

Key Herbs: Blue Vervain, Chamomile (English and Roman), **Aloe vera**, **Cats Claw (Uña de Gato, Gambier)**, **Licorice**, **Wild Yam**, Devil's Claw, Ginger, Pau d' Arco, Psyllium, Slippery Elm, Venus Fly Trap and Yucca

Key Nutrients: Magnesium, Omega-3 Essential Fatty Acids, **Probiotics**, **Iron**, **L-Glutamine** and Lipase Enzymes

Croup

See also *Cough (spastic)*

A spasmodic laryngitis, especially in infants, is called croup. Symptoms include difficulty breathing and a hoarse metallic cough. *Antispasmodic Formulas* are helpful, or single herbs like blue vervain, catnip and small doses of lobelia. *Topical Analgesic Formulas* may be rubbed onto the throat and chest for added relief, but should probably be diluted with olive oil (or another vegetable oil) when applied to infants.

Therapies: Hydration

Formulas: Antispasmodic and Topical Analgesic

Key Herbs: Blue Vervain, **Catnip**, **Fenugreek**, **Lobelia**, Mullein, Pine (White), Rosemary and Thyme

Key Nutrients: Omega-3 Essential Fatty Acids, Vitamin E and Zinc

Cushing's Disease

Cushing's disease is characterized by elevated adrenal glands, meaning that the adrenal glands are overactive and overproducing adrenal hormones. Symptoms include excess cortisol, low blood sugar, poor wound healing, lowered immune response, thinning hair, muscle wasting, abdominal fat and high blood pressure.

In this disease, licorice root and other supplements that enhance adrenal function should be avoided. Adaptogens like eleuthero root, schizandra berries and rhodiola can be used to calm down elevated adrenal function. Therefore, a good *Adaptogen Formula* may be helpful. B-complex vitamins, kava kava and blue vervain may also be beneficial.

This is a serious illness requiring competent medical help.

Therapies: Affirmation and Visualization and Stress Management

Formulas: Adaptogen

Key Herbs: Blue Vervain, Chamomile (English and Roman), **Eleuthero (Siberian ginseng)**, **Holy Basil**, Hops, Lavender and Passionflower

Key Nutrients: Vitamin B-Complex

Cuts

See also *Bleeding (external)*

Styptics are herbs, usually astringents, that have the power to stop bleeding and speed the healing of cuts. Some of the herbs that have this property include bayberry, calendula, capsicum and yarrow, which can be poured directly into cuts and followed by applying pressure. *Styptic/Hemostatic Formulas* can also be used on cuts.

To prevent infection in cuts, you can apply a *Topical Antiseptic Formula*. The herbs in these formulas should speed healing and prevent scarring, too. To prevent scarring you can also apply vitamin E and helicrysum or lavender essential oil.

Therapies: Poultice

Formulas: Styptic/Hemostatic and Topical Antiseptic

Key Herbs: Bayberry, Capsicum (Cayenne), **Calendula**, **Yarrow**, Goldenseal, Grindelia (Gumweed), Lavender, Lomatium, St. John's wort, Tea Tree, White Oak and Yerba Santa

Key Nutrients: Vitamin E and Colloidal Silver

Cystic Breast Disease

See also *Breast Lumps*

The formation of benign fluid-filled sacs in the breast tissue is called cystic breast disease. If you have lumps in the breast they should be tested to determine if they are benign or malignant before choosing a course of therapy.

If the lumps are benign, start by avoiding caffeine. Caffeine contributes to this problem and all forms should be avoided, including coffee, tea, cola drinks and possibly chocolate.

There is a need to improve lymphatic drainage from the breast tissue, so *Lymphatic Drainage Formulas* should be used internally. A *Lymphatic Drainage Formula* in liquid form can also be applied topically to the breasts. A few drops of poke oil can also be massaged into the breasts, but this should be done under the supervision of a qualified professional herbalist (*findanherbalist.com*) or naturopath.

A colon and liver cleanse is appropriate using *Blood Purifier* or *General Detoxifying Formula*. These will also help to improve lymphatic drainage and reduce fluid-filled sacs.

There may also be a problem with low thyroid and a lack of iodine. In this case, *Hypothyroid Formulas* or iodine supplements may be helpful.

Excess estrogens and xenoestrogens, in particular, can contribute to cystic breast disease. Use the therapy Avoid Xenoestrogens and use foods and herbs containing phytoestrogens to reduce excess estrogen stimulation.

Since the liver breaks down excess estrogens, supplements that enhance liver detoxification can also be helpful. Indole-3-carbinol, a substance found in cruciferous vegetables like cabbage, broccoli and cauliflower, is very helpful for breaking down excess estrogens. It is also available in supplement form. A *Hepatoprotective Formula* may also be helpful in breaking down xenoestrogens.

Therapies: Avoid Caffeine, Avoid Xenoestrogens, Fresh Fruits and Vegetables, Healthy Fats and Stress Management

Formulas: Lymphatic Drainage, Blood Purifier, General Detoxifying, Hyperthyroid, Phytoestrogen and Hepatoprotective

Key Herbs: Chamomile (English and Roman), **False Unicorn (Helonias)**, Gentian, Hydrangea and Oregon Grape

Key Nutrients: Indole-3 Carbinol (DIM), Magnesium, Digestive Enzymes, Omega-3 Essential Fatty Acids, Vitamin A, Vitamin C, Vitamin D, **Vitamin E** and Zinc

Cystic Fibrosis

Cystic fibrosis is a hereditary disease that appears in early childhood and involves a generalized disorder of the exocrine glands. Symptoms include faulty digestion due to a deficiency of pancreatic enzymes, difficulty breathing and excessive loss of salt in the sweat.

Natural remedies may not offer a cure, but they can ease symptoms. For starters, high quality, nutrient-packed foods need to be eaten. Use the Eliminate Allergy-Causing Foods and Colon Cleanse therapies. Also increase antioxidants and good fats and consider adopting a Gut-Healing Diet as outlined in the *Therapies Section*. *Digestive Enzyme Formulas* will help to thin mucous and improve digestive function. For additional natural help one should work with a qualified alternative health practitioner.

Therapies: Colon Cleanse, Eliminate Allergy-Causing Foods, Fresh Fruits and Vegetables, Gut Healing Diet, Healthy Fats and Mineralization

Formulas: Digestive Enzyme

Key Herbs: Alfalfa, **Blue Vervain**, Fenugreek, Marshmallow, Papaya, Spirulina and Thyme

Key Nutrients: Vitamin B-12, **Protease Enzymes**, **N-Acetyl Cysteine**, Digestive Enzymes, Vitamin B-Complex, **Probiotics** and Colloidal Minerals

Cystitis

See *Interstitial Cystitis*

Cysts

Cysts are closed sacs with distinct membranes that are usually fluid filled. They form abnormally in a cavity or other structure of the body. Detoxification is essential for eliminating cysts. General cleansers like *Blood Purifier* and *General Detoxifying Formulas* can be taken internally. The Poultice therapy using a blend containing plantain can help to break up cysts. The Castor Oil Pack therapy is also good for breaking up cysts.

Therapies: Aromatherapy, Colon Cleanse and Poultice

Formulas: Blood Purifier and General Detoxifying

Key Herbs: Chickweed, **Plantain**, **Red Clover**, Gentian, Kelp, Poke Root, Red Root, Safflowers and Yellow Dock

Key Nutrients: Protease Enzymes, Vitamin A and Vitamin D

Dandruff

See also *Fungal Infections (Yeast Infections, Candida albicans)* and *Leaky Gut Syndrome*

Dandruff is caused by extreme dryness of the scalp, which results in white flakes. Jojoba oil rubbed into the scalp may relieve dandruff problems. Coconut oil may also be applied to the scalp. Increase intake of essential fatty acids.

Adding tea tree, rosemary or other essential oils to one's shampoo to stimulate circulation to the scalp can also relieve dandruff. Dandruff can be related to stress, so B-complex vitamins and *Relaxing Nervine Formulas* may be helpful.

In some cases, dandruff may be linked to yeast overgrowth in the intestinal tract or intestinal inflammation and Leaky Gut Syndrome. If this is the case, *Antifungal Formulas*, probiotics, digestive enzyme supplements or *Intestinal Toning Formulas* may be helpful.

Therapies: Aromatherapy, Friendly Flora, Healthy Fats and Stress Management

Formulas: Relaxing Nervine, Antifungal and Intestinal Toning

Key Herbs: Black Walnut, **Tea Tree**, Kelp, Pau d' Arco and Rosemary

Key Nutrients: Omega-3 Essential Fatty Acids, Vitamin E, Digestive Enzymes, Vitamin B-Complex, Selenium and Zinc

Debility

See also *Convalescence*

Debility is a general weakness of the body brought on by prolonged illness or general poor health. *Adaptogen* and *Superfood Formulas* can be helpful (along with basic supplementation) for overcoming debility.

Therapies: Affirmation and Visualization, Healthy Fats and Mineralization

Formulas: Adaptogen, Energy-Boosting and **Superfood**

Key Herbs: Barley, **Bee Pollen**, Ginseng (American), Ginseng (Asian, Korean), Slippery Elm and Spirulina

Key Nutrients: Digestive Enzymes, Co-Q10, Omega-3 Essential Fatty Acids and Colloidal Minerals

Defensiveness

See *Irritability* and *Anger (excessive)*

Dehydration

See also *Diabetes*

Dehydration is a lack of water in the tissues of the body. Although water needs to be consumed to overcome dehydration, sometimes water is not being properly taken up and utilized by the tissues. When this happens, the person drinks water, urinates excessively and is still thirsty. This can be an early warning sign of diabetes and other blood sugar problems.

Licorice root and *Adrenal Tonic Formulas* can help the body stay more hydrated. If the problem is related to blood sugar, then *Blood Sugar Reducing Formulas* may help. Medical diagnosis should be sought to determine if diabetes is a factor.

Mineral electrolytes like potassium help the body hold onto moisture. These can be lost during exercise. Electrolyte supplements or herbal *Mineral Formulas* can be taken to restore mineral balance and help the body hold onto moisture.

Therapies: Hydration, Low Glycemic Diet and Mineralization

Formulas: Blood Sugar Reducing, Mineral and Adrenal Tonic

Key Herbs: Kelp, **Licorice** and Nopal (Prickly Pear)

Key Nutrients: Potassium, Vitamin B-12 and Magnesium

Dementia

See also *Alzheimer's Disease* and *Memory and Brain Function*

Dementia is a loss of cognitive and intellectual function, without the loss of perception. Symptoms include disorientation, impaired memory and judgment, and a loss of intellectual capacity. It may be caused by toxins causing free radical damage or diseases of the brain. Antioxidants and good fats help to protect the brain as a person ages. *Brain and Memory Tonic Formulas* can also help to prevent dementia and even help reverse it in some cases. Also consider Heavy Metal Detoxification in cases of dementia. Seek appropriate professional assistance.

Therapies: Fresh Fruits and Vegetables, Healthy Fats, Heavy Metal Cleanse and Low Glycemic Diet

Formulas: Brain and Memory Tonic

Key Herbs: Bacopa (Water Hyssop), **Ginkgo**, **Rosemary**, Gotu kola and Sage

Key Nutrients: Omega-3 Essential Fatty Acids, **Vitamin B-Complex**, **Magnesium**, **Alpha Lipoic Acid**, DHA and **L-Arginine**

Denture Sores

Denture sores are abrasions or ulcerations on the gums or gingiva as a result of improperly fitted dental appliances. Aloe vera, chamomile and vitamin E are all remedies that can be applied directly to the gums to reduce inflammation and promote healing. *Topical Vulnerary* and *Topical Analgesic Formulas* may also be helpful.

Therapies: Compress

Formulas: Topical Vulnerary, Topical Analgesic and Anti-Inflammatory

Key Herbs: Aloe vera, Clove, **Chamomile (English and Roman)**, Tea Tree and Turmeric

Key Nutrients: Vitamin E

Depression

See also *Grief and Sadness*, *Hypothyroid*, *Inflammatory Bowel Disorders (Colitis, IBS)*, *Post Partum Depression*, *Seasonal Affective Disorder* and *PMS Type D*

Are you singing the blues? If you are, you are not alone because statistics suggest that one out of ten Americans are depressed. Unfortunately, the most popular treatment for depression is prescription drugs, which only work in about one-third of the cases.

Depression is a misunderstood, misdiagnosed and often mistreated condition, so let's identify some of the causes of depression and offer some natural alternatives to prescription drugs.

Once named melancholia, shamans and sages felt that bad thoughts or demons caused the disorder. Our modern understanding of depression comes from research done on chemicals called neurotransmitters. Here's how these chemicals work.

The area where two nerves meet and exchange information is referred to as a synapse. This synaptic region is filled with fluid in which neurotransmitters travel and transmit information from one nerve to another. As one nerve releases a neurotransmitter, the other nerve has its receptor that will then accept and process the information.

Once the receptor has been stimulated by this chemical message, the neurotransmitter may be returned to the originating nerve for recycling or it may be destroyed. Destruction of neurotransmitters involves converting them into substances that can be absorbed into the bloodstream and eliminated in the urine. Various enzymes, such as monoamine oxidase (MAO) accomplish this task.

The nerves must replenish their supply of neurotransmitters in order to send the next message. This can be accomplished by reabsorbing the previously released neurotransmitters (a process called reuptake) or by manufacturing a new supply. Neurotransmitters are created from amino acids using vitamins and minerals.

Modern scientists believe that during depression there may be an imbalance of neurotransmitters, either a depleted supply or excess. Some of the neurotransmitters believed to be involved in depression include serotonin, norepinephrine and dopamine. When the supply of one of these chemicals is depleted, the nerve is unable to send signals properly. When the chemical is present in excess, the message is over-sent.

Today's antidepressant drugs are all designed to alter neurotransmitters in some fashion. In the 1940s, tricyclic drugs, better known as MAOIs (monoamine oxidase inhibitors) came to market. These drugs inhibited the enzyme mentioned earlier that breaks down some of these neurotransmitters. Although this approach worked for some, it had serious side effects for others, including death. In some cases individuals who were depressed ended up with anxiety and vice versa.

In 1988, Prozac, a SSRI (Selective Serotonin Reuptake Inhibitor) was introduced to the market. In no time 22 million Americans were taking the drug. With the fad popularity of Prozac, more antidepressant drugs soon appeared on the scene.

Antidepressants such as Wellbutrin and Zyban work by inhibiting the reuptake of serotonin and dopamine. Effexor inhibits serotonin, norepinephrine and dopamine. SSRIs such as Prozac, Paxil and Zoloft cause more of the serotonin to remain in the synapses for extended periods of time.

These drugs all have numerous side effects. For starters, they mask the real causes of depression, which relate to diet, exercise, stress and unresolved emotional issues. Instead of making appropriate life-style adjustments or dealing with life's issues, patients are given a false sense of reality and often feel detached and indifferent to family, friends and environment.

These drugs may also contribute to joint pain, abnormal blood cell counts, sexual dysfunction and altered appetite/weight. An overdose or faulty interaction with other drugs can also cause a SSRI to induce hallucinations, irregular heartbeat and seizures. As an odd irony, depression is one of the common side effects of these drugs.

A common cause of depression is prescription medication. Your busy family physician may overlook the fact that the antibiotic or antihistamine you are taking could be the cause of your being down and out. Diuretics, beta-blockers, hormone replacement therapies, painkillers, *Sleep Formulas*, Tagamet and Zantac can all create the imbalance of neurotransmitters that may color your days gray. You can see the importance of educating yourself about the medications and supplements you use.

It is also important to recognize the difference between feeling a little blue because of grief, losses or setbacks and having serious depression. There's a general belief in our society that we're supposed to be happy all the time or something is wrong with us. If we're down or feeling sad then we need to get a positive attitude. This is ridiculous.

It is perfectly normal and healthy to experience sadness, grief and even some depression when bad things happen to us. Depression allows us to pull into ourselves, introspect on our life, reevaluate our situation and hopefully make constructive changes. This is why one of the best things you can do if you are feeling depressed is to find someone to talk to, whether it's a counselor, a minister or a trusted friend. Talk therapy is just as effective as drugs and can actually "cure" a person's depression, not just mask it.

General Therapy for Depression

Unfortunately, when we're feeling depressed we don't take the best care of ourselves. We may binge out on junk food, fail to get needed exercise or otherwise ignore the body's needs. So, if you are depressed, start taking better care of yourself. Eat a healthier diet, get some fresh air, sunshine and physical activity (such as taking a walk outdoors), and make sure you're getting a good night's sleep.

To work on the emotional side of the depression, keep a journal and/or talk to a friend or trusted advisor who can be a sounding-board for you to work through what's bothering you. Aromatherapy using oils such as bergamot, rose, pine and rosemary can help lift your spirits. Flower essences can also help.

Also consider a few basic nutritional supplements. A deficiency of amino acids or B-complex vitamins will result in a deficiency of neurotransmitters. Tyrosine and phenylalanine will both elevate levels of norepinephrine, seen to improve mood in depression and anxiety case studies. Tryptophan (and its derivative 5-HTP) will increase serotonin levels.

Amino acids are derived from vitalized protein. Overcooked meat is not a good source of amino acids. Furthermore, many people have problems with protein digestion. Algae supplements containing blue-green algae, spirulina or chlorella can be beneficial here, along with protease enzyme supplements and high quality vegetable or animal protein sources.

B-complex has remarkable results for many sufferers because the B-vitamins are critical to the synthesis of neurotransmitters. Dr. Peter D'Adamo reports that he has successfully treated depression, hyperactivity and Attention Deficit Disorder in many people with the O blood type with high doses of folic acid and B12. One should always make sure to incorporate B-complex when taking a single B vitamin.

Essential fatty acids are also important to nerve function and may help depression and other nervous system disorders. So make sure to take some omega-3 fatty acids, fish liver oils and other good fats.

You can always start by trying one of the *Antidepressant Formulas* listed in this book. If that doesn't work, you may need more specific herbs and supplements. The remedies that work best for you will depend on what is causing your depression. So, consider the following.

Stress

Stress can bring us down and make us feel tired and depressed. If your depression was preceded by a lot of stress, use the Stress Management therapy, including taking supplements to help you cope with it. Stress-related depression usually couples a high state of anxiety and nervousness with fatigue, loss of interest in life, reduced sex drive and a general feeling that "I just can't cope!" If this fits you, try taking an *Adaptogen Formula* to bring down levels of cortisol and stress hormones. *Adrenal Tonic Formulas* may also be helpful if you feel completely "burned-out."

If you feel particularly nervous and tense, consider using kava kava. Kava targets the limbic system in the brain, relaxing muscles. It helps promote a calm, mentally alert state coupled with a feeling of well-being. A *Relaxing Nervine Formula* where kava kava is a key ingredient can be helpful for depression associated with tension.

Low Thyroid

The thyroid plays an important role in mood regulation. Hypothyroidism is often overlooked as a possible cause of depression. If you have fatigue, problems losing weight, dry skin, low body temperature and/or high cholesterol levels, low thyroid may be a contributing factor to your depressed feelings.

If low thyroid is a factor, feeding the thyroid gland with a *Hypothyroid Formula* (or herbs like kelp and dulse) may help. However, the most common cause of low thyroid in modern times is Hashimoto's thyroiditis, which is an autoimmune disorder. So, if you suspect low thyroid is a factor, try the recommendations found under the heading Hashimoto's.

Colon Problems

Hashimoto's and other autoimmune conditions have links to the intestinal tract. This is also true in many cases of depression. Folk medicine has long recognized a connection between the digestive function and depression. Constipation was thought to produce melancholy in traditional Western medicine. Recent research shows there is scientific validity to this point of view, as the bowel produces more serotonin than the brain.

In recent years, St. John's wort has been widely touted as a natural product for mild to moderate depression. St. John's wort does have antidepressant action, but works best on depression associated with anxiety and problems with the gastrointestinal tract. This is because St. John's wort helps to regulate the nerves of the digestive tract.

Using digestive enzyme supplements and probiotics to help heal the intestinal membranes will be very helpful in many cases of depression. Consider doing the Colon Cleanse therapy or taking one of the *General Detoxifying* and *Gentle Laxative Formulas*. Getting rid of toxins in this manner can help a person feel "lighter" and more energized. Also consider therapy for Leaky Gut Syndrome.

Liver Issues

The liver is charged with the responsibility of breaking down toxins in the body. When the liver is overwhelmed in its task, a person can feel tired and overwhelmed, thus contributing to depression. *Liver Tonic Formulas* may be helpful when this is a factor in depression. Bupleurum is a major Chinese herb that is said to "dredge" the liver of anger and sadness, which can help to improve mood.

Since 1976 s-adenosyl l-methionin (SAM-e) has elevated mood, eliminated suicidal tendencies and improved intellectual performance. This improvement was noted in approximately 80% of the cases. This is as effective as clomipramine and amitriptyline. SAM-e also aids liver detoxification.

Hormonal Imbalances

Depression associated with PMS, pregnancy, the aftermath of childbirth and menopause is typically hormonally related. An herb that is often helpful in these cases is black cohosh. It is also a good antidepressant for women who feel trapped or anyone who feels like they are wrestling with darkness, like the cartoons with the "black cloud" following a person around. Damiana is another mood elevator, which can treat depression in both men and women caused by low reproductive hormones.

Seasonal Depression

Many people get depressed in winter, a condition known as Seasonal Affective Disorder. One of the causes of this may be a lack of vitamin D3, which is produced in the skin in response to sunlight. Taking 2000 IU of vitamin D3 daily can cause significant improvement in seasonal depression. Calendula and St. John's wort may also helpful for seasonal depression.

Grief and Loss

When depression is due to a recent tragedy in one's life, such as the death of a loved one, breakup of a relationship, loss of a job or other difficulties, remedies for grief will be helpful. Lemon balm is a good herb for lifting depression associated with grief. Roses also have a heart-healing effect in depression brought on by grief. Rose can be used as a tincture or glycerite of the petals, a flower essence or used in aromatherapy. Two of the best remedies for depression brought on by sadness are mimosa and albizia. These have a very uplifting effect on a broken heart.

Age-Related Depression

As a person ages, they may become depressed. This may be associated with dementia or the early stages of Alzheimer's disease. Ginkgo has been helpful for this type of depression. Ginseng and gotu kola may also be helpful. All of these herbs are common key ingredients in *Brain and Memory Tonic Formulas.*

Getting off Antidepressants

For individuals who have already been subject to synthetic antidepressants, it is essential that you wean yourself gradually from these drugs while transitioning to other therapies. Sometimes the sudden loss of said chemicals can contribute to a deeper and more disturbing condition for the depression sufferer. This should ideally be done under professional supervision.

While transitioning, it is vital to keep the bowel and liver in good condition in order to aid in the elimination of wastes and to support the rest of the body with a good diet and good health habits. A remedy that may be helpful in transitioning is 5-HTP. As a precursor to serotonin, 5-HTP aids in balancing mood and regulating sleep patterns. It can up-regulate serotonin levels in a manner similar to SSRIs.

Therapies: Affirmation and Visualization, Colon Cleanse, Deep Breathing, Exercise, Friendly Flora, Gut Healing Diet, Healthy Fats, Hydration, Low Glycemic Diet and Stress Management

Formulas: Antidepressant, Relaxing Nervine, Adaptogen, Adrenal Tonic, Gentle Laxative, General Detoxifying, Hypothyroid, Liver Tonic and Brain and Memory Tonic

Key Herbs: Bupleurum, Calendula, **Ashwaganda**, **Black Cohosh**, **Borage**, **Damiana**, **Mimosa (Albizia, Silk Tree)**, **Rose flower essence**, Eleuthero (Siberian ginseng), Ginkgo, Ginseng (American), Ginseng (Asian, Korean), Gotu kola, Kava-kava, Lemon Balm, Motherwort, Muira Puama, Oat seed (milky), Passionflower and St. John's wort

Key Nutrients: 5-HTP, Folate (Folic Acid, Vitamin B9), L-Glutamine, Melatonin, Vitamin D, Vitamin B-6 (Pyridoxine), **Vitamin B-12**, Vitamin B-3 (Niacin), **SAM-e**, Omega-3 Essential Fatty Acids, **Magnesium**, Probiotics, Omega-3 Essential Fatty Acids, Betaine Hydrochloric Acid (HCl), DHA and Iron

Dermatitis

See also *Diaper Rash, Eczema, Hypothyroid, Poison Ivy or Oak* and *Rashes and Hives*

Inflammation of the skin is known as dermatitis. Although this problem may be the result of the skin being exposed to an irritant (such as exposure to poison ivy), it is often a sign of deeper health issues, particularly with the colon and liver. Eczema is a form of chronic dermatitis.

Traditional herbal remedies for diseases involving irritation to the skin include *Blood Purifier Formulas.* These formulas contain herbs like burdock, red clover and yellow dock, which have been used to "clean up" the internal environment of the body (blood and lymph) to reduce irritation to the skin.

Essential fatty acids are very important to healthy skin, and deficiencies can lead to irritation and dryness of the skin. Lack of bile flow can also be the cause of a lack of fatty acids to keep the skin smooth and moist. *Cholagogue Formulas* stimulate the flow of bile and aid the digestion of fats. Lipase enzyme supplements may also help with fat metabolism. Since the thyroid is involved in fat metabolism, low thyroid may also be a contributing factor in skin problems.

Topical Vulnerary and *Anti-Itch Formulas* may also be helpful for dermatitis. See related conditions for more suggestions.

Therapies: Aromatherapy, Colon Cleanse, Epsom Salt Bath, Fresh Fruits and Vegetables, Friendly Flora, Healthy Fats and Stress Management

Formulas: Blood Purifier, Cholagogue, Topical Vulnerary, Anti-Itch and **Skin Healing**

Key Herbs: Chamomile (English and Roman), Coptis (Chinese Goldenthread), **Aloe vera**, **Yucca**, Gotu kola,

Grindelia (Gumweed), Milk Thistle, Nettle (Stinging), Oregon Grape, Pau d' Arco, St. John's wort and Wild Yam

Key Nutrients: Pantothenic Acid (Vitamin B5), Omega-3 Essential Fatty Acids, MSM, Probiotics, Vitamin B-12, Vitamin C, Zinc, Lipase Enzymes, Vitamin A and Vitamin D

Diabetes

See also *Cardiovascular Disease (Heart Disease)*, *Hyperinsulinemia (Metabolic Syndrome* and *Syndrome X)*

Diabetes is a problem with insulin, a hormone produced by the pancreas that enables the cells of the body to utilize glucose or "blood sugar"—their major source of fuel. There are two types of diabetes.

In Type I (insulin dependent) diabetes, the pancreas has been damaged or destroyed and doesn't produce the necessary insulin. It is believed that this damage is the result of an autoimmune response. Insulin production may be as low as 4 units (versus the normal 31) in this type of diabetes. People with Type I diabetes must have regular insulin shots and constant monitoring of insulin levels to keep them as close to the normal 31 as possible. Supplements that reduce insulin resistance can reduce the need for insulin in this type of diabetes, but they will not restore normal pancreatic function.

In Type II (insulin resistant) diabetes, the pancreas has no trouble producing insulin. The problem is that the cells of the body develop resistance to insulin, so the pancreas produces more insulin in order to overcome the cells' resistance. Insulin levels may exceed 100 units (versus the normal 31). Type II develops slowly, over the course of years. It is really a long-term, severe case of Hyperinsulinemia, also known as Metabolic Syndrome or Syndrome X.

Insulin or oral hypoglycemic medications may be necessary to stabilize a Type II diabetic, but changes in lifestyle and nutrition can stabilize and even cure this condition.

Both types of diabetics should avoid high glycemic carbohydrates and eat a diet with a balanced intake of fats, proteins and low glycemic carbohydrates. Exercise and weight loss are also very helpful in overcoming insulin resistance in cells. *Blood Sugar Reducing Formulas* containing herbs like bitter melon, nopal, devil's club, huckleberry, cinnamon and jambul can reduce insulin resistance. This can reduce the need for insulin or other drug medications.

There are a number of nutrients that help overcome insulin resistance and can be helpful in Type II diabetes. Chromium, zinc and vanadium are all important minerals for blood sugar regulation. Omega-3 essential fatty acids help membranes become more permeable to insulin and sugar. Alpha lipoic acid has also been helpful in lowering insulin resistance in diabetics.

To get blood sugar under control rapidly, go on a temporary diet of nothing but non-starchy vegetables like zucchini, beans, leafy greens like chard and turnip greens, onions and so forth, while taking *Blood Sugar Reducing Formulas* and nutrients. Once blood sugar levels have stabilized, one can start to gradually introduce high quality fats and animal proteins back into the diet. All starchy and sugary foods, however, should be strictly avoided, including fruits, grains, potatoes, carrots and beets.

After a few months on this diet it may be possible to reintroduce whole grains, whole fruits and starchy vegetables back into the diet, but all refined sugars and grain products should continue to be strictly avoided. *Adaptogen Formulas* can also be used during this dietary transition to help stabilize the glands.

Since diabetes also involves a deterioration of circulation, herbs that help cardiovascular disease are also important in diabetes. *Antioxidant* and *Cardiovascular Stimulant Formulas* are very helpful to diabetics. Single herbs like garlic, hawthorn and ginkgo can reduce circulation-related side effects.

Diabetes is a serious disorder. So, seek appropriate medical assistance and monitor the condition regularly.

Therapies: Affirmation and Visualization, Dietary Fiber, Exercise, Fresh Fruits and Vegetables, Gut Healing Diet, Healthy Fats, Low Glycemic Diet and Stress Management

Formulas: Blood Sugar Reducing, Adaptogen, Antioxidant and Cardiovascular Stimulant

Key Herbs: Bilberry (Blueberry, Huckleberry), **Bitter Melon**, **Cinnamon**, **Devil's Club**, **Nopal (Prickly Pear)**, Fenugreek, Garlic, Ginkgo, Ginseng (American), Ginseng (Asian, Korean), Goldenseal, Gymnema, Hawthorn, Holy Basil, Jambul, Maitake, Olive and Thuja

Key Nutrients: Alpha Lipoic Acid, Chromium, L-Carnitine, Vitamin B-12, Vitamin B-3 (Niacin), Vitamin B-6 (Pyridoxine), Omega-3 Essential Fatty Acids, MSM, **Magnesium**, DHEA, DHA, Co-Q10, **Vitamin D**, Zinc, Fiber, Betaine Hydrochloric Acid (HCl) and Proanthocyanidins

Diabetic Retinopathy

See also *Diabetes*

Diabetic retinopathy is caused by damage to the retina due to complications of diabetes. Antioxidants can help to prevent and possibly heal this condition. Some of the best remedies to consider include bioflavonoids and vitamin C, alpha lipoic acid, proanthocyanidins, and bilberries. Good fats may also be helpful. Consider an *Antioxidant Formula* or a *Vision Supporting Formula*.

Therapies: Fresh Fruits and Vegetables, Healthy Fats and Low Glycemic Diet

Formulas: Antioxidant and **Vision Supporting**

Key Herbs: Bilberry (Blueberry, Huckleberry) and Ginkgo

Key Nutrients: Bioflavonoids, **Vitamin C**, Proanthocyanidins, **Alpha Lipoic Acid** and **Omega-3 Essential Fatty Acids**

Diaper Rash

See also *Dermatitis*

Diaper rash is a form of contact dermatitis (inflammation of the skin) that is common in infants and young children where there is prolonged exposure to urine-soaked or soiled diapers and the chemicals found in disposable diapers.

Apply a *Topical Vulnerary* salve when changing diapers to prevent diaper rash. You can also soothe diaper rash by applying aloe vera gel to the rash or sprinkling slippery elm powder into the fresh diaper when changing. Be sure to change diapers promptly after a child wets or soils them.

A fiery-looking diaper rash is typically caused by yeast infections. The infant may also have thrush. Probiotics are beneficial in this case. Open the capsules and put the sweet tasting powder into the baby's mouth. Probiotic powder can also be sprinkled in the diaper to help prevent diaper rash. *Antifungal Formulas* may be helpful in this case.

Therapies: Friendly Flora

Formulas: Topical Vulnerary and Antifungal

Key Herbs: Aloe vera, Cornsilk, **Calendula** and **Slippery Elm**

Key Nutrients: Probiotics and Chlorophyll

Diarrhea

See also *Giardia*, *Infection (bacterial)*, *Inflammatory Bowel Disorders (Colitis, IBS)* and *Parasites (general)*

Excessively loose, watery and frequent bowel movements are a sign that the bowels are trying to eliminate toxic irritants. The best approach to treating this condition naturally is to use agents that absorb toxins in the digestive tract such as *Fiber Blend Formulas*. For severe diarrhea, activated charcoal is the best choice. Be careful not to use too much activated charcoal, however, as it is so effective it can actually cause constipation. For diarrhea in infants, slippery elm or marshmallow are good choices. You can also use an *Anti-Diarrhea Formula*.

When diarrhea is extremely watery, astringents may be needed to tone bowel tissue and halt fluid loss. Some of the herbs that can be used for this purpose include blackberry root, bayberry or white oak bark, although almost any astringent may help.

For diarrhea caused by infectious organisms, garlic and goldenseal are good antimicrobial remedies that can be helpful. Look for an *Antibacterial Formula* with these herbs as primary ingredients.

Diarrhea may also be due to parasites or giardia. So, if diarrhea develops after foreign travel or drinking possibly contaminated water, get checked for parasites. *Antiparasitic Formulas* are needed if parasites are a problem. However, many times antiparasitic herbs may not be strong enough and antiparasitic drugs may be needed.

Probiotics can be helpful for both treating and preventing diarrhea from infectious microbes. When traveling, taking digestive enzyme supplements or *Digestive Enzyme Formulas* and probiotics can help prevent diarrhea.

Constant diarrhea is a symptom of inflammation in the bowels. Diarrhea alternating with constipation can be a sign of poor digestion and/or a spastic colon. In the case of a spastic colon, magnesium may be helpful. For poor digestion use *Digestive Enzyme* and/or *Digestive Tonic Formulas*.

After a bout with diarrhea it is always good to take probiotics as well as minerals to replace lost mineral electrolytes. If diarrhea is severe or persistent, seek medical attention.

Therapies: Friendly Flora and Gut Healing Diet

Formulas: Anti-Diarrhea, Fiber Blend, Antibacterial, Digestive Enzyme, Digestive Tonic and Antiparasitic

Key Herbs: Agrimony, Atractylodes, Bayberry root bark, Boswellia, Cherry (Wild), Cinnamon, Clove, Codonopsis, **Andrographis**, **Blackberry root**, **Goldenseal**, **Red Raspberry**, **Slippery Elm**, **Yellow**

Dock, Erigeron (Fleabane), Garlic, Ginger, Irish moss, Jambul, Kudzu, Lady's Mantle, Marshmallow, Myrrh, Psyllium, Shatavari, Thuja, White Oak and Wild Yam

Key Nutrients: Charcoal (Activated), Zinc, Vitamin B-3 (Niacin), **Probiotics**, Potassium, Magnesium, Bromelain, Colloidal Minerals and Fiber

Dieting

See *Weight Loss (aids for)*

Digestion (poor)

See also *Hiatal Hernia* and *Wasting*

Poor digestion leads to an inability to properly break down food into usable nutrients. Symptoms include pain, bloating, gas, cramping and/or heartburn. This is usually due to a deficiency of stomach acid or digestive enzymes. When poor digestion becomes chronic and severe it can lead to weight loss, an inability to develop muscle mass, wasting, pallor and fatigue.

Taking digestive enzyme supplements is the first step towards correcting this problem. *Digestive Enzyme Formulas* are a good place to start. It is also a good idea to try to stimulate the body's natural digestive secretions. *Digestive Tonic* or *Digestive Bitter Tonic Formulas* can help with this. When a person is elderly, herbs like American ginseng, saw palmetto, licorice root and astragalus can help to restore good digestion when taken with digestive enzyme supplements.

Chronically poor digestion may be caused by a hiatal hernia. This is a mechanical and stress-related problem that needs to be fixed before digestive powers can be restored.

It takes water to digest food, especially proteins, so if you are dehydrated digestion will be poor. Try drinking two glasses of water and taking a pinch of salt 20-30 minutes prior to meals.

Therapies: Gall Bladder Flush, Hiatal Hernia Correction and Hydration

Formulas: Digestive Enzyme, Digestive Bitter Tonic and Digestive Tonic

Key Herbs: Astragalus, Atractylodes, Blue Vervain, Chamomile (English and Roman), **Dandelion**, **Gentian**, **Oregon Grape**, Ginseng (American), Goldenseal, Horehound, Horseradish, Marshmallow, Orange Peel, Papaya, Rosemary, Safflowers, Saw Palmetto and Turmeric

Key Nutrients: Lactase Enzymes, Bromelain, Protease Enzymes, Probiotics, Magnesium, **Digestive Enzymes**, Colloidal Minerals and Lipase Enzymes

Diphtheria

See also *Contagious Diseases*

Diphtheria is an infectious disease caused by a bacteria (*Corynebacterium diphtheriae*) that affects mucus membrane linings. The microorganism produces a toxin that causes degeneration of the nerves, heart and other tissues. Diphtheria can cause anemia and fatigue if left untreated and may result in high levels of toxicity. It is important to stay hydrated to flush toxins. An inhalation of moist steam with a small amount of essential oils for the respiratory system, such as pine or eucalyptus, may also be helpful. It is wise to seek medical attention. Since this is a bacterial infection, *Antibacterial* and *Goldenseal & Echinacea Formulas* may be helpful.

Therapies: Hydration and Sweat Bath

Formulas: Antibacterial and Goldenseal & Echinacea

Key Herbs: Black Cohosh, Blue Vervain, Cordyceps, **Echinacea**, **Garlic**, Lobelia and Pine (White) essential oil

Key Nutrients: Colloidal Silver

Disks (bulging or slipped)

See also *Backache (Back Pain, Lumbago)*

Problems with spinal disks are often due to poor posture, incorrect lifting and other mechanical stresses. Chiropractic care, improved posture and stretching exercises can be helpful.

Goldenseal extract can be applied topically over the spine to help disks heal. *Topical Analgesic Formulas* can also be applied to the back where there are disk problems to ease pain. *Joint Healing Formulas* may also be used to promote healing.

Therapies: Mineralization and Stress Management

Formulas: Topical Analgesic and Joint Healing

Key Herbs: Boswellia, **Solomon's Seal**, Goldenseal, Lobelia, Thyme, Turmeric and Willow

Key Nutrients: MSM, Chlorophyll, Vitamin A, Vitamin D, Digestive Enzymes and **Bromelain**

Dislocation

A dislocation is the displacement of a body part, such as an internal organ or the bones in a joint, from its proper position. Dislocations should be mechanically corrected by a professional therapist, but *Joint Healing Formulas* and *Tissue Healing Formulas* can be taken internally to speed healing. herbal *Analgesic Formulas* and *Anti-Inflammatory Formulas* may be helpful for easing pain. If the area is accessible to topical applications, you can use a *Poultice Formula*, *Topical Analgesic Formula* and/or *Topical Vulnerary Formula* using the Poultice or Compress therapies.

Therapies: Compress, Mineralization and Poultice

Formulas: Joint Healing, Tissue Healing, Analgesic, Anti-Inflammatory, **Topical Analgesic**, Topical Vulnerary and Poultice

Key Herbs: Solomon's Seal, Lobelia and Mullein

Key Nutrients: MSM

Diverticulitis (Diverticuli)

See also *Inflammatory Bowel Disorders (Colitis, IBS)*

Diverticuli are abnormally formed pockets in the bowel. When they become inflamed, the afflicted person has diverticulitis.

Fiber Blend Formulas can be very helpful for diverticuli. Very soft fibers like marshmallow and slippery elm are preferred over fibers like bran and psyllium. Make sure to drink plenty of water and stay well hydrated while taking the fiber. When diverticuli are inflamed (diverticulitis) it is best to avoid fiber and use Intestinal Toners. *Gentle Laxative Formulas* may be used to help keep the stool soft and moving properly, but *Stimulant Laxative Formulas* should be avoided with diverticulitis.

Anti-Inflammatory Formulas or herbs like chamomile and cat's claw can reduce irritation in diverticulitis. Black walnut and cat's claw can help to tone and strengthen the bowel tissue. Medical attention is required in severe cases.

Therapies: Dietary Fiber and Hydration

Formulas: Fiber Blend, **Intestinal Toning**, Gentle Laxative and Anti-Inflammatory

Key Herbs: Chamomile (English and Roman), **Black Walnut**, **Cats Claw (Uña de Gato, Gambier)**, Ginger, Marshmallow, Slippery Elm and Wild Yam

Key Nutrients: Probiotics, Fiber and Omega-3 Essential Fatty Acids

Dizziness (Vertigo)

See also *Circulation (poor)* and *Hypoglycemia*

A loss of the sense of balance, vertigo can be caused by an ear infection or damage to the inner ear. Other possible causes include poor circulation, low blood sugar and nerve damage. Seek professional help to determine the cause.

The remedies that help will depend on the cause. Possibilities to consider include ginger, ginkgo biloba, licorice root, he shou wu and *Adaptogen Formulas*. In some cases, *Brain and Memory Tonic Formulas* might help.

Therapies: Low Glycemic Diet and Stress Management

Formulas: Adaptogen and Brain and Memory Tonic

Key Herbs: Black Cohosh, Cordyceps, **Ginger**, **Ginkgo**, Eleuthero (Siberian ginseng), Gotu kola, Hawthorn, He Shou Wu (Ho Shou Wu, Fo-Ti), Licorice, Linden, Mistletoe and Peppermint

Key Nutrients: Vitamin B-12, Omega-3 Essential Fatty Acids, L-Glutamine and Vitamin B-Complex

Down Syndrome

Down Syndrome is a genetic defect characterized by slow physical development and moderate to severe mental retardation. We are not aware of any cures for Down Syndrome, but some of the basic supplements and therapies mentioned in the Introduction may be helpful in promoting better overall health and improving comorbid conditions in someone with Down Syndrome.

Therapies: Fresh Fruits and Vegetables, Friendly Flora and Mineralization

Formulas: Digestive Enzyme, Digestive Bitter Tonic and Adaptogen

Key Herbs: Ashwaganda, Ginseng (American), Ginseng (Asian and Korean)

Key Nutrients: Omega-3 Essential Fatty Acids, Co-Q10, Vitamin B-Complex and Probiotics

Dropsy

See *Edema (Dropsy, Water Retention, Swelling)*

Drug Detox or Withdrawal

See *Addictions (drugs)*

Duodenal Ulcers

See also *Ulcers*

An ulceration of the first part of the small intestine. *Ulcer Healing Formulas* can be helpful. See Ulcers for more suggestions.

Therapies: Dietary Fiber

Formulas: Ulcer Healing

Key Herbs: Aloe vera and **Licorice**

Dysentery

See also *Diarrhea*

Dysentery is a severe form of diarrhea characterized by frequent watery stools, often with blood and mucus. Symptoms include pain, fever and dehydration. See *Diarrhea* for more information.

Therapies: Dietary Fiber, Friendly Flora and Hydration

Key Herbs: Bayberry, Coptis (Chinese Goldenthread), **Blackberry root**, **Goldenseal**, Garlic, Kudzu, Psyllium, Quassia, Slippery Elm bark and White Oak bark

Key Nutrients: Probiotics and **Charcoal (Activated)**

Dysmenorrhea (Painful Menstruation)

See also *Cramps (menstrual)* and *PMS (general)*

Painful menstruation or pain during menses is called dysmenorrhea. Native people felt that cramping is nature's way of exercising muscles for childbirth, so minor cramping was considered normal. For excessive pain, remedies that decongest pelvic circulation or relax muscle spasms can be helpful.

As a general remedy for menstrual problems consider using a *Female Hormonal Balancing* or a *PMS Relieving Formula*. Also follow the Avoid Xenoestrogens therapy and stay adequately hydrated.

When pain is dull, it is probably congestive pain caused by a lack of good blood flow in the pelvic region. Pelvic decongestants will help. Two of the best herbs for this purpose are ginger and yarrow. The Castor Oil Pack therapy can be used over the lower abdomen to ease congestive pain.

Liver congestion is often involved in congestive menstrual pain. Formulas that encourage liver detoxification like *Liver Tonic* or *Blood Purifier Formulas* may be helpful.

When the pains are sharp and cramping they are probably due to muscle spasms. Antispasmodics such as black cohosh, kava kava, lobelia and wild yam can be helpful. Magnesium is also helpful for menstrual cramping. Use a *Menstrual Cramp* or *Antispasmodic Formula*. Peppermint, clary sage and lavender essential oils applied topically will also help spasmodic pain.

Dysmenorrhea can also be due to unresolved emotional trauma such as rape, sexual abuse or shame surrounding menstrual functions. Flower Essences and Emotional Healing Work may be necessary when this has been the case.

Therapies: Aromatherapy, Avoid Xenoestrogens, Colon Cleanse, Emotional Healing Work, Flower Essences, Fresh Fruits and Vegetables and Hydration

Formulas: Female Hormonal Balancing, **Menstrual Cramp**, PMS Relieving, Antispasmodic, Liver Tonic and Blood Purifier

Key Herbs: Black Haw, Blue Cohosh, Chastetree (Vitex), **Black Cohosh**, **Cramp Bark**, **Jamaican Dogwood**, **Wild Yam**, Dong Quai, False Unicorn (Helonias), Ginger, Ginseng (Asian, Korean), Kava-kava, Lavender, Lavender essential oil, Lobelia, Milk Thistle, Myrrh, Partridge Berry (Squaw Vine), Passionflower, Peppermint essential oil and Yarrow

Key Nutrients: Bromelain, SAM-e and **Magnesium**

Dyspepsia

See also *Gastritis*, *Indigestion* and *Small Intestinal Bacterial Overgrowth (SIBO)*

Impaired gastric function due to some disorder of the stomach is called dyspepsia. Symptoms include pain and sometimes nausea or burning. herbal *Antacid Formulas* may be helpful for temporary relief of burning pains. *Carminative Formulas* may be helpful in easing belching or intestinal gas. *Digestive Bitter Tonic Formula* are very helpful for this condition and should be taken 15-20 minutes prior to meals with one or two large glasses of water.

Therapies: Hiatal Hernia Correction and Hydration

Formulas: Antacid, Carminative, **Digestive Bitter Tonic** and **Catnip & Fennel**

Key Herbs: Alfalfa, Aloe vera, Angelica, Chamomile (English and Roman), **Catnip**, **Fennel**, Fenugreek, Garlic, Ginger, Goldenseal, Jambul, Papaya and Thyme

Key Nutrients: Calcium, Probiotics, Omega-3 Essential Fatty Acids, Magnesium, Digestive Enzymes, Vitamin B-Complex and **Betaine Hydrochloric Acid (HCl)**

Ear Infection or Earache

See also *Allergies (food), Fungal Infections (Yeast Infections* and *Candida albicans)*

An earache is the result of inflammation, often due to infection in the ear. The irritation or infection can happen in the outer ear canal (otitis externa or swimmer's ear), in the middle ear behind the eardrum (otitis media) or in the inner ear (otitis interna). An inner ear infection causes the sudden onset of vomiting, vertigo, and loss of balance.

Children are more prone to earaches than adults. Part of the reason that children are prone to ear infections is that their ear passages are small, so an amount of fluid/mucus that would not cause a problem in an adult can cause severe problems in a child.

There is evidence that ear infections are often allergy induced. The allergy is usually toward cow's milk and/or an infant formula, but wheat is another common allergen. The allergy causes irritation to the mucous membranes, which results in swelling. This causes constriction of the Eustachian tube, a tube between the middle ear and the throat. This tube allows for equalization of pressure on both sides of the eardrum and for drainage of fluid from the inner ear. When this tube is swollen, pressure builds up in the inner ear and causes pain.

Antibiotics are typically used to treat ear infections, but they are often ineffective and contribute to problems in the intestinal tract that weaken the immune system and create more lymphatic stagnation. Thus, antibiotics perpetuate the tendency toward earaches.

Parents are often afraid to treat earaches naturally for fear that the ear infection will cause permanent hearing loss. This is simply not the case. There is no scientific evidence that antibiotics do anything for 99% of people with ear infections but can in 1% of the population shorten the duration of pain and infection. The trade off, however, is normally more frequent earaches.

There are many very effective natural remedies for earaches and ear infections. Garlic oil is very effective for ear infections. Warm the oil to body temperature and place a few drops in the ear. You can also rub some of the oil down the side of the neck to improve lymphatic drainage. Even better, use one of the *Ear Drop Formulas*, which contain garlic mixed with other herbs like mullein flower and St. John's wort.

For adults or older children, cut a clove of raw garlic, put a little olive oil on it, and place it on the outside of the ear (sort of like a hearing aid). This will rapidly eliminate infection, stimulate lymphatic drainage and relieve the pain.

Another highly effective therapy is to bake or steam an onion and place a few drops of the onion juice into the ear. (Make certain it has cooled to body temperature first.) You can also cut the cooked onion in half and place it over the ear while it is still warm. In most cases, the onion or onion juice almost instantly relieves the pain and eases the inflammation and infection.

Essential oils like lavender, thyme and tea tree oil can be diluted in olive oil (1 drop of essential oil to 20 drops of olive oil) and used as ear drops. Lobelia is also useful as ear drops to reduce pain. Make sure that anything you put in the ear is warmed to body temperature first!

Where children have frequent ear infections, eliminate the possibility of food allergies and yeast infections. Eyebright is very effective at preventing the Eustachian tubes from swelling, or opening them after they are swollen. It is the herbal equivalent of tubes in the ears. The herb works best as a tincture of the fresh plant, but large doses of the dried powder may also be effective. Taken regularly, *Allergy-Reducing Formulas* that feature eyebright as a major ingredient can also be taken internally to reduce these reactions. Osha is another ingredient in these formulas that can be helpful in reducing the allergic reactions that cause earaches, especially when due to dairy products.

Internally, *Echinacea Blend* and *Goldenseal & Echinacea Formulas* can be used internally to help fight infection and reduce inflammation in earaches. Herbs that promote lymphatic drainage such as *Lymphatic Drainage Formulas* can also be helpful.

Therapies: Aromatherapy, Colon Cleanse, Eliminate Allergy-Causing Foods and Eliminate Gluten

Formulas: Ear Drop, Allergy-Reducing, Echinacea Blend, Goldenseal & Echinacea and Lymphatic Drainage

Key Herbs: Andrographis, **Eyebright**, **Garlic**, **Mullein flowers**, Echinacea, Lavender essential oil, Lobelia, Osha, Spilanthes, St. John's wort, Tea Tree essential oil and Thyme essential oil

Key Nutrients: L-Glutamine and Digestive Enzymes

Eczema

See also *Itching, Dermatitis, Leaky Gut Syndrome, Rashes and Hives* and *Skin Care (general)*

Eczema is a very common skin condition that usually involves a rash, itching, redness and flaking of the skin. Acute inflammation of the skin is known as dermatitis and usually occurs when the body comes in contact with an irritating substance (such as poison ivy). Eczema is a chronic form of dermatitis, or in other words, a chronic inflammation of the skin.

All inflammatory diseases happen when damaged cells release histamine and bradykinin into surrounding fluids. This causes capillary pores to dilate, allowing fluid and protein to enter the tissue spaces. Tissues become red, swollen, hot and painful. In both eczema and dermatitis, the skin becomes irritated, resulting in red and itchy skin.

In eczema, the skin is repeatedly irritated and inflamed which causes the upper layer of the skin (epidermis) to thicken as skin cells multiply rapidly. This creates a scaly effect on the surface of the skin. Oil glands become obstructed and the skin becomes dry. The scaly skin inhibits elimination through the skin, causing toxins to become trapped under the skin. This causes itching, which leads the person to scratch. Scratching breaks the epidermal layer so the skin develops a broken and cracked appearance.

Eczema is caused by the body being hypersensitive to certain irritants, so it is closely related to allergic asthma, hayfever and food allergies. These conditions are actually caused by an immune system that is overburdened with toxins. Simply put, the body is being overwhelmed by more irritants than it can effectively handle.

This may explain why children are extremely prone to eczema. Almost thirty percent of all newborn babies may develop this condition, which affects about one in eight young children. It often occurs on the scalp or the cheeks, but can spread over other parts of the body, making children itchy and miserable. Although 75% outgrow this condition by their mid-teens, we wonder if it disappears simply because their immune system is too depressed to manifest it. Adults who had eczema as children will remain prone to dry skin in later years and to occasional flare-ups of skin inflammation.

Diet can be very important in treating eczema. A good place to start is to avoid foods that are incompatible with your blood type. Some of the common allergenic foods that may contribute to skin irritation include wheat, dairy, corn, orange juice, coffee, black tea, soda pop and sugar.

Eczema is often treated medically with corticosteroid drugs that mimic the anti-inflammatory action of the adrenal hormone cortisol.

People with eczema often suffer from adrenal exhaustion (with a corresponding deficiency in the production of cortisol). This helps explain why excessive inflammation is present and why eczema can flare up under stress. Stress depletes the adrenals. This is why *Adrenal Tonic Formulas* may be useful for people with eczema.

So, along with using the techniques listed under the Stress Management therapy, you can use herbs that support adrenal function and have a cortisol-like action. Both licorice root and yucca have this effect. Licorice, however, should be avoided with weeping eczema.

Blood Purifier Formulas are a traditional herbal approach to conditions like eczema, especially when used in conjunction with good fats like omega-3. Look for blood purifiers that contain herbs like burdock, chickweed, dandelion, gotu kola, pau d'arco and red clover. If there are problems with fat metabolism, *Cholagogue Formulas* may be beneficial, too.

Fat soluble vitamins like A and D are often helpful along with good fats. Sometimes the thyroid is involved because the thyroid hormones are essential to fat metabolism. So, if there are signs of low thyroid, a *Hypothyroid Formula* may help. The seaweeds like kelp and dulse found in many of these formulas also have trace minerals that promote healthy skin.

Since eczema is a chronic form of dermatitis or skin inflammation, *Anti-Inflammatory Formulas* can also be helpful. *Allergy-Reducing Formulas* may also be helpful in blocking histamine reactions that are causing the skin inflammation.

Finally, eczema can have roots in the nervous system. Too much intellectual activity in the head, without enough engaging in artistic or physical activities can make one's neurosensory system over stimulated, a condition known as neurodermatitis. If eczema isn't responding to physical treatments, consider using flower essences and doing Emotional Healing Work, to balance out nervous system activity by healing unresolved emotional wounds. See *Skin Care (general)* for more information on the connection between the nervous system and the skin.

Therapies: Colon Cleanse, Dietary Fiber, Drawing Bath, Eliminate Allergy-Causing Foods, Emotional Healing Work, Fast or Juice Fast, Fresh Fruits and Vegetables, Friendly Flora and Healthy Fats

Formulas: Adrenal Tonic, **Blood Purifier**, Cholagogue, Hypothyroid, Anti-Inflammatory, Allergy-Reducing and **Skin Healing**

Key Herbs: Aloe vera, Black Walnut, Bloodroot, Blue Flag, Borage, Coptis (Chinese Goldenthread), **Burdock**, **Dandelion**, **Red Clover**, Gotu kola, Grindelia (Gumweed), Licorice, Myrrh, Nettle (Stinging), Pau d' Arco, Pleurisy Root, Poke Root, Turmeric, Violet and Yucca

Key Nutrients: Pantothenic Acid (Vitamin B5), **Omega-3 Essential Fatty Acids**, Colloidal Minerals, Digestive Enzymes, Vitamin B-Complex, Zinc and Betaine Hydrochloric Acid (HCl)

Edema (Dropsy, Water Retention, Swelling)

See also *Injuries* and *Congestive Heart Failure*

The first thing to try when a person has general edema is a *Diuretic Formula*. In choosing an appropriate formula, keep in mind that there are two major classes of diuretic herbs. The first are those that stimulate the kidneys to work harder. These could also be called irritating diuretics. Juniper berry is one of the stronger herbs in the class. Other stimulating diuretics include buchu and uva ursi. These formulas are contraindicated when the kidneys are inflamed.

Another class of diuretics are herbs that nourish and improve kidney function without stimulating kidney activity. These are known as non-irritating diuretics. They include nettles, goldenrod, dandelion leaf and cornsilk. These remedies are useful for kidney inflammation and problems where the kidneys are not filtering wastes from the body effectively.

In addition to selecting a *Diuretic Formula* that is appropriate for the situation, it's also helpful to use a *Lymphatic Drainage Formula*. This will help the lymphatics pull fluid out of the tissue spaces for elimination.

Believe it or not, drinking more water and using all natural sea salt can actually help to relieve water retention. Detoxification of the liver and bowel can also help. So, consider using *General Detoxifying Formulas* as well.

Tissues hold water when they are damaged through inflammation, so acute swelling is typically the result of some type of tissue injury, irritation or infection. See *Injuries* for information.

When water retention is more general and/or chronic, it is usually a problem with lymphatic drainage and kidney function, although it can also be a cardiac problem known as Congestive Heart Failure. In this case, medical assistance should be sought. Look up Congestive Heart Failure for information on helpful natural therapies.

Therapies: Exercise, Hydration and Mineralization

Formulas: Anti-Inflammatory, Tissue Healing, **Diuretic**, Lymphatic Drainage, Cardiac Tonic and General Detoxifying

Key Herbs: Cleavers (Bedstraw), Cornsilk, **Buchu**, **Dandelion leaf**, **Goldenrod**, **Juniper Berry**, **Nettle (Stinging)**, Hawthorn, Horsetail, Lady's Mantle, Parsley, Prickly Ash and Uva ursi

Key Nutrients: Potassium and Magnesium

Electromagnetic Pollution

In modern society, we are constantly exposed to electromagnetic radiation from computers, microwave ovens, radar, TV sets, digital clocks and other electrical items. Cell phones are another growing source of electromagnetic pollution. While the research is not yet clear, evidence suggests there may be a link between electromagnetic pollution and cancer.

Minimize your exposure to these energy fields by keeping digital clocks at least three feet away from your head while sleeping, keeping some distance between yourself and computers and TV sets (such as not using a laptop computer on your lap) and wearing a headset when using a cell phone.

There are a number of devices in the marketplace that are reported to help reduce the negative effects of electromagnetic pollution, such as Wayne Cook's Diodes. However, simply carrying a small magnet in your left pocket seems to have a similar effect.

If you are exposed regularly to electromagnetic pollution, make sure you get plenty of antioxidant nutrients. You can also take an *Immune Stimulating Formula* or use single herbs like bee pollen, cordyceps and barley grass. These remedies seem to boost the body's ability to deal with electromagnetic pollution.

Therapies: Fresh Fruits and Vegetables

Formulas: Immune Stimulating

Key Herbs: Barley, Cordyceps, **Bee Pollen** and Spirulina

Key Nutrients: Vitamin C

Emotional Sensitivity

See also *Adrenals (exhaustion, weakness or burnout)* and *Anxiety or Panic Attack*

Sometimes people feel overly sensitive emotionally. There are several reasons for this. The first, and most common, is a high level of stress that is depleting the adrenal glands. When this happens, this emotional sensitivity is coupled with feelings of fatigue, mental confusion, restless sleep, disturbed dreams and/or a loss of sex drive. In this case *Adrenal Tonic Formulas* will probably help. In more serious adrenal exhaustion, DHEA is a supplement to consider as well.

When a person is in a high state of anxiety, due to chronic stress, they will feel shaky inside and unable to cope with life. They may even tremble (that is, have shaky hands). *Adaptogen Formulas* reduce the output of stress hormones and can help a person feel less anxious and shaky and restore the feeling that they can cope with life. Using the techniques under the Stress Management therapy can also be helpful.

People with highly sensitive nervous systems may benefit from *Nerve Tonic Formulas*, increased mineral intake (particularly calcium, magnesium and potassium) and good fats in the diet (omega-3 essential fatty acids). If little things bother you a lot and you tend to fidget, fuss over details, worry about the small stuff and feel nervous a lot, use these nerve-enhancing remedies.

Kava kava is an excellent single herb for reducing anxiety, especially when a person has a lot of muscle tension. Chamomile is a good remedy for emotionally sensitive children (and sometimes adults), who make a lot of fuss over small things.

Women who are delicate and extremely sensitive may have excess estrogen. Balancing hormones with *Female Hormonal Balancing Formulas* containing chaste tree berries may help. Pulsatilla is often used as a homeopathic remedy for this as well.

Emotional sensitivity may be linked to feelings of excessive fear or the inability to stand up for oneself. Often this is linked to being abused as a child, which makes one hyper-vigilant and alert to danger. Emotional Healing Work and Flower Essences may be helpful in working on these unresolved emotional wounds.

Therapies: Emotional Healing Work, Flower Essences, Healthy Fats, Low Glycemic Diet, Mineralization and Stress Management

Formulas: Adaptogen, Adrenal Tonic and Female Hormonal Balancing

Key Herbs: Chamomile (English and Roman), **Ashwaganda**, **Pulsatilla**, Eleuthero (Siberian ginseng), Kava-kava and Wild Yam

Key Nutrients: Omega-3 Essential Fatty Acids, Calcium, **Magnesium**, Potassium, DHEA, Silicon and Pantothenic Acid (Vitamin B5)

Emphysema

See also *Chronic Obstructive Pulmonary Disorder (COPD)*

Emphysema is a chronic lung condition involving a loss of elasticity of the alveoli, the tiny air sacs in the lungs. It is usually caused by smoking. The alveoli eventually collapse, causing drowning in lung fluid. Symptoms include labored breathing, wheezing and a husky cough. This is a serious condition requiring appropriate medical assistance.

In addition to following a general program for improving health, a number of specific herbs may be helpful in emphysema. Mullein is very helpful when taken in doses

of about 6 capsules per day for at least six months. It has a slow, cumulative effect in helping the lungs become more moist and supple. Horsetail can also be used to help restore elasticity to lung tissue. Astragalus and cordyceps are Chinese herbs that are also very nourishing to the lungs and supportive of this condition. Look for *Lung and Respiratory Tonic Formulas* that contain these herbs.

Since there is a lot of structural damage to lung tissue in this condition, it may also be helpful to use remedies that help soothe and moisten tissue while promoting healing. Look for herbal *Mineral* or *Tissue Healing Formulas* that contain slippery elm, marshmallow, plantain, horsetail and nettles.

Antioxidants are also important for this condition. Consider *Antioxidant Formulas*, while increasing antioxidants in the diet. Also consider taking good fats (omega-3 supplements) and the fat soluble vitamins A and D.

Therapies: Affirmation and Visualization, Fresh Fruits and Vegetables, Healthy Fats, Heavy Metal Cleanse and Stress Management

Formulas: Lung and Respiratory Tonic, Mineral, Tissue Healing and Antioxidant

Key Herbs: Capsicum (Cayenne), Coltsfoot, **Horsetail**, **Mullein**, Echinacea, Fenugreek, Garlic, Grindelia (Gumweed), Licorice, Lobelia, Marshmallow, Plantain and Thyme

Key Nutrients: Co-Q10, Chlorophyll, **Omega-3 Essential Fatty Acids**, Vitamin A, Vitamin D and Pantothenic Acid (Vitamin B5)

Endometriosis

A common cause of pelvic pain, endometriosis is a disorder where endometrial tissue is found outside of the uterus. This tissue responds to hormonal changes in the menstrual cycle just like the uterine lining. It falls apart at the same time the uterine lining sheds, causing menstruation. This can cause internal bleeding that causes surrounding tissues to become swollen and inflamed. It may even cause scar tissue.

Medical treatment for endometriosis can range from using non-steroidal anti-inflammatory drugs (NSAIDs like ibuprofen) to ease the pain of surgically removing the endometrial tissue or undergoing a complete hysterectomy. Medical treatment can also involve using birth control pills or other synthetic progestins (progesterone-mimics) to counteract the estrogen stimulation of these tissues.

About 10 to 20 percent of adult women have endometriosis. No one is sure why this uterine tissue is growing outside the womb, but some researchers believe the high incidence of it may be due to the influence of xenoestrogens. Xenoestrogens are environmental chemicals that mimic the action of estrogen. This excess estrogen stimulation promotes the growth of estrogen-sensitive tissues such as the uterine lining and breasts.

So, the first thing women with endometriosis should do is follow the Avoid Xenoestrogens therapy.

Fat cells make estrogen, so if you are overweight, get on a program to lose weight. This will also reduce estrogen production.

Herbal remedies can help balance hormones, too. Chaste tree berries can help to normalize levels of estrogen and progesterone in the body by regulating hormones from the pituitary. Look for a Female Hormone Balancing Formula where chaste tree is a principle ingredient.

Because progesterone and estrogen compete for receptor sites (which is why synthetic progesterone is used by the medical community to treat endometriosis), women with endometriosis could try using progesterone creams to enhance progesterone levels. False unicorn also has a progesterone-like effect.

Supplements that break down excess estrogens in the liver, such as indole-3 carbinol, may also be helpful. A good *Blood Purifier* or *Liver Tonic Formula* may be helpful.

Endometriosis is often painful. In Chinese medicine pain is a symptom of blocked chi, and in this case it may also be thought of as blocked blood or blood stagnation. A very good therapy for easing the pain and breaking up the stagnation is the Castor Oil Pack. This topical application of castor oil boosts the immune system, reduces inflammation, pain and swelling and can help the body detoxify.

Because there is inflammation associated with endometriosis, an *Anti-Inflammatory Formula* may be helpful, especially when taken around the time of the period. An herbal *Analgesic Formula* may also be helpful for easing pain. Also, since this disease is characterized by abnormal tissue growth, a standardized extract of paw paw may also be helpful.

Medical science believes that endometriosis is incurable without surgery, but many women have found relief from this problem naturally by adopting a healthier diet, using appropriate supplements and working with their emotions and stress. Symptoms of endometriosis will disappear naturally with menopause, so even if natural means don't offer a complete cure, they may allow a woman to be symptom-free and maintain the integrity of her reproductive organs by avoiding drugs and surgery.

Therapies: Avoid Xenoestrogens, Castor Oil Pack, Colon Cleanse, Fresh Fruits and Vegetables and Healthy Fats

Formulas: Female Hormonal Balancing, Blood Purifier, Liver Tonic, Anti-Inflammatory and Analgesic

Key Herbs: Alfalfa, Bayberry, **False Unicorn (Helonias)**, Gentian, Pau d' Arco and Paw Paw

Key Nutrients: Omega-3 Essential Fatty Acids, Vitamin A, **Vitamin D** and Vitamin E

Endurance (lack of)

See also *Adrenals (exhaustion, weakness or burnout), Anemia, Fatigue, Hypothyroid* and *Nervous Exhaustion (Enervation)*

A lack of stamina and endurance can result from glandular imbalances such as low thyroid or adrenal weakness. It can also be due to anemia, stress, lack of sleep and poor metabolism. For starters, try *Energy-Boosting Formulas*. If this doesn't help, look through the related conditions to see what might be causing the problem or seek professional assistance in determining the underlying causes.

Therapies: Fresh Fruits and Vegetables, Hiatal Hernia Correction, Hydration, Low Glycemic Diet and Mineralization

Formulas: Energy-Boosting

Key Herbs: Bee Pollen, **Eleuthero (Siberian ginseng)**, **Ginseng (American)**, **Ginseng (Asian, Korean)**, Horny Goat Weed (Epimedium) and Licorice

Key Nutrients: Digestive Enzymes and Colloidal Minerals

Energy (lack of)

See *Fatigue*

Enteritis

See also *Inflammatory Bowel Disorders (Colitis, IBS)*

Enteritis is an inflammation of the intestines, often the ileum, marked by diarrhea. See *Inflammatory Bowel Disorders*.

Enuresis

See *Incontinence (urinary)*

Conditions

Environmental Pollution (protection from)

See also *Chemical Poisoning* and *Heavy Metal Poisoning*

Pollutants from the environment are a growing health concern. People who work in polluted areas or with toxic chemicals of any kind (dry cleaners, beauty salons, labs, etc.) should consider taking remedies to protect their body from these pollutants. *Hepatoprotective Formulas* containing herbs like milk thistle and schizandra will help the liver process these chemicals and protect the body from them. *Liver Tonic Formulas* may also be helpful.

Fiber Blend Formulas can also be taken to bind toxins in the digestive tract for elimination. It is also important to drink adequate amounts of pure water. A periodic cleanse (once or twice a year) using fiber and a *General Detoxifying Formula* is also helpful.

Therapies: Colon Cleanse, Dietary Fiber, Fresh Fruits and Vegetables, Friendly Flora, Healthy Fats and Hydration

Formulas: Liver Tonic, **Hepatoprotective**, Fiber Blend and General Detoxifying

Key Herbs: Milk Thistle, Lycium (Wolfberry, Gogi), Schisandra (Schizandra) and Turmeric

Key Nutrients: Alpha Lipoic Acid, Omega-3 Essential Fatty Acids, N-Acetyl Cysteine and Probiotics

Epilepsy

See also *Seizures*

Epilepsy refers to disorders marked by disturbed electrical rhythms of the central nervous system. Episodes of excess firing in the neurons may create convulsions or a clouding of consciousness.

If there has been a blow or other trauma to a person's head, a cranial adjustment may be helpful. This can relieve pressure on the brain.

GABA is an inhibitory neurotransmitter that calms brain activity. It may be helpful in some cases of epilepsy. *Brain Calming Formulas* may also be helpful. Good fats are also important for healthy brain function.

Appropriate professional help should be sought for this problem.

Therapies: Healthy Fats

Formulas: Brain Calming

Key Herbs: Blue Vervain, **Scullcap (Skullcap)**, Lobelia and Passionflower

Key Nutrients: GABA, **Magnesium**, **Omega-3 Essential Fatty Acids**, **Vitamin B-Complex** and **Vitamin B-12**

Epstein Barr Virus

See also *Chronic Fatigue Syndrome (CFS)*

Chronic infection with the Epstein-Barr virus creates severe lack of energy, lymphatic swelling, muscle aches and sleep disturbances. There is no magical treatment for this condition, but there are a number of types of herbal remedies that may assist in recovery.

First of all, because this is a viral condition, *Antiviral Formulas* may help the body get rid of the viral component. *Immune Stimulating Formulas* can boost immune responses and enhance energy levels, too. Important herbs to look for in these formulas include echinacea, lomatium, elderberry and cat's claw (una de gato).

It is very important with conditions like Epstein Barr to practice good general health practices, such as eating a healthy diet and getting adequate rest and relaxation. For sleep disturbances try herbal *Sleep Formulas*. Stress Management therapy may be necessary as it is very important to relax and give the body time to heal.

Various herbs can help with symptomatic relief as well. To reduce swollen lymph nodes, for instance, one can use *Lymphatic Drainage* or *Echinacea Blend Formulas*. For muscle aches, try herbal *Analgesic Formulas*. Since fatigue is a big part of the picture, *Energy-Boosting Formulas* may also be helpful.

Therapies: Affirmation and Visualization, Eliminate Allergy-Causing Foods, Healthy Fats and Stress Management

Formulas: Antiviral, Immune Stimulating, Lymphatic Drainage, Energy-Boosting, Echinacea Blend, Analgesic and Sleep

Key Herbs: Ashwaganda, Black Walnut, **Cats Claw (Uña de Gato, Gambier)**, **Lomatium**, Echinacea, Elder, Eleuthero (Siberian ginseng), Licorice, Maca, Mullein, Olive and Pau d' Arco

Key Nutrients: Probiotics, MSM, Magnesium, Digestive Enzymes, Pantothenic Acid (Vitamin B5) and Potassium

Erectile Dysfunction

See also *Arteriosclerosis (Atherosclerosis, Hardening of the Arteries)*, *Diabetes* and *Testosterone (low)*

Erectile dysfunction (ED) affects almost half of American males. When Viagra® was released, one million prescriptions were filled. But, there are natural alternatives to drugs like Viagra®.

It is important to understand that erections are dependent on a strong supply of blood to the penis. Narrow or clogged arteries cause insufficient supply of blood to produce an erection. One major cause of ED is arteriosclerosis of the penile artery.

Diabetes can also cause ED because high blood sugar levels cause narrowing of blood vessels. According to Dr. Hugo Rodier, M.D., candy, soda pop and other sugar-laden treats should come with a warning label—"Caution: May Cause Erectile Dysfunction."

Other possible causes of erectile dysfunction include exposure to xenoestrogens, side effects of pharmaceutical drugs and poor diet and lifestyle. In some cases ED may be due to relationship problems which require counseling.

A natural approach to the treatment of ED should start by checking all medications for warnings. Then, depending on the man's general health, it might include improving circulation, regulating blood sugar and/or balancing hormones with Male Reproductive Tonic Formulas.

If hardening of the arteries is a problem, use *Cardiovascular Stimulant Formulas* to increase circulation. Where high blood pressure is involved, *Hypotensive Formulas* may also be helpful.

A supplement that can be helpful for ED and hypertension is the amino acid, l-arginine. Five grams of l-arginine daily has helped many men with ED and high blood pressure.

If diabetes is a problem, reduce refined carbohydrates in the diet and eat more good quality fats. Take a good *Blood Sugar Reducing Formula*. Also consider taking chromium, magnesium and zinc.

Environmental estrogens or xenoestrogens are reducing male testosterone levels. Men who want to stay virile need to become aware of the sources of xenoestrogens and make efforts to minimize their exposure. They should also take remedies to enhance testosterone, such as *Male Aphrodisiac* or *Male Glandular Tonic Formulas* that contain herbs like ginseng, maca, muira puama, and tribulus.

Stress can cause temporary ED, so if a man is under a lot of stress, he may want to take some *Adaptogen Formulas* to reduce the output of stress hormones. He may also want to get some relationship counseling, use Flower Essences Therapy and/or do Emotional Healing Work.

Therapies: Avoid Xenoestrogens, Emotional Healing Work, Exercise, Flower Essences, Healthy Fats and Stress Management

Formulas: Cardiovascular Stimulant, Hypotensive, **Male Aphrodisiac**, Male Glandular Tonic, Blood Sugar Reducing and Adaptogen

Key Herbs: Ashwaganda, **Damiana**, **Horny Goat Weed (Epimedium)**, Eleuthero (Siberian ginseng), Ginkgo, Ginseng (American), Ginseng (Asian, Korean), Maca, Muira Puama, Nettle (Stinging) root, Rhodiola, Shatavari, Tribulus and Yohimbe

Key Nutrients: DHEA, **L-Arginine**, **Omega-3 Essential Fatty Acids**, Vitamin E, Zinc, Chromium and **Magnesium**

Estrogen (low)

See also *PMS Type D*

When a woman's estrogen levels are low, herbs may help to balance her hormones. Herbs and foods containing phytoestrogens may be helpful, which include soy and other beans and legumes, green leafy vegetables, whole grains, black cohosh, hops and licorice root. Look for *Female Hormonal Balancing* or *Phytoestrogen Formulas*. Bioidentical hormones may be necessary for severe cases.

Formulas: Female Hormonal Balancing and **Phytoestrogen**

Key Herbs: **Black Cohosh**, **Licorice**, Flax Seed and Red Clover

Key Nutrients: Vitamin B-6 (Pyridoxine)

Exercise

See also *Body Building*

Herbs can be a helpful adjunct to exercise programs. There are herbal formulas specifically formulated to support exercise programs. They are listed under herbal *Exercise Formulas*. However, there are other herbs that can help exercise, too.

Adaptogens have been shown to improve athletic performance and stamina, so consider a good *Adaptogen Formula* for enhancing your exercise program. Some *Energy-Boosting Formulas* may also be helpful during exercise. Men may benefit from *Male Glandular Tonic Formulas*, if the goal is to build greater muscle mass.

After exercise, *Topical Analgesic Formulas* can be used to relieve sore muscles. A tea made with safflowers will also help to neutralize lactic acid buildup and ease sore muscles.

Therapies: Healthy Fats, Hydration, Low Glycemic Diet and Mineralization

Formulas: Energy-Boosting, **Exercise**, Topical Analgesic, Male Glandular Tonic and Adaptogen

Key Herbs: Barley, Bee Pollen, **Cordyceps**, **Eleuthero (Siberian ginseng)**, Rhodiola and Safflowers

Key Nutrients: Omega-3 Essential Fatty Acids and Potassium

Eye Infections

See also *Conjunctivitis (Pink Eye)* and *Stye*

There are a number of herbs that can be helpful for eye infections, including goldenseal, eyebright and chamomile. One can make a tea out of any of these herbs or an herbal *Eye Wash Formula* and apply it as a compress, eye drops or an eyewash. Be sure to strain the tea thoroughly and allow it to cool before using it in the eyes.

Goldenseal & Echinacea Formulas taken internally can also be helpful. See related conditions for more suggestions.

Therapies: Compress

Formulas: Eye Wash and Goldenseal & Echinacea

Key Herbs: Chamomile (English and Roman), **Goldenseal** and Eyebright

Key Nutrients: Vitamin A

Eye Problems

See *Cataracts, Conjunctivitis (Pink Eye), Eye Infections, Eyes (red or itching), Glaucoma, Macular Degeneration* and *Stye*

Eyes (red or itching)

See also *Allergies (respiratory)* and *Rhinitis*

Eyes can become red due to stress or irritation. When they are red and itchy, it is typically an allergic reaction. An herbal *Eye Wash Formula* can be used topically to ease the redness. The alkaloids in goldenseal were once used in a popular over-the-counter eye drop that promised to take the redness away from tired and sore eyes. A chamomile or green tea bag can be used as a compress. For allergy-related problems see Rhinitis or Allergies (respiratory).

Therapies: Compress, Fresh Fruits and Vegetables, Hydration and Stress Management

Formulas: Eye Wash

Key Herbs: Chamomile (English and Roman), **Goldenseal**, Eyebright and Tea (Green or Black)

Key Nutrients: Vitamin A and Vitamin C

Eyesight

See also *Conjunctivitis (Pink Eye)* and *Eye Infections*

When we see something beautiful, we often think of it as a feast for the eyes, but the eyes also need proper nourishment from our diet. Eye health is not isolated from general health. In fact, most eye diseases are signs of deeper health problems, such as stress, free radical damage, diabetes and circulatory disorders. Poor nutrition plays a major role in creating the health problems that lead to a deterioration of eye health.

For instance, antioxidant nutrients that counteract free radical damage are essential to healthy eyes. Many eye disorders such as macular degeneration, cataracts and glaucoma are probably caused by free radical damage to the eyes. One cause of this damage can be the ultraviolet radiation present in natural light, but chemical toxins, cardiovascular inflammation and blood sugar problems are also contributing factors.

The beautiful colors of many fruits and vegetables are both pleasing and nourishing to the eyes. That's because the purples, yellows, greens, blues, reds and other bright colors found in the plant kingdom are signs of the presence of antioxidants. If you want to keep your eyes healthy, it is very important to "eat the rainbow" by including lots of brightly colored fruits and vegetables in your diet. You can also consider using antioxidant supplements.

Certain antioxidants called carotenoids are particularly critical to eye health. One of these is beta-carotene, which is a precursor to the formation of vitamin A. Two other carotenoids are also essential for healthy eyes. These are lutein and zeaxanthin. Lutein is a yellow pigment found in green leafy vegetables like kale, chard and spinach. It is also found in egg yolks and animal fats. Lutein is found in the macula (the center of the retina) and has been shown to counteract free radical damage caused by blue and ultraviolet light. It protects against macular degeneration and inhibits the formation of cataracts (the number one cause of blindness in the elderly). Zeaxanthin has similar properties. It is also a yellow pigment found naturally in green vegetables, eggs and yellow corn that protects the macula from light-damage. It also inhibits cataract formation.

Several antioxidant vitamins are also essential to eye health, including vitamins A, E and C. vitamin A is extremely critical to eye health. In fact, another name for vitamin A is retinol (showing its relationship to protecting the retina of the eye). A deficiency of vitamin A is known to cause blindness.

Vitamin A keeps fats in the eye from oxidizing and prevents the eye from dehydrating by helping with tear formation. Carrots are high in beta-carotene, the precursor to vitamin A, which explains why they have a reputation as being good for the eyes. However a few studies suggest that about 35% of people can't convert beta-carotene to vitamin A, so supplementing with vitamin A or Cod Liver Oil might be necessary.

Vitamin E is found in both the retina and the lens. Adequate intake of this fat-soluble vitamin reduces the risk of cataract formation. It also works with bioflavonoids to inhibit macular degeneration.

Vitamin C is also critical to eye health because it helps protect the capillaries nourishing the eye tissue. It reduces pressure in glaucoma (the second leading cause of blindness), reduces cataract formation and helps rebuild the cornea when it has been damaged.

Other antioxidants that protect the eyes include anthocyanidins, found in blueberries and bilberries, silymarian from milk thistle and quercitin from onions. The amino acid taurine is found in high quantities in the retina. It is depleted by diabetes and is low in vegan diets. It helps protect the retina against UV radiation.

The eyes, like the brain, need good fats to be healthy, too. Omega-3 essential fatty acids, especially DHA, are critical to eye health. DHA helps with communicating information from the eyes to the brain. Good fats also lubricate the eyes and keep them from drying out. The fat-soluble vitamins like A and E protect these fats from oxidation.

Poor nutrition isn't the only reason why eyesight deteriorates. Eyes need exposure to natural sunlight and artificial lighting plays a part in our diminishing eye health. Stress, and more particularly, eye strain, also plays a big role in vision problems.

In fact, the major reason myopia (nearsightedness) is becoming increasingly common is the amount of time people are spending doing close-up work like reading and working on computers. Constantly staring at these nearby objects strains the eyes, which need to regularly shift their focus from looking at nearby objects to objects in the distance, to stay relaxed. The eye strain caused by working at computer terminals and other close-up work creates muscle tension that inhibits the eyes from relaxing and seeing in the distance.

A final, but extremely important aspect of general eye health is protecting the eyes from injury. It is very important when working with chain saws, weed-eaters and other power tools to wear protective eye gear. About 2,000 cases of eye injury occur daily, and most of these could be prevented with protective eye wear.

Therapies: Compress, Fresh Fruits and Vegetables, Healthy Fats and Hydration

Formulas: Vision Supporting and Antioxidant

Key Herbs: Bilberry (Blueberry, Huckleberry), Hawthorn, Lycium (Wolfberry, Gogi) and Milk Thistle

Key Nutrients: Vitamin A, N-Acetyl Cysteine, **Zeaxanthin**, **Lutein**, **Vitamin C**, Vitamin E, Proanthocyanidins and DHA

Failure to Thrive

Failure to thrive is a problem when infants don't gain weight and develop properly. This is often a digestive problem, so changing the mother's diet (if nursing) or the infant's formula can be helpful. It may also help to mix a small amount of plant enzymes with food. A little bit of black strap molasses and some gruel made with slippery elm can also be beneficial.

Formulas: Digestive Enzyme

Key Herbs: Marshmallow and Slippery Elm

Key Nutrients: Lactase Enzymes, Omega-3 Essential Fatty Acids, DHA and **Digestive Enzymes**

Fat Cravings

See also *Gall Bladder (sluggish or removed)*

When a person craves fats constantly, he or she is probably not getting enough essential fatty acids in their diet, or not digesting and metabolizing fats correctly. The body needs good fats and, contrary to popular opinion, good fats are essential to health. Good fats include organic butter from grass-fed cows, coconut oil, olive oil, avocados, flax seeds, chia seeds, hemp seeds, walnuts, macadamias, deep ocean fish, and fat from grass-fed animals. *Digestive Enzyme* and *Cholagogue Formulas* can help the body digest fats better.

Therapies: Gall Bladder Flush and Healthy Fats

Formulas: Digestive Enzyme, **Cholagogue** and Digestive Bitter Tonic

Key Herbs: Barberry, **Chickweed**, **Fringe Tree**, Dandelion and Gentian

Key Nutrients: Omega-3 Essential Fatty Acids and Lipase Enzymes

Fat Metabolism (poor)

See also *Gall Bladder (sluggish or removed)*, *Hypothyroid*, *Weight Loss (aids for)* and *Fatty Liver Disease*

The inability to properly or adequately digest and assimilate lipid or fat-containing foods is common in individuals who have had their gallbladders removed. This is because the body no longer stores adequate amounts of bile, which is necessary to emulsify or break down fats.

There may also be a problem utilizing fats in the body. This is often associated with the liver, but can also be due to the thyroid, spleen, prostate or uterus. Having the uterus or prostate removed can create problems with fat metabolism, since these organs are involved in the production of hormones that help with the combustion of fats.

If you have a problem digesting fats, start by taking *Digestive Enzyme* or *Cholagogue Formulas*. You may also want to try the Gall Bladder Flush therapy. Lipase enzymes are especially important for digesting fats.

Low thyroid will cause problems with fat metabolism, so get your thyroid checked. If it is low, try a *Hypothyroid Formula*. You may also need thyroid medication.

Because the reproductive glands are involved in fatty acid metabolism, a *Liver Tonic Formula* may be beneficial. In particular, *Liver Tonic Formulas* containing burdock and chickweed can be particularly helpful.

Therapies: Gall Bladder Flush

Formulas: Digestive Enzyme, **Cholagogue**, Hypothyroid and Liver Tonic

Key Herbs: Burdock, Chickweed, Cinnamon, **Artichoke**, **Fringe Tree** and Stone Breaker

Key Nutrients: L-Glutamine, **Digestive Enzymes** and **Lipase Enzymes**

Fatigue

See also *Adrenals (exhaustion, weakness or burnout)*, *Anemia*, *Depression*, *Hashimoto's Disease (Thyroiditis)*, *Hypoglycemia*, *Hypothyroid* and *Insomnia*

Fatigue is a symptom that something is wrong with energy production in the body. Many systems are involved in energy production, so it is important to identify which systems need support. So, consider all the related conditions listed above.

For starters, you can try an *Energy-Boosting Formula* as a general aid. Remember, though, that using stimulants like caffeine or capsicum doesn't actually build energy. Stimulants cause the body to dip into its energy reserves, which means that over time, they deepen fatigue. It then takes more and more of the stimulant to have an effect. So, if you're tired, avoid stimulants and figure out what's causing the lack of energy and correct it.

One of the major causes of fatigue is a simple lack of sleep. The body rebuilds its energy reserves through rest. If we do not get 8-9 hours of sleep each night, we can wind up with a sleep debt that results in low energy levels. The person suffering from a lack of sleep further depletes their energy by using stimulants and a vicious cycle of energy loss ensues.

If you aren't getting enough sleep, use a *Sleep Formula* or look up Insomnia to learn how to enjoy a better night's rest. Furthermore, taking herbs that help you relax will increase your energy as relaxed muscles are able to store more energy. Tense muscles are exhausted muscles. Magnesium, kava kava and *Relaxing Nervine Formulas* can all be helpful here.

Another major cause of fatigue is low thyroid. When low thyroid is the problem, the person may be cold, have difficulty losing weight, and have problems with dry skin. *Hypothyroid Formulas* may be of help, but this problem may require other remedies. See Hypothyroid and *Hashimoto's Disease*.

When the adrenals are involved in the fatigue, the person may have symptoms like a quivering tongue, dark circles under their eyes and restless sleep. *Adrenal Tonic* or *Adaptogen Formulas* should be helpful. See Adrenals.

Low blood sugar will cause fatigue in the afternoons or sudden fatigue a few hours after eating. The nose or limbs will suddenly go cold and the person may have difficulty concentrating. Licorice root or *Energy-Boosting Formulas* may be of benefit here. Dehydration will also cause fatigue and increase the craving for sugary foods.

When the pituitary is out of balance, it will upset the general balance of the glandular system. Herbs that help the pituitary as a cause of fatigue include alfalfa, spirulina and bee pollen.

Anemia may also be a cause of fatigue. If you are pale and get cold or tired easily, try an *Iron Formula*. Sixty percent of Americans have a mild to severe B12 deficiency. This can create fatigue, insomnia, tingling in the fingers and toes and poor digestion.

When fatigue is accompanied by a run-down immune system, frequent infections and general weakness, *Immune Stimulating* and *Adaptogen Formulas* may be helpful.

Fatigue associated with depression may be resolved with *Antidepressant Formulas*. Fatigue after eating is an indication of poor digestion and the need for *Digestive Enzyme Formulas*.

Therapies: Fresh Fruits and Vegetables, Hydration and Low Glycemic Diet

Formulas: Hypothyroid, **Adaptogen**, **Adrenal Tonic**, **Energy-Boosting**, Iron, Immune Stimulating, Sleep, Antidepressant, Digestive Enzyme and Relaxing Nervine

Key Herbs: Capsicum (Cayenne), Codonopsis, Cordyceps, **Ashwaganda**, **Bee Pollen**, **Eleuthero (Siberian ginseng)**, Damiana, Ginseng (American), Ginseng (Asian, Korean), Gotu kola, Guarana, Jujube, Kelp, Maca, Muira Puama, Oat, Rhodiola and Spirulina

Key Nutrients: L-Carnitine, L-Glutamine, **Iron**, Vitamin B-6 (Pyridoxine), Vitamin B-3 (Niacin), Pantothenic Acid (Vitamin B5), Melatonin, Magnesium, Digestive Enzymes, Co-Q10, Chlorophyll, Vitamin C, 5-HTP, **Vitamin B-Complex** and **Vitamin B-12**

Fatty Liver Disease

The accumulation of fat in the liver of people who drink little or no alcohol is called nonalcoholic fatty liver disease. It is common and in most people causes no signs or symptoms. For some people, however, it can lead to inflammation, scarring of the liver and eventually liver failure. It is probably related to a diet of refined carbohydrates and processed oils. Essential fatty acid supplements should be avoided by people with fatty liver disease.

Some herbs that may be helpful in getting rid of fat in the liver include chickweed, milkweed and burdock. Look for Cholagogue, *Liver Tonic* and *Hepatoprotective Formulas* containing these herbs. Take these herbs with lipase enzyme supplements and *Fiber Blend Formulas* and go on the Low Glycemic Diet therapy. Supplementing with the amino acid choline and doing the Gall Bladder Flush therapy can also be helpful.

Therapies: Dietary Fiber, Fast or Juice Fast, Gall Bladder Flush, Gut Healing Diet and Low Glycemic Diet

Formulas: **Cholagogue**, Liver Tonic, Hepatoprotective and Fiber Blend

Key Herbs: Chickweed, **Burdock**, **Milk Thistle** and Stone Breaker

Key Nutrients: Digestive Enzymes, Iodine, **L-Carnitine** and Lipase Enzymes

Fatty Tumors or Deposits

See also *Fat Metabolism (poor)* and *Fatty Liver Disease*

These are abnormal growths that are mostly composed of lipid or fatty material. Herbs that have been used historically to break up these deposits include burdock, chickweed and red clover. *Blood Purifier Formulas* containing these herbs may be helpful.

Thyroid problems could also contribute to the development of these deposits. Consider *Hypothyroid Formulas*.

Digestive Enzyme and *Cholagogue Formulas*, which aid with digestion and metabolism of fats, may also be useful. Lipase enzyme supplements are also important.

Therapies: Gall Bladder Flush

Formulas: Blood Purifier, Hypothyroid, Digestive Enzyme and Cholagogue

Key Herbs: Burdock and **Chickweed**

Key Nutrients: Lipase Enzymes and **Iodine**

Fear (excessive)

See also *Adrenals (exhaustion, weakness or burnout)* and *Anxiety Disorders*

Fear is the emotion we feel when situations arise that we perceive have a great potential for pain or loss. Fear can arise from potentially painful or traumatizing situations, but it can also arise in positive situations where there is a lot at stake (such as starting a new relationship or a new business).

Fear strongly affects the systems that regulate body functions, such as the glandular system (particularly the adrenal glands and thyroid) and the nerves. It activates the parasympathetic nervous system and the adrenal glands to produce a heightened state of energy and tension. This response primes the body to be ready for optimal action, not just to "fight or flee," but to be able to physically perform to the best of our abilities.

In dangerous situations fear is a useful emotion. It can prompt us to be alert and careful and help us make choices that keep us safe.

However, some fears have no basis in any real danger. Children are born with only a few natural fears. Most fears are learned from parents and other adults. That is, children sense when their parents are afraid of something and they adopt the same fear. Many fears are rooted in experiences that wounded the person emotionally. For example, many adults are afraid of making mistakes because past mistakes caused them pain. Children have no such fear.

Any fear that is not based in an actual danger, that is, something that can cause you actual physical or psychological harm, is not a healthy fear. If other people are able to do something safely and it frightens you, then the fear is likely based in emotional wounds or unrealistic thought processes. These are the fears that people need to overcome if they want to improve their lives.

What overcomes these unhealthy fears is the ability to take action in spite of them. When the energy produced by the fear response is channeled into action, it fulfills its purpose and fuels us for maximum performance. Courage is the ability to take action in spite of our fear. Both the hero and the coward feel fear on the battlefield, but the hero is able to do what he needs to do in spite of his fear. Courage is the ability we have to allow our mind to override the anxiety and stress we feel, make the best choice we can, and then take appropriate action.

When the energy of fear is channeled into constructive action through exercising courage, it builds excitement and self-confidence. People who are able to overcome their fears and take calculated risks develop strong "wills," instead of "won'ts." These people develop the confidence that they can handle what life brings to them and rise above it. This allows them to lead more exciting lives, achieving the status of the "hero." Those who are unable to take action in the face of fear are allowing cowardice to keep them stuck in mediocrity.

The Flower Essences, Affirmation and Visualization, and Emotional Healing Work therapies can all help a person overcome unreasonable fears. Aromatherapy with essential oils like bergamot, frankincense, lavender, sandalwood and ylang ylang can also be helpful for calming fear.

Keeping blood sugar stable with the Low Glycemic Diet therapy also reduces fear. Staying well hydrated can help a person feel more relaxed in difficult circumstances, as dehydration interferes with brain function.

Interestingly, traditional systems of medicine associate fear with the kidneys. In Traditional Chinese Medicine, the water element is associated with fear and is connected to the kidneys, urinary bladder and adrenal glands. Because adaptogens calm stress hormones, they can also help to reduce fears. B-complex vitamins and vitamin C can help to reduce feelings of stress and fear, as well. In cases of long term stress, an *Adrenal Tonic Formula* may be helpful. *Kidney Tonic Formulas* may help.

Therapies: Affirmation and Visualization, Aromatherapy, Deep Breathing, Emotional Healing Work, Flower Essences, Hydration, Low Glycemic Diet and Stress Management

Formulas: Kidney Tonic, Adaptogen and **Adrenal Tonic**

Key Herbs: Chamomile (English and Roman), **Borage**, Ginseng (American), Lavender essential oil, Licorice and St. John's wort

Key Nutrients: Vitamin B-Complex, Vitamin C and GABA

Fever

See also *Infection (bacterial)* and *Infection (viral)*

Most of the time fevers are generated by the immune system as part of its effort to fight infection. Unless the fever is very high (104 or higher) or lasts more than a day or two, it is not a cause for serious concern.

In most cases, the fever will go down as soon as the bowel is cleared. This is most easily done by taking an enema. A solution of herbal tea or a liquid herbal product added to water will make the enema more effective.

There are also many herbs that can be used in the enema solution to make it more effective. *Catnip & Fennel Formulas*, yarrow, elderflower, peppermint, chamomile and garlic make good enema solutions for both children and adults.

Herbs that promote perspiration can also be used internally to bring down fevers. Ideally, these should be taken as warm teas or as extracts taken with warm water. Some of the herbs that have proven useful here include yarrow, peppermint, chamomile, catnip, ginger and capsicum. Yarrow is particularly helpful for serious fevers when taken in the form of a hot tea, but it tastes better when combined with peppermint and other more pleasant tasting herbs. You can also use a *Sudorific* or *Cold and Flu Formula* that contains these herbs as primary ingredients.

Boneset is a good herb for fever associated with the flu where the bones ache. Garlic (especially raw garlic) is another herb that can help with fevers, especially when caused by bacterial infection or respiratory infection.

Generally speaking, sour herbs like lemon, lycium (gogi or wolfberries), acai, mangosteen and elderberries, contain antioxidants that will reduce fever and inflammation in the body. So, you can also look for *Antioxidant Formulas* that have these sour tasting herbs in them.

Historically, white willow bark was used for fever and inflammation. It is a usually a major ingredient in herbal *Analgesic Formulas*, which may also be helpful for fevers accompanied by muscle aches and headaches. However, we do not recommend using willow to reduce fevers as this is actually suppressing immune activity that is fighting the infection.

Essential oils like chamomile, lemon, lavender, peppermint, rosemary and thyme, can be used topically as an aromatherapy application for fevers. Dilute them in water, then moisten a wash cloth with the aromatic water and gently sponge off the fevered person.

If the fever is high and does not respond to these remedies within a couple of hours, seek medical attention. Also seek medical attention for a persistent low fever or a fever that doesn't respond to natural remedies after a day or so.

Therapies: Aromatherapy, Colon Cleanse, Colon Hydrotherapy, Hydration and Sweat Bath

Formulas: Catnip & Fennel, Cold and Flu, Antioxidant, Analgesic and **Sudorific**

Key Herbs: Borage, Bupleurum, Capsicum (Cayenne), Catnip, Chamomile (English and Roman), **Blue Vervain**, **Boneset**, **Elder flowers**, **Yarrow**, Devil's Claw, Feverfew, Garlic, Ginger, Horehound, Isatis, Lavender, Lemon Balm, Lycium (Wolfberry, Gogi), Osha, Peppermint, Pleurisy Root, Rosemary essential oil, Sweet Annie (Ching-Hao), Thyme essential oil, Turmeric, Violet and Willow

Fever Blisters

See *Cold Sores (Fever Blisters)*

Fibroids (uterine)

See also *Fibrosis*

Fibroids are abnormal growths of connective tissue, usually benign, that are found in the uterus or breast. Fibroids may form as large elevated scars after large infected wounds. Excess levels of estrogen in the body usually cause fibroids. High levels of estrogen are often the result of xenoestrogens found in pesticides and plastics.

Symptoms of uterine fibroids include heavy menstrual bleeding, abdominal bloating, menstrual cramps, and spotting between periods. Anemia may result from loss of blood, and there may be abdominal pain, pain during intercourse, painful urination, or constipation. Since symptoms are often obscure, it is important to get an accurate medical diagnosis.

Factors that increase the risk of uterine fibroids are too much caffeine, too much of the wrong kinds of fats in the diet, deficiencies of essential fatty acids, hormone imbalances, underactive thyroid, birth control pills and X-rays. Obesity and family history of fibroids further increase the tendency for them to develop.

Commercial meat and dairy products typically contain hormones that aggravate fibroids. Soft plastic containers (like plastic milk bottles) leech xenoestrogens into food that contribute to fibroids. Pesticide residues on commercially grown produce also stimulate estrogen receptor sites and aggravate the condition. Coffee contributes heavily to fibroid growth. All of these should be avoided or eliminated.

Progesterone cream massaged into the abdomen may help by shifting the balance between estrogen and progesterone. Herbs that help balance estrogen and progesterone like chaste tree and false unicorn may also be helpful for uterine fibroids. It is possible that some *Female Hormonal Balancing Formulas* could also be helpful.

Yarrow has been helpful in breaking up fibroids in many cases. It is also a good herb for arresting the heavy bleeding that sometimes accompanies uterine fibroids. *Uterine Tonic Formulas* can also be helpful for the heavy bleeding.

Fibroids can be related to congestion in the liver, so a cleanse of the liver and colon may be of help. Use a *General Detoxifying* and *Fiber Blend Formulas* for this. Indole-3 carbinol helps break down excess estrogens by stimulating liver detoxification. It is found naturally in cruciferous vegetables.

The uterus helps the body metabolize fats, and having it removed can cause permanent problems with fat metabolism, which can lead to weight and heart problems. A woman's uterus serves many important functions and she should do her best to keep it her entire life. Using some of the remedies described here, it is possible to get rid of uterine fibroids without having a hysterectomy.

Therapies: Avoid Xenoestrogens and Colon Cleanse

Formulas: General Detoxifying, Fiber Blend, Phytoestrogen, Uterine Tonic, Female Hormonal Balancing and Blood Purifier

Key Herbs: Chastetree (Vitex), **Yarrow**, Dong Quai and False Unicorn (Helonias)

Key Nutrients: Indole-3 Carbinol (DIM), Omega-3 Essential Fatty Acids, Digestive Enzymes, Vitamin E and Iodine

Fibromyalgia Syndrome (FMS)

See also *Autoimmune Disorders*, *Epstein Barr Virus* and *Small Intestinal Bacterial Overgrowth (SIBO)*

Fibromyalgia Syndrome (FMS) can cause severe pain and impair deep sleep. It is a stress-related autoimmune disorder, and many of the symptoms mimic those of chronic fatigue syndrome (CFS) and arthritis.

Symptoms of fibromyalgia include painful, tender and recurrent aches in various points all over the body. There is a persistent, but diffused pain in the structural system (bones and muscles), accompanied by fatigue, headaches, general weakness, irritable bowel, poor sleep patterns, digestive problems, and nervous system problems (depression and anxiety).

Modern medicine hasn't identified the cause of FMS, but it is likely caused by diet and lifestyle factors, as evidenced by the fact that many people have experienced relief from FMS by making diet and lifestyle changes. While there is no magic bullet formula or secret recipe of things to do to cure FMS, working on the suspected causes will probably bring relief, if not complete recovery.

Nutrition should be a person's first concern in overcoming FMS. A mild food diet consisting primarily of fresh vegetables with some fruits has led to a reduction in joint stiffness and pain in many FMS suffers. These foods contain antioxidants which reduce inflammation and tissue damage.

Sugar, refined carbohydrates, processed vegetable oils, shortening, margarine and processed, packaged foods should be avoided. In addition, FMS sufferers usually benefit from some specific supplements, including (in order of importance) magnesium, iodine, omega-3 essential fatty acids and antioxidants.

Magnesium is essential for the synthesis of adenosine triphosphate (ATP), the energy powerhouse for cells. Deficiencies of magnesium causes cells to resort to using anaerobic pathways to produce energy, which leads to lactic acid formation and pain in the muscles. Magnesium ions are also essential to helping muscles relax, so deficiencies lead to muscle stiffness.

Supplements containing magnesium with malic acid have been beneficial for FMS. This combination aids in the production of ATP in the muscles and helps reduce muscle pain and stiffness. It also helps reduce fatigue in people suffering from FMS.

Iodine is an essential nutrient for the thyroid gland and many FMS sufferers also have a dysfunctional thyroid. Dr. David Brownstein, author of *Iodine: Why You Need It, Why You Can't Live Without It*, claims that iodine supplements alone have cured fibromyalgia. This helps explain why several natural healers independently discovered that black walnut was helpful for FMS. Black walnut, especially concentrated black walnut, is a good source of natural iodine. It is also antimicrobial, antiparasitic, and mildly detoxifying.

Hypothyroid Formulas that contain iodine-rich seaweeds like dulse, kelp, bladderwrack and Irish moss can supply iodine in a natural form. These and other seaweeds can be purchased in bulk and added to soups and stews.

For some people, a high-potency iodine supplement called Iodoral can be helpful.

Omega-3 essential fatty acids are essential for the health of nerve fibers and aid in the production of chemical messengers resulting in reduced inflammation and pain. Most modern diets are deficient in omega-3 fatty acids, so supplements containing them may also be helpful.

FMS sufferers who are having a hard time eating as many vegetables and fruits as they should will find it helpful to supplement their diets with antioxidant nutrients. *Antioxidant Formulas* can add additional protection against the oxidative stress that is a part of the FMS pattern. People who suffer from FMS tend to be low in enzymes. This is due to the high level of enzyme inhibitors and the lack of raw and enzyme-rich foods in most modern diets. Supplementing enzymes with *Digestive Enzyme Formulas* or other digestive enzyme products is important for people suffering from just about any chronic health problem. In most cases, these people also have a hiatal hernia that needs to be corrected.

One of the biggest contributing factors to FMS and its related conditions may be chronic intestinal inflammation and leaky gut syndrome. Intestinal inflammation can be caused by enzyme deficiency, poor digestion, environmental toxins, yeast or bacterial infections, parasites or synthetic drugs. The inflammation causes the intestines to become excessively porous, which allows toxins from the digestive tract to easily enter the bloodstream, causing irritation and inflammation of tissues.

Regular use of a *Fiber Blend Formula* can reduce intestinal inflammation and aid in the repair of leaky gut. Uña de gato is one of the best herbal remedies available for toning up intestinal membranes and reducing gut leakage. Kudzu and Intestinal Toners can also help tone up intestinal walls.

A yeast or parasite cleanse may also be needed. It is very probable that environmental toxins play a role in FMS. However, harsh cleansing is usually contraindicated in these situations because it will aggravate symptoms. What is needed is gentle detoxification, starting with fiber to help bind toxins in the gut.

In addition to the fiber, a small amount of a supplement to help cleanse the liver and aid its detoxification process is also helpful. Taking just one capsule of a *Blood Purifier* or *Hepatoprotective Formula* is all that is needed. These formulas will encourage the liver to break down chemicals in the system. The fiber will help bind and remove them. As your body gets stronger, you can take more.

Heavy metal toxicity may play a role in some of the problems associated with FMS. If this is a problem, try adding one capsule of a *Heavy Metal Cleansing Formula* per day along with six to eight capsules of sodium alginate (algin), a mucilaginous fiber from kelp that binds heavy metals in the intestines for elimination.

FMS is most common in hardworking perfectionists. K.P. Khalsa, RH(AHG), has noted that FMS sufferers are usually high achieving women that are burning the candle at both ends and in the middle, too. From this point of view, FMS can be considered a health collapse related to chronic stress.

The adrenal glands are responsible for helping the body cope with stress. They synthesize cortisol to control inflammation and balance blood sugar in times of crisis. They also produce hormones like epinephrine (adrenaline) to give us the energy we need to face challenges.

Chronic stress depletes the adrenal glands, which makes it difficult for the body to control pain and inflammation. Adrenal exhaustion also leads to a collapse of a person's drive and energy and produces fatigue coupled with restless and disturbed sleep patterns.

To overcome adrenal exhaustion, it is necessary to avoid refined carbohydrates (particularly sugar), alcohol and caffeinated beverages. An *Adrenal Tonic Formula* will help to rebuild the adrenal glands and restore energy levels and sleep. Rebuilding the adrenals will also help to reduce pain and inflammation throughout the body.

Of course, it also helps to learn to deal with stress more effectively. People suffering from FMS should learn to pace themselves by setting realistic goals and balancing work with rest and recreation. Taking breaks when one is tired, getting a good night's sleep and allowing time in one's life for relaxing activities is a must. Consider stretching, meditation, yoga, tai chi, relaxing baths or long walks in nature.

You will probably want to consult with a qualified professional herbalist (*findanherbalist.com*) or naturopath to help you customize a program for FMS. Many people with FMS have found relief through natural healing, but recovery can take time and dedication to lifestyle changes.

Therapies: Affirmation and Visualization, Dietary Fiber, Fresh Fruits and Vegetables, Gut Healing Diet, Healthy Fats, Heavy Metal Cleanse, Hiatal Hernia Correction, Hydration and Stress Management

Formulas: Antioxidant, Anti-Inflammatory, Adrenal Tonic, Digestive Enzyme, Antispasmodic, Analgesic and Hypothyroid

Key Herbs: Cats Claw (Uña de Gato, Gambier), **Ashwaganda**, **Black Walnut**, Kava-kava, Kudzu, Licorice, Lobelia and Yucca

Key Nutrients: 5-HTP, SAM-e, Protease Enzymes, **Probiotics**, MSM, **Magnesium**, **Digestive Enzymes**,

Omega-3 Essential Fatty Acids, DHA, Iodine and Indole-3 Carbinol (DIM)

Fibrosis

See also *Fibroids (uterine)*

Fibrosis is the abnormal formation of fibrous tissue in a part of the body, such as the lungs, breast or uterus. protease enzyme supplements, taken between meals can help to break down this fibrous tissue. Vitamin E may also be helpful.

Therapies: Castor Oil Pack

Key Herbs: Devil's Claw, Licorice, Mullein, Plantain and Red Clover

Key Nutrients: Digestive Enzymes, Vitamin E and **Protease Enzymes**

Fingernail Biting

Nail biting may be due to nervousness, parasites or mineral deficiencies. *Relaxing Nervine Formulas* or vitamin B-complex may help calm the nerves. Herbal *Mineral Formulas*, horsetail or colloidal mineral supplements may supply missing minerals. An *Antiparasitic Formula* will help remove parasites. Seek professional assistance to determine the underlying cause.

Therapies: Mineralization and Stress Management

Formulas: Relaxing Nervine, Mineral and Antiparasitic

Key Herbs: Horsetail

Key Nutrients: Colloidal Minerals and **Vitamin B-Complex**

Fingernails (weak or brittle)

Weak or brittle fingernails are a sign of a lack of silica and other trace minerals. Herbal *Mineral Formulas* containing herbs like dulse or horsetail may be of help. Colloidal mineral supplements may also be of help. Making Bone Broth, as described in the *Therapies Section*, is one of the best ways to get these extra minerals naturally.

Therapies: Bone Broth and Mineralization

Formulas: Mineral

Key Herbs: Horsetail and **Kelp**

Key Nutrients: Colloidal Minerals, **Digestive Enzymes** and Silicon

Flatulence

See *Gas and Bloating*

Floaters

Floaters are small black specks that appear to dance or float across the visual field. Possible causes include an unhealthy diet, excessive eye strain and inadequate rest. A generally good diet is helpful, along with extra doses of vitamin A, zinc, vitamin C and magnesium. An eyewash or compress over the eyes using a tea made from an herbal Eyewash Formula may also be helpful.

Therapies: Compress, Fresh Fruits and Vegetables and Low Glycemic Diet

Formulas: Eye Wash

Key Herbs: Bayberry, Chamomile (English and Roman), Eyebright and Goldenseal

Key Nutrients: Magnesium, **Vitamin A**, **Vitamin C**, Vitamin D and Zinc

Flu (Influenza)

Also known as influenza, the flu refers to viral infections accompanied by nausea, vomiting, diarrhea, fever, malaise, body pain, and respiratory symptoms. The media is constantly warning people about flu epidemics to scare people into getting vaccines, but the truth is that very few people die of the flu. Most of the people who die of the flu are elderly or have compromised immune systems.

Furthermore, there are thousands of strains of the flu and any flu shot contains only a few strains that might be active that year. So, it's perfectly possible to get a strain of the flu that wasn't in the vaccine. For this reason we do not recommend flu vaccinations.

Besides, there are numerous effective natural remedies for the flu. For prevention, simply wash your hands frequently. You can also diffuse essential oils into the home or office or make a spray of antimicrobial essential oils to take with you.

During flu season, take something to boost the immune system, such as astragalus, *Immune Stimulating* or *Mushroom Blend Formulas*. If you do get the flu, take an *Antiviral Formula*. It also helps to drink plenty of water and use the Sweat Bath therapy.

Several single herbs are also good for the flu. Elderberry and elderflowers are great antiviral remedies for the flu. The combination of elderflower and peppermint is a great flu remedy. Add yarrow to this blend if there is fever present. These are often found in *Sudorific Formulas*.

Boneset is a good remedy for flu that causes muscle aches and pains. Ginger and peppermint can be helpful for settling digestive upset.

The Colon Hydrotherapy and the Sweat Bath therapy can speed recovery from the flu. So can resting in bed and drinking lots of fluids.

Therapies: Colon Hydrotherapy, Hydration and Sweat Bath

Formulas: Immune Stimulating, Mushroom Blend, Antiviral, **Sudorific** and **Cold and Flu**

Key Herbs: Astragalus, Capsicum (Cayenne), Catnip, Cinnamon, **Andrographis**, **Boneset**, **Osha**, Echinacea, Elder, Garlic, Ginger, Hyssop, Isatis, Lemon, Lemon Balm, Olive, Peppermint, Pleurisy Root, Red Raspberry, Spilanthes, Thyme, Usnea and Yarrow

Key Nutrients: Vitamin A and Vitamin D

Foot Odor

Severe foot odor is a good indication of the need to do some cleansing. Improve the diet, do the Colon Cleanse therapy and perhaps the Drawing Bath therapy. You can even soak your feet in a pan containing water and Epsom salts.

Therapies: Colon Cleanse, Colon Hydrotherapy, Drawing Bath and Epsom Salt Bath

Formulas: General Detoxifying

Key Nutrients: Chlorophyll

Fractures

See *Broken Bones*

Free Radical Damage

See also *Aging (prevention)*

Experts suggest that about 50-80% of all chronic and degenerative diseases, including heart disease, cancer, diabetes, arthritis, macular degeneration, Alzheimer's and dementia are caused by oxidative stress, also known as free radical damage. Free radical damage also causes the cosmetic problems we associate with aging, dry skin, wrinkles, age spots and so forth. Read about Fresh Fruits and Vegetables in the *Therapies Section* for more information. Herbs and supplements listed below have antioxidant properties.

Therapies: Fresh Fruits and Vegetables

Formulas: Antioxidant

Key Herbs: Barley, Bilberry (Blueberry, Huckleberry), **Açaí**, **Lycium (Wolfberry, Gogi)**, **Mangosteen**, Ginkgo, Rosemary and Tea (Green or Black)

Key Nutrients: Co-Q10, Chlorophyll, Vitamin A, Vitamin C, Vitamin D, Vitamin E, Zinc, **Alpha Lipoic Acid**, L-Carnitine, Proanthocyanidins, Zeaxanthin, Lutein and Lycopene

Frigidity

See *Sex Drive (low)*

Frostbite (prevention)

Sprinkle tiny amounts of capsicum in socks or gloves to prevent frostbite. If skin irritation occurs, add a little baby powder or corn starch to buffer the capsicum.

Key Herbs: Capsicum (Cayenne)

Fungal Infections (Yeast Infections, Candida albicans)

See also *Athlete's Foot, Jock Itch, Thrush* and *Vaginal Discharge*

There are many positive benefits of yeast. Yeast helps bread to rise. Yeast creates the fermentation process that allows brewers to make beer and wine. Yeast microorganisms are a type of fungus, like mushrooms. They are present in the soil as part of the microbial mix needed for soil health. Yeasts are also included in the dozens of species of microorganisms that inhabit our intestines. This blend of microbes are known collectively as the intestinal microflora, and are critical to health. So, yeast can be very beneficial under the right conditions.

Under the wrong conditions, however, yeast can create problems with our health. When an imbalance of yeast and bacteria occurs this is known as dysbiosis. Yeast or fungal infections, particular overgrowth of a strain of yeast known as *Candida albicans*, can be a problem for many people living in modern Western society. Obvious yeast infections include thrush, vaginal yeast infections, athlete's foot, jock itch and nail fungus. Some doctors and healers believe that dysbiosis can be a factor in other health problems, including chronic sinus problems, frequent colds and flu, earaches, swollen lymph nodes, fatigue, reduced immunity, brain fog, leaky gut syndrome and more.

Dysbiosis occurs primarily because of overuse of antibiotics (and other drugs such as birth control pills, NSAIDs and chemotherapy agents) that upset the balance of intestinal microflora by killing the friendly bacteria. Other substances that have negative effects on our intestinal flora include alcohol, chlorinated drinking water, MSG, nitrates, and sulfates.

When friendly flora are disrupted, yeast or harmful strains of bacteria often proliferate, which can weaken overall immunity. Once the bacteria or yeast grows out of control, it secretes substances that weaken the integrity of the intestines (resulting in intestinal inflammation and leaky gut syndrome) and are absorbed into the blood stream, weakening the immune system and causing us to crave more sugar. Since both yeast and bacteria feed on sugar, it's almost like they hijack the body and make us want to perpetuate the environment that sustains their existence.

Determining If You Have a Dysbiosis:

Candida often becomes a "catch-all" diagnosis because the symptoms are vague and the medical test not very accurate. Many people think they have yeast overgrowth even though they have done extensive yeast cleanses, making this an over-diagnosed condition in the alternative health community.

Here is a little quiz to help you determine if dysbiosis may be contributing to your health problems. If you answer "yes" to any of the following questions, make a check on the line on the left. If you check five or more, you may have a problem with yeast overgrowth.

_____ Do you generally feel fatigued or have low energy?

_____ Do you experience food sensitivities or food allergies?

_____ Do you have nail fungus, athlete's foot or jock itch?

_____ Do you have recurrent vaginal yeast infections?

_____ Have you taken broad spectrum antibiotics recently?

_____ Do you crave sugar or sweets (candy, soda pop, etc.)?

_____ Do you often have gas, bloating or indigestion?

_____ Do you crave refined white flour (bread, pasta, baked goods)?

_____ Have you been on birth control pills for 6 months or more?

_____ Do you experience brain fog, mental confusion or mental fatigue?

If you do appear to have a problem with dysbiosis, here are some steps to getting it under control.

Step One: Modify the Diet

Yeast and bacteria love carbohydrates—especially simple sugars. So, you need to get all simple carbohydrates out of the diet for a period of time. For two to four weeks eliminate all simple sugars and refined grain products from your diet. Simple sugars include table sugar (sucrose), glucose, fructose, corn syrup and even natural sugars like honey, brown sugar and fruit juices. Refined grain products include white flour, white rice, corn chips and breakfast cereals. You'll need to start reading labels carefully to do this because sugars and refined grains are added to most prepackaged foods.

It is also important to avoid alcohol because it too is converted to sugar in the body. In fact, if your problem is severe, you may wish to avoid even whole grains, most fruit and starchy foods like potatoes for at least the first two weeks. However, severely restricting carbohydrates can cause ketosis. Candida prefers ketones over sugar as seen in the common yeast infections of diabetic ketosis.

Use the Low Glycemic Diet therapy and include some good fats in your diet. A particularly good fat for fighting candida is coconut oil because it contains a medium chain saturated fatty acid called caprylic acid that helps control yeast.

Step Two: Improve General Digestive and Intestinal Health

Yeast and bad bacteria get out of control when the environment becomes conducive to their growth. So, if we want to get them back under control, we need to change the environment of the digestive tract. Normally, the hydrochloric acid and enzymes found in our stomach help keep these microbes in check. Consider taking digestive enzyme supplements and, if you are over 50, betaine hydrochloric acid (HCl) supplements. Digestive secretions can be stimulated by taking Digestive Bitters 15-20 minutes before meals. It will also help to relieve the gas and bloating common in people with dysbiosis. Taking protease enzyme supplements between meals will also help to regulate digestive microbes, including both unfriendly bacteria and fungus.

Also look at the recommendations under Inflammatory Bowel Diseases and Leaky Gut Syndrome. Many times symptoms that have been associated with yeast are actually symptoms of bacterial overgrowth in the small intestines or poor digestion. Improving digestion, eating a better diet and using fermented foods to balance friendly flora are often all that is needed.

Step Three: Use Antifungal and Antimicrobial Agents to Reduce Yeast Overgrowth

After cutting off the yeast's food supply and altering the digestive environment to make it hostile for yeast growth, we can knock it down using antifungal herbs and supplements. Some of the herbs helpful for reducing yeast overgrowth include garlic, oregano leaf, pau d'arco, spilanthes and usnea. These are key ingredients in *Antifungal Formulas*.

Essential oils are also powerful allies in dealing with yeast infections. *Antifungal* essential oils include tea tree, lavender, thyme, clove, and oregano. These can be used in baths, diffused into the room or diluted with vegetable oil to apply topically in cases of fungal infections on the skin or nails.

Step Four: Repopulate the Body with Friendly Bacteria (Probiotics)

The final step in taming the yeast is to repopulate the intestines with friendly bacteria or probiotics. Naturally fermented foods such as yoghurt, raw sauerkraut and miso are good dietary sources of these friendly microbes to take after cleansing, but you will probably want to also take probiotic supplements.

Therapies: Aromatherapy, Colon Cleanse, Colon Hydrotherapy, Dietary Fiber and Friendly Flora

Formulas: Digestive Bitter Tonic, Digestive Enzyme and **Antifungal**

Key Herbs: Chaparral, **Barberry**, **Oregano**, **Pau d' Arco**, **Usnea**, Garlic, Lavender essential oil, Olive, Paw Paw, Poke Root, Shiitake, Spilanthes, Tea Tree, Thuja and Yarrow

Key Nutrients: Probiotics, Digestive Enzymes, Protease Enzymes and **Betaine Hydrochloric Acid (HCl)**

Gall Bladder (sluggish or removed)

See also *Gall Stones*

Sluggish activity of the gall bladder will result in poor digestion of fats. It will also make it difficult for the body to eliminate excess cholesterol. Clay-colored or greasy stools that float are symptoms of sluggish gall bladder function. Herbs that stimulate gall bladder function are called cholagogues and include remedies like fringetree, artichoke, celandine, Culver's root and barberry. These are some of the key ingredients in *Cholagogue Formulas*. Lipase enzyme supplements are also helpful for problems with digesting fats. When people have had their gall bladder's removed, supplementing with lipase enzymes and ox bile and/or taking *Cholagogue Formulas* can be very helpful in maintaining their health.

Therapies: Gall Bladder Flush

Formulas: Cholagogue

Key Herbs: Blue Flag, Buckthorn, Burdock, Celandine, **Artichoke**, **Barberry**, **Fringe Tree**, **Turmeric**, **Wild Yam**, Culver's root, Dandelion, Gentian, Jambul, Milk Thistle, Stone Breaker and Yellow Dock

Key Nutrients: Lipase Enzymes

Gall Stones

See also *Circulation (poor)*

Deposits resembling small rocks that form in the gallbladder are called gall stones. They are usually composed primarily of cholesterol. If they are large or numerous enough, they may cause severe abdominal pain. Besides doing the Gall Bladder Flush therapy, drinking more water and taking fiber is very helpful, especially if you use a *Cholagogue Formula*. Taken over time, herbs like fringetree, turmeric and barberry can help to improve gall bladder function and may help to flush out stones without surgery. Consult with a professional herbalist (*findanherbalist.com*) for assistance.

Therapies: Dietary Fiber, Gall Bladder Flush and Hydration

Formulas: Cholagogue and Fiber Blend

Key Herbs: Celandine, **Barberry**, **Fringe Tree**, **Turmeric**, **Wild Yam**, Khella, Lemon juice, Milk Thistle and Stone Breaker

Key Nutrients: Magnesium, Digestive Enzymes and Lipase Enzymes

Gangrene

Gangrene is localized death of the skin and underlying soft tissue due to lack of blood supply. This is a serious illness and medical attention should be sought. Colloidal silver liquid and gel have been proven in scientific studies to halt the progression of gangrene and often prevent the need for amputation. Apply the gel topically. Other remedies that may be helpful include taking echinacea and other antimicrobial herbs internally and applying tea tree essential oil topically. Alternating soaks with ice water and warm water to stimulate circulation to the afflicted areas can also be helpful.

Therapies: Fresh Fruits and Vegetables and Low Glycemic Diet

Formulas: Antibacterial, **Echinacea Blend** and Goldenseal & Echinacea

Key Herbs: Capsicum (Cayenne), **Echinacea**, **Garlic (raw)**, **Thuja**, **Usnea**, Goldenseal, Tea Tree and Wild Indigo (Baptista)

Key Nutrients: Colloidal Silver, **Vitamin C** and MSM

Gas and Bloating

See also *Belching, Hiatal Hernia, Ileocecal Valve, Lactose Intolerance* and *Small Intestinal Bacterial Overgrowth (SIBO)*

Intestinal gas is created by the action of friendly flora on foods we eat. Some amount of gas production is normal. Excessive gas is usually due to imbalances in the friendly flora or problems with digesting certain foods. Digestive enzyme supplements can help reduce intestinal gas. Taking fiber or probiotics sometimes temporarily increases intestinal gas by altering intestinal microbes.

Bloating is an abnormal feeling of fullness in the gastrointestinal tract caused by excessive gas that builds up pressure in the abdomen. Bloating puts pressure on the stomach and contributes to the development of a hiatal hernia. It may even cause stress on the heart. Where bloating is frequent, the ileocecal valve is probably swollen and inflamed and needs to be closed (See Ileocecal Valve).

Herbs used to relieve gas and bloating are called carminatives. These herbs relieve intestinal gas by increasing blood flow to the abdominal cavity. Most of the gas produced in the intestines is actually absorbed into the bloodstream and excreted through the lungs. *Carminative* herbs aid this process. They also aid digestion to slow gas production.

Examples of carminative herbs include catnip, chamomile, fennel, ginger and peppermint. These are some of the key herbs in *Carminative Formulas*. Catnip & Fennel Formulas are used to help colic and gas in infants and small children, but they work for adults, too.

Where bloating is severe and accompanied by foul belching, there is putrefaction taking place in the digestive tract. Activated charcoal can be very helpful for relieving this condition. It also helps to take digestive enzyme supplements. If gas and bloating occurs after consuming dairy products, it is a sign of lactose intolerance. In this case probiotics and lactase enzyme supplements will help.

Gas and bloating can also be caused by an excess of bacteria in the small intestines, called small intestinal bacterial overgrowth (SIBO). Increasing HCl and taking *Antibacterial Formulas* can be helpful.

Severe gas and bloating can also be a sign of an open ileocecal valve. Closing this valve can bring rapid relief. See *Ileocecal Valve* for more information.

Therapies: Aromatherapy, Colon Cleanse, Colon Hydrotherapy, Dietary Fiber, Friendly Flora, Gut Healing Diet and Hiatal Hernia Correction

Formulas: Carminative, Catnip & Fennel and Antibacterial

Key Herbs: Black Pepper, Blessed Thistle, Bupleurum, Cardamom, Catnip, Cilantro/Coriander, Cinnamon, Clove, **Angelica**, **Anise**, **Barberry**, **Chamomile (English and Roman)**, **Gentian**, **Ginger**, **Peppermint**, **Thyme**, Fennel, Papaya, Rosemary and Triphala

Key Nutrients: Lactase Enzymes, Probiotics, **Digestive Enzymes**, Charcoal (Activated) and **Betaine Hydrochloric Acid (HCl)**

Gastritis

See also *Acid Indigestion (Heartburn, Acid Reflux), Indigestion, Leaky Gut Syndrome* and *Small Intestinal Bacterial Overgrowth (SIBO)*

Gastritis is an inflammation of the stomach. It is caused by a combination of factors, including stress, rapid eating, alcohol and tobacco use, NSAIDs and dehydration. It can also be caused by an overgrowth of bacteria in the small intestines giving rise to excessive gas and pressure on the stomach. Headaches and constipation are also commonly associated with gastritis. A person may feel dull and drowsy after eating, but have difficulty falling asleep at bedtime.

To correct gastritis, the diet should be simple, consisting primarily of meat and vegetables. Simple sugars and starchy foods should be avoided (especially if there is gas and bloating). Digestive enzyme supplements and betaine hydrochloric acid (HCl) supplements may be helpful to take with meals.

Taking a *Digestive Bitter Tonic Formula* about 15-20 minutes prior to meals along with a glass or two of water, then avoiding liquids with meals, can also be helpful. Dehydration decreases downward motility of the digestive organs, but liquids should primarily be consumed between meals.

Remedies to reduce stress, especially when eating, are helpful. *Goldenseal & Echinacea* or herbal *Antibacterial Formulas* may also be helpful.

Soothing mucilaginous herbs like aloe, licorice, marshmallow and slippery elm can also soothe stomach irritation. Meadowsweet not only helps to neutralize acid burning, it also eases pain and inflammation.

Therapies: Colon Hydrotherapy, Gut Healing Diet and Hydration

Formulas: Digestive Bitter Tonic, Digestive Enzyme, Goldenseal & Echinacea and Antibacterial

Key Herbs: Aloe vera, **Goldenseal**, **Licorice**, Marshmallow, Meadowsweet, Slippery Elm and St. John's wort

Key Nutrients: Digestive Enzymes, Calcium and Betaine Hydrochloric Acid (HCl)

Gastroesophageal Reflux Disease (GERD)

See *Acid Indigestion (Heartburn, Acid Reflux)*

Generalized Anxiety Disorder

See *Anxiety Disorders*

Giardia

See also *Parasites (general)*

A single celled organism, giardia (Giardia lambila) is the most common cause of waterborne disease in the United States. It is picked up by drinking contaminated water. Because giardia form cysts that are not destroyed by chlorination they must be filtered from water.

Symptoms of giardia infection include diarrhea, gas, upset stomach or stomach cramps, nausea and/or greasy stools that tend to float. Symptoms usually appear 7-14 days after exposure. Goldenseal is a good herbal remedy for giardia. Consider using it as a single, or in a *Goldenseal & Echinacea Formula*. Activated charcoal can be helpful for the diarrhea. Be sure to drink plenty of water and replace electrolytes like potassium. If symptoms are severe, seek medical attention.

Therapies: Hydration

Formulas: Goldenseal & Echinacea

Key Herbs: Andrographis, **Goldenseal**, Echinacea and Thuja

Key Nutrients: Charcoal (Activated) and Potassium

Gingivitis (Bleeding Gums, Gum Disease, Pyorrhea)

See also *Cardiovascular Disease (Heart Disease)*

When bacteria get into spaces between the teeth and gums, they can cause inflammation (gingivitis) and a breakdown of the gum tissue. This leads to bleeding of the gums. Pyorrhea is a discharge of pus or an advanced form of periodontal disease associated with a discharge of pus and loose teeth.

A thorough cleaning by a dental hygienist is highly recommended. It is also absolutely essential that the teeth be brushed and flossed several times daily.

There are herbal remedies that can help to heal the gums. For starters, after cleaning the teeth, brush with a mixture of black walnut, white oak bark and goldenseal powders. Leave some of the powder on your gums for 5-10 minutes (or even overnight) and then rinse. These herbs fight infection, strengthen tooth enamel and gums, and contract tissues to arrest bleeding. Other herbs that can be applied topically to the gums to reduce bleeding and inflammation include bayberry root bark and calendula.

There are specific *Dental Health Formulas* some herbalists have created which can be applied topically or used as a mouth rinse. Key herbs in these formulas include cloves, myrrh and spilanthes, all of which help to fight infection. One could also apply a *Goldenseal & Echinacea* extract or a *Topical Antiseptic Formula* to the gums.

Gum disease is not just a localized problem. People with gingivitis have a higher risk of cardiovascular inflammation. This means that one should also treat the problem systemically.

First, one needs to increase mineral intake. Using colloidal mineral supplements as a mouth wash will also help to stop bleeding. Swallow the colloidal minerals after swishing them around in your mouth so that you increase mineral levels in the body as well. Vitamin D3 also helps to boost the immune system and help mineralize the teeth.

Increase antioxidants in the diet and avoid high glycemic foods. One of the best antioxidants for this problem is Co-Q10, which helps reduce gum inflammation and cardiovascular inflammation. Vitamin C also reduces the inflammation and helps the gums to heal.

Therapies: Fresh Fruits and Vegetables, Low Glycemic Diet and Mineralization

Formulas: Topical Antiseptic and Goldenseal & Echinacea

Key Herbs: Bayberry, Bloodroot, Bloodroot, Calendula, Clove, **Black Walnut**, **Myrrh**, **Propolis**, **Spilanthes**, **White Oak**, Echinacea, Goldenseal, Tea Tree and Usnea

Key Nutrients: Zinc, Vitamin D, Vitamin C, Colloidal Minerals, **Co-Q10**, Vitamin K, Folate (Folic Acid and Vitamin B9)

Glands (swollen lymph)

See also *Congestion (lymphatic)* and *Tonsillitis (Adenoids)*

The lymphatic system contains lymph nodes that filter lymphatic fluid to remove infectious microbes and toxins. When these glands become irritated, they swell. This happens in the neck, throat, armpits, groin and chest where these nodes are located. Swollen lymph nodes are usually present in respiratory congestion, earaches, sore throats and breast swelling.

Use *Lymphatic Drainage Formulas* for lymphatic swelling. Some of the key herbs to look for in these formulas include cleavers, red clover, ocotillo and red root. Be sure to drink plenty of water and get some moderate exercise, as movement increases lymph flow. *Topical Antiseptic Formulas* can be massaged into swollen lymph nodes to further aid drainage. You can also dilute essential oils like tea tree or thyme with a vegetable oil and massage this into the swollen glands. Garlic oil can be massaged into swollen lymph nodes too, but the smell isn't as pleasant.

Therapies: Aromatherapy, Exercise and Hydration

Formulas: **Lymphatic Drainage** and Topical Antiseptic

Key Herbs: Burdock, Cleavers (Bedstraw), **Echinacea**, **Red Root**, Garlic, Lobelia, Ocotillo, Oregon Grape, Red Clover, Tea Tree essential oil, Thyme essential oil and Violet

Key Nutrients: Vitamin A, Vitamin D and Vitamin K

Glaucoma

See also *Free Radical Damage*

Glaucoma is a serious eye disease characterized by abnormally elevated fluid pressure within the eye. This is caused by a tiny mesh in the eye that allows fluid to drain and become clogged. The clogging is usually due to free radical damage causing debris in the lymph. Untreated, this pressure can damage the retina and destroy the optic nerve, resulting in loss of vision or blindness. In fact, glaucoma is the most common cause of blindness.

Risk factors for this disease include people of African ancestry, people with diabetes, high blood pressure, severe myopia (nearsightedness) or a family history of glaucoma, and those taking corticosteroid preparations. Other contributing factors include diabetes, food allergies, excess caffeine, adrenal exhaustion, liver and thyroid problems and arteriosclerosis.

To prevent glaucoma, take plenty of antioxidants. Bilberry is a good antioxidant for the eyes and is typically a main ingredient in *Vision Supporting Formulas*, which can help keep eyes healthy as people age. Supplements to consider include N-acetyl cysteine, vitamins A, C, D3 and E and the antioxidants lutein and zeaxanthin, which are found in many *Vision Supporting Formulas*.

If you have glaucoma, seek medical attention. You can also use remedies for preventing it to help support medical treatment. Remedies that relax the eye and allow the drain to open may also be helpful. One such remedy that may be effective, but is legal in only a few states, is cannabis. It is possible that kava kava, lobelia or an *Antispasmodic Formula* could have a similar effect.

Therapies: Avoid Caffeine, Eliminate Allergy-Causing Foods, Low Glycemic Diet and Stress Management

Formulas: Vision Supporting and Antispasmodic

Key Herbs: Bilberry (Blueberry, Huckleberry), **Lobelia** and Kava-kava

Key Nutrients: N-Acetyl Cysteine, **Magnesium**, **Vitamin A**, **Vitamin C**, Vitamin D, Vitamin E, Lutein and Zeaxanthin

Goiter

See also *Hyperthyroid (Grave's Disease)*, *Hashimoto's Disease (Thyroiditis)* and *Hypothyroid*

A goiter is an enlargement of the thyroid gland that can be seen as a swelling in the neck. This can result from insufficient intake or utilization of iodine or from Hashimoto's disease. Use a *Hypothyroid Formula* or take seaweeds like dulse and kelp. An iodine supplement can also be used. See related conditions for more ideas.

Formulas: Hypothyroid

Key Herbs: Black Walnut and Kelp

Key Nutrients: Iodine and **Selenium**

Gonorrhea

See also *Infection (bacterial)*

Gonorrhea is a sexually transmitted bacterial infection that causes inflammation of the genital mucous membranes. Symptoms of gonorrhea in men include painful urination and a thick discharge from the penis. Women

may have no initial symptoms at all, but painful urination and vaginal discharge, along with abnormal menstrual bleeding, are typical symptoms. In advanced states the disease can cause fever, muscle aches and inflamed joints. It can also cause infertility.

Seek medical attention for this condition. You can also use herbs with antibacterial action in addition to antibiotics. Be sure to repopulate the colon with probiotics following the antibiotics.

Formulas: Antibacterial

Key Herbs: Echinacea, Garlic, Goldenseal and Wild Indigo (Baptista)

Key Nutrients: Probiotics

Gout

See also *Arthritis*

Gout is a metabolic disease characterized by excessive amounts of uric acid in the blood and deposits of uric acid crystals in the joints. Uric acid is a byproduct of protein and fructose metabolism and is filtered from the blood by the kidneys.

Animal protein consumption should be reduced and when it is consumed, a betaine hydrochloric acid (HCl) supplement with pepsin in it should be taken with it. Soda pop, and any drink sweetened with fructose should be avoided completely. Make sure you are drinking sufficient amounts of pure water to flush metabolic waste from the body. Complex carbohydrates such as fresh fruits, dark green vegetables and other antioxidant foods should be increased in the diet. Black cherry juice and lemon water are also helpful for flushing the acid out of the system.

A tea made with nettles and alterative herbs like alfalfa, red clover, cleavers and dandelion can help to neutralize the acid. You can also consider *Diuretic* or *Joint Healing Formulas* which have these herbs as key ingredients.

Therapies: Fresh Fruits and Vegetables and Hydration

Formulas: Diuretic and Joint Healing

Key Herbs: Alfalfa, Burdock, Celery seed, **Gravel root**, **Nettle (Stinging)**, Dandelion, Devil's Claw, Lemon juice, Red Clover and Safflowers

Key Nutrients: Chlorophyll, Omega-3 Essential Fatty Acids and Potassium

Grave's Disease

See *Hyperthyroid (Grave's Disease)*

Grief and Sadness

See also *Shock*

Everyone experiences the pain of loss and heartbreak at some point in their life. When we lose someone or something that brought us joy and pleasure, we experience grief. Grief begins as a shock to the system. In shock, the blood retreats from the skin and moves into the internal organs. In the grieving process, this creates a swelling sensation in our chest we call "heartbreak." If the pain is intense enough it actually feels like our heart is going to "burst."

If you've ever seen a person go into shock, you'll see the color drain from their face, making them look pale. They also feel "cold." Their eyes glaze over and they feel numb. They become cold and clammy. This is exactly the opposite energetic state to that of being "in love," which causes blood to flow more readily to the surface of the skin, making the person rosy, warm and radiant. Love opens us up to greater connection. Shock is a state of being withdrawn and closed down.

When a grieving person is able to acknowledge their pain, they will start sobbing. Sobbing is more than just shedding tears; it involves the whole body. The convulsive shaking of the body associated with sobbing can also lead to wailing, moaning or even screaming. These actions empty the lungs (which creates a release of endorphins that helps the person feel better). It also forces redistribution of the blood so a person can feel again.

The emptying of the lungs is symbolic of the "letting go" associated with grieving. Grieving is a releasing of what we have lost, a breaking of the attachment or desire we felt. Sighing (which also involves a long slow exhale) is a milder form of the same energy.

Grieving can also involve anger. Feeling deeply hurt often brings out feelings of anger. The grieving person may be mad at the person who left them or even blame God for taking the person away from them.

When a person is unable to fully grieve and let go, they can become congested, particularly in the lungs. In traditional Chinese medicine it was recognized that prolonged sorrow damages the energy of the lungs. A person who is unable to fully grieve may cough because they need to "get something off their chest." Their lungs may fill up with fluid resulting in pneumonia, or they may shed tears internally in the form of post nasal drip. This is why formulas that support the respiratory system, such as *Lung and Respiratory Tonic Formulas*, may be helpful for the grieving person.

Healthy grief is an expression of love. It is healthy to express grief when we have lost someone or something important to us. Grieving helps us to accept our loss, to rediscover peace and joy, and then to move forward.

During a time of loss, people will often reach out to the grieving person, offering comfort and help. This is a wonderful thing, but it cannot replace the grieving process. One still has to go through the process of releasing pain and letting go of that which has been lost.

In other words, receiving help is good, but a person still needs to experience the sighing, sobbing or wailing that allows the pain to be released from the body. When a person doesn't allow themselves to do this, they may become addicted to the comfort and sympathy of others, seeking it like an addict seeks a drug. This places responsibility for their healing outside of themselves, which means they become perpetually stuck in seeking sympathetic allies to try to heal their grief.

Sometimes the suffering a person feels leads them to conclude that it is dangerous to experience love and vulnerability. So, they close down their hearts to avoid feeling close to anyone or anything, hoping to avoid experiencing future grief or sorrow.

Unfortunately, closing one's self off to pain also closes one off to the joy that comes from love and connection. It causes one to become "hard of heart" and experience a lack of empathy and compassion for others. A person with a closed heart will become inflexible, rigid and judgmental.

Heart problems, such as hardening of the arteries, high blood pressure and heart attacks can all be signs of a person who has closed their heart to try to avoid having to feel grief or pain. A closed heart not only prevents one from experiencing loving connections with others, it also reduces one's ability to experience joy, happiness and pleasure in one's life. Diabetes and blood sugar problems can also be signs of a closed heart and the inability to experience the "sweetness" of love.

Seeking counseling or assistance from a minister or a friend may be necessary when one has undergone a lot of grief. Aromatherapy and Flower Essences therapy may be helpful during this process. Lemon balm essential oil or tea can help lift feelings of sadness. If the grief has resulted in depression, consider using an *Antidepressant Formula*.

Rose as a flower essence, tea of the petals or essential oil can be helpful for comforting the heart and helping a person open up to love again. Nervous system support with B-complex vitamins and vitamin C can be helpful. If anxiety or insomnia are problems use *Relaxing Nervine* or *Sleep Formulas*.

Therapies: Affirmation and Visualization, Aromatherapy, Emotional Healing Work and Flower Essences

Formulas: Lung and Respiratory Tonic, Relaxing Nervine, Sleep and Antidepressant

Key Herbs: Borage, Bupleurum, Chamomile (English and Roman), **Lemon Balm**, **Mimosa (Albizia, Silk Tree)**, **Rose essential oil**, Myrrh, Night Blooming Cereus (Cactus) and Oat seed (milky)

Key Nutrients: Vitamin B-Complex and Vitamin C

Gum Disease

See *Gingivitis (Bleeding Gums, Gum Disease, Pyorrhea)*

Hair (graying)

Gray hair is associated with aging and is typically the result of mineral deficiencies, as minerals help to add color to the hair. It can also be a sign of declining hydrochloric acid production (resulting in poor protein digestion and mineral absorption). A lack of B-complex vitamins may also contribute to this problem. He shou wu has a reputation in China as an herb that can prevent or reverse graying if taken regularly.

Therapies: Mineralization

Formulas: Mineral

Key Herbs: He Shou Wu (Ho Shou Wu, Fo-Ti)

Key Nutrients: Pantothenic Acid (Vitamin B5), Colloidal Minerals, Vitamin B-Complex, Zinc, Selenium and **Copper**

Hair (loss or thinning)

See also *Hair Care (general)*, *Hashimoto's Disease (Thyroiditis)* and *Hypothyroid*

Loss of hair or baldness may be caused by hormonal imbalances such as low thyroid, lack of protein in the diet, stress and poor circulation to the scalp. Appropriate remedies depend on the underlying causes.

One of the most common causes (especially in women) is low thyroid. In this case, an iodine supplement, kelp or a *Hypothyroid Formula* may be of help. However, most low thyroid problems are an autoimmune disorder called Hashimoto's. See that listing for ideas on how to work with this condition.

Lack of adequate protein in the diet or difficulty in digesting and assimilating protein is another common cause. If your diet is low in protein, increase consumption of protein-rich foods. If you have a hard time digesting them, take a *Digestive Bitter Tonic Formula*, a *Digestive Enzyme Formula* and/or a betaine hydrochloric acid (HCl) supplement.

Stress can cause hair to thin. If you are under a lot of stress, try using a *Relaxing Nervine Formula* and/or an *Adaptogen Formula* to ease your stress.

Minerals can also aid hair growth. Consider using colloidal minerals or mineral rich herbs like those found in herbal *Mineral Formulas*. Horsetail, nettles, rosemary and sage have all proven helpful for improving the health of hair, along with skin and fingernails.

Sage and rosemary essential oils can also be used topically on the scalp to encourage circulation to the scalp. Simply add a few drops to your shampoo.

For men who are experiencing balding, try using maca, muira puama or a *Male Glandular Tonic Formula* to balance your hormones. The herbs in *Prostate Formulas* may also be of help.

These are basic suggestions. Each case must be evaluated individually to determine the underlying cause.

Therapies: Mineralization

Formulas: Hypothyroid, Adaptogen, Mineral, Male Glandular Tonic, Prostate, Digestive Bitter Tonic and Relaxing Nervine

Key Herbs: Horsetail, **Rosemary**, **Sarsaparilla**, Eleuthero (Siberian ginseng), Kelp, Khella, Maca, Muira Puama, Nettle (Stinging) and Sage

Key Nutrients: Iron, Protease Enzymes, Co-Q10, Colloidal Minerals, Zinc, Iodine, Digestive Enzymes, **Betaine Hydrochloric Acid (HCl)**, Vitamin B-12 and Silicon

Hair Care (general)

See also *Hair (graying)* and *Hair (loss or thinning)*

Healthy hair requires protein, trace minerals and good circulation to the scalp. herbal *Mineral Formulas* can improve the general health of hair, as can colloidal mineral supplements. Horsetail and nettles are two single herbs that are rich in minerals for healthy hair. Essential oils like rosemary, sage and tea tree oil, added to a natural shampoo can stimulate circulation to the scalp. Chamomile has been used as a rinse to help blonde hair, too.

Therapies: Aromatherapy and Mineralization

Formulas: Mineral

Key Herbs: Chamomile (English and Roman), **Rosemary**, **Tea Tree**, Horsetail, Nettle (Stinging) and Sage

Key Nutrients: Colloidal Minerals, Digestive Enzymes, Omega-3 Essential Fatty Acids, Vitamin B-Complex, Vitamin E and Zinc

Halitosis (Bad Breath)

See also *Belching* and *Sinus Infection*

Halitosis is a bad odor from the mouth. Sinus infections, oral diseases, cigarette smoking and poor digestion can all contribute to halitosis. Start by cleaning the teeth. Essential oils like clove and peppermint can be added to water and used as a mouthwash. Propolis can also be used as a mouthwash and helps to fight infection. If the bad odor is caused by foul belching, use remedies to aid digestion such as *Digestive Enzyme Formulas* or digestive enzyme supplements. Colon cleansing may also be helpful. Chlorophyll is a very good natural deodorizer and can reduce body odor in general, including bad breath.

Therapies: Colon Cleanse

Formulas: Digestive Enzyme

Key Herbs: Cardamom, Clove, **Coptis (Chinese Goldenthread)**, **Peppermint**, Lavender, Parsley and Propolis

Key Nutrients: Vitamin B-3 (Niacin), **Digestive Enzymes** and **Chlorophyll**

Hangover

See also *Addictions (alcohol)* and *Hypoglycemia*

A hangover is a set of acute symptoms such as headache, nausea and/or vomiting as a result of recent, excessive consumption of alcohol. Alcohol is dehydrating and causes blood sugar swings (hypoglycemia). One can reduce the negative effects of alcohol by consuming about twice the amount of water as alcoholic beverages and by using alcohol with meals so that there are proteins and fats available to keep blood sugar stable.

Hepatoprotective Formulas containing herbs like milk thistle, can help the liver detoxify the alcohol and reduce the tendency to hangovers. Other supplements that can help with liver detoxification of alcohol include milk thistle, kudzu, n-acetyl-cysteine and B-complex vitamins.

Therapies: Hydration

Formulas: Hepatoprotective

Key Herbs: Borage, **Milk Thistle**, Kudzu, Licorice and St. John's wort

Key Nutrients: Vitamin B-Complex and N-Acetyl Cysteine

Hardening of the Arteries

See *Arteriosclerosis (Atherosclerosis, Hardening of the Arteries)*

Hashimoto's Disease (Thyroiditis)

See also *Grave's Disease*

Hashimoto's Disease is the most common cause of hypothyroid (low thyroid). It is an autoimmune disease in which the immune system attacks the tissue that produces the thyroid hormone. Since 90% of the people who have been diagnosed with low thyroid have antibodies to thyroid tissue in their blood, this is the most common cause of low thyroid.

Conventional medicine has no effective treatments for this disease other than to replace the hormones that are not being made because of the damage to the thyroid. Most herbalists simply try to strengthen the thyroid with iodine or iodine-rich herbs. However, none of this is effective because Hashimoto's is not a disease of the thyroid, it is a disease of the immune system.

Most doctors rely primarily on blood levels of TSH to determine thyroid function. However, TSH can remain within normal ranges even when the thyroid is being attacked by the immune system.

Several studies have shown a link between autoimmune thyroid disorders and gluten intolerance. The molecular structure of gliadin in gluten closely resembles that of the thyroid gland. When gliadin passes the protective barrier of the gut and enters the bloodstream, the immune system tags it for destruction. These antibodies to gliadin (and possibly the other 100 protein structures in wheat) also cause the body to attack thyroid tissue by molecular mimicry.

Based on this finding and clinical experience, here is a seven step program developed by Thomas Easley to treat Hashimoto's naturally.

Step 1: Don't Eat Gluten!

Avoid all gluten bearing grains. Antibodies to gliadin can show up in the blood up to six months after eating gluten, so you need to be very strict about this. It may also help to avoid all other grains and legumes for a few months while the gut heals. The GAPS diet (*gapsdiet.com*) may be helpful.

Step 2: Heal the Gut

Avoid all toxins that inhibit nutrient absorption and inflame the gut including acid reflux medications, NSAIDS and birth control medications. Increase stomach acid by taking Betaine HCl or 1 tablespoon of Apple Cider Vinegar before meals. Drink 3-6 cups of bone broth a day. Take one capsule of black walnut three times a day to help heal mucus membranes. It also helps to eat fermented vegetables (sauerkraut, kimchi, etc.) several times a day and take probiotics with every meal.

Seventy-percent of the immune tissue in the body is found in or around the gut. This tissue is called the GALT, or gut-associated lymphoid tissue. When the gut lining becomes compromised, undigested food particles can leak out of the gut and create an immune response. The immune system can then mistake food proteins for body organs. This immune confusion results from what is referred to as molecular mimicry.

Thyroid hormones play a big role in regulating the tight junctions of the intestinal membrane and help govern GALT function. This means that you can't have a healthy thyroid without a healthy gut and you can't have a healthy gut without a healthy thyroid. This is why if you have an elevated TSH with low T4 and T3, prescription thyroid medication (like Armour Thyroid) might be necessary for a short time to allow the gut to heal.

Step 3: Supplement with Selenium

The exacerbation of Hashimoto's disease by iodine almost always occurs in the presence of a selenium deficiency. Selenium by itself has been shown in several studies to reduce thyroid antibodies, showing a lessening of the immune attack on the thyroid. Take one capsule a day of a selenium supplement that supplies 200 mcg of selenium preferably in the form of L-selenomethionine, sodium selenate, selenodiglutathione and Se-Methyl L-Selenocysteine. This can improve thyroid function and balance immune excess.

Step 4: Supplement with Vitamin D

Vitamin D is produced from cholesterol when your skin is exposed to the sun. Vitamin D deficiency is very common and most people don't have adequate levels. People with Hashimoto's should try to slowly increase their blood level to the therapeutic level of 70 ng/ml.

Healthy people that don't have any absorption or conversion issues might get adequate vitamin D blood levels from 2,000-5,000 mcg a day of D3. Most people need to do much higher doses of D3 to get blood levels in the therapeutic range. Vitamin D3, like all fat soluble vitamins, absorbs best when taken with a fatty meal. Vitamin D also works best when balanced with vitamins K, E and A.

Step 5: Iodine

Dr. David Brownstein published the theory that supplemental iodine in large doses could help Hashimoto's disease. Iodine loading test show that about 70% of the people coming to me do have a mild iodine deficiency. Af-

ter you have been taking selenium and vitamin D for 2 weeks you can start taking one-half of a capsule of Iodoral (an iodine supplement) per day. Don't take a higher dose without doing an iodine loading test.

If done correctly, supplementing with iodine can be beneficial to people with Hashimoto's disease. If done incorrectly it can make the immune system hyperactive and worsen the disease.

Step 6: Use Botanicals that Balance Immune Function

Astragalus and ashwagandha have a strong balancing action on the immune system and the thyroid. An easy way to use these is to put 2 ounces each of astragalus and ashwaganda into three quarts of water in a crockpot. Turn the crockpot on low. Drink one cup four times a day and refill the crockpot every night. Every three days add more herbs. Every two weeks dump everything and start a fresh batch.

Step 7: Use Armour Thyroid if Needed

If your thyroid tests show function is low, you may need to take Armour Thyroid while you are working on the other steps. Armour Thyroid is the most well known brand of desiccated porcine thyroid. It is available by prescription only. You should never take any form of desiccated porcine thyroid without doctor supervision and regular blood testing. Unfortunately, many doctors are resistant to prescribing Armour Thyroid because of misinformation by pharmaceutical reps promoting Synthroid. You may have to hunt around for a doctor who will be willing to write a prescription for you.

Therapies: Affirmation and Visualization, Eliminate Gluten, Friendly Flora, Gut Healing Diet, Heavy Metal Cleanse and Stress Management

Formulas: Gentle Laxative and Fiber Blend

Key Herbs: Black Walnut, **Ashwaganda**, **Astragalus**, Eleuthero (Siberian ginseng), Licorice and Saw Palmetto

Key Nutrients: Co-Q10, Vitamin E, Zinc, **Selenium**, **Vitamin D**, Vitamin K and Iodine

Hay fever

See *Allergies (respiratory)*, *Rhinitis* and *Allergic*

Headache (cluster)

See also *Migraine* and *Headache (general)*

Cluster headaches are severe and often occur after a person falls asleep. The burning, sharp pain typically occurs on one side of the head, often around the eye. There is often swelling under or around the eye (or eyes), tearing, red eyes, runny nose and a flushed face.

Cluster headaches may be due to a lack of oxygen from congested sinuses or other problems. They may also be a sign of problems with the hypothalamus, hormonal imbalances, digestive disorders, nerve dysfunction, structural issues or stress.

Massaging a small amount of capsicum extract or a *Topical Analgesic Formula* on the temples may offer some relief. Also consider doing some colon cleansing and screening for food allergies. Make sure you stay well hydrated. Chiropractic care or craniosacral therapy may also be helpful. If you have problems with cluster headaches, work with your natural health care advisor to try to identify the underlying causes.

Therapies: Colon Cleanse, Eliminate Allergy-Causing Foods and Hydration

Formulas: Topical Analgesic and Digestive Bitter Tonic

Key Herbs: Barberry, Capsicum (Cayenne), Celandine and **Scullcap (Skullcap)**

Key Nutrients: Magnesium, Vitamin B-12 and Iron

Headache (general)

See also *Headache (tension)*, *Migraine* and *Pain (general remedies for)*

Headaches are a symptom of an imbalance in the body, or some type of interference with normal body processes. While an analgesic can temporarily suppress the pain, if you want long-term relief from chronic headaches, you need to start identifying what might be throwing your body out of balance.

For starters, dehydration can cause headaches. Bathed in a saline solution, the brain is the most hydrated organ in the body. Even a slight decrease in the water level of the brain affects neurotransmitters that can trigger headaches. This may be why caffeine, alcohol and exercise trigger headaches; they all increase water loss.

So, a good place to start in eliminating chronic headaches is to increase your water intake. If you have a headache, try drinking two or three glasses of water. Often this will result in an immediate reduction in pain. Make certain you drink at least one half-ounce of water per pound of body weight per day to stay properly hydrated.

Foods and Beverages to Avoid

While increasing your water intake, try reducing consumption of caffeinated beverages (tea, coffee, ener-gy drinks and soda) and alcohol. These beverages are all known to trigger headaches. If you consume them, increase your water intake even more. It is also wise to avoid MSG, aspartame (Nutri-Sweet®), aged meats and cheeses and foods containing nitrates (bacon, hot dogs, cured lunch meats) as these substances have also been known to trigger headaches.

Certain foods trigger what might be considered a brain "allergy." Histamine is a neurotransmitter in the brain and is also released during allergic reactions. In some people, certain foods appear to trigger excess histamine production, causing migraines. Common foods that may cause this reaction include: chocolate, processed and pickled foods, smoked fish, chicken livers, figs, avocados, bananas, citrus fruits, nuts, peanut butter, onions, dairy products and gluten-bearing grains like wheat, oats, barley and rye.

If you suffer from frequent headaches, especially migraines, it may be helpful to keep a food journal. Record what you eat throughout the day and the time you eat it. Also, record the times when you experience headaches. This can help you identify food triggers that may be making your head ache.

Relax and Relieve the Pain

Since muscle tension is the most common cause of headaches, find ways to reduce your stress and relax. If you work at a computer, take a break periodically to stretch and do some self-massage on your neck and shoulders.

You can also try relaxing the muscles in your neck and shoulders by rubbing an extract of lobelia mixed with an extract of capsicum into the muscles. Follow this up with a *Topical Analgesic Formula*. You can also try applying magnesium oil topically. These topical applications and self-massage can often permanently relieve a tension headache in less than 1/2 hour. Laying down and practicing Deep Breathing therapy after doing this self-massage will increase its effectiveness.

You may find that the services of a massage therapist or chiropractor will be helpful, too. Having a massage is a great way to reduce stress and tension and can help reduce the frequency of headaches. Chiropractors often relieve headaches by adjusting the vertebrae in the upper back and neck to release pressure on nerves.

If you're under a lot of stress, take some supplements to help your body relax more, such as a *Relaxing Nervine Formula*. B-complex vitamins and magnesium may also be helpful for tension induced by stress.

Fatigue and insomnia are known to increase muscle tension, which increases your risk of getting a pain in your head. Try a *Sleep Formula* or some kava kava to help you relax the tension in your body and get the sleep you need.

Ease the Eye and Neck Strain

Many people get headaches from working too much at the computer. As people strain to look at the screen, their head leans forward, causing the muscles in their upper back and neck to strain trying to hold the head up against the weight of gravity. This creates upper back, shoulder and neck tension, which can ultimately result in a "splitting" headache. Eye strain can also cause headaches.

The solution is simple. Make sure your work or reading area is well lit. Have your eyes checked regularly and wear glasses if needed. Take breaks from close work, letting your eyes look up and focus across the room every 15 minutes. It also helps to stretch the neck and shoulders backwards to help relax the muscles. Be aware of your posture and try to keep your head erect.

Kudzu can help headaches caused by tension in the neck. Black cohosh can also be helpful for these types of headaches.

If you just want some symptomatic relief, try using an herbal *Analgesic Formula* or a *Migraine/Headache Formula* with willow bark as a primary ingredient. Willow is a source of salycilates and is useful for easing headaches in much the same manner as aspirin does.

Therapies: Affirmation and Visualization, Aromatherapy, Colon Cleanse, Colon Hydrotherapy, Compress, Deep Breathing, Fast or Juice Fast, Hydration and Stress Management

Formulas: Analgesic, Topical Analgesic, Relaxing Nervine and Sleep

Key Herbs: Black Cohosh, Capsicum (Cayenne), **Jamaican Dogwood**, **Willow**, Kava-kava, Kudzu, Linden, Lobelia, Sage, Stillingia and Thyme

Key Nutrients: Vitamin B-Complex, **Magnesium**, 5-HTP and Potassium

Headache (migraine)

See *Migraine*

Headache (sinus)

See also *Congestion (sinus)*

Sinus headaches are the result of sinus infections and are felt in the sinus areas (below and above the eyes). Not all headaches felt in this area are related to the sinuses, however. It is only a sinus headache when there is infection present. Along with taking something for infection, such as an *Antibacterial Formula* or a *Goldenseal & Echinacea* product, the herbs fenugreek and thyme have proven beneficial. Look for a good *Decongestant Formula* or *Sinus Decongestant* with these herbs as primary ingredients.

Therapies: Colon Cleanse

Formulas: Antibacterial, Goldenseal & Echinacea, Decongestant, Sinus Decongestant and Topical Analgesic

Key Herbs: Fenugreek, St. John's wort and Thyme

Key Nutrients: Digestive Enzymes, Vitamin A and **Vitamin D**

Headache (tension)

See also *Headache (general)*

If you have a tension headache, it is generally felt equally on both sides of the head. The pain may be dull or squeezing, with a sensation that the head is in a tight band or a vice. You will also typically have tension and even soreness in your neck and shoulders.

The quickest way to ease a tension headache is to drink a lot of water and massage your neck and shoulders to ease the tension as described under Headaches (general). Anything that helps your body relax is going to help you ease the pain of a tension headache, such as a *Relaxing Nervine Formula*, kava kava, passionflower, lavender, valerian or hops. Emptying the contents of a magnesium capsule onto your tongue is another way to relax tension quickly.

Tension headaches may arise from the digestive system and from being constipated. If you've got digestive upset, acid indigestion or your bowels aren't moving regularly, take something to clear out your gastrointestinal tract, like a *Stimulant Laxative* or a *General Detoxifying Formula*. Often the headache will go away as soon as the digestive tract is clear. If you suffer from frequent tension headaches, try doing the Colon Cleanse therapy.

Therapies: Aromatherapy, Colon Cleanse, Deep Breathing, Hydration and Stress Management

Formulas: Relaxing Nervine, Analgesic, Stimulant Laxative and General Detoxifying

Key Herbs: California Poppy, **Black Cohosh**, **Blue Vervain**, **Scullcap (Skullcap)**, Eleuthero (Siberian ginseng), Hops, Kava-kava, Khella, Lavender, Lobelia, Mistletoe, Passionflower, Periwinkle (Lesser), Skunk Cabbage, Valerian and Wood Betony

Key Nutrients: Magnesium, Vitamin B-Complex and L-Arginine

Hearing Loss

See also *Ear Infection or Earache* and *Tinnitus (Ringing in the Ears)*

Hearing loss is common among the elderly and middle-aged folks, but today's youth are starting to experience hearing problems that used to belong only to the older generation. So, while Baby Boomers are now reaping the consequences of listening to rock 'n roll at loud volumes when they were young, today's youth are rapidly, yet sadly, joining their ranks. Ear buds, exotic car audio systems and high-output home theater components crank out tunes at unprecedented volume levels, and most people are completely unaware of the damage they are inflicting on their delicate ears. Hearing specialists say they're also seeing more people in their 30s and 40s, many of them among the first Walkman users, who suffer from pronounced tinnitus, an internal ringing, whooshing or humming in the ears.

Of all the factors contributing to hearing loss, loud noise is generally the most common. Fortunately, this is something over which we have a lot of control. Noise levels are measured in decibels, or "dB" for short. The higher the decibel level, the louder the noise. Our hearing system can be injured not only by a loud blast but also by prolonged exposure to high noise levels. Sounds of 85 to 90 dB and higher can cause permanent hearing loss.

To get an idea of the decibel level of various sounds, here are a few examples: Sounds over 120 dB can be acutely painful, such as a jet plane taking off or a siren (120 dB), a jackhammer (130 dB), firearms (140 dB) and fireworks at three feet (150 dB). Prolonged exposure to the following extremely loud sounds can also create hearing problems: a passing motorcycle (90 dB), a hand drill (100 dB), small gas engines like lawn mowers and snow blowers (106 dB) and a chain saw (110 dB). 110 dB is the maximum output of most MP3 players.

In contrast, a vacuum cleaner or busy traffic is only 70 dB, and most kitchen appliances and hair dryers are between 80-90 dB. A typical conversation is only 60 dB.

If you have to raise your voice to be heard, can't hear someone three feet from you, have difficulty discerning speech after leaving a noisy area, or have pain or ringing in your ears after exposure to noise, your hearing has probably been damaged, so get your ears checked. Meanwhile, here are some natural remedies that may help.

The ear is often referred to as the most energy-hungry organ of the body. All parts of the ear require high quantities of nutrients to function properly and to avoid degenerative problems such as hearing loss or tinnitus. Only if the right minerals and enzymes are present can the nerves successfully fire the precise signals at millisecond intervals required to accurately transmit sound.

The delicate balance of the hearing system can be upset by:

Insufficient oxygen due to poor circulation in the inner ear

A deficiency in the trace minerals needed for enzyme activity

A toxic overload being carried by the body

Excessive free radical activity

The electrical stability of the cochlea depends on the presence of minerals such as magnesium and calcium, as well as a correct balance of necessary enzymes, fatty acids and amino acids. The tiny hair-like cells called cilia are the final stage of sound transmission before the charge is relayed to the auditory nerve. Slight disturbances in the equilibrium of enzymes can lead to the death of some of the cilia.

This means adequate trace minerals are needed for ear health. Antioxidants can also protect the ears, just like they help protect the eyes. Herbs that may be helpful for the ears include: lobelia (used as ear drops), ginkgo (taken internally) and St. John's wort (used internally and as ear drops). Helichrysum essential oil may also be helpful.

Therapies: Fresh Fruits and Vegetables, Hydration and Mineralization

Formulas: Antioxidant

Key Herbs: Ginkgo, **St. John's wort** and Lobelia

Key Nutrients: Magnesium, Calcium, Colloidal Minerals, Folate (Folic Acid and Vitamin B9)

Heart (weakness)

See also *Cardiac Arrest (Heart Attack)*, *Cardiovascular Disease (Heart Disease)* and *Congestive Heart Failure*

When the heart has been stressed or weakened by disease, there are herbs and nutrients that can be used to strengthen it. *Cardiac Tonic Formulas* are based on herbs like hawthorn, arjuna, night-blooming cerus and lily of the valley, which can encourage a stronger heartbeat and improve cardiac function. Good fats and nutrients like magnesium, l-carnitine and Co-Q10 may also be helpful. Consult with a qualified herbalist (*findanherbalist.com*) or natural doctor to help determine which supplements would be best.

Therapies: Fresh Fruits and Vegetables and Healthy Fats

Formulas: Cardiac Tonic

Key Herbs: Astragalus, Capsicum (Cayenne), **Arjuna**, **Hawthorn**, Eleuthero (Siberian ginseng), Ginkgo, Night Blooming Cereus (Cactus) and Tribulus

Key Nutrients: Magnesium, Co-Q10, Omega-3 Essential Fatty Acids, L-Carnitine and Vitamin B-1 (Thiamine)

Heart Attack

See *Cardiac Arrest (Heart Attack)*

Heart Disease

See *Cardiovascular Disease (Heart Disease)*

Heart Fibrillation or Palpitations

See also *Hiatal Hernia*

Rapid, irregular contractions of the heart muscle are called heart palpitations or fibrillations. Symptoms can include an irregular or rapid heart rate, skipped heartbeats, shortness of breath, and chest discomfort. They may be caused by anxiety, lack of exercise, high blood pressure, diabetes, hyperthyroid or other problems. Many of the best herbal remedies for this problem are toxic botanicals that are not readily available, such as lily of the valley, so professional assistance should be sought. However, one of the best natural solutions is to make sure the person has adequate amounts of minerals, especially magnesium, potassium and calcium. *Cardiac Tonic* and *Cardiovascular Stimulant Formulas* may offer some help. Herbs to look for in these formulas include hawthorn, motherwort, night blooming cereus and passionflower. A hiatal hernia can sometimes put stress on the heart and cause palpitations. Consult with a professional herbalist (*findanherbalist.com*) or natural health care provider for more assistance and have the condition monitored by a medical doctor.

Therapies: Affirmation and Visualization, Hiatal Hernia Correction and Stress Management

Formulas: Cardiac Tonic and Cardiovascular Stimulant

Key Herbs: Astragalus, Bugleweed, California Poppy, Capsicum (Cayenne), **Hawthorn**, **Lily of the Valley**, **Motherwort**, Eleuthero (Siberian ginseng), Lemon Balm, Linden, Night Blooming Cereus (Cactus), Passionflower and Valerian

Key Nutrients: L-Carnitine, Iron, Vitamin B-12, Calcium, **Potassium**, **Magnesium**, Co-Q10, Chlorophyll, Vitamin B-Complex and Vitamin E

Heart Rate (irregular)

See *Arrhythmia (Irregular Heartbeat)*

Heart Rate (rapid)

See *Tachycardia*

Therapies: Deep Breathing

Heart Valves

Heart valve problems may be present at birth or can be caused by infections, heart attacks or some other damage to the heart. There are three basic problems that can occur. First, the valve may not close tightly, allowing blood to leak back through the valve. This is called regurgitation. Second, if the valve doesn't open wide enough to allow for normal blood flow, this is called stenosis. The third and most common heart valve problem occurs in the mitral valve. Sometimes it doesn't close tightly, allowing regurgitation. This is called mitral valve prolapse.

Heart valve conditions should be monitored by a medical doctor. There are some herbs and nutrients that may be helpful, too. A cactus, called night blooming cereus, is a particularly good remedy for mitral valve prolapse and other valvular problems. Look for a *Cardiac Tonic Formula* that contains this herb and hawthorn, which is also helpful for valvular insufficiency.

Therapies: Mineralization

Formulas: Cardiac Tonic

Key Herbs: Hawthorn, **Night Blooming Cereus (Cactus)** and Ginkgo

Key Nutrients: Magnesium

Heartburn

See *Acid Indigestion (Heartburn, Acid Reflux)*

Heavy Metal Poisoning

See also *Lead Poisoning* and *Mercury Poisoning*

Rome may not have been built in a day, but it was destroyed by heavy metal poisoning in its water supply! The Roman aqueduct system and the plumbing in it's famous public baths and the residences of Rome's ruling class were incredible for their time. However, the lead pipes in the water system caused neurological disorders that led to the decadent behavior which caused the Roman Empire to collapse.

Today, heavy metals and other toxic substances in our environment are bringing about a similar decline in the mental (and physical) health of society. Learning disabilities and behavioral problems are rampant, and a new category of diseases, autoimmune disorders, have been increasing at an alarming rate. These include rheumatoid arthritis, chronic fatigue, type I diabetes, fibromyalgia, lupus, Lou Gehrig's disease, myasthenia gravis and multiple sclerosis. Besides being a major factor in autoimmune diseases, heavy metals play a role in cancer, heart disease, dementia, Alzheimer's, reduced immunity and mental illness.

Ideally, we should do all we can to avoid them, so here are some important tips for reducing your exposure to these health-destroying elements.

Purify your water! Make sure your water pipes have no lead, avoid lead-based painted objects, and don't store liquids in lead crystal containers. Be especially cautious of imports from China, as they often have lead contamination.

Buy and prepare fresh, organic food as much as possible. Keep the chemicals in your life, especially cleaning chemicals, to a minimum.

Avoid cooking with aluminum pans or using anything that is aluminum with your food, especially acidic foods like citrus.

Read labels—many processed foods, including iodized salt and baking powder, may contain aluminum as an anti-caking agent. Antiperspirant deodorants always contain aluminum; use a natural deodorant or enzyme solution instead.

Insist on composite fillings from your dentist, not mercury/silver amalgams. Avoid unnecessary vaccinations as they contain heavy metals.

You can also periodically do a "cleanse" to pull heavy metals from the body. This is especially important for people who work around a lot of chemicals or are starting to develop signs of neurological problems.

A good heavy metal cleanse would include a *Heavy Metal Cleansing Formula* and some type of fiber to bind heavy metals in the intestines. Sodium alginate (algin), a mucilaginous fiber from kelp, is very good at binding heavy metals. Essential fatty acids are also helpful for a heavy metal cleanse.

In serious cases, oral or intravenous chelation may be helpful for getting heavy metals out of the body. Drawing baths and foot soaks can also be helpful.

Therapies: Drawing Bath, Epsom Salt Bath and Heavy Metal Cleanse

Formulas: Heavy Metal Cleansing and Fiber Blend

Key Herbs: Cilantro/Coriander herb, **Milk Thistle** and Psyllium

Key Nutrients: N-Acetyl Cysteine, **Alpha Lipoic Acid**, Sodium Alginate (Algin), Omega-3 Essential Fatty Acids and Iodine

Hemochromatosis

When a person has too much iron in the blood the condition is commonly known as hemochromatosis. Primary hemochromatosis refers to accumulating to much iron because of a genetic mutation. Secondary hemochromatosis is iron overload from any other (non-genetic) cause like excessive iron consumption, multiple blood transfusions, lack of iron binding capacity and zinc deficiencies. Nutrients that help the body utilize iron better may be helpful, including folate, vitamin B6 and vitamin B12. Another option may be an *Iron Formula*, as the nutritional cofactors in iron-rich herbs can sometimes help the body utilize iron more efficiently.

Formulas: Iron

Key Herbs: Alfalfa, Nettle (Stinging) and Yellow Dock

Key Nutrients: Zinc, Vitamin B-6 (Pyridoxine), Vitamin B-12, Folate (Folic Acid, Vitamin B9) and Chlorophyll

Hemorrhage

See *Bleeding (external)* and *Bleeding (internal)*

Hemorrhoids

See also *Varicose Veins*

A hemorrhoid is a mass of dilated veins in the rectum that cause painful bowel eliminations. It is important to keep the stool soft with a *Fiber Blend Formula* and plenty of water and to keep the bowels moving using a *Gentle Laxative Formula* or perhaps even a *Stimulant Laxative Formula* (for a short period, such as two weeks).

A good natural treatment is to mix a *Topical Vulnerary Formula* (salve) with white oak bark powder and apply the mixture topically. You can also use astringent herbs like white oak or collinsonia internally.

Hemorrhoids are in indication that blood vessels, in general, need toning. It is common for an individual with hemorrhoids to have other varicosities like varicose veins. When this is the case, *Vascular Tonic Formulas* containing herbs like butcher's broom and horsechestnut can be helpful.

Conditions

Therapies: Dietary Fiber, Fresh Fruits and Vegetables and Hydration

Formulas: Topical Vulnerary, Fiber Blend, Gentle Laxative and Vascular Tonic

Key Herbs: Aloe vera, Bilberry (Blueberry, Huckleberry), Butchers Broom, Cherry (Wild), Chickweed, **Collinsonia (Stoneroot)**, **Horse Chestnut**, **White Oak**, Goldenseal, Horsetail, Marshmallow, Milk Thistle, Poke Root, Psyllium, Slippery Elm, St. John's wort, Witch Hazel and Yellow Dock

Key Nutrients: Digestive Enzymes, Vitamin E and Fiber

Hepatitis

Hepatitis is inflammation of the liver. Hepatitis A is an infectious hepatitis that can be transmitted through poor sanitary conditions, and food handlers or child care workers not washing their hands. Hepatitis B or serum hepatitis is passed through a blood transfusion or other contact with blood. Hepatitis C is also infectious and viral in nature. Hepatitis can also be caused by chemicals, poor diet and other lifestyle factors that damage the liver. Seek appropriate medical assistance when dealing with hepatitis, as it is a very serious condition.

Natural remedies that may be helpful include herbs with hepatoprotective properties such as milk thistle and schizandra. A good *Hepatoprotective Formula* should contain these and other herbs that protect the liver. SAM-e and vitamin C can be helpful taken internally. Since most cases are viral-related, an *Antiviral Formula* may also aid in recovery.

To allow the liver to rest when recovering from hepatitis, fast, or eat only mild foods, and drink plenty of water. Avoid spices, alcohol, caffeine and all chemicals.

Therapies: Avoid Caffeine, Fast or Juice Fast, Fresh Fruits and Vegetables and Hydration

Formulas: Hepatoprotective, Liver Tonic and Antiviral

Key Herbs: Astragalus, Bupleurum, **Andrographis**, **Milk Thistle**, **Reishi (Ganoderma)**, Dandelion, Elder, Lycium (Wolfberry, Gogi), Oregon Grape, Rehmannia, Schisandra (Schizandra), Shiitake and Yellow Dock

Key Nutrients: SAM-e, Vitamin C, **N-Acetyl Cysteine** and Betaine Hydrochloric Acid (HCl)

Hernias

See also *Hiatal Hernia*

The protrusion of an organ through connective tissue or the wall of a cavity by which it is normally enclosed is called a hernia. There are many types of hernias, depending on where the weakness in the abdominal cavity occurs. Medical attention should be sought, but *Tissue Healing Formulas* may help strengthen the connective tissue to aid in the healing of a hernia.

Therapies: Mineralization

Formulas: Tissue Healing

Key Herbs: Red Raspberry

Herniated Disks

See *Disks (bulging or slipped)*

Herpes

See also *Chicken Pox* and *Cold Sores (Fever Blisters)*

Herpes is a name for any of several inflammatory viral diseases characterized by blister-like sores. *Herpes simplex* can cause cold sores or fever blisters around the mouth or genital area. Herpes zoster is responsible for chicken pox and shingles. *Antiviral Formulas* can be helpful in treating herpes infections naturally. A variety of single herbs with antiviral properties may also be helpful, including black walnut (topically for outbreaks), cat's claw, isatis and propolis. Research suggests that l-lysine is involved in the immune system and its ability to fight the herpes simplex virus. This makes it useful as a remedy for cold sores, canker sores, fever blisters and genital herpes. However, it only works if the diet is low in arginine. Enhancing the immune system in general by supplementing with probiotics and using a *Mushroom Blend* or an *Immune Stimulating Formula* may also be helpful. Since stress tends to weaken the immune system and promote outbreaks, Stress Management therapy is also important.

Therapies: Friendly Flora and Stress Management

Formulas: Antiviral, Immune Stimulating and Mushroom Blend

Key Herbs: Bitter Melon, Black Walnut, Cats Claw (Uña de Gato, Gambier), **Lemon Balm**, **St. John's wort**, Isatis, Propolis, Shiitake and Spilanthes

Key Nutrients: L-Lysine, Zinc and Probiotics

Hiatal Hernia

See also *Ileocecal Valve* and *Small Intestinal Bacterial Overgrowth (SIBO)*

In a hiatal hernia the stomach pushes upward through the opening in the diaphragm for the esophagus. This can cause acid reflux, put stress and pressure on the heart, create poor digestive function and generally weaken the body. The instructions for dealing with this problem are found under Hiatal Hernia Correction in the *Therapies Section*. The remedies listed here may also be helpful.

Therapies: Deep Breathing, Hiatal Hernia Correction and Stress Management

Formulas: Antispasmodic

Key Herbs: Black Haw, Catnip, **Dandelion flower essence**, **Lobelia**, Dandelion root and Slippery Elm

Key Nutrients: Digestive Enzymes

Hiccups

Hiccups are involuntary, spasmodic contractions of the diaphragm causing a quick inhalation of air that makes a strange sound. *Antispasmodic Formulas* and herbs like lobelia may relax the spasms associated with hiccups.

Formulas: Antispasmodic

Key Herbs: Catnip, **Cramp Bark** and Lobelia

Key Nutrients: Magnesium

High Blood Pressure

See *Hypertension*

High Cholesterol

See *Cholesterol (high)*

HIV (AIDS)

See *Acquired Immune Deficiency Syndrome (AIDS)/HIV*

Hives

See *Rashes and Hives*

Hoarseness

See *Laryngitis (Hoarseness)*

Hodgkin Lymphoma (Hodgkin's Disease)

See *Hodgkin Lymphoma (Hodgkin's Disease)*

Hormone Replacement

See *Estrogen (low)*, *Hypothyroid* and *Testosterone (low)*

Hot Flashes

See also *Menopause*

Hot flashes are a complex symptom associated with menopause and the most common menopausal problem. There is an initial feeling of discomfort followed by a sensation of heat moving toward the head. The face becomes red, which is followed by sweating and fatigue.

Night sweats are simply hot flashes that occur at night and cause heavy perspiration.

Although the exact cause of hot flashes is not fully understood, there is some evidence that hot flashes occur via the hypothalamus, a part of the brain that sends signals to the pituitary gland to activate various hormones. The hypothalamus also regulates the body temperature.

When the hypothalamus senses there is a need for more estrogen it sends the gonadotropin-releasing hormone (GNRH) to the pituitary. GNRH stimulates the release of the follicle-stimulating hormone (FSH). During a woman's childbearing years, FSH stimulates the development of an egg follicle, which releases estrogen. The hypothalamus senses the increased estrogen level and stops producing GNRH.

During menopause, when there is no viable egg to develop, there is no estrogen response from the ovaries. So, the hypothalamus increases production of GNRH to try to increase estrogen. The low estrogen can cause epinephrine to release from the adrenals, which stimulates the hypothalamus and resets the body's internal thermostat. This doesn't just create the sensations of heat, it can also cause the heart to speed up, resulting in feelings of anxiety and a pounding sensation in the chest.

After awhile the hypothalamus learns to adjust to lower levels of estrogen and stops trying to stimulate the ovaries. But until this happens, hot flashes may be a problem.

Fortunately, there are ways to help balance hormones to reduce the severity of hot flashes, if not eliminate them entirely. Different women will respond to different remedies, so if the first thing you try doesn't work, don't be discouraged. Try some other approaches.

For starters, heat and substances that dilate arteries (coffee, chili and alcohol) can all aggravate hot flashes, as can smoking and sugar consumption. Stress and adrenal fatigue also contribute to increased problems with hot flashes. Establishing basic health practices, like a good diet, exercise and adequate sleep is also important to minimizing problems with hot flashes.

The second approach is to use a *Menopause Balancing Formula*. These formulas contain herbs like black cohosh and chaste tree (vitex) to help regulate hormones.

Many women find these herbs effective, but they are not the only remedies that can help. Since the adrenal glands produce estrogens, adrenal exhaustion may be a factor in hot flashes and other menopausal symptoms. Pantothenic acid and/or an *Adrenal Tonic Formula* may also be helpful. Adaptogens like eleuthero root may also help, and are often found in *Menopause Balancing Formulas*. Ashwaganda is another potentially helpful adaptogen.

Essential oils with estrogen-stimulating effects can also be helpful. These include clary sage, pink grapefruit and geranium. Lavender essential oil can also be helpful for hot flashes because of its relaxing effects. Mix a few drops of these oils with a little water in a small spray bottle and mist this around your face when you are having a hot flash. Essential oils directly affect the hypothalamus via the sense of smell, so this can help to instantly reset your body thermostat and cool you down.

Increasing your intake of good fats containing omega-3 and omega-6 essential fatty acids can also be helpful. Evening primrose oil is also frequently used for female problems like hot flashes.

Therapies: Avoid Xenoestrogens, Fresh Fruits and Vegetables, Healthy Fats, Low Glycemic Diet and Stress Management

Formulas: Menopause Balancing and Adrenal Tonic

Key Herbs: Ashwaganda, **Black Cohosh**, **Chastetree (Vitex)**, **Damiana**, Eleuthero (Siberian ginseng), Lavender essential oil, Licorice and Sage essential oil

Key Nutrients: Pantothenic Acid (Vitamin B5) and Omega-3 Essential Fatty Acids

Hyperactivity

See *Attention Deficit Disorder (ADD, ADHD)*

Hyperinsulinemia (Metabolic Syndrome, Syndrome X)

See also *Diabetes* and *Weight Loss (aids for)*

Research has brought to light a previously hidden cause of many modern illnesses. Dubbed Metabolic Syndrome or Syndrome X, this condition involves high levels of insulin in the blood or hyperinsulinemia. This syndrome is the precursor to type 2 diabetes, which occurs when cells become resistant to the action of insulin.

High levels of insulin in the blood are primarily caused by consuming too many simple carbohydrates, especially sugar. However, excess consumption of refined flour, bread, and grains like rice, corn and potatoes contributes to the problem. When too much sugar enters the blood stream, the blood sugar level spikes, which causes insulin to be released from the pancreas to move this sugar out of the blood stream and into the cells for utilization or storage.

The excess sugar is stored as fat, which is why hyperinsulinemia causes weight gain. It also is a major contributing factor to increased levels of inflammation in the body, which can cause high blood pressure and arteriosclerosis. In fact, excess insulin is a bigger risk factor for cardiovascular disease than excess cholesterol.

Hyperinsulinemia also disrupts sodium metabolism, increasing water retention. By depressing neurotransmitters in the brain, Syndrome X contributes to depression. In women, 75% of all cases of polycystic ovarian syndrome are also related to too much insulin.

In the initial stages, producing too much insulin causes a rapid lowering of blood sugar levels, which causes hypoglycemia or low blood sugar. This increases the craving for sweets and stresses other hormone systems. It interferes with the conversion of thyroid hormone T-4 to T-3, which can result in functional hypothyroidism. Another negative effect is a rise in cortisol production from the adrenals. This reduces our ability to cope with stress, lowers our immune response and eventually exhausts our adrenals. Excess cortisol also contributes to aging.

If you want to know if you have Syndrome X, you could have lab tests run to check your insulin levels. (Fasting levels of insulin should be below 10 units.) However, there is an easier way—measure your waist and hips.

Abdominal obesity is a major indicator of excess insulin production. So, grab a tape measure and check your circumference at the navel and at the widest part of your hips. In men, if your waist measurement is larger than your hips, you've got Syndrome X. In women, the waist should be less than 80% of the hip measurement.

Another indicator of Syndrome X is your triglyceride and HDL levels in routine blood tests. If your triglyceride level is greater than 150 or your HDL level is less than 35, you're having problems with excess insulin production and insulin resistance.

The primary cause of hyperinsulinemia is a high carbohydrate, low protein diet and a lack of good dietary fats. So, using the Low Glycemic Diet therapy is the major way to combat this problem. Other contributing factors include:

Too many omega-6 essential fatty acids in the diet, with insufficient omega-3.

Sedentary life-styles and lack of exercise.

Deficiencies of dietary chromium and magnesium. Deficiencies of zinc, manganese, vanadium, B-vitamins and vitamin A may also be involved.

Besides going on a low glycemic diet, the following are also helpful in overcoming hyperinsulinemia.

Resistance exercise trains muscles to take up glucose without the need for insulin, thereby decreasing insulin requirements. After just five days without exercise insulin resistance increases. Exercise like weight lifting done to the point that it makes muscles burn a little, is causing muscle tissue to take up sugar without insulin. Thus, a program of muscle building exercise at least three times per week will reduce insulin levels.

A second key is changing the kinds of fats one consumes. Transfatty acids, found in margarine and vegetable oils increase cellular resistance to insulin. Most vegetable oils are high in omega-6 fatty acids, but deficient in omega-3 fatty acids, which decrease insulin resistance. Switch from vegetable oils and hydrogenated fats (fries, chips, pastries, bagels, etc.) to high quality fats like olive oil, butter, nuts and fish.

A third secret is to use herbs and supplements that lower insulin levels. Chromium, magnesium and zinc all help the body utilize sugar. It also helps to take a *Blood Sugar Reducing Formula*. For additional supplement ideas, see diabetes.

Therapies: Exercise and Low Glycemic Diet

Formulas: Blood Sugar Reducing

Key Herbs: Bitter Melon, **Cinnamon**, Dandelion, Ginseng (American), Ginseng (Asian, Korean), Juniper Berry, Licorice, Nopal (Prickly Pear) and Turmeric

Key Nutrients: Omega-3 Essential Fatty Acids, Chromium, **Magnesium**, Zinc, Vitamin B-Complex, Vitamin A, **Alpha Lipoic Acid** and Vitamin C

Hypertension

See also *Arteriosclerosis (Atherosclerosis, Hardening of the Arteries), Cardiovascular Disease (Heart Disease), Hyperinsulinemia (Metabolic Syndrome, Syndrome X)* and *Weight Loss (aids for)*

When there is excessive arterial tension, the heart has to pump harder in order for blood to reach the extremities of the body. This results in high blood pressure. When this happens, most people start taking high blood pressure medication prescribed by their doctor.

How many people do you know who have cured high blood pressure by taking prescription medications? Probably none. That's because high blood pressure isn't caused by a deficiency of high blood pressure medications, and the medicine prescribed isn't designed to cure hypertension. In fact, the whole issue of hypertension is a perfect example of the major shortcoming of modern Western medicine. Modern medicine focuses on symptom management, but does little to address the root causes of most diseases, including high blood pressure.

High blood pressure is a problem associated with lifestyle. It is virtually unknown in undeveloped areas of the world where people are living on their traditional diets. For example, high blood pressure is not found in Africa among natives living a traditional lifestyle, even among the elderly. In contrast, a high percentage of Americans have this problem (about 60 million).

Hypertension greatly increases the risk of other diseases. Research done by insurance companies has shown that even slight increases in blood pressure can result in decreased survival rates. It increases the risk of heart attack, stroke, and kidney failure. Clearly, solving the problem of high blood pressure is important, but 90% of all cases are treated with drugs that only address the symptoms.

About 80% of all hypertension cases involve mild to moderate symptoms and can be effectively managed with dietary and lifestyle changes accompanied by herbs and dietary supplements. For example, all of the following have been scientifically demonstrated to reduce blood pressure: consuming sufficient amounts of pure water, using the Dietary Fiber therapy, losing weight, moderating salt consumption, eliminating caffeine, alcohol and tobacco, exercising, consuming omega-3 essential fatty acids and balancing the intake of calcium and magnesium. These are all options individuals can experiment with to find out what works for them. In addition, they can examine the specific causes of hypertension and choose other supplements and diet and lifestyle changes that address their individual situation.

High blood pressure is a symptom of other imbalances, not a disease in itself, so to understand how to work with it, we first need to understand what blood pressure is all about. Blood pressure consists of the systolic pressure and the diastolic pressure. The systolic is the pressure exerted by the contraction of the heartbeat moving blood through the blood vessels. The diastolic is the resting pressure, the pressure remaining in the blood vessel in between heartbeats.

Blood pressure is expressed with the systolic reading first, followed by the diastolic reading. Normal blood pressure is considered 90/60 to 130/90, but research shows that 115-125/70-80 is optimal for health and longevity.

The dynamics of blood pressure are fairly straightforward. Your body has about 100,000 miles of blood vessels. The larger vessels have muscular walls that can expand and contract to increase or decrease the diameter of the blood vessels. The diastolic pressure is the pressure needed to maintain full blood vessels. In other words, the blood vessel is like a pipe carrying liquid, which must expand or contract to match the volume of liquid it is carrying.

If air pockets get into the water pipes of your home, water doesn't flow freely to your faucet. Instead, it sputters and spurts. Likewise, if the diameter of the blood vessel "pipes" were allowed to be bigger than the volume of blood they were carrying, then air pockets would form and disrupt circulation. Thus, the body has a built in system of pressure regulation to keep its "pipes" full.

If the blood vessels contract or get smaller in diameter, the diastolic pressure will rise. This also means that the heart has to increase its pressure to push the blood through the smaller pipes, so there will be a corresponding rise in the systolic pressure.

This increase in pressure has negative consequences on health. It forces the heart to work harder, which wears it out faster. It increases the risk of forming blood clots in the circulatory system, which increases the risk of myocardial infarction, strokes and thrombosis. It can cause blood vessels to "blow" from the pressure, causing an aneurism. It can also damage the kidneys, eyes, brain and other organs.

Furthermore, arterial plaque never forms in veins (which are areas of low pressure). Arterial plaque only forms in areas of the circulatory system subject to high pressures. In fact, plaque formation may be a protective mechanism to shore up blood vessels so they can handle the higher pressure.

It's clear that if we want to get rid of hypertension, we need to help the blood vessels relax so that less pressure is required to move blood through the cardiovascular system.

Coupled with changes in diet and lifestyle, herbal remedies can help with the underlying causes of high blood pressure. You can start by using one of the many *Hypotensive Formulas* that are specifically designed to help with this problem, but you can also examine what the underlying causes are and work on them. Here are some factors to consider.

Water Retention and Kidney Function

When the tissues of the body are filled with fluid, this will put pressure on the blood vessels, again constricting blood flow. The kidneys also have an influence on the heart, so problems with the kidneys can also cause the blood pressure to rise. Kidney issues are often an undiagnosed issue behind blood pressure problems.

Where fluid retention is a problem, use an herbal *Diuretic Formula* to help lower blood pressure. Where kidney weakness is an issue, consider a *Kidney Tonic Formula*. Reducing table salt consumption and replacing it with an all-natural sea salt can also help reduce fluid retention and blood pressure.

Dehydration

Water retention may not be the only issue with fluids that contribute to high blood pressure. In his book, *You're Not Sick, You're Thirsty*, Dr. F. Batmanghelidj, MD, explains how dehydration causes an increase in blood pressure. In fact, it's fairly easy to see if you understand that the diastolic pressure is dependent on the volume of blood in the circulatory system. If a person becomes dehydrated, it reduces the volume of blood in their blood vessels, which causes them to contract and increases the pressure.

This seems an extremely plausible explanation as to why people tend to experience an increase in blood pressure as they age, because it is well established that most people become more and more dehydrated as they age. (It's why people tend to get "shriveled" and "wrinkled" with age—they're drying out.)

Based on this understanding, Dr. Batmanghelidj also explains why the current medical approach to hypertension doesn't work. As the body becomes increasingly dehydrated, it tries harder to hang onto salt and water, which causes people to develop edema. Unfortunately, people are given diuretics to try to flush out the water and told to avoid salt. This is 100% opposite of what people actually need to do.

Instead, they need to increase water intake and make sure they are getting adequate amounts of a natural salt. The water and salt will hydrate the body, increase the volume of blood, and help the "pipes" expand to allow for the increased amount of fluid they are carrying. Dr. Batmanghelidj recommends drinking one-half ounce of pure water per pound of body weight per day and taking a pinch of salt with the water.

Excess Weight

Excess weight alone can increase blood pressure simply because there are blood vessels the heart has to pump blood through. There is also a link between excess insulin production, which contributes to excess weight and imbalances in messenger chemicals that cause arterial constriction. If you have excess weight start following the suggestions in this book found under weight loss.

Hardening of the Arteries

Arterial plaque creates obstructions in the blood vessels. Like hard water deposits in a water pipe, these deposits reduce the size of blood vessels and restrict blood flow. As a result, more force is needed to get the blood through the narrower pipes.

When hardening of the arteries is the cause of high blood pressure, *Cardiac Tonic* and *Cardiovascular Stimulant Formulas* can be helpful. For additional suggestions see *Arteriosclerosis*.

Vasoconstriction

Blood vessels have muscular walls that can either tense or relax. When they tense, there is vasoconstriction. It's very similar to the problem asthmatics have when the bronchial pipes constrict, reducing the flow of air into the lungs. They begin gasping for oxygen. Vasoconstriction does the same thing to the arteries. The constricted artery walls limit the flow of blood, and the heart pumps harder trying to force the life-giving blood through the constricted vessels. There are several root causes of vasoconstriction, each with its own remedies.

Stress

In response to stress, real or perceived, the sympathetic nervous system becomes more active and the body tenses. We've all felt the results of this fight-or-flight response when someone suddenly startled us and adrenaline started pumping. The heart started beating harder and blood pressure rose as the body went on red alert. This sensation is due to the release of a hormone and neurotransmitter called epinephrine (or adrenaline).

Adaptogens can modulate the output of stress hormones and may be very helpful for stress related hypertension. So, if you feel like you're under a lot of stress, try an *Adaptogen Formula* and perhaps a *Relaxing Nervine Formula* as well.

Nerve receptors that react to epinephrine are called adrenergic receptors. There are two types, alpha and beta. When the beta adrenergic receptors are stimulated, they cause blood vessels to contract and the heart to beat harder. Perhaps you've heard of beta blockers. These are drugs that help to lower blood pressure, and they work by blocking these beta adrenergic receptor sites.

Lobelia contains a compound called lobeline which acts as a natural beta blocker. It combines well with capsicum and a small amount of black cohosh to reduce cardiac stress and angina, improve circulation to the heart, and lower blood pressure caused by tension. Other nervines like linden flowers, kava kava and passion flower may also help. So, a good *Antispasmodic Formula* with lobelia as a major ingredient, used in conjunction with a Cardiovascular Tonic Formula, can also be an aid to lowering stress-related blood pressure.

Caffeine and Other Stimulants

Caffeine stimulates the sympathetic nervous system and causes the release of more epinephrine. So excessive caffeine consumption increases stress responses and raises blood pressure. Other substances that trigger a sympathetic nervous reaction and stress response include alcohol, tobacco, chocolate, cheese, sugar, alcoholic beverages, and cured pork products such as ham and sausages. All of these substances can contribute to hypertension and should be avoided or severely restricted in the diet. If you need extra energy try an herbal *Energy-Boosting Formula* instead.

Magnesium Deficiency

Contrary to what most people believe, the number one mineral deficiency in most Americans is not calcium; it is magnesium. When muscles contract, calcium ions flow into the muscle cells; as the muscle relaxes, there is an exchange of magnesium for calcium. In other words, calcium helps muscles contract and have tone, while magnesium helps muscles relax.

This is why calcium channel blockers are sometimes used to lower blood pressure. These drugs block calcium from entering the muscle tissues, causing them to be more relaxed. Taking extra magnesium usually creates the same results. It helps blood vessels relax and increases blood flow.

Hyperinsulinemia or Syndrome X

High insulin levels in the blood due to the consumption of refined carbohydrates causes inflammation in the blood vessels, which constricts blood flow. Simple sugars also react with proteins to reduce elasticity, causing blood vessels to lose flexibility. Eliminating simple carbohydrates from the diet can be very helpful for preventing and reversing high blood pressure. Also consider using *Blood Sugar Reducing Formulas*.

Healing the Endothelial Lining

All of the thousands of miles of blood vessels in your body are coated with a lining, just one cell thick, known as the endothelial lining. The endothelial cells make a gas called nitric oxide, which dilates the blood vessels, reducing pressure. Nitric oxide also keeps platelets from sticking to the blood vessel wall, suppresses the formation of arterial plaque and can reduce arterial plaque that has already formed. This is why Dr. Sherry A. Rogers, MD and author of *The High Blood Pressure Hoax!*, believes that dysfunction of the endothelial lining is a primary factor in high blood pressure.

Nitroglycerine pills, which are often used to treat angina, work by stimulating a nitric oxide response in the endothelial lining. We can do the same thing using a simple nutrient, the amino acid l-arginine. Research shows that about 5 grams (5,000 mg) of l-arginine per day can help to control high blood pressure and improve cardiovascular health.

The fat-soluble vitamins A, D, E and K are all essential for protecting cardiovascular health. This is because it isn't regular dietary cholesterol that "sticks" to your arteries; it's oxidized cholesterol that winds up forming arterial plaque. Fat-soluble vitamins keep cholesterol from oxidizing and fats from turning rancid, which protects your cardiovascular system. Supplementing with l-arginine not only helps endothelial dysfunction (ED), it also helps Erectile Dysfunction. Drugs like Viagra® and Cialis® were originally developed as drugs for high blood pressure. They work by increasing nitric oxide responses. Interestingly enough, many of the "male-enhancing" herbs do the same thing, such as yohimbe and horny goat weed (epimedium).

There are also herbs that help the endothelial lining and create vasodilation. Hawthorn and ginkgo have both been found to dilate peripheral blood vessels and improve blood flow to the extremities, thus reducing hypertension. Numerous studies have also shown that garlic can reduce blood pressure 10 to 15 points when taken regularly. Besides having a vasodilative effect, it also decreases blood cholesterol and triglycerides. Onions also have this effect, as do many pungent spices and herbs, which can all be safely consumed as part of the regular diet. These are common ingredients in *Cardiac Tonic* and *Cardiovascular Stimulant Formulas*.

For more information on selecting the remedies that are right for you, consult with a qualified herbalist (*findanherbalist.com*) or natural healer. However, do not discontinue blood pressure medications abruptly. Try using appropriate herbs, supplements and lifestyle changes in conjunction with blood pressure medications. As your blood pressure improves, you can work with your doctor to gradually reduce the dose and possibly eliminate the need for the medication entirely.

Therapies: Affirmation and Visualization, Avoid Caffeine, Deep Breathing, Dietary Fiber, Fresh Fruits and Vegetables, Healthy Fats, Low Glycemic Diet and Stress Management

Formulas: Cardiac Tonic, Cardiovascular Stimulant, Antispasmodic, Blood Purifier, Relaxing Nervine, Adaptogen, Diuretic, Kidney Tonic, Blood Sugar Reducing, Antispasmodic, Weight Loss and **Hypotensive**

Key Herbs: Black Cohosh, Capsicum (Cayenne), **Arjuna**, **Blue Vervain**, **Hawthorn**, **Linden**, **Mistletoe**, **Motherwort**, Eleuthero (Siberian ginseng), Garlic, Ginkgo, Ginseng (American), Ginseng (Asian, Korean), Khella, Kudzu, Lobelia, Maitake, Nopal (Prickly Pear), Olive leaf, Passionflower, Reishi (Ganoderma) and Shatavari

Key Nutrients: Alpha Lipoic Acid, N-Acetyl Cysteine, **Magnesium**, Co-Q10, Selenium, **L-Arginine**, Omega-3 Essential Fatty Acids, Calcium, Potassium, Vitamin C, Vitamin B-3 (Niacin), Chromium and Sodium Alginate (Algin)

Hyperthyroid (Grave's Disease)

See also *Adrenals (exhaustion, weakness or burnout), Autoimmune Disorders* and *Hashimoto's Disease (Thyroiditis)*

Although the percentage of people with hyperthyroid (high thyroid) is much lower than the people who suffer from hypothyroid (low thyroid), about 2.5 million Americans have a hyperthyroid disorder. The most common hyperthyroid disorder is Grave's disease, which is an autoimmune disorder.

In hyperthyroid disorders, the thyroid gland is producing too much thyroid hormone. This over stimulates metabolism. You can think of this as having the thermostat set too high or racing the engine on your car. As a result, fuel burns too quickly, which results in weight loss, intolerance to heat, hyperactivity and restlessness. Some of the specific symptoms associated with Grave's disease include bulging eyes, rapid pulse rate (90-160), heart palpitations, tremors, restlessness and anxiety, lack of periods, muscle weakness and impaired sleep.

The reason why heart rate is linked with thyroid function is because the heart prefers fatty acids over carbohydrates for fuel. So, when fat burning is hot, the heart is over stimulated. When fat burning is slow, the heart tends to beat more slowly, too.

Hyperthyroid disorders are a serious medical condition and need proper medical attention. The rapid heartbeat can over-stress the heart and circulation, resulting in life-threatening effects. This is why it is essential that a physician monitor someone with a hyperthyroid condition, even if the patient is opting to try a natural approach. Medication may be needed to lower the heart rate and inhibit the thyroid while you work on removing the underlying health problems.

While it is important to have proper medical monitoring of a hyperthyroid condition, medical treatments for hyperactive thyroid conditions leave much to be desired. While drugs can be used to inhibit thyroid function, physicians usually convince the patient to destroy the thyroid gland with radioactive iodine.

This therapy is designed to literally "fry" the thyroid gland. The radioactive iodine is taken up by the thyroid gland, causing it to be destroyed. Thereafter, the person will have to take medications for low thyroid, as their thyroid gland will no longer function properly. Clearly, this should be the last option if other remedies fail to bring the condition under control.

There are herbs that mildly inhibit thyroid function. These plants contain substances known to bind to TSH receptor sites in the thyroid, inhibiting them and reducing thyroid output. These include bugleweed and lemon balm. These herbs form the basis for *Hyperthyroid Formulas*. Other herbs that can be helpful include motherwort and mistletoe, which can also be used to calm the heartbeat.

However, simply inhibiting the thyroid (even with herbs) isn't correcting the underlying problem or cause. The underlying problem is an immune attack on the thyroid. Nutritional deficiencies combined with food allergies and stress is most likely what starts the immune over activity. See *Autoimmune Disorders* for more suggestions.

Since the heart is affected, a *Cardiac Tonic Formula*, or even just hawthorn berries can be taken to help protect the heart. Hawthorn has a cooling (anti-inflammatory) effect as well. Co-Q10, l-carnitine and magnesium can also protect the heart. Magnesium can help calm the heart and reduce high blood pressure.

In Grave's disease the problem is linked to immune function. *Mushroom Blend Formulas* have a balancing effect on immune responses and may be helpful. Antioxidants generally have a cooling effect on metabolism. Reducing heat and irritation to the body also helps to calm down the overactive immune responses.

People with Grave's disease and hyperthyroid disorders are often under a lot of stress. They may tend to "burn the candle at both ends." It is very important with this condition to relax as much as possible. One should not push themselves with hyperthyroid conditions. Use the techniques listed under Stress Management therapy and take *Adaptogen* and/or *Relaxing Nervine Formulas* to assist with staying calm and relaxed.

The adrenals tend to work with and balance the thyroid. People with hyperactive thyroid function also tend to have adrenal problems. The stress hormone, cortisol, is an anti-inflammatory, so hyperthyroidism may be a sign of excess stress, accompanied by adrenal weakness. In this case, the immune calming effect of the adrenal hormone, cortisol, is reduced. In this case, licorice root, an *Adrenal Tonic* or *Adaptogen Formula* may help.

Diet can also play a role in helping to balance an overactive thyroid. High carbohydrate diets, coupled with low protein and/or fat intake, tend to elevate thyroid function. So, a properly balanced diet with correct proportions of fats, proteins, and low glycemic carbohydrates is helpful.

Cruciferous vegetables, such as cabbage, broccoli and cauliflower tend to have an inhibiting effect on the production of thyroid hormones, primarily when eaten raw. Soy also has a thyroid inhibiting effect. These foods can be consumed freely.

Hyperthyroid patients may actually be deficient in iodine. If your body is saturated with iodine, it would not take up radioactive iodine, so the fact that the medical profession can use radioactive iodine to kill the thyroid suggests the tissues are not properly saturated with iodine. However, one needs to be very careful with this, as excess iodine will also overstimulate the thyroid. A little bit of iodine containing seaweeds like kelp or dulse can be helpful, but monitor the person's reaction carefully. Do NOT take iodine supplements unless medical testing reveals the person is low in iodine.

Many of the same dietary therapies that are helpful for Hashimoto's Disease can also be helpful for Grave's Disease. Also look under Autoimmune Disorders for more ideas about how to work on calming the overactive immune responses in Grave's disease.

Again, hyperthyroid conditions can be serious and life-threatening, so the situation should be monitored by a physician to make certain the therapy is working, even when the person chooses to go the natural route.

Therapies: Avoid Caffeine, Fresh Fruits and Vegetables, Heavy Metal Cleanse, Hiatal Hernia Correction, Hydration and Stress Management

Formulas: Hyperthyroid, Adaptogen, Mushroom Blend, Cardiac Tonic, Antioxidant, Adaptogen, Relaxing Nervine and Adrenal Tonic

Key Herbs: Bugleweed, Lemon Balm, Motherwort, Eleuthero (Siberian ginseng), Hawthorn, Hops, Licorice and Mistletoe

Key Nutrients: L-Carnitine, **Magnesium**, Co-Q10, Vitamin B-Complex and Betaine Hydrochloric Acid (HCl)

Hypochondria

A hypochondriac is a person with abnormal or excessive interest in diseases, who fears they have conditions that they do not have. This may actually be a sign of moderate liver disfunction, which presents itself as many vague and fleeting symptoms and a general feeling that a person is "not well." So, the person might first try taking a *Liver Tonic* or a *Hepatoprotective Formula*.

If a person has a fear of infection, they can infuse essential oils like oregano, peppermint, rosemary, tea tree and thyme into their home, which kills airborne germs. They could also consider *Nerve Tonic* or *Adaptogen Formulas* to calm their feelings of stress and anxiety. If the person feels a sense of nervous exhaustion, milky oat seed is particularly helpful. Affirmation and Visualization therapy, where the person affirms or pictures themselves as healthy, whole and protected would also be helpful.

Therapies: Affirmation and Visualization

Formulas: Liver Tonic, Hepatoprotective and Adaptogen

Key Herbs: Oat seed (milky), Oregano essential oil, Peppermint essential oil, Rosemary essential oil, Tea Tree essential oil and Thyme essential oil

Key Nutrients: Vitamin B-Complex

Hypoglycemia

See also *Addictions (sugar and refined carbohydrates), Hyperinsulinemia (Metabolic Syndrome* and *Syndrome X)*

Hypoglycemia is low blood sugar. When blood sugar gets low, it results in dizziness, weakness, inability to concentrate, cold nose or fingers, irritability, mood swings and fatigue. The hypoglycemic person tends to experience an energy slump in the middle of the afternoon. There also tends to be a constant craving for sugar and simple carbohydrates. Hypoglycemia is one of the symptoms of hyperinsulinemia.

Start by following the Low Glycemic Diet therapy. Start the day by eating a good breakfast with protein and good fats (like eggs). Do not eat carbohydrates (breakfast cereals, pastries, bread, etc.) for breakfast. Eat small, regular meals containing some protein and a little high quality fat (like some nuts) throughout the day. Eating small meals with some protein in them throughout the day is very beneficial.

There are a couple of *Hypoglycemic Formulas* you could try. You could also try an *Energy-Boosting Formula* that contains herbs like bee pollen, he shou wu, licorice or spirulina. Supplements that help regulate blood sugar, such as alpha lipoic acid and chromium, can also be helpful. Omega-3 fatty acids and other good fats may be helpful as well.

Therapies: Healthy Fats and Low Glycemic Diet

Formulas: Energy-Boosting and Hypoglycemic

Key Herbs: Bee Pollen, Burdock, Cinnamon, **Licorice**, **Spirulina**, Eleuthero (Siberian ginseng), He Shou Wu (Ho Shou Wu, Fo-Ti), Juniper Berry and Safflowers

Key Nutrients: Chromium, L-Glutamine, Alpha Lipoic Acid, Digestive Enzymes and **Omega-3 Essential Fatty Acids**

Hypotension

See also *Adrenals (exhaustion, weakness or burnout)*

While not as readily recognized as high blood pressure, low blood pressure can also be a serious problem. Low blood pressure can result in fatigue, fainting or dizziness. Low blood pressure may be the result of blood loss, but can also be due to glandular problems, particularly adrenal fatigue.

Since this problem is often due to adrenal weakness, *Adrenal Tonic Formulas* may be helpful. Adaptogens can lower high blood pressure and raise low blood pressure by also modulating adrenal function.

Capsicum and garlic tend to normalize blood pressure, so *Cardiovascular Stimulant Formulas* containing these herbs may also be helpful. As a single herb, shepherd's purse is one of the best vasoconstrictive herbs for tightening blood vessels. Nettle leaf can also help to raise low blood pressure.

Formulas: Adaptogen, Adrenal Tonic and **Cardiovascular Stimulant**

Key Herbs: Capsicum (Cayenne), **Ginseng (American)**, **Licorice**, **Nettle (Stinging)**, **Shepherd's Purse**, Garlic, Ginseng (Asian, Korean), Hawthorn and Nettle (Stinging)

Key Nutrients: Omega-3 Essential Fatty Acids and Vitamin B-Complex

Hypothyroid

See also *Hyperthyroid (Grave's Disease)* and *Hashimoto's Disease (Thyroiditis)*

Sitting at the base of the neck is a butterfly shaped gland called the thyroid. This important endocrine gland helps regulate metabolism, the rate at which the body burns fuel. It can be likened to the gas pedal on your car. When the thyroid is hyperactive, the body's engine races, burning hot and fast. When the thyroid activity is low, the body engine sputters, runs slowly and stalls.

A malfunctioning thyroid gland can be the cause of many health problems. For hypothyroid, the most important symptoms are: feeling cold and fatigue. If you are tired and get cold easily, especially when others feel hot, it is very likely you have low thyroid function. Other important symptoms of low thyroid are excess weight, difficulty losing weight, dry skin and thinning hair (hair loss). Blood tests do not always reveal thyroid problems, since most doctors are looking only at TSH levels. People can have a thyroid problem with TSH levels in normal range.

An easy way to check for possible thyroid problems is to take your temperature every morning before you get out of bed for 3-7 days. If your body temperature is consistently below normal (98 degrees), you probably have a low thyroid.

Thyroid problems are extremely common. About 5 million people suffer from low thyroid (hypothyroidism) in the United States. Worldwide, it has been estimated that as many as one and a half billion people are at risk for thyroid disorders. Thyroid problems are much more common in women than they are in men. About 90% of the people with thyroid disorders are women.

So, why are thyroid disorders so prevalent? While the exact reasons aren't clear, there are a number of causal factors to consider.

First, iodine is essential to the production of thyroid hormones. This nutrient, while found in abundance in sea foods, is not found in high concentrations in plants or animals raised inland. Furthermore, fluoride, chlorine and bromide are all found in the same group as iodine on the periodic table of elements. This means they can displace iodine in the body, so the chlorination of water supplies and the use of fluorides may be a contributing factor. Drugs, corticosteroids, aspirin (salicylates) and anticoagulants can depress thyroid activity.

To understand how to deal effectively with low thyroid using natural substances, it is necessary to know a little bit about how the body produces thyroid hormones. The hypothalamus, a stalk of the brain, is the master regulator of most of the body's major endocrine hormones. When the hypothalamus detects the need for thyroid hormones, it produces the thyroid-releasing hormone (TRH). TRH travels to the pituitary gland where it stimulates the release of the thyroid stimulating hormone, TSH or thyrotrophin.

TSH travels through the blood stream and binds to receptor sites in the thyroid gland. It stimulates the thyroid to produce two hormones, thyroxin (T4) and tri-iodotyrosine (T3).

In response to TSH, T4 and T3 are released in a ratio of about 4:1 (4 times more T4 than T3). T3 is the more active form. T4 is a storage form of the hormone. T4 is converted to T3 in peripheral tissues, with 20% conversion in the liver and 20% in the intestines.

The thyroid can also produce relatively inactive reverse T3 (RT3). During times of grief, trauma and illness, the body produces more RT3 and less T3, presumably to conserve energy and force us to slow down.

The primary job of these thyroid hormones is to regulate metabolism and to help burn fuel, especially fats. The thyroid acts much like a metabolic thermostat. When the thyroid output is low, the fats tend to be stored instead of burned, resulting in weight gain. Since the body burns fat primarily to keep warm, the body temperature tends to be low. The skin is usually dry, again due to a lack of proper fat metabolism, because fats are what keep the skin moist and supple. Reproductive hormones may also be thrown out of balance (since they are made of fat) and energy levels tend to be low because the metabolism is slow.

The most common cause of thyroid problems is Hashimoto's disease, which is not really a disease of the thyroid gland, but rather a problem with the immune system. Since 90% of all hypothyroid problems in modern society are due to this autoimmune condition, try the therapies listed under Hashimoto's disease first.

If Hashimoto's is not the cause of the low thyroid (that is, a person tests negative for TPO and thyroglobulin antibodies), the first thing to try is increasing one's intake of dietary iodine. Adding foods rich in natural iodine to the diet will often improve thyroid function. While the primary use of iodine is in the thyroid gland, it may have other functions. For example, iodine is also concentrated around the nipples in female breast tissue and is critical to breast health. Iodine is also important for the immune system and helps the body fight infection.

Iodine is a very rare nutrient in land plants but is common in fish and sea vegetables like kelp, dulse, bladderwrack, and Irish moss. Sea vegetables (especially kelp) can be sprinkled on food or added to soups, stews, etc. They add a pleasant salty taste to foods. Liquid dulse is another great source of natural iodine. Herbal *Hypothyroid Formulas* are usually based on these herbs. Other herbs that help promote thyroid health include ashwaganda, black walnut, he shou wu, nettles and saw palmetto. These herbs may also be found in *Hypothyroid Formulas.*

Natural Sea Salt is a good way to get extra iodine in the diet to stimulate the thyroid. Cruciferous vegetables and soy have a thyroid inhibiting effect, but it is very mild, so eating these foods in moderation should have little effect.

Even if levels of thyroid hormones are low, one can still have thyroid problems if the liver and other tissues are not converting T4 into T3 properly. Weak adrenals may contribute to this problem, so *Adrenal Tonic Formulas* or licorice root may have indirect benefits to the thyroid by supporting the adrenal glands.

Eating a properly balanced diet (especially reducing simple carbohydrates) will also aid this conversion. Some supplements that can indirectly help the thyroid by aiding the liver include *Liver Tonic Formulas* and SAM-e taken with MSM.

Formulas: Hypothyroid, Adrenal Tonic and Liver Tonic

Key Herbs: Bladderwrack, **Ashwaganda**, **Black Walnut**, He Shou Wu (Ho Shou Wu, Fo-Ti), Kelp, Licorice, Nettle (Stinging) and Saw Palmetto

Key Nutrients: Iodine, SAM-e, MSM, Omega-3 Essential Fatty Acids, **Selenium**, **Zinc** and Betaine Hydrochloric Acid (HCl)

Hysteria

See also *Adrenals (exhaustion, weakness or burnout), Hypoglycemia* and *Nervous Exhaustion (Enervation)*

Hysteria is a neurotic condition where there is no recognizable organic disease, but there can be symptoms mimicking various diseases. The person is calm but aloof and may become very emotional (laughing or crying) for no apparent reason. This emotional state is almost like a second personality and there may be a forgetting of what happened in this other state when the normal personality reasserts itself. There is emotional instability with a marked craving for sympathy.

Hysteria may be a sign of adrenal or nervous exhaustion due to chronic stress. Stress Management therapy, along with *Adrenal Tonic Formulas* or *Nerve Tonic Formulas* may be helpful. It may also be a sign of unresolved trauma requiring Emotional Healing Work and Flower Essences Therapy. Blood sugar problems (hypoglycemia) can also be a cause of mood swings like those found in hysteria.

Therapies: Affirmation and Visualization, Emotional Healing Work, Flower Essences, Healthy Fats, Low Glycemic Diet and Stress Management

Formulas: Relaxing Nervine and Adrenal Tonic

Key Herbs: Aloe vera, Blue Cohosh, Chamomile (English and Roman), **Black Cohosh**, **Scullcap (Skullcap)**, Lavender, Passionflower, Peppermint, Rosemary, Shatavari and Thyme

Key Nutrients: Vitamin B-Complex

IBS

See *Irritable Bowel Syndrome (IBS)*

Ileocecal Valve

See also *Hiatal Hernia*

The ileocecal valve is the valve between the small intestine and the large intestine. This valve may become so irritated and inflamed it cannot shut properly. This causes a leakage of material from the colon back into the small intestine which weakens the body. It often causes serious gas and bloating.

Massage to the area helps. To locate the ileocecal valve draw an imaginary line from your navel (belly button) to the right hip. The ileocecal valve is located about halfway along that line. Massage the area in a clockwise motion to close the valve.

Dietary Fiber therapy, especially with soothing mucilaginous herbs like aloe vera and slippery elm, may be helpful. Also consider taking digestive enzyme supplements. A *Carminative Formula* may help with the gas and bloating. Problems with the ileocecal valve are often found with a hiatal hernia and a video demonstration of how to work on it is included in the hiatal hernia videos found on *modernherbalmedicine.com* and *youtube.com.*

Therapies: Dietary Fiber

Formulas: Carminative and Intestinal Toning

Key Herbs: Aloe vera, Marshmallow and Slippery Elm

Key Nutrients: Digestive Enzymes

Impetigo

See also *Infection (bacterial)*

Impetigo is an inflammatory skin disease caused by a contagious staph or strep infection. It is characterized by isolated pustules, usually around the nose and mouth. These pustules become crusted and rupture. *Antibacterial* or *Goldenseal & Echinacea Formulas* may be helpful, especially if applied topically. So can antiseptic essential oils like tea tree oil or *Topical Antiseptic Formulas* with black walnut, echinacea and/or goldenseal.

Therapies: Compress

Formulas: Antibacterial, Goldenseal & Echinacea and **Topical Antiseptic**

Key Herbs: Black Walnut, **Echinacea**, **Tea Tree**, Goldenseal and Usnea

Key Nutrients: Vitamin A and Vitamin D

Impotency

See *Erectile Dysfunction*

Incontinence (urinary)

Incontinence is the inability to retain urine through the loss of sphincter control in the bladder. Increasing mineral intake in order to improve muscle tone may be helpful. Stay well hydrated in order to keep urine diluted so it doesn't irritate the bladder. Herbs for the kidneys with an astringent or tonic action, such as agrimony, horsetail and uva ursi are particularly helpful. Also consider a *Kidney Tonic Formula*. Kegel exercises, which strengthen the pelvic floor, can be helpful, as can Sitz Baths.

Therapies: Hydration and Mineralization

Formulas: Kidney Tonic

Key Herbs: Agrimony, Buchu, Cornsilk, Cranberry, **Horsetail**, **Uva ursi**, Juniper Berry and St. John's wort

Key Nutrients: Colloidal Minerals

Indigestion

See also *Acid Indigestion (Heartburn, Acid Reflux)* and *Gastritis*

Indigestion is simply a dysfunction of the digestive process that leaves food incompletely digested. This can cause discomfort in the stomach, a heavy feeling in the stomach after meals, gas, bloating, belching, and bad breath. Generally speaking, indigestion is a need for more digestive enzymes or betaine hydrochloric acid (HCl). In addition to supplements that supply enzymes, *Digestive Bitter Tonic Formulas* can be taken 15-20 minutes prior to meals to stimulate digestive secretions. They should be taken with a large glass of water. A small pinch of natural salt, taken with the water, can also be helpful in stimulating digestion. *Digestive Bitter Tonic Formulas* typically combine bitter herbs (such as dandelion and gentian) with aromatic herbs (like catnip, chamomile, fennel and peppermint). These herbs not only stimulate digestive secretions, they

also tend to promote downward motility of the digestive tract (to ease belching and reflux) and ease gas and bloating.

Therapies: Hydration

Formulas: Digestive Enzyme and **Digestive Bitter Tonic**

Key Herbs: Alfalfa, Artichoke leaf, Blessed Thistle, Blue Vervain, Bupleurum, Cardamom, Catnip, Clove, **Chamomile (English and Roman)**, **Dandelion**, **Gentian**, Fennel, Lemon Balm, Papaya, Peppermint, Rosemary, Safflowers and Thyme

Key Nutrients: Digestive Enzymes and Betaine Hydrochloric Acid (HCl)

Infection (bacterial)

See also *Antibiotics (alternatives to)*, *Carbuncles*, *Conjunctivitis (Pink Eye)*, *Diphtheria*, *Gingivitis (Bleeding Gums, Gum Disease, Pyorrhea)*, *Gonorrhea*, *Impetigo*, *Lyme Disease*, *Pertussis (Whooping Cough)*, *Staph Infections*, *Strep Throat*, *Syphilis*, *Tetanus*, *Tuberculosis (Consumption* and *Scrofula)*

Herbs can be very helpful for fighting bacterial infections. Here are some of the options.

Crushed raw garlic is an extremely powerful antibacterial agent against most infection-causing bacteria. Garlic oil can also be effective, whereas encapsulated garlic products are not very strong infection fighters.

Echinacea is also quite effective at treating bacterial infections. *Echinacea Blend Formulas* contain several species and are often more effective than one species by itself. Echinacea is commonly combined with goldenseal, which is helpful for infections on the mucus membranes, in *Goldenseal & Echinacea Formulas*, which are available from many companies. Oregon grape and coptis are alternatives to goldenseal.

For more severe bacterial infections, echinacea combines well with herbs like wild indigo, usnea and thuja. These herbs may be found in some *Antibacterial Formulas*.

For bacterial infections of the skin you can use antimicrobial herbs as a Compress or Poultice as discussed in the *Therapies Section*. *Topical Antiseptic Formulas* are available for this purpose. You can also apply essential oils like rosemary, thyme and tea tree oil topically.

After using antibiotics, even herbal ones, it can be helpful to take probiotics to enhance friendly bacteria in the intestines. Digestive enzyme supplements taken between meals can also help with bacterial infections in the gastrointestinal tract. See specific bacterial infections for more information.

Bacterial infections can be hard to treat. You may wish to consult with a professional herbalist (*findanherbalist.com*).

Therapies: Aromatherapy, Compress, Friendly Flora and Poultice

Formulas: Antibacterial, **Goldenseal & Echinacea**, Echinacea Blend and Topical Antiseptic

Key Herbs: Coptis (Chinese Goldenthread), **Echinacea**, **Oregon Grape**, **Tea Tree**, **Thuja**, **Usnea**, **Wild Indigo (Baptista)**, Elder, Garlic, Goldenseal, Oregano, Propolis, Reishi (Ganoderma), Rosemary and Thyme

Key Nutrients: Digestive Enzymes, **Probiotics**, Vitamin A, Vitamin C and Vitamin D

Infection (fungal)

See *Fungal Infections (Yeast Infections, Candida albicans)*

Infection (viral)

See also *Chicken Pox, Colds (remedies for), Epstein Barr Virus, Herpes, Measles, Mumps* and *Shingles*

The plant kingdom contains many antiviral agents that can be used to help viral infections from colds and influenza (flu) to herpes, shingles and other chronic viral infections. Some of the potent antivirals in the plant kingdom include elderberry, garlic, oregano, St. John's wort, thuja and thyme. Vitamin C and zinc can also be helpful for boosting the immune system in fighting viral infections. See specific viral conditions for more specific suggestions.

Therapies: Aromatherapy

Formulas: Antiviral, Cold and Flu and Immune Stimulating

Key Herbs: Aloe vera, Astragalus, **Lemon Balm**, **St. John's wort**, Echinacea, Elder, Garlic, Lemon, Olive, Oregano, Osha, Propolis, Thuja, Thyme and Yarrow

Key Nutrients: Vitamin C, L-Lysine, Zinc, **Vitamin A**, Vitamin D and Proanthocyanidins

Infertility

See also *Cholesterol (low)*

The inability to conceive a baby may be due to multiple factors, so it is wise to seek professional help to determine the exact cause of the problem. Poor general health, a lack of essential nutrients and excessive stress can all be contributing factors.

Start by eating a healthy diet, including getting adequate amounts of vitamin, protein and essential fatty acids. During times of high stress, reproductive functions shut down to prevent babies from being born during times when there are not enough resources to care for them. So, if you're under a lot of stress, practice the techniques listed under the Stress Management therapy.

Low cholesterol can be a factor in infertility in both men and women. A low percentage of body fat can also be a factor, especially in women. Extreme athletic training has been known to cause periods to stop in women, too.

In men, low sperm counts can be caused by exposure to xenoestrogens. Herbs like ginseng, maca, horny goat weed and tribulus have been helpful for increasing sperm counts, sperm health and/or general fertility in men. A *Male Glandular Tonic* or a *Male Aphrodisiac Formula* may be helpful.

In women, low thyroid, irregular periods and hormonal imbalances can be a factor. Herbs like dong quai, maca, false unicorn and partridge berry have been helpful for balancing hormones and regulating periods. For women, a *Female Aphrodisiac* or a *Female Hormonal Balancing Formula* may be helpful.

Therapies: Avoid Xenoestrogens, Healthy Fats, Low Glycemic Diet and Stress Management

Formulas: Male Glandular Tonic, Male Aphrodisiac, Female Aphrodisiac and **Female Hormonal Balancing**

Key Herbs: Damiana, **Ginseng (American)**, Dong Quai, Eleuthero (Siberian ginseng), False Unicorn (Helonias), Ginseng (Asian, Korean), Horny Goat Weed (Epimedium), Maca, Partridge Berry (Squaw Vine), Shatavari and Tribulus

Key Nutrients: Colloidal Minerals, L-Carnitine, L-Arginine, Omega-3 Essential Fatty Acids and Vitamin E

Inflammation

See also *Free Radical Damage*

Inflammation is the body's normal response to any kind of tissue damage. When you cut, bruise, burn, bump, scrape or break some part of your body, inflammation sets in. Inflammation also occurs from chemical and microbial damage (toxins and infection). So, no matter how the body gets injured, inflammation is going to be the body's primary response to the damage.

"Itis" is the Latin term for inflammation, which is characterized by heat, swelling, redness and pain at the site of injury. Many traditional names for diseases are simply naming the location of the heat, swelling, redness and pain. Thus, appendicitis is inflammation of the appendix; bronchitis is inflammation of the bronchials; tonsillitis, inflammation of the tonsils, and so forth. When you consider all the itises there are—arthritis, tendonitis, bursitis, colitis, dermatitis, gingivitis, conjunctivitis, diverticulitis, sinusitis, etc.—it is clear that inflammation is involved in a lot of health problems.

Normally, inflammation resolves itself naturally, and the injuries heal. However, when healing isn't completed, tissues become chronically inflamed. A slow process of deterioration ensues, resulting in the development of chronic and degenerative diseases, including cardiovascular disease, arthritis, obesity and mental deterioration, to name just a few. The fact is that just about any chronic disease probably involves inflammation.

We've already established that inflammation starts with tissue damage. To understand why inflamed tissues don't heal, we need to understand the normal process of inflammation, which works like this:

When the tissues are initially damaged, there is a release of histamine, which is followed by a release of bradykinin, serotonin and other chemical mediators. These dilate capillary pores and initiate inflammation by allowing fluid and protein to enter the tissue spaces (creating swelling). This is the first phase of inflammation.

In the second phase, chemical messengers are released to further open blood vessels so white blood cells can reach the damaged area. This causes further swelling. At this stage, if the inflammation is in the respiratory tract, histamine and leukotrienes will cause bronchial constriction and increased mucus production to flush toxins from mucus membranes. Pain receptors are also activated at this stage.

During the third phase, white blood cells use free radicals to destroy microbes and cellular debris. Healthy cells need adequate levels of antioxidants in order to protect themselves from these free radicals. If antioxidant levels are too low, healthy tissues will get damaged causing inflammation to spread.

Once white blood cells have completed their cleanup of the area, a healing phase is initiated. Cortisol from the adrenals is secreted to shut down production of the chemical messengers that mediate the inflammatory process. Macrophages clean up the remaining debris and a regenerative cycle begins as chemical messengers are released to stimulate tissue repair.

In chronic inflammation, the body gets stuck in the earlier phases and is never able to complete the healing phase of the inflammatory process. Meanwhile, the free radical activity in phase three causes more and more cells to get damaged, causing the inflammatory fires to spread.

It's like a forest fire, which starts when dry, dead plant material catches fire and gets hot enough to ignite even green trees and plants.

So, here are the factors that cause inflammation to become chronic. First, inflammation can't heal if there is a lack of nutrients needed for the healing and repair phase. Second, chronic tissue irritation from environmental toxins and poor diet continually re-irritate tissues, preventing healing. Third, adrenal fatigue from chronic stress (which shuts down cortisol production), prevents initiation of the healing phase. Finally, lack of adequate lymphatic drainage prevents the removal of excess fluid from the tissues.

Now that we understand what the inflammatory process is, we can understand what we can do to put out the fires of chronic inflammation. Here are seven keys to locking up the inflammation arsonist in your body.

Key #1 is to detoxify. Your body can't heal if it is constantly being re-inflamed by environmental toxins. So, start by avoiding chemicals as much as possible (food additives, pesticide residues, cleaning solutions, etc.). Buy organic food wherever possible and use natural household cleaning and personal care products. A good cleanse will help eliminate toxins already in the body.

Key #2 is to eat the right kinds of fats. The chemical messengers that mediate the inflammatory process are made from omega-6 and omega-3 essential fatty acids (EFA). A ratio of two parts omega-6 EFA to one part omega-3 EFA is important in order to keep inflammation in check. That's because many of the chemical messengers that promote the healing process are made from omega-3 EFA. If there are too many omega-6 EFAs and not enough omega-3 EFAs, then the body will be unable to heal properly and chronic inflammation will ensue.

Key #3 is to avoid simple carbohydrates. Refined sugars and grains cause spikes in insulin production. High levels of insulin inhibit the conversion of essential fatty acids to anti-inflammatory chemical messengers. The result is chronic inflammation.

Key #4 is to improve lymphatic drainage. One of the major effects of inflammation is the pooling of lymphatic fluid in the spaces around the cells. The only way this fluid can be removed is via the lymphatic system. This is one of the little known secrets to reducing chronic inflammation. The lymph system has no pump, so moderate exercise (walking, swimming, bouncing up and down on a mini-trampoline, etc.) and Deep Breathing therapy are needed to encourage lymphatic drainage and reduce inflammation. When lymph glands are congested, a *Lymphatic Drainage Formula* will also improve lymph drainage.

Key #5 is to use antioxidant nutrients. Inflammation and oxidative stress go hand-in-hand. An adequate level of antioxidant nutrients will help reduce both oxidative stress (free radical damage) and control inflammation.

Key #6 is to support the adrenal glands. The adrenals produce the hormone cortisol, which keeps inflammation in check. Corticosteroid drugs mimic this hormone. Chronic stress, caffeine and sugar exhaust these important glands and reduce their ability to control inflammation. A Nervous Fatigue Formula or an *Adrenal Tonic Formula* can help rebuild the adrenal glands and keep chronic inflammation in check. Also, yucca and licorice root are two herbs that have cortisol-like action.

Key #7 is to use natural anti-inflammatory remedies. Nature has supplied us with many natural remedies that reduce chronic inflammation and promote tissue healing. These include, Devil's claw, yucca, MSM, willow bark, turmeric, boswellia, Solomon's seal and several others.

Using these seven keys, we can keep inflammation from damaging our health.

Therapies: Avoid Caffeine, Colon Cleanse, Fresh Fruits and Vegetables, Gut Healing Diet, Healthy Fats, Low Glycemic Diet and Stress Management

Formulas: Anti-Inflammatory, Antioxidant, Lymphatic Drainage, General Detoxifying and Adrenal Tonic

Key Herbs: Bupleurum, Chamomile (English and Roman), **Boswellia**, **Devil's Claw**, **Turmeric**, **Yucca**, Feverfew, Holy Basil, Licorice, Mangosteen, Myrrh, Rose, Solomon's Seal, St. John's wort, Tea (Green or Black) and Yarrow

Key Nutrients: N-Acetyl Cysteine, Omega-3 Essential Fatty Acids, **MSM**, Glucosamine, Co-Q10, Digestive Enzymes, Zinc, Alpha Lipoic Acid, Proanthocyanidins and Bromelain

Inflammatory Bowel Disorders (Colitis, IBS)

See also *Celiac Disease*, *Colitis* and *Leaky Gut Syndrome*

The term Inflammatory Bowel Disease (IBD) is a broad term referring to any disease characterized by inflammation in the gastrointestinal tract. The two most common types of these diseases are Crohn's and ulcerative colitis. Both of these conditions can make your life miserable with symptoms such as diarrhea, abdominal cramps, rectal bleeding, fever, joint pain, loss of appetite and fatigue, not to mention fistulas and complications that can require surgery to remove part or all of the colon. The Centers for Disease Control (CDC) estimates that about 1.4 million Americans suffer from IBD, and 10% of those are children.

The main difference between Crohn's disease and ulcerative colitis is the location and nature of the inflammation. Crohn's can affect any part of the gastrointestinal tract, from mouth to anus, although most cases start in the ileum. Ulcerative colitis is restricted to the colon and the rectum. Microscopically, ulcerative colitis is restricted to the epithelial lining of the gut, while Crohn's disease affects the entire wall of the bowel.

People who live in Western countries have a higher risk for developing IBD than people in other countries. However, as countries industrialize and adopt Western diets and lifestyles, IBD increases. So, there is definitely a lifestyle cause.

Smokers are at higher risk of developing Crohn's disease, whereas they are at lower risk of developing ulcerative colitis. Research has linked long-term oral contraceptive use to a higher risk of both ulcerative colitis and Crohn's. Other drugs, such as isotretinoin (Accutane), could also play a role. Pain-relieving NSAIDs (like ibuprofen) can worsen IBD symptoms but are not thought to increase the risk of getting the disease initially.

Studies report a possible link to over consumption of foods high in omega-6 polyunsaturated fatty acids, which suggests a lack of omega-3 essential fatty acids may be involved.

A big factor may be the balance of bacteria in the gastrointestinal tract. Healthy intestines contain trillions of good bacteria or friendly flora. These organisms play a role in digesting certain foods (especially dairy), protecting the body from infection and regulating the immune responses.

Antibiotics and other drugs can disrupt the balance of these intestinal bacterial, as can infections with harmful bacteria such as salmonella and campylobacter. Both of these bacteria have been associated with IBD. They are ingested in contaminated food and are responsible for thousands of cases of food poisoning each year.

Since stress can trigger these bowel disorders, it's possible they may have emotional triggers, too. Adrenal fatigue results in lower levels of cortisol, which controls inflammation. Also, stress can be a factor in the regulation of the immune system, which may aggravate the autoimmune factor in intestinal inflammation.

The following measures have helped many people bring Crohn's disease and ulcerative colitis under control.

Adopt a Paleo Diet

Just a few thousand years ago, practically all human beings lived on what has been called the hunter-gatherer or paleo diet. These people simply collected the foods nature provided, which means they ate wild game and fish, raw milk and wild plant foods. Grain was not a significant part of this diet, and what grains and seeds were consumed were typically soaked and/or fermented before consumption. In addition, foods were not sterilized, so people had a wider range of gut microflora (probiotics) than people do today.

As mankind learned to farm, diets changed. Today, we consume a large amount of grain and simple sugars. The meat and dairy products we consume are also raised on grain instead of grass. Dairy products are no longer whole and raw. Naturally fermented foods and other foods containing probiotics are not consumed. These changes in diet are probably the underlying cause of all of these diseases of the intestines.

The place to start is to avoid all gluten-bearing grains, including wheat (bulgur, durum flour, farina, graham flour, semolina), barley (malt, malt flavoring and malt vinegar), rye, triticale, spelt and kamut. This is an absolute necessity when working with Celiac disease, but is also important for any IBD.

Usually rice, corn, amaranth, buckwheat, millet and quinoa will be okay because they don't contain gluten. However, some people have found that in the beginning stages of therapy, it can be helpful to avoid all grains to give the intestines a better chance to heal. Many people also find it's a good idea to avoid all legumes (beans, soy products, lentils and peas) as well.

It may also be necessary to avoid all dairy products. Some people will do all right with cultured dairy like yoghurt and cheese, but many people have to eliminate all dairy foods.

It is also important to avoid eating refined sugars of all kinds and may even be helpful to eliminate honey, maple syrup and sugary fruits. In addition, people with IBD and IBS should avoid products sweetened with manitol, sorbitol and xylitol.

Ideally, the diet should include servings of meat from grass-fed animals, eggs from pasture-raised chickens, wild-caught fish and game, and lots of vegetables, particularly non-starchy ones like zucchini, greens (such as mustard greens, beet greens, Swiss chard and kale), broccoli, cauliflower and cabbage. Good fats, like butter from grass-fed cows, coconut oil and avocados are also acceptable.

Use Natural Anti-inflammatories

Consuming soothing mucilaginous herbs has proven helpful in treating all types of inflammatory bowel disorders. A good remedy to consider is aloe vera juice. A double-blind, randomized trial examined the effectiveness and safety of aloe vera in the treatment of mild-to-moderate cases of IBS. Researchers gave 30 patients 100 milliliters of

oral aloe vera and 14 patients 100 milliliters of a placebo twice daily for 4 weeks.

Results with the aloe vera were: clinical remission in 9 patients, improvement in 11 patients and a positive response in 14 patients. The results for the placebo were just 1 clinical remission, 1 improvement and 2 positive responses.

Another good herbal remedy for soothing the intestinal tract is slippery elm. It is best used in bulk form and made into gruel. Combine one teaspoon of the powder with one teaspoon of honey and two cups of boiling water. Stir well. Flavor with cinnamon and drink one or two cups twice a day. Bulk slippery elm may also be blended with juice or nut milks if honey can't be tolerated.

It can also help to take a good *Anti-Inflammatory Formula* containing herbs like turmeric, boswellia, chamomile and licorice. Although all of these ingredients may be helpful for IBD, one of them, boswellia, has been clinically proven to do so. A 1997 study of people with ulcerative colitis found that 82% of those who took 350 milligrams of boswellia extract three times daily experienced remission.

Manage Stress

Stress often acts as a trigger for IBD, IBS and Celiac disease. This is why nervine herbs can also help to manage them. Look for a good *Relaxing Nervine Formula* where chamomile is a key ingredient. Chamomile is helpful here because it calms the nerves, regulates digestion and reduces inflammation.

Coffee, cola drinks, energy drinks, black tea and other sources of caffeine should be avoided. Caffeine stresses the adrenal glands and can increase feelings of anxiety, as well as inflammation. Also avoid stimulant drugs and alcohol.

Learn the skills listed under the Stress Management therapy. Practice breathing exercises to relax. Massage, yoga, regular exercise and meditation can also be helpful. Also consider using biofeedback, hypnotherapy or guided imagery to use the mind/body connection to heal the gut. You may even want to consider psychotherapy or cognitive behavioral therapy to work on emotional conflicts that can exacerbate symptoms.

Use Probiotics

A healthy digestive system contains thousands of species of friendly bacteria and people who live closer to the earth tend to have more species than people living in more sterile environments. It is very likely that the disruption of the friendly flora has a lot to do with the development of Crohn's, Celiac, colitis and IBS.

Research shows that probiotic supplements can be helpful with IBD. For example, a University of Alberta study examined 34 people with mild-to-moderate active ulcerative colitis who were unresponsive to conventional treatment. The researchers gave them a probiotic supplement providing a total of 3,600 billion bacteria a day for 6 weeks. At the end of the study, 18 people (53%) demonstrated remission and an additional 8 people (24%) had a favorable response.

In another study, researchers at the University of Dundee analyzed bacteria from rectal biopsies of patients with active ulcerative colitis and healthy control subjects. There were significantly less bifidobacterium numbers in the Ulcerative Colitis biopsies, suggesting that these probiotic bacteria might play a protective role against the disease. In a further study, 18 people with active Ulcerative Colitis were given a bifidobacterium supplement or a placebo for one month. Sigmoidoscopy, biopsy, and blood tests showed significant improvement in the probiotic group compared with the placebo group. While you can buy probiotic supplements, increasing consumption of cultured foods, especially naturally fermented vegetables, is more beneficial.

Omega-3 Fatty Acids

Some studies have found that omega-3 fatty acids may reduce inflammation in people with ulcerative colitis. A critical analysis published in the *American Journal of Clinical Nutrition* looked at controlled trials published from 1966 to 2003 concerning IBD and omega-3 fatty acids. Although the researchers concluded that more research is needed, three studies found that omega-3 fatty acids reduced the need for corticosteroids.

In other research conducted at the Cleveland Clinic, an oral supplement containing fish oil, soluble fiber, and antioxidants (vitamins C and E with selenium) was given to adults with mild-to-moderate Ulcerative Colitis. In the study, 86 patients with Ulcerative Colitis consumed 18 ounces of the supplement or a placebo each day for 6 months. Patients taking the oral supplement had a significantly lower rate of need for prednisone over 6 months compared with the placebo group. Both groups showed significant and similar improvement in clinical and histological responses.

Additional Tips

A high fiber diet may also be beneficial for some, but during the active stages of the illness, raw fruits, vegetables, seeds and nuts will irritate the digestive system. A Fiber Supplement based primarily on slippery elm and marshmallow could be beneficial. Intestinal Toners are formulas that contain herbs that can help damaged intestinal membranes to heal. Enzyme supplements may be helpful, too.

Therapies: Avoid Caffeine, Bone Broth, Eliminate Gluten, Fast or Juice Fast, Fresh Fruits and Vegetables, Friendly Flora, Gut Healing Diet, Healthy Fats, Low Glycemic Diet and Stress Management

Formulas: Anti-Inflammatory, Relaxing Nervine, Fiber Blend, **Intestinal Toning** and Digestive Enzyme

Key Herbs: Aloe vera, Black Walnut, Catnip, Coptis (Chinese Goldenthread), **Boswellia, Calendula, Cats Claw (Uña de Gato, Gambier), Chamomile (English and Roman), Plantain**, Kudzu, Licorice, Marshmallow, Slippery Elm, St. John's wort, Wild Yam and Yellow Dock

Key Nutrients: Probiotics, Magnesium, Digestive Enzymes, Omega-3 Essential Fatty Acids, Vitamin B-Complex, Bromelain and Chondroitin

Influenza

See *Flu (Influenza)*

Injuries

See also *Abrasions*, *Cuts* and *Wounds and Sores*

Many herbs can promote faster healing of injuries. Some of the best are comfrey, white oak bark and yarrow. Many essential oils, including lavender and tea tree oil also help injuries heal more quickly. To prevent infection use a *Topical Antiseptic Formula*.

To promote faster healing use a *Topical Vulnerary Formula*. For pain, use a *Topical Analgesic Formula*. Herbs can be applied as salves or as a Compress or Poultice as discussed in the *Therapies Section*. The Bach Flower Rescue Remedy is also helpful applied topically for injuries. It can also be taken internally to help treat shock. Besides topical remedies, a *Tissue Healing Formula*, vitamin C, zinc and/or colloidal mineral supplements can be taken internally to speed healing.

Therapies: Compress, Flower Essences, Mineralization and Poultice

Formulas: Topical Antiseptic, Topical Analgesic, **Topical Vulnerary** and **Tissue Healing**

Key Herbs: Bayberry, **Comfrey**, Goldenseal, Marshmallow, Mullein, Tea Tree essential oil, White Oak and Yarrow

Key Nutrients: MSM, Colloidal Minerals, Vitamin C, Zinc and Bromelain

Insect Bites

See *Bites* and *Stings*

Therapies: Compress and Poultice

Insects

See also *Bites* and *Stings*

Aromatherapy can be used as a natural method insect repellant. Oils that may be helpful include peppermint, rosemary, lemon grass, citronella and tea tree oil. Garlic, taken internally, also helps to repel insects.

Therapies: Aromatherapy

Key Herbs: Pennyroyal essential oil, **Rosemary essential oil**, Garlic, Peppermint and Tea Tree essential oil

Key Nutrients: Vitamin B-1 (Thiamine)

Insomnia

See also *Adrenals (exhaustion, weakness or burnout)*, *Hypoglycemia, Stress* and *Tension*

You may recognize the perils of financial debt, but did you know that you can also build up debt when it comes to sleep? Getting shortchanged occasionally on your sleep isn't a serious problem, but when it happens night after night, you build up a backlog of needed sleep. This sleep debt adversely affects your mood, health and safety.

The average person needs around eight and one-half hours of sleep every night. You might need a little less or a little more, but you need this sleep every day, just like you need water and oxygen every day. Losing just one hour of sleep per day (seven hours instead of eight, for instance) builds up a "sleep debt."

It's not just the quantity of sleep that you need, it's also the quality of that sleep. You need several hours of REM (rapid eye movement) sleep every night to be healthy. This is the sleep where you dream. When catching up on sleep-debt, your body will often "compress" sleep patterns to catch up on this much-needed REM sleep.

You also need a certain amount of deep sleep. During the deepest stages of sleep, your body releases growth hormone to stimulate tissue repair and regeneration. This means that if you don't get enough good quality sleep, it will adversely affect your physical health.

For instance, sleep debt makes you more likely to catch a cold or the flu. In fact, sleep deprivation can actually cause flu-like symptoms without an infection. Sleep debt even makes you more prone to heart disease and stroke.

Lack of sleep also affects your mood and your performance. It makes it harder for you to concentrate, which means you're not as productive at work. Sleep debt can make you irritable or depressed and otherwise affect your mood. You even age more quickly when you don't get enough sleep.

Another major problem with sleep debt is that it causes you to be more accident prone. About 100,000 automobile accidents occur due to sleep deprivation every year resulting in 1500 deaths and about $12.5 billion dollars in damages. Numerous industrial accidents are also caused by a lack of sleep. The famous Exxon Valdez oil spill in Alaska was not caused by alcohol as most people think. In the trial, it was found that sleepiness was the actual cause. It cost $2 billion dollars to clean up that spill and Exxon was fined $5 billion.

The bad news is that one-half of all Americans suffer from some degree of insomnia and about one-third suffer from life-disrupting insomnia. So a large percentage of the population is suffering from sleep debt and/or poor quality sleep.

Tips on Getting a Good Night's Sleep

There are many factors that contribute to sleep problems, so if you're having trouble falling asleep, staying asleep or sleeping soundly, it's important to examine your lifestyle and determine what you can do to get the sleep you need. You may even need to experiment a little to determine what will help you get the sleep you need. To get you started, here are a dozen tips for getting a better night's sleep. Pick one or two to work on at a time and see if they make a positive difference in your sleep patterns.

Sleep Tip #1: Schedule Sleep

Your body has an internal "clock" that helps engage periods of sleep and wakefulness. If you can get on a schedule that allows you to get to bed at roughly the same time each night and wake up at the same time each morning, it will ease both falling asleep and waking up. When your sleep schedule is thrown off (such as during international travel), you can help to "reset" this biological clock by taking melatonin at bedtime to help you get a new sleeping rhythm.

Sleep Tip #2: Get to Bed Early

In Chinese medicine, it is believed that certain meridians (or energy flows) are active at certain times of the day. According to this theory, the gall bladder and liver meridians are active from around 11 PM to 1 AM and 1 AM to 3 AM respectively. This is the peak time for your body to detoxify if you are asleep by 11 PM. If you are not asleep when the gallbladder meridian becomes active, you may get a surge of nervous energy that inhibits sleep. This will be followed by feeling sluggish and tired the next morning.

Generally speaking, if you can get to bed by about 10:30 you'll sleep more soundly and wake more refreshed. If you regularly stay up late and have a hard time getting out of bed in the morning, consider taking a *Hepatoprotective* or *Liver Tonic Formula* to support the health of your liver.

Sleep Tip #3: Avoid Late Night Stimulation

In the evening, avoid activities that get your adrenaline pumping. This includes watching exciting TV shows or movies, listening to loud stimulating music or even reading thrilling novels. It's also not a good idea to exercise before bedtime. Instead, pick evening activities that help you wind down, such as listening to relaxing music, reading uplifting books or sharing a massage with your partner.

Sleep Tip #4: Create a Relaxing Atmosphere

Seek to make your bedroom a place that is conducive to rest, not work or recreation. Remove TVs, computers, cell phones and other distractions from your sleep area and keep your bedroom uncluttered. Most importantly, don't work or keep work materials in your sleep area. Also, keep electrical equipment, including digital clocks at least three feet away from your bed to minimize electromagnetic influences while you sleep.

If you have a hard time relaxing at night, try taking some nervine herbs in the evening. Hops, valerian, passionflower, scullcap and kava kava are all herbs that can help you relax and get to sleep. Kava kava is a good herb to use if your body is tense and you suffer from anxiety. Magnesium taken before bed can also help your muscles relax.

Choose a good *Sleep Formula* that combines a number of herbs and nutrients that help you sleep. You'll typically want to take the remedy about 30-60 minutes before bedtime.

Sleep Tip #5: Don't Eat Late

It is hard for your body to fall asleep when it is digesting a heavy meal, so try to eat dinner at least two hours and preferably four hours before bedtime. Don't eat sugary snacks before sleeping, as this creates blood sugar problems that can wake you up at night. Also, avoid all stimulants, including spicy foods in the evening. They interfere with quality of sleep. It is okay to eat a small snack of nut butter, cheese or some other high protein food before bed if you suffer from hypoglycemia (See Tip #10).

Sleep Tip #6: Make Your Sleep Area Dark

The natural way to fall asleep is for your body to convert a neurotransmitter called serotonin into melatonin. Melatonin puts you to sleep. Your pineal gland starts converting melatonin to serotonin when it gets dark. Even the LED lights from electric clocks or "on" lights from electronic equipment will inhibit this process and help contribute to keeping you awake.

Unfortunately, with the advent of electric lights, we extend our "day" into the evening hours. This prevents us from falling asleep naturally. Watching TV, staring at a computer screen and artificial light all inhibit sleep. So, make your bedroom as dark as possible and as the time for sleep approaches, turn off the TV and computer and get into a darkened room. You may even want to try wearing a sleep mask.

If darkening the room doesn't work, try taking 5-HTP about one hour before bedtime. 5-HTP is a precursor to serotonin, which will increase production of melatonin when you turn out all the lights and make your bedroom as dark as possible.

Sleep Tip #7: Breathe Deeply

Oxygen is very important to sound sleep. Many people find that cracking a window open to let in a little fresh air results in a better night's sleep. If you snore at night, it's a sign that you have constricted airways that are inhibiting the amount of oxygen you are getting while you are sleeping. So, not only does snoring contribute to insomnia in anyone who sleeps with you, it also interferes with the quality of your own sleep.

If you snore really loudly, you may have a problem with sleep apnea. See sleep apnea for more information.

Factors that can contribute to both snoring and sleep apnea include excess weight, swollen lymph nodes, sinus congestion or any inflammation of the mucus membranes. A *Sinus Decongestant Formula* may help shrink swelling of inflamed mucus membranes, reduce sinus congestion and swollen lymph nodes and otherwise help to open respiratory passages. Food and respiratory allergies may be a factor, so screen yourself for allergy-causing foods. High doses of vitamin C (2,000-3,000 milligrams per day) along with Hydration therapy can help to counteract histamine reactions if allergies are a factor. Weight loss and colon cleansing are also helpful.

Sleep Tip #8: Quiet Your Mind

If you're one of those people who lie awake at night unable to get your mind to "shut up" so you can go to sleep, here are some suggestions for quieting your mind for a better night's sleep. First, before going to bed, get a pad of paper and write down your to-do list for the next day. This helps you "get it off your mind" so you can relax. It may also help to have a journal that you write in each evening, allowing you to express things on paper so you can let go of them.

A second technique to quiet your mind is to breathe deeply as you lie in bed and focus on relaxing your body. Starting with your toes and working your way up to your head, tense your muscles and then let them relax. Imagine them sinking into the bed. Focus your mind on your breathing or mentally recite a positive statement such as "I am relaxed" or "All is well."

If you're still having trouble getting your mind to quiet down, GABA or passion flower may be helpful. Take these supplements about one hour before bedtime. If you are easily distracted by small things (such as a dripping faucet or other small noises), try taking about 400 milligrams of magnesium. It's best to empty a magnesium capsule or two under your tongue or use a magnesium supplement in liquid form. If you put the powders from the capsules in your mouth, let the magnesium sit there for ten to fifteen seconds before washing it down with some water.

Sleep Tip #9: Reduce Your Stress Level

Since stress is a major factor in sleep problems, reducing your stress level during the day can help you sleep better at night. If you are tired during the day but have poor quality of sleep at night, you may be suffering from adrenal exhaustion. Symptoms of tired adrenals include fatigue, mental confusion and emotional sensitivity during the day, followed by restless sleep with disturbing dreams. You may also need to wake up frequently to urinate.

In this situation, an *Adaptogen Formula* taken during the day may be helpful. In more serious cases, such as post-traumatic stress disorder, an *Adrenal Tonic Formula* may be helpful.

In addition, it is very important for people suffering from too much stress to avoid sugar and caffeine, as these make the problem worse. You may need to reduce your workload, or at least make more time for rest and relaxation.

A good therapy for people who are under a lot of stress is using Epsom Salt Bath therapy. Lavender, bergamot, rose, ylang ylang and patchouli are good essential oils to use here. Light a few candles, put on some relaxing music and turn out the lights, then soak in the warm bath for 15-20 minutes. This can really reduce nervous stress and prepare you for a better night's sleep.

Sleep Tip #10: Balance Your Blood Sugar

If you wake up in the middle of the night thinking about your problems and unable to get back to sleep, this can be a sign of blood sugar problems. What is happening is that your blood sugar is dropping too low in the middle of the night and your adrenal glands are firing off stress hormones (adrenaline and cortisol) to elevate your blood sugar. Avoiding sugar, white flour products, alcohol and caffeine will help. Eat a small protein-rich snack at bedtime, such as a couple of tablespoons of almond butter, peanut butter or cottage cheese or a few raw walnuts.

Bed-wetting in children can often be a sign of blood sugar problems or dehydration. If you have a child with bed-wetting problems, try keeping them away from refined carbohydrates and giving them licorice root to stabilize their blood sugar levels. Magnesium and cornsilk may also be helpful for bed-wetting.

Sleep Tip #11: Stay Hydrated

Not drinking enough water can make you feel anxious and tense. Proper hydration calms the brain and promotes better sleep. Try drinking at least 1/2 ounce of pure water per pound of body weight per day. In other words, two quarts (64 ounces) is the right amount of water for a 128 pound person.

If you have a problem with waking up to urinate, drink more water during the day, but not a lot of water in the evening. You may also need to take something to strengthen your kidneys, such as a *Kidney Tonic Formula* or work on your adrenals and blood sugar.

Sleep Tip #12: Be Physically Active

A sedentary lifestyle will also cause problems with sleep. We need physical activity and rest, so if you work at a desk job and then watch TV when you get home, you may need to become more physically active in order to sleep better. Take a walk, dance, swim, ride a bike, lift weights or otherwise engage your muscles 15-20 minutes per day to improve your sleep.

Waking up frequently at night (not to urinate), can result from an elevation of cortisol levels. If you go to sleep fine, but wake up regularly for no reason, taking L-theanine or phosphatidylserine before bed can help. This can also be due to blood sugar problems and a small protein snack (almond butter, natural cheese, etc.) before bedtime may also be helpful.

Therapies: Avoid Caffeine, Eliminate Allergy-Causing Foods, Epsom Salt Bath, Hydration, Low Glycemic Diet and Stress Management

Formulas: Hepatoprotective, Liver Tonic, **Sleep**, Sinus Decongestant, **Adaptogen**, Adrenal Tonic and Kidney Tonic

Key Herbs: Blue Vervain, Chamomile (English and Roman), **California Poppy**, **Corydalis**, **Passionflower**, **Scullcap (Skullcap)**, Eleuthero (Siberian ginseng), Hops, Kava-kava, Linden, Lobelia, Mimosa (Albizia, Silk Tree), Motherwort, Oat seed (milky), Reishi (Ganoderma) and Valerian

Key Nutrients: 5-HTP, **Melatonin**, Calcium, Magnesium, Vitamin B-Complex, Vitamin D, **GABA**, Vitamin C, Folate (Folic Acid, Vitamin B9) and Potassium

Interstitial Cystitis

See also *Bladder (ulcerated)* and *Bladder (irritable)*

Interstitial cystitis is inflammation of the urinary bladder. This can be caused by infectious organisms, see UTI's for more detail. Remedies to reduce inflammation and soothe irritation in the urinary passages are helpful. Look for *Diuretic* or *Kidney Tonic Formulas* that contain soothing herbs like marshmallow, cornsilk, horsetail and parsley. Mullein root is also helpful. Avoid warming herbs like juniper and uva ursi. Be sure to drink plenty of water to dilute toxins in the urine, thus reducing irritation to the bladder.

Therapies: Fresh Fruits and Vegetables, Gut Healing Diet, Healthy Fats and Hydration

Formulas: Kidney Tonic and Diuretic

Key Herbs: Agrimony, Celery, Cleavers (Bedstraw), **Cornsilk**, **Pipsissewa**, Gravel root, Horsetail, Hydrangea, Irish moss, Marshmallow, Mullein, Parsley, Shepherd's Purse and Spilanthes

Key Nutrients: Omega-3 Essential Fatty Acids, Probiotics, L-Arginine, Quercitin and **MSM**

Irregular Heart Rate

See *Arrhythmia (Irregular Heartbeat)*

Irritability

See also *Anger (excessive)*

Irritability is the tendency to be easily annoyed and angered, often over insignificant things. Irritability can be related to congestion in the liver, blood sugar problems like hypoglycemia or hormonal imbalances. Some of the remedies one might try include *Liver Tonic* or *General Detoxi-*

fying Formulas to clear out the liver, *Adaptogen Formulas* to reduce stress and balance blood sugar and *Relaxing Nervine Formulas* to calm the nerves. See Anger for more ideas.

Therapies: Affirmation and Visualization, Avoid Caffeine, Colon Cleanse, Emotional Healing Work, Flower Essences and Hydration

Formulas: Liver Tonic, General Detoxifying, Adaptogen and **Relaxing Nervine**

Key Herbs: Blue Vervain, **Chamomile (English and Roman)**, **Mimosa (Albizia, Silk Tree)**, Lavender and St. John's wort

Key Nutrients: SAM-e, Magnesium, Vitamin C and Potassium

Irritable Bowel Syndrome (IBS)

See also *Inflammatory Bowel Disorders (Colitis, IBS), Leaky Gut Syndrome* and *Small Intestinal Bacterial Overgrowth (SIBO)*

Inflammatory bowel disease (IBD) and irritable bowel syndrome (IBS) are quite different. Unlike IBD, IBS does not cause inflammation, ulcers or other damage to the bowel. In IBS, the digestive system looks normal but doesn't work as it should. Symptoms of IBS, once referred to as "spastic colon," include painful cramping, bloating, gas, mucus in the stool, diarrhea and constipation. However, IBS can have root causes similar to IBD, so look under Inflammatory Bowel Disorders for additional information. IBS is frequently caused by holding too much stress in the stomach. Most people with IBS are anal retentive and have an inability to "let go" of emotions. Lobelia and a fresh tincture of catnip can help with the physical tension, but Emotional Healing Work and Stress Management therapy are often necessary to get to the root of the problem. Try using an Intestinal Toner to soothe digestive irritation or an *Antispasmodic Formula* to ease intestinal cramps.

Therapies: Bone Broth, Eliminate Allergy-Causing Foods, Emotional Healing Work, Fast or Juice Fast, Gut Healing Diet, Hydration and Stress Management

Formulas: Antispasmodic and **Intestinal Toning**

Key Herbs: Chamomile (English and Roman), Cramp Bark, **Catnip**, Lobelia and Wild Yam

Key Nutrients: Magnesium

Itching

See also *Chicken Pox, Poison Ivy or Oak* and *Rashes and Hives*

Itching is an irritating sensation on the surface of the skin that compels one to scratch the area affected. It is common in allergic reactions and is a sign of irritants affecting the skin.

To ease itching and prevent scarring when a person is itching due to rashes, exposure to poison ivy or oak, chicken pox or other afflictions of the skin, the afflicted person can use any of the following herbs in the Compress, Poultice or Drawing Bath therapies can be used with herbs like burdock, comfrey, goldenseal, yellow dock, chickweed, linden and Oregon grape.

Mixing tea tree oil with vitamin E, one can also make a topical application for chicken pox and other irritations. Aloe vera gel can also be applied topically to soothe itching.

Blood Purifier Combinations can be taken internally to ease itching.

Therapies: Compress, Drawing Bath, Fresh Fruits and Vegetables, Healthy Fats and Poultice

Formulas: Topical Vulnerary, **Anti-Itch** and Blood Purifier

Key Herbs: Burdock, Comfrey, **Aloe vera**, **Chickweed**, **Grindelia (Gumweed)**, **Yellow Dock**, Goldenseal, Linden, Oregon Grape and Tea Tree

Key Nutrients: MSM, Vitamin E and Vitamin B-Complex

Itching (rectal)

See also *Hemorrhoids* and *Parasites (general)*

Rectal itching may be a sign of parasites. It can also be a sign of hemorrhoids. Try doing a parasite cleanse or apply white oak bark or another astringent herb mixed with a *Topical Vulnerary Formula* in salve or ointment form. You can also mix the herbs with vitamin E to apply topically.

Formulas: Topical Vulnerary and Antiparasitic

Key Herbs: Black Walnut, Collinsonia (Stoneroot) and White Oak

Key Nutrients: Vitamin E

Itching Ears

See also *Allergies (food), Fungal Infections (Yeast Infections* and *Candida albicans)*

An irritating sensation of the ears that compels one to scratch is often a sign food allergies.

Therapies: Eliminate Allergy-Causing Foods

Key Herbs: Garlic, Pau d' Arco and Tea Tree

Key Nutrients: Probiotics and **L-Glutamine**

Jaundice (adults)

See also *Hepatitis*

Jaundice is caused by a buildup of bilirubin in the blood. This causes a yellowing of the skin. Several blood or liver disorders can cause jaundice, including hepatitis. Seek medical attention for an accurate diagnosis and treatment. Herbs and herbal formulas for the liver may be helpful, but hey should be used under professional supervision and after a diagnosis has been made.

Therapies: Dietary Fiber, Fast or Juice Fast and Fresh Fruits and Vegetables

Formulas: Hepatoprotective, Liver Tonic and Cholagogue

Key Herbs: Alfalfa, Artichoke, Butchers Broom, **Dandelion**, **Milk Thistle**, Fringe Tree, Gotu kola, Lemon, Oregon Grape, Safflowers, St. John's wort, Wild Yam and Yellow Dock

Key Nutrients: Charcoal (Activated), Vitamin C and **SAM-e**

Jaundice (infants)

It is common for newborn infants to have a small amount of jaundice. Exposure to 5-10 minutes of sunlight per day is helpful. Safflower tea or activated charcoal mixed with water can also be given to infants to help clear up jaundice.

Key Herbs: Safflowers

Key Nutrients: Charcoal (Activated)

Jet Lag

See also *Fatigue* and *Insomnia*

Fatigue and irritability after a long flight on an airplane is called jet lag. It is especially a problem when a person crosses several time zones creating a disruption of the circadian rhythms of the body. Melatonin is a good remedy for helping a person get to sleep after time zone changes.

herbal *Sleep Formulas* may also be helpful. To help with fatigue, try an *Energy-Boosting Formula. Adaptogen Formulas* can ease the stress of jet travel.

Formulas: Sleep, Energy-Boosting and **Adaptogen**

Key Herbs: Bee Pollen, **Eleuthero (Siberian ginseng)**, Ginseng (Asian, Korean), Licorice and Spirulina

Key Nutrients: Melatonin

Jock Itch

See also *Fungal Infections (Yeast Infections, Candida albicans)*

Jock itch is a fungal infection that affects the folds of skin in the thigh area. Signs are persistent itching and eruptions of small red bumps or flaking skin. It is more common in men. *Antifungal Formulas* or herbs like pau d'arco may be applied topically to the affected areas. Essential oils like tea tree or lavender can be diluted in olive oil (or another similar vegetable oil) and carefully applied to affected areas. It can also help to take probiotics and *Antifungal Formulas* internally. Keep skin in the thigh area dry.

Therapies: Friendly Flora and Low Glycemic Diet

Formulas: Antifungal

Key Herbs: Pau d' Arco, Garlic, Lavender essential oil, Tea Tree essential oil and Thuja

Key Nutrients: Probiotics

Kidney Infection

See also *Infection (bacterial)*

When there is an infection in the kidneys, try taking a *Urinary Infection Fighting Formula* that includes herbs like buchu, goldenseal, echinacea or uva ursi. Stay well hdyrated and eat a simple diet of devoid of heavy proteins and simple sugars. A little bit of fasting, to take the stress of the kidneys, may even be helpful. Seek medical attention if the condition persists. While urinary tract infections can be treated effectively with herbs, kidney infections are serious and should be treated medically with herbs used as adjuncts.

Therapies: Fast or Juice Fast and Hydration

Formulas: Urinary Infection Fighting and Goldenseal & Echinacea

Key Herbs: Buchu, Cranberry, **Echinacea**, **Goldenseal**, **Pipsissewa**, **Uva ursi**, Kava-kava and Yarrow

Kidney Stones

Deposits resembling small rocks that form in the kidneys are called kidney stones. If they are large or numerous enough, they may cause severe back pain, blood in the urine, or interfere with the elimination of urine. Most (80%) of kidney stones are made of calcium oxalate and are the result of minerals solidifying out of too-concentrated urine.

People in primitive societies rarely develop kidney stones. So modern diets and lifestyles contribute to this problem. If you are prone to kidney stones, start by drinking more water. This helps keep the minerals in the urine well-diluted so they don't precipitate. You should also avoid foods that increase urinary oxalate significantly including nuts, chocolate, tea, and peanuts. Caffeine, carbonated beverages, table salt and animal protein all increase the risk of forming kidney stones.

Magnesium and vitamin B6 help the body to convert oxalate into other substances. Calcium supplements should be avoided by persons with a history of kidney stones. People who consume plenty of fiber and potassium have a lower risk of forming kidney stones. Fruits and vegetables are high in fiber and potassium.

Several herbs have been used traditionally to aid the passing of, and inhibit the formation of, kidney stones. These include gravel root (Joe-Pye weed), hydrangea, nettles and lemon. These remedies are often combined in *Lithotriptic Formulas*. Fresh lemon juice in pure water is very helpful in dissolving and passing stones. One very useful folk remedy for passing kidney stones is to juice four fresh lemons and put the juice in one gallon of distilled water. Fast, drinking only the lemon water, until the stones have passed.

This program can be even more effective when hydrangea or gravel root are taken along with the lemon water, as both of these herbs will help dissolve the stones. At the very least, they help to dissolve the rough edges of the stones so they will pass more easily.

Marshmallow root can also be taken to soothe urinary passages, thus helping the stones to pass. *Antispasmodic* herbs such as lobelia or kava kava can be taken, especially when there is severe pain, as they will relax urinary passages and help the stones pass more easily. High doses of magnesium (2-3,000 milligrams) may also be helpful when passing stones. Agrimony helps with the pain of kidney stones passing.

Here's a sample program for helping to pass kidney stones. The exact supplements and amounts required will vary from person to person and from situation to situation. This is only a general guideline. These supplements should be taken while fasting and drinking lemon water as described above.

Hydrangea or a Lithotriptic Formula—1-2 capsules every two hours

Magnesium—400 mg capsules every two hours

Marshmallow—1 capsule every two hours

Kava Kava—1 capsule every two hours

These measures are effective and have worked for many people. However, always seek medical attention for kidney stones, as this can be a potentially serious condition if the stone blocks a urinary passage for an extended period of time.

Therapies: Avoid Caffeine and Hydration

Formulas: Lithotriptic

Key Herbs: Bitter Melon, **Hydrangea**, **Kava-kava**, **Lemon juice**, Erigeron (Fleabane), Goldenrod, Gravel root, Khella, Lobelia, Marshmallow, Stone Breaker and Uva ursi

Key Nutrients: Magnesium, Vitamin B-6 (Pyridoxine) and Potassium

Labor and Delivery

See also *Pregnancy (herbs and supplements for)* and *Pregnancy (herbs and supplements to avoid during)*

There are a number of herbal remedies that can ease labor and delivery. Using a Pregnancy Formula or an appropriate *Uterine Tonic Formula* (one that is not contraindicated during pregnancy) can strengthen the uterus and prepare the woman's body for childbirth. *Pre-Delivery* formulas are taken starting about five or six weeks before the due date to further prepare the body for childbirth.

Antispasmodic herbs such as lobelia and black cohosh have been taken during labor to reduce the pain from contractions. Blue cohosh has been used to help induce labor and to strengthen contractions during labor. However, there is some evidence that it can be harmful to the unborn baby, so use it only under professional supervision.

A mixture of bayberry and capsicum extracts in a little apple cider vinegar has been used to help stop bleeding after the birth. Shepherd's purse has also been used for this purpose.

Consult with a midwife or professional herbalist (*findanherbalist.com*)for assistance in selecting herbs appropriate for pregnancy, labor and delivery.

Formulas: Pregnancy Tonic, **Pre-Delivery** and Uterine Tonic

Key Herbs: Bayberry, Black Cohosh, Blue Cohosh, Capsicum (Cayenne), Dong Quai, Lobelia, Partridge Berry (Squaw Vine), Red Raspberry and Shepherd's Purse

Key Nutrients: Magnesium, Chlorophyll and Vitamin C

Lactose Intolerance

See also *Gas and Bloating*

Lactose intolerance results in bloating and gas after eating dairy products due to the inability to break down the lactose or milk sugar in dairy products that have not been cultured. Lactase is the enzyme that helps break down this sugar. The best remedy is to take lactase enzyme supplements and probiotics. One can also take a *Carminative Formula* for the gas.

Therapies: Friendly Flora and Gut Healing Diet

Formulas: Carminative

Key Herbs: Fennel, Ginger and Peppermint

Key Nutrients: Lactase Enzymes and **Probiotics**

Laryngitis (Hoarseness)

Laryngitis is an inflammation of the larynx or voice box that causes a complete or partial loss of voice. Sage and licorice tea, sipped slowly or used as a gargle is a good remedy. One can also apply herbs like capsicum and lobelia topically to the throat and follow this up with a *Topical Analgesic Formula*. Collinsonia is good for laryngitis brought on by straining the voice and is a useful remedy for singers and public speakers.

Formulas: Topical Analgesic

Key Herbs: Capsicum (Cayenne), Clove, **Collinsonia (Stoneroot)**, **Licorice**, **Sage**, Marshmallow and Yerba Santa

Key Nutrients: Zinc

Lead Poisoning

See also *Heavy Metal Poisoning*

Lead is one of the most toxic metals known. Many years have passed since our society was made aware of the damage that exposure to lead-based paints was doing to our health, especially to young children who suck on and chew anything they can get their hands on.

When lead reaches toxic levels in the body, it can damage the kidneys, liver, heart and nervous system. The body can't tell the difference between lead and calcium, so pregnant women, children and other people who are deficient in calcium absorb lead more easily, with infants and children affected most severely. Possible symptoms of lead poisoning include anxiety, arthritis, confusion, chronic fatigue, behavioral problems, juvenile delinquency, hyperactivity, learning disabilities, metallic taste in the mouth, tremors, mental disturbances, loss of memory, mental retardation, impotence, reproductive disorders, infertility, liver failure and death.

Exposure to lead can come from food that is grown near roads or factories, lead-based paint, hair products, food from lead-soldered cans, imported ceramic products (especially from Mexico and China), lead crystal glassware, ink on bread bags, batteries in cars, bone meal, insecticides, tobacco, lead pipes, and lead solder in water pipes. If you suspect you could have lead pipes or lead solder in your water system, have the water tested.

Remedies that can help eliminate lead from the body include n-acetyl cysteine, sodium alginate (algin), lobelia and *Heavy Metal Cleansing Formulas*. Seek medical assistance if you think you have lead poisoning. See Heavy Metal Poisoning for additional suggestions.

Therapies: Heavy Metal Cleanse

Formulas: Heavy Metal Cleansing

Key Herbs: Kelp

Key Nutrients: N-Acetyl Cysteine, Sodium Alginate (Algin), **Zinc**, **Iodine** and **Alpha Lipoic Acid**

Leaky Gut Syndrome

See also *Fungal Infections (Yeast Infections, Candida albicans)*, *Inflammatory Bowel Disorders (Colitis, IBS)*, *Parasites (general)* and *Small Intestinal Bacterial Overgrowth (SIBO)*

Leaky gut is a byproduct of intestinal inflammation. When the intestinal membranes become inflamed, they lose structural integrity. This allows partially digested food stuffs and irritants to enter the blood stream

Just imagine for a minute that your sewer or septic system started backing up into your kitchen. It's not a pleasant thought, is it? Yet, many people have a similar problem happening right inside their own bodies because of this excess intestinal permeability.

Numerous physical and "mental" health problems have been linked with this leakage in the intestines, including ADHD, autism, depression, allergies, asthma and skin diseases like eczema and psoriasis. Leaky gut syndrome may also be a factor in autoimmune diseases like Hashimoto's thyroiditis, arthritis, chronic fatigue and fibromyalgia.

The intestinal inflammation that causes leaky gut is brought on by a combination of factors. These include drugs (e.g. antibiotics, birth control pills, NSAIDs, chemotherapy agents), infections, parasites, food allergies, and chemicals. Enzyme deficiencies and a high carbohydrate diet are also contributing factors.

The intestines do not absorb nutrients correctly when they are inflamed, which can cause fatigue and bloating. Leaking toxins also burden the liver, which acts as a second line of defense to eliminate substances absorbed from the intestines that the body doesn't want in the general circulation.

When large, undigested food particles are absorbed because of the excessive porousness in the membranes, they trigger immune reactions. This can hypersensitize the immune system, resulting in allergic and autoimmune reactions. The inflammation also damages carrier proteins that help nutrients to be assimilated. This can cause nutritional deficiencies. Finally, the damaged intestinal membranes also allow bacteria, viruses and yeast to pass more readily into the system to damage other organs and systems.

Reducing intestinal inflammation and rebuilding damaged intestinal membranes to stop gut leakage can help numerous health problems. Here are seven steps you can take to reduce intestinal inflammation, promote healing and stop intestinal leakage.

Step One is to avoid intestinal irritants, such as food allergens, food additives, drugs and chemicals. A great way to do this is by adopting a GAPS, Paleo or Specific Carbohydrate Diet.

Step Two is to improve digestion and increase stomach acid by taking a betaine hydrochloric acid (HCl) supplement (and possibly a digestive enzyme supplement). You could also take a little raw apple cider vinegar at the beginning of a meal to increase stomach acid. *Digestive Bitter Tonic Formulas* can also be used to increase stomach acid. Take them about 15-20 minutes prior to meals with a large glass of water.

Step Three is to eliminate harmful organisms from the digestive tract. If parasites or bacterial overgrowth is part of the problem, these harmful organisms need to be eliminated as part of the process. See Parasites and Small Intestinal Bacterial Overgrowth (SIBO). Fungal Infections may occasionally be a problem as well.

Step Four is to bind intestinal toxins and improve colon transit time. If small intestinal bacterial overgrowth (SIBO) isn't a problem, consider taking a *Fiber Blend Formula* first thing in the morning before breakfast. Make sure to take it with plenty of water. If SIBO is a problem, fiber will not be helpful.

Colon transit time is the length of time it takes for material to travel from one end of the alimentary canal to the other. In a healthy colon, this should be about 18-24 hours. To test your own colon transit time, eat a food that "dyes" the stool (like beets or liquid chlorophyll) and see how long it takes for the color to show up in the stool being eliminated. If it takes more than a day, then you have a sluggish colon transit time.

Just drinking plenty of water and taking a *Fiber Blend* formula will usually improve colon transit time, but you may need magnesium, vitamin C or an herbal laxative. Try taking a *Stimulant Laxative Formula* for a short period of time (while taking the fiber) until your colon is moving more rapidly. Then switch to a *Gentle Laxative Formula* for maintenance. Stimulant Laxatives should not be used on a long term basis. If you find it difficult to have a bowel movement without stimulant laxatives and *Gentle Laxative Formulas* aren't strong enough, then try taking high doses of vitamin C (3-5,000 mg per day) and magnesium (800-1200 mg per day). Vitamin C also helps tone the intestinal membrane and promote healing.

Step Five is to reduce intestinal inflammation. Up to this point, we've focused on helping to "clean out" the intestines. It's also important to reduce the intestinal inflammation to promote tissue regeneration and repair. The following herbs are some of the best for reducing intestinal inflammation: aloe vera, cat's claw, chamomile, licorice, wild yam and St. John's wort, as all of these herbs are good at reducing the inflammation and promoting healing. You can also try an Anti-inflammatory Formula.

Step Six is to plug the "leaks," meaning to restore the integrity of the intestinal membranes. This is our primary goal in the whole process, but in this step we focus on remedies that repair and rebuild the tissues. To achieve this we look to Intestinal Toners. *Tissue Healing Formulas* can also be helpful in reducing inflammation and promoting repair. The amino acid l-glutamine and vitamin C are helpful nutrients in promoting repair. There is considerable evidence that taking l-glutamine can aid the gut in its role of protecting against viral, bacterial and food-borne antigen invaders.

Step Seven is to repopulate the colon with friendly bacteria or probiotics. One way to repopulate the colon with friendly bacteria is to eat fermented foods with live cultures, such as yoghurt or raw sauerkraut. Another way is to take probiotic supplements.

People are often amazed at how many health problems disappear (and how much better their overall health and energy is) when they heal their intestinal tract by reducing inflammation and putting a halt to gut leakage.

Therapies: Bone Broth, Colon Cleanse, Dietary Fiber, Eliminate Allergy-Causing Foods, Fast or Juice Fast, Fresh Fruits and Vegetables, Friendly Flora, Healthy Fats and Hydration

Formulas: Fiber Blend, Stimulant Laxative, **Gentle Laxative**, Antifungal, Antibacterial, Antiparasitic, **Intestinal Toning**, Tissue Healing, Anti-Inflammatory and **Digestive Bitter Tonic**

Key Herbs: Aloe vera, Chamomile (English and Roman), **Black Walnut**, **Calendula**, **Cats Claw (Uña de Gato, Gambier)**, **Kudzu**, **Triphala**, Erigeron (Fleabane), Licorice, Plantain, Sarsaparilla, St. John's wort and Wild Yam

Key Nutrients: L-Glutamine, **Probiotics**, **Digestive Enzymes**, Omega-3 Essential Fatty Acids, Fiber, Magnesium, Vitamin C and **Betaine Hydrochloric Acid (HCl)**

Leg Cramps

See *Cramps (leg)*

Lesions

See also *Abscesses*, *Acne (Pimples, Blackheads)*, *Boils*, *Wounds and Sores* and *Moles*

A lesion is an area of pathologically altered tissue such as an injury, abscess, boil, mole, pimple, rash or wound. Look up the specific type of problem for suggested remedies.

Leucorrhea (Vaginal Discharge)

See also *Vaginitis*

Leucorrhea is a whitish discharge from the vaginal area and uterus, usually the result of an estrogen imbalance or chronic bacterial or fungal infection. It is associated with inflammation of the vagina (vaginitis). If bacterial in nature try a 10% solution of povidone iodine in water as a douche or take garlic, a *Goldenseal & Echinacea Formula* or an *Antibacterial Formula* internally. For fungal issues, consider pau d'arco or an *Antifungal Formula*. Supplementing with probiotics may be helpful. One can also douche with a tea made of calendula or pau d'arco. One can also add one drop of tea tree oil to one pint of water for a douche as well.

Therapies: Friendly Flora

Formulas: Antibacterial, Goldenseal & Echinacea and Antifungal

Key Herbs: Calendula, **Tea Tree essential oil**, Garlic, Lady's Mantle and Pau d' Arco

Key Nutrients: Probiotics, Vitamin A, Vitamin D and Iodine

Leukemia

See also *Cancer (natural therapy for)*

A cancer involving a proliferation of abnormal white blood cells (leukocytes). In addition to the general protocols listed under cancer, it is important to use remedies that add the lymphatic system, such as a good *Lymphatic Drainage Formula*. Seek medical attention for this serious health problem.

Therapies: Fresh Fruits and Vegetables and Heavy Metal Cleanse

Formulas: Anticancer, Lymphatic Drainage and Mushroom Blend

Key Herbs: Burdock, **Wild Indigo (Baptista)**, Pau d' Arco and Red Clover

Key Nutrients: Protease Enzymes and Vitamin C

Lice

The following have been used to control head lice, an insect that can infest the hair and scalp. Mix essential oils or some paw paw herb powder with shampoo and wash the hair, leaving the shampoo in the hair for about 5-10 minutes before rinsing.

Key Herbs: Black Walnut, Cinnamon, **Tea Tree essential oil**, False Unicorn (Helonias), Oregano and Paw Paw

Ligaments (torn or injured)

See also *Sprains*

A torn ligament is similar to a sprain, but more serious. Torn ligaments cause severe swelling, bruising and pain, and may require surgical intervention. So, seek medical assistance. Herbs that help tissues to heal, such as arnica, comfrey and calendula can all be helpful applied topically using the Compress or Poultice therapies. Increasing mineral intake and/or taking an herbal *Mineral* or *Tissue Healing Formula* internally will also help.

Therapies: Compress, Mineralization and Poultice

Formulas: Mineral and Tissue Healing

Key Herbs: Arnica, Calendula, **Comfrey**, **Solomon's Seal** and Plantain

Key Nutrients: Vitamin C and **MSM**

Liver (fatty)

See *Fatty Liver Disease*

Liver Detoxification

See also *Chemical Poisoning* and *Heavy Metal Poisoning*

Technological society has created a new challenge to our health—environmental toxicity. Each day we are exposed to hundreds of chemicals. When these chemicals enter our body through our lungs, digestive tract or skin, the body has to break them down and eliminate them to protect our health.

The good news is that the body has systems for doing this. In particular, an amazing organ called the liver has numerous enzyme systems that process various kinds of toxins for elimination. So, we can handle a certain amount of chemical exposure and remain healthy. The bad news is that our modern lifestyle puts a great deal of stress on the liver, which means it isn't always able to keep up with its job.

The liver needs nutrients in order to process these toxins. Vitamins, minerals, amino acids and other nutrients are needed to construct and activate the enzyme systems that break down chemicals in the body. The junk-food diet of many people in modern civilization doesn't provide the raw materials the body needs to get rid of these toxins.

As a result, the liver may be unable to protect the body from these chemicals, which contributes to the development of many forms of disease. For example, some of the ailments that may involve environmental toxins include: allergies, asthma, autism, autoimmune disorders (like lupus, MS, arthritis, etc.), birth defects, cardiovascular disease, cancer, chronic headaches, fatigue, hormonal imbalances, kidney diseases, learning disabilities (ADHD, mental retardation, memory loss, senility, etc.), liver disease, neurological disorders, obesity and skin disorders (eczema, rashes and psoriasis). It's a long list, but the truth is that almost all chronic ailments probably involve some irritation to the system from chemical toxicity.

The liver is an amazing organ. It filters everything coming from the digestive tract and plays the dual role of processing nutrients for utilization and processing toxins for elimination. In its detoxification role, the liver deals with normal by-products of metabolism (i.e. cholesterol, hormones, cellular waste), toxins produced by microbial infections, drugs and other chemicals and toxins that were previously stored in fatty tissue.

To process these toxins, the liver has numerous enzymes, which convert toxins into water soluble compounds that can be flushed from the system. It does this in two steps: phase one detoxification and phase two detoxification. In phase one detoxification, about 50 different enzymes will create an electrical charge on the toxins by adding or removing an electron. In phase two, six different detoxification pathways will attach these electrically charged toxins to another compound. These six pathways are acylation, glucuronidation, glutathione conjunction, methylation, sulfation and acetylation. These six phase, dual detoxification systems make the toxin water soluble so it can be removed from the body via the urine or bile.

When a person has a strong liver, they can drink alcohol, caffeinated beverages or take medications and the effects of these substances will be relatively short-lived. A person who has sluggish detoxification will find that the effects of these substances is relatively long lasting. Another sign of sluggish detoxification is having difficulty getting to sleep at night, and then waking up with a sort of groggy, "drugged" feeling. One may also experience a bloated and stuffy feeling under the right rib cage or readily experience light-headedness, dizziness or headaches when smelling chemicals.

Sometimes phase one detoxification is working fine, but phase two detoxification pathways are sluggish. When this is the case, taking supplements that enhance phase one detoxification can make you feel sick. This is probably the cause of the "healing crisis" which occurs in natural medicine when someone consumes healthy foods and supplements and starts to feel sick. What is happening is that phase one detoxification is being increased, but phase two systems can't keep up with the toxic load.

Part of the problem here is that phase one detoxification produces free radicals (superoxide radicals, to be precise). The intermediate metabolites produced by phase one detoxification can also be free radicals (radical oxygen intermediates). If these compounds are not processed rapidly enough through phase two, they start causing irritation and inflammation to tissues. This can also happen when the body doesn't have enough antioxidants to neutralize these free radicals. Symptoms of this problem include headaches, stomach pain, nausea, fatigue, dizziness and "brain fog" during detoxification, fasting or weight loss. Toxemia during pregnancy is also a sign of sluggish phase two detoxification.

Of course, even if you don't have any of the symptoms above, but are exposed to any kind of chemicals on a regular basis in your job, it would be wise to support your liver's ability to detoxify. Examples of people who may wish to consider regular liver support include dry cleaners, painters, construction workers, lab technicians, beauticians, people who handle agricultural chemicals (like farmers and landscapers) and carpet cleaners.

Many factors can inhibit your liver's ability to detoxify. These include certain drugs, low thyroid, liver diseases, insulin resistance (diabetes) and nutritional deficiencies. Fortunately, there are several things you can do to support your liver's detoxification systems. For starters, because both phase one and phase two detoxification require a variety of vitamins, minerals and amino acids, attention should be paid to basic good nutrition.

Obviously, a diet of whole, nutrient-rich foods is optimal. Processed foods are not only low in the vitamins and minerals the liver needs to detoxify, but they also contain chemical additives that contribute to its workload. Many people take a good multi-vitamin and mineral daily to help make certain the body has the nutrients it needs. A good whole food supplement can also supply the liver with nutrients it requires for detoxification. You should seek professional guidance to determine which herbs and supplements may be helpful for you.

Therapies: Fast or Juice Fast, Fresh Fruits and Vegetables, Gall Bladder Flush and Hydration

Formulas: Hepatoprotective, General Detoxifying and Liver Tonic

Key Herbs: Blue Flag, **Bupleurum**, **Dandelion**, **Milk Thistle**, **Turmeric**, Culver's root, Garlic, Lycium (Wolfberry, Gogi), Rehmannia, Reishi (Ganoderma) and Schisandra (Schizandra)

Key Nutrients: Alpha Lipoic Acid, **Vitamin B-Complex**, **Indole-3 Carbinol (DIM)**, **N-Acetyl Cysteine**, Magnesium, Vitamin A, Vitamin C, MSM, SAM-e and L-Glutamine

Liver Spots

See *Age Spots*

Lockjaw

See *Tetanus*

Lou Gehrig's Disease (Amyotrophic Lateral Sclerosis)

See also *Autoimmune Disorders* and *Multiple Sclerosis (MS)*

Lou Gehrig's disease is a rare, fatal, progressive degenerative condition that usually begins in middle age and is characterized by increasing and spreading muscular weakness leading to paralysis. It is also called amyotrophic lateral sclerosis. It is an autoimmune disorder and a very difficult condition to treat. It is very similar to MS, but there are high levels of iron in the tissue causing highly rapid oxidative damage.

Professional assistance should be sought, but there are some natural therapies that may be helpful. For starters, since there is oxidative damage taking place in the tissues, antioxidant herbs and nutrients may be helpful. Anti-inflammatory Formulas and good fats, especially omega-3 essential fatty acids, may also be of benefit. It will also be helpful to follow the general guidelines for Multiple Sclerosis and Autoimmune Disorders.

Therapies: Affirmation and Visualization, Fresh Fruits and Vegetables and Healthy Fats

Formulas: Antioxidant and Anti-Inflammatory

Key Herbs: Ashwaganda, Ginseng (American), Ginseng (Asian, Korean) and Sarsaparilla

Key Nutrients: Colloidal Minerals, Digestive Enzymes, **Omega-3 Essential Fatty Acids**, Vitamin C, Vitamin E and **Vitamin D**

Lumbago

See *Backache (Back Pain, Lumbago)*

Lungs (congestion)

See *Congestion (lungs)*

Lupus

See also *Autoimmune Disorders*

Lupus is a chronic inflammatory and autoimmune disease that attacks multiple organs. It affects the skin in many people creating a butterfly rash over the face. Immune stimulants should be avoided and general therapies for autoimmune diseases should be applied. This is a serious illness and professional assistance should be sought.

There are a number of natural remedies that may be helpful, however. For starters, levels of DHEA tend to be low in people with lupus. You can supplement with DHEA and/or strengthen the adrenal glands with *Adrenal Tonic Formulas*. It is also useful to calm stress levels with *Adaptogen Formulas*.

Licorice root, wild yam and yucca are single herbs that may help to ease pain and inflammation. Look for Anti-inflammatory and herbal *Analgesic Formulas* that contain these herbs.

Follow the general guidelines for Autoimmune Disorders, paying close attention to the health of the digestive tract, a diet high in antioxidant nutrients and Hydration therapy.

Therapies: Fresh Fruits and Vegetables, Gut Healing Diet, Hydration and Low Glycemic Diet

Formulas: Adrenal Tonic, Adaptogen, Anti-Inflammatory and Analgesic

Key Herbs: Barley grass, Black Walnut, Chastetree (Vitex), Cordyceps, **Astragalus**, **Yucca**, Garlic, Licorice and Wild Yam

Key Nutrients: Protease Enzymes, **Probiotics**, **Omega-3 Essential Fatty Acids**, DHEA, Vitamin B-Complex, Vitamin C, Zinc, **Vitamin D**, **Betaine Hydrochloric Acid (HCl)** and Indole-3 Carbinol (DIM)

Lyme Disease

Lyme disease is most commonly a tick-borne illness. It is a bacterial infection that can be difficult to eradicate and become very debilitating. Medical attention should be sought, as it is easily cured with antibiotics in the early stages. Once the disease is established it is much harder to work with. It requires antibacterial agents to get rid of the bacteria. Teasel root provides symptomatic relief in some cases, but is not a cure. It is probably wise to seek medical attention and take antibiotics, but herbs and natural therapies could be used to support medical treatment.

Therapies: Gut Healing Diet and Stress Management

Formulas: Antibacterial and Immune Stimulating

Key Herbs: Andrographis, Black Walnut, Boneset, **Cats Claw (Uña de Gato, Gambier)**, **Stillingia**, **Sweet Annie (Ching-Hao)**, Echinacea, Garlic, Isatis, Lomatium, Sarsaparilla and Usnea

Key Nutrients: Vitamin A, Vitamin C, **Vitamin D**, Zinc and Vitamin B-6 (Pyridoxine)

Lymph Nodes or Glands (swollen)

See also *Congestion (lymphatic)*

Herbs that promote increases lymphatic flow can help to reduce swollen lymph nodes or lymph glands. These include echinacea, red root, red clover, burdock and cleavers. Take a *Lymphatic Drainage Formula* or a *Blood Purifier Formula* containing these herbs as key ingredients. If infection is present, echinacea and wild indigo can be helpful. Use an *Antibacterial Formula* with these herbs and some of the lymph-moving remedies listed above. Topically, lobelia extract, poke oil or a *Topical Analgesic Formula* can be helpful.

Therapies: Colon Cleanse, Compress and Hydration

Formulas: Lymphatic Drainage, Blood Purifier, Antibacterial and Topical Analgesic

Key Herbs: Burdock, **Echinacea**, **Poke Root oil**, **Red Clover**, **Red Root**, Lobelia, Mullein and Wild Indigo (Baptista)

Lymphoma

See also *Cancer (natural therapy for)*

Lymphoma is a type of cancer involving cells of the immune system, called lymphocytes. There are many different types of lymphomas, including Hodgkin lymphoma. The lymphocytes become cancerous and travel through the lymph system causing swelling of the lymph nodes. They may also collect in other organs such as the spleen. Professional assistance should be sought for this serious condition.

Herbs that encourage lymphatic drainage, including mullein, red clover and red root have all been used to aid in the recovery from lymphomas. Consider a good *Lymphatic Drainage Formula* containing these herbs. Keeping the colon healthy is beneficial. Digestive enzyme supplements taken between meals on an empty stomach may also be helpful. Since this is a form of cancer, look under Cancer for additional suggestions about natural therapies.

Therapies: Colon Cleanse

Formulas: Lymphatic Drainage, Immune Stimulating and Mushroom Blend

Key Herbs: Poke Root, **Red Root**, **Venus Fly Trap**, Mullein and Red Clover

Key Nutrients: Digestive Enzymes, **Vitamin A**, **Vitamin D** and **Vitamin C**

Macular Degeneration

See also *Free Radical Damage*

The macula is the center of the retina and when this part of the retina starts to deteriorate, a person experiences a loss of central vision in one or both eyes. This degeneration of the macula is also caused by inflammation and free radical damage. High blood pressure and hardening of the arteries increases the risk of developing macular degeneration.

As with other eye diseases, increasing dietary antioxidants is an important step to preventing macular degeneration. Avoid cigarette smoke (including second-hand smoke) and protect the eyes from UV radiation with hats or sunglasses.

Antioxidant supplements can definitely prevent and possibly even reverse macular degeneration. Consider using a *Vision Supporting Formula*. Bilberry, as a single herb, is especially helpful for preventing macular degeneration.

Therapies: Fresh Fruits and Vegetables and Healthy Fats

Formulas: Vision Supporting

Key Herbs: Bilberry (Blueberry, Huckleberry) and **Ginkgo**

Key Nutrients: Zeaxanthin, **Lutein**, **Omega-3 Essential Fatty Acids**, **Vitamin A**, **Vitamin C**, **Vitamin D**, **Zinc**, Folate (Folic Acid and Vitamin B9)

Malaria

Malaria is an acute or chronic disease caused by parasites that invade the red blood cells. It is transmitted from an infected person to an uninfected person by the bite of a mosquito. Symptoms include chills, fever, mass destruction of red blood cells and the parasitic release of toxic substances. An extract of sweet annie called artemisinin and cinchona have been used to treat this condition. Medical attention should be sought.

Key Herbs: Andrographis, **Sweet Annie (Ching-Hao)** and Echinacea

Key Nutrients: Vitamin A and Probiotics

Mania

See also *Bipolar Mood Disorder (Manic Depressive Disorder)*

When a person has an abnormally elated mental state, characterized by euphoria, risk taking, setting unreasonable goals and expectations for themselves, and exaggerated feelings of self importance, they are exhibiting mania. This can be accompanied by excessive talkativeness, impatience, hyperactivity and a loss of sleep. In severe cases, mania can have psychotic features. When mania alternates with depression, a person has bipolar mood disorder, also known as manic-depressive disorder.

No one knows the cause of mania, but it may be the result of imbalances in neurotransmitters (serotonin, dopamine, etc.) or unresolved emotional wounds. From a natural point of view, there are many things we can do to help someone who gets manic from time to time.

One of the first steps to maintaining a stable mood is to maintain a stable blood sugar level. When blood sugar goes high, we tend to get more manic because our brain is over stimulated. Following the Low Glycemic Diet therapy and avoiding stimulants, like caffeine, can be helpful. It is important to start the day with protein for breakfast and to obtain adequate protein from the diet to keep the brain stable. L-tyrosine, an amino acid found in red meat, is often very helpful. It can be taken as a supplement or obtained naturally in the diet by consuming some type of grass-fed, organic red meat daily (preferably for breakfast). Spirulina or other algae supplements can also supply amino acids to help stabilize mood.

Feeding the brain and nerves with a *Brain and Memory Tonic* or a *Nerve Tonic Formula* may be helpful. Also consider B-complex vitamins. Lemon balm is a particularly useful herb for balancing mania and depression, as it helps stabilize the mood.

Emotional Healing Work or Flower Essences therapy can be used to help people work through the underlying traumas that contribute to mood swings. If the situation is severe, seek appropriate assistance in the form of counseling and/or medical help.

Therapies: Avoid Caffeine, Emotional Healing Work, Flower Essences and Low Glycemic Diet

Formulas: Brain and Memory Tonic

Key Herbs: Lemon Balm and Spirulina

Key Nutrients: Vitamin B-Complex

Manic Depressive Disorder

See *Bipolar Mood Disorder (Manic Depressive Disorder)*

Mastitis

See also *Breasts (swelling and tenderness)*

Mastitis is an infection in the breast that can occur during breast feeding, causing inflammation and tenderness. Using the Poultice therapy with ingredients like slippery elm, plantain, mullein and/or echinacea is often helpful. Poke root oil can be massaged into the breasts, but should be avoided if the woman is breast-feeding. *Lymphatic Drainage Formulas*, taken internally, can improve lymphatic flow in the breasts and *Antibacterial Formulas* can be used to fight the infection. If the problem does not clear up in a day or two, it is best to seek the advice of a medical doctor.

Therapies: Hydration and Poultice

Formulas: Lymphatic Drainage and Antibacterial

Key Herbs: Echinacea, **Poke Root**, Lobelia, Mullein, Red Clover, Slippery Elm and Wild Indigo (Baptista)

Measles

Measles is an acute, contagious viral disease that begins with inflammation of mucus membranes, conjunctivitis and cough. This is followed on the third or fourth day by an eruption of distinct circular red spots. Internally, *Blood Purifier Formulas* can help to speed recovery. In children less than two years old supplementing with 200,000 IU of vitamin A, two days in a row reduced mortality significantly. Drawing Bath therapy is very effective in easing itching and discomfort.

Therapies: Drawing Bath

Formulas: Blood Purifier

Key Herbs: Black Cohosh, Burdock, Catnip, **Isatis**, **Oregon Grape**, **Yarrow**, Goldenseal and Pleurisy Root

Key Nutrients: Vitamin A

Melanoma (Skin Cancer)

See *Cancer (natural therapy for)*

Memory and Brain Function

See also *Alzheimer's Disease* and *Dementia*

Body builders take extra protein and nutrients to help them build their muscles because it is well established that the right diet and nutritional supplements can enhance athletic performance. So, why should the brain be any different?

When we're "working out" (learning something new) to build our mental muscle, shouldn't we think about optimum nutrition for the mind? Of course we should. The brain simply functions better when you give it the right raw materials to work with in the first place.

In fact, your brain is the most chemically sensitive organ in your body and nutritional problems tend to show up in your thoughts and mood before they show up as physical illness. So, let's begin by learning how to give the brain what it needs.

Get Water on the Brain

Your brain is 70% water and is very sensitive to dehydration. A mere 2% drop in body water can trigger problems like fuzzy short-term memory and trouble with basic math. Dehydration can also make it difficult for you to focus on a printed page or a computer screen. So, start your journey to a better brain by drinking adequate quantities of pure water.

Become a Fat Head

We sometimes call a person who is dull of thinking a "fat head," but it's really the smart people who are "fat heads." If you remove the water from the brain, 50% of what is left is fat. That's why children who receive plenty of good fats in the womb and earlier childhood have better brain development. The bottom line is that low fat diets are harmful to the brains of both developing children and adults.

Not just any fats will do, however. You need the right kinds of fats to become a smart "fat head." What your brain primarily needs is more omega-3 essential fatty acids, which are deficient in most American diets. One of these omega-3 fatty acids is DHA, the most abundant phospholipid in the brain. It is highest in the frontal cortex and critical to the developing brains of infants.

Deficiencies in DHA result in reduced learning ability in both children and adults. Low levels also result in a reduction of brain serotonin levels, which can lead to depression. Deficiencies have also been associated with ADHD and Alzheimer's disease.

So, to be smart increase your intake of DHA and other good fats. Deep ocean-fish and grass fed meats are good sources of brain-healthy fats. So are dark green leafy vegetables, omega-3 eggs and certain nuts and seeds (like walnuts, macadamia nuts, flax seeds and hemp seeds).

Amino Acids Aid Intelligence

Brain cells talk to each other by sending messages via chemicals called neurotransmitters. All neurotransmitters are built from amino acids, the building blocks of protein. So, not only do low fat diets reduce your brain power, so do low protein diets. Without adequate levels of amino acids from proteins, you brain cells can't communicate properly with each other.

Studies have shown that children who start the day with a traditional breakfast that contains high protein foods like eggs, perform better in school than children who eat sugar-sweetened breakfast cereals. It's the same for adults.

This doesn't mean you need to eat bacon and eggs for breakfast to stay smart, but it does mean you should have some kind of high quality protein at the beginning of your day. If you don't have time for eggs or meat, try a protein shake or fruit smoothie made with a protein powder.

A great way to get more amino acids is to take an algae supplement like spirulina, blue-green algae and chlorella. These are all great vegetarian sources of amino acids and help to balance blood sugar levels, increase energy, stabilize mood and increase mental clarity.

B Vitamins are an A+ for Your Brain

Synthesizing neurotransmitters from amino acids takes other nutrients, particularly B vitamins. They are found naturally in most complex carbohydrates like fruits, vegetables and whole grains. They are missing, however, from refined carbohydrates like white sugar, white flour and white rice, which is why most Americans aren't getting enough B's to keep their brains working at the A+ level.

To better the "grade" your brain gets, try taking B-complex. They calm your nerves and clarify your thoughts. Together with vitamin C, they will also reduce your stress level, help you feel calmer and give you better energy at the same time.

Ban Sugar for a Better Brain

If you want a clear, sharp mind it's best to avoid refined carbohydrates like refined sugar and white flour products. These foods spike your blood sugar and then allow it to drop dramatically a couple of hours later. This is bad for the brain, since the amount of sugar reaching your brain affects your memory, focus and mental clarity.

When your blood sugar is too high, your brain is over stimulated, which will make you hyperactive and irritable. You'll feel agitated, excitable and restless, but have difficulty concentrating. When your blood sugar is too low, your brain won't function properly. You'll feel sluggish and lethargic or angry and irrational.

So, for example, eat complex carbohydrates like fresh fruits, vegetables and whole grains for breakfast instead of processed cereals, white toast, pancakes or waffles (covered with sugar-laden jam or syrup) and fruit juices. Complex carbohydrates will give you a more stable brain, which will make your mind clear and sharp instead of muddled and confused.

If you crave sugar, try using xylitol as a sweetener instead of refined sugar. It doesn't spike your blood sugar and actually helps reduce carbohydrate cravings. You can also take licorice root to help stabilize your blood sugar levels and reduce sugar cravings.

Herbal Brain Boosters

Besides basic good nutrition, there are some specific herbs that have been shown to help your brain function better. These include ginkgo, gotu kola, bacopa, rosemary and sage. *Brain and Memory Tonic Formulas* typically combine herbs like these and can be helpful for enhancing learning and slowing memory loss in aging.

Additional Tips

Hardening of the arteries will impair blood flow to the brain and reduce cognitive function. People with reduced blood flow to the brain often get sleepy when they sit for long periods and have problems with being absent minded. *Cardiovascular Stimulant Formulas* are helpful in these cases.

Toxins can seriously damage the brain, especially fat-soluble toxins (such as petrochemical solvents) and heavy metals like mercury, aluminum and lead. In addition, drugs and alcohol do serious damage to the brain. So, to keep your mind clear and active avoid as many chemicals as possible, don't use drugs, and minimize the consumption of alcohol. To further avoid chemicals, don't use aluminum cookware, purify your drinking water, use non-toxic household cleaning products and personal care items, and read labels carefully.

Therapies: Colon Cleanse, Fresh Fruits and Vegetables, Healthy Fats, Heavy Metal Cleanse, Hydration, Low Glycemic Diet and Mineralization

Formulas: Brain and Memory Tonic, Cardiovascular Stimulant and Heavy Metal Cleansing

Key Herbs: Ashwaganda, Blessed Thistle, Cordyceps, **Bacopa (Water Hyssop)**, **Ginkgo**, **Gotu kola**, **Holy Basil**, **Rosemary**, Hawthorn, Lemon Balm, Rhodiola and Sage

Key Nutrients: Vitamin B-12, **Omega-3 Essential Fatty Acids**, **DHA**, **Vitamin B-Complex**, Folate (Folic Acid, Vitamin B9), Vitamin B-1 (Thiamine) and Magnesium

Ménière's Disease

See also *Tinnitus (Ringing in the Ears)*

Ménière's disease affects the inner ear. The cause of Ménière's remains unknown, although it usually begins between the ages of 30 and 50. In Ménière's disease, a part of the inner ear, called the endolymphatic sac, becomes swollen. This disrupts a person's sense of balance.

A person with Ménière's disease will often have a combination of sensorineural hearing loss, dizziness (vertigo), ringing in the ear (tinnitus), and sensitivity to loud sounds. This type of hearing loss should be managed by a doctor and audiologist. Some people with Ménière's disease report mild symptoms, but for others the symptoms are more severe, transient and even permanent.

There is no specific natural therapy for Ménière's disease, but gingko and some of the remedies listed under Tinnitus may be helpful.

Key Herbs: Ginkgo

Key Nutrients: Potassium

Meningitis

Inflammation of the membranes that surround the brain and spinal cord is called meningitis. This is often caused by a bacteria or virus, but can also be caused by adverse reactions to vaccines. It is a serious condition for which medical attention should be sought. Herbs can be used as complimentary therapies with professional guidance.

Formulas: Antiviral, Antibacterial and Anti-Inflammatory

Key Herbs: Isatis, Echinacea, Goldenseal, Gotu kola, St. John's wort and Yarrow

Key Nutrients: Vitamin C

Menopause

See also *Aging (prevention)*, *Hot Flashes* and *Osteoporosis*

Menopause has been called the "change of life," but it's really the second change of life women undergo. The first was puberty, when hormonal shifts transformed her from being a girl to being an adult woman. Traditionally, a girl's first period was seen as her passage from being a child to being a woman.

Menopause is a second hormonal shift that transforms a woman's body from the childbearing years into the wise-woman (or elder) years. At menopause, periods cease because the ovaries no longer produce fertile eggs.

Just as the hormonal shifts during puberty may cause discomfort or problems, so might the hormonal shifts during menopause. So, although menopause is a natural process, ninety percent of all women experience some menopausal symptoms. In most cases, however, it's not necessary for women to turn to synthetic hormone replacement or synthetic drugs to ease these symptoms. There are plenty of natural remedies that can help.

Common Menopausal Problems

To understand how to make menopause marvelous instead of uncomfortable, it is necessary to understand some of the common problems women experience during menopause and the potential problems of medical solutions. Besides the cessation of periods, common menopausal symptoms include hot flashes, night sweats, vaginal dryness, breast tenderness and mood swings. It's also common for many women to experience some bone loss (osteoporosis), thinning of hair and the development of more facial hair, and some weight gain.

Emotional changes can also occur with menopause, including irritability, depression or anxiety. There may be difficulty concentrating, mental confusion and memory lapses.

In modern times, doctors began to routinely prescribe synthetic hormone replacement for women going through menopause to ease menopausal symptoms. However, these drugs are not without their side effects.

In July 2002, a study of 16,000 women on a common hormone-replacement drug, Prempro®, revealed some serious side effects. There was an increased risk of breast cancer and heart attack in women taking these hormones. Specifically, the stroke rate was 41% higher, breast cancer was 26% higher and the rate of blood clots doubled. So, although the synthetic hormones did reduce the rate of hip fractures, the increased risks in other areas made routine use of these medications unwise.

These synthetic hormones have other side effects, too. The side effects of synthetic progesterone can include weight gain, hair loss, low energy, depression, water retention, migraine headaches, reduced sex drive and skin problems. In fact, it has been found that one-half of all women who take synthetic hormone replacement quit after one year because they are unable to tolerate the side effects.

The good news is that women living in traditional cultures did not experience as many problems with menopause. So, it is possible to reduce or eliminate menopausal symptoms by creating a healthier lifestyle and using natural herbs and supplements. Since it is hormonal changes that create the physiological and psychological shifts you experience at menopause, it helps to start by understanding a little bit about the two types of hormones that make you a woman—estrogen and progesterone.

Understanding Estrogens

Estrogen, of course, is the hormone that dominates in the female body, just like testosterone dominates in men. The word estrogen is derived from the Latin *oestrus* and Greek *oistros*, words that refer to the time of the month when a female is fertile and ready to mate. *Gen* means to generate or produce, so the word estrogen refers to a compound that makes a woman ovulate and become fertile.

What most women don't understand is that estrogen isn't a single compound. There are, in fact, many forms of estrogen.

For starters, a woman's body produces three primary forms of estrogen: estrone (E1), estradiol (E2) and estriol (E3). As if that's not enough, there are also phytoestrogens (estrogen-like compounds found in plants) and xenoestrogens (chemical pollutants that have estrogenic effects).

Estrogens are involved in a lot more than just ovulation. There are over 300 tissues in the body with estrogen receptor sites, and estrogens play a role in 400 functions of the body. These include bone density, mood, eye health, muscle strength, energy production, temperature regulation, intestinal function, libido and even brain function (which is also why men and women think differently and even have different sensory perceptions).

Estradiol (E2)

Estradiol is the strongest estrogen and the main form of estrogen produced by a woman's body during her childbearing years. Estradiol is produced in the ovaries under the influence of the follicle-stimulating hormone (FSH) from the pituitary. FSH causes an egg-bearing follicle to mature, producing E2.

E2 is the estrogen that stimulates breast development, so it is increased E2 that causes many of the changes a woman experiences during puberty. After menopause, when eggs are no longer maturing, the ovaries stop producing E2. The decline in levels of E2 causes many of the changes associated with menopause.

High levels of E2 increase the risk of uterine and breast cancer. However, E2 also has many benefits.

E2 helps absorption of minerals (which help to build bone). E2 also decreases LDL, increases HDL and balances triglycerides, which reduces a woman's risk of heart disease. It also makes tissues more insulin-sensitive, which reduces diabetes. Low levels of E2 can cause fatigue, problems sleeping, memory problems, increased risk of blood clots and depression.

Estrone (E1) and Estriol (E3)

E1 is the main form of estrogen produced after menopause. It can be formed in the adrenal glands, liver and fat cells, as well as the ovaries. During a woman's fertile years the ovaries convert E1 to E2. After menopause this conversion stops.

E3 is a milder estrogen that does not stimulate the breast tissue or uterine lining like E1 and E2 do. Because of this E3 protects the intestinal tract, vaginal lining and the breasts. E3 is even used to treat breast cancer in other countries. Asian and vegetarian woman have higher levels of E3 and lower rates of breast cancer.

Balancing Estrogen After Menopause

Many of the symptoms women experience after menopause are the result of declining levels of estrogens. However, when the ovaries stop producing E2 a woman still continues to produces estrogens through the adrenals, liver and fat cells. So, here are three natural ways a woman can enhance her estrogen after menopause.

For starters, the body has a natural way of storing estrogen to ease the transition to menopause, increasing fat cells. It is common for women to experience a slight weight gain (5-10 pounds) just prior to entering menopause. This is nature's way of storing extra estrogen to be prepared for the hormonal shift. So, ladies, don't fight it or worry about it, accept it gracefully because it will make menopause easier.

Secondly, since the adrenal glands are a major source of estrogens after menopause, having healthy adrenal glands is vital to having a trouble-free change of life. Unfortunately, many women enter menopause suffering adrenal fatigue from sugar and caffeine consumption and chronic stress. Remedies that support the adrenals like *Adrenal Tonic Formulas*, pantothenic acid and B-complex vitamins can help to build the adrenals and reduce menopausal discomfort.

Finally, many natural foods and herbs contain plant-based estrogens called phytoestrogens. Women whose diets contain phytoestrogen-rich foods have fewer menopausal problems. Beans (not just soybeans) are great sources of phytoestrogens, as are whole grains and dark green, leafy vegetables.

There are also herbal remedies that contain phytoestrogens. These can be found in *Phytoestrogen Formulas*. You can also take a *Menopause Balancing Formula*, which can help to naturally balance your hormones.

Avoid Xenoestrogens

Women of all ages who want to protect their health should avoid xenoestrogens, the third type of estrogenic compound. These environmental pollutants that mimic estrogen cause abnormal changes in breast and uterine tissue, contributing to the development of breast lumps, breast cancer, uterine fibroids and endometriosis. They may also contribute to mood swings, cramps or heavy bleeding, thinning hair, hot flashes and weight gain. The American Geriatric Society also reports that post menopausal women with higher levels of circulating estrogen also experience greater cognitive decline.

Understanding Progesterone

Progesterone is made by the ovaries before menopause and by the adrenal glands after menopause. This hormone helps to lay down new bone, relieve depression, enhance sex drive, and support thyroid function. Because it competes with estrogen for receptor sites, it also helps prevent over-stimulation of estrogenic processes, reducing the risk of fibrocystic breasts, breast cancer and other estrogen-dependent cancers.

After menopause, women also experience a decline in progesterone production. Increasing progesterone levels after menopause can help balance blood sugar levels, prevent blood clotting and maintain bone health. Two herbs that are very good at enhancing progesterone and helping to balance estrogen and progesterone levels are chaste tree berries and false unicorn. These are often found in *Menopause Balancing Formulas*. Natural progesterone is also available in a cream form for topical application. Many women, both pre- and post-menopausal, find that using a progesterone cream improves their overall health. It may be a good idea to get a saliva hormone test before using natural hormone replacements to see if you really need them.

Other Factors to Consider

In a culture that places such high value on youthfulness (and often views menopause as a "tragedy"), it's understandable that many women feel sadness, grief or stress at the onset of a transition that's often seen as the end of that youthfulness. This is coupled with other stresses of middle-aged life—children growing up and becoming more independent, health challenges, and difficulties with finances and career. All of these stresses serve to exacerbate these hormonal imbalances and aggravate the symptoms of menopause. Flower Essences Therapy and Emotional Healing Work may help.

Other lifestyle-related sources of hormonal imbalance during menopause include a poor diet and lack of exercise. Studies done at Harvard Medical School, as well as in

Scandinavia, showed that women who engaged in regular exercise experienced fewer and less intense hot flashes.

See related conditions for additional suggestions on dealing with specific problems like hot flashes and osteoporosis.

Therapies: Avoid Xenoestrogens, Emotional Healing Work, Flower Essences, Healthy Fats and Stress Management

Formulas: Menopause Balancing, Adrenal Tonic and Phytoestrogen

Key Herbs: Chamomile (English and Roman), **Black Cohosh**, **Chastetree (Vitex)**, **Red Clover**, Dong Quai, False Unicorn (Helonias), Peppermint, Shatavari and St. John's wort

Key Nutrients: L-Glutamine, DHEA, Colloidal Minerals, Digestive Enzymes, Omega-3 Essential Fatty Acids, **Vitamin B-Complex**, Vitamin E, Pantothenic Acid (Vitamin B5) and **Vitamin D**

Menorrhagia (Heavy Menstrual Bleeding)

See also *Fibroids (uterine)*

Excessive menstrual bleeding or menorrhagia is often caused by excess estrogens or xenoestrogens. It may be due to uterine fibroids, too. Get an appropriate medical diagnosis if the problem is persistent and doesn't respond to natural remedies. If the problem is fibroids, look under that section for more assistance.

Yarrow, tienchi ginseng, shepherd's purse and bayberry are all possibilities for reducing the bleeding. You can take them internally or use them as a douche. A *Uterine Tonic Formula* can tone up the uterus and further help to reduce the blood loss.

Chaste tree or false unicorn may help to increase progesterone and reduce estrogens. Nettles are nourishing to make up for the loss of blood. An *Iron Formula* can also be helpful for this.

Therapies: Affirmation and Visualization, Avoid Xenoestrogens, Fresh Fruits and Vegetables, Healthy Fats, Hydration, Low Glycemic Diet, Mineralization and Stress Management

Formulas: Uterine Tonic, **Iron**, Female Hormonal Balancing and Uterine Tonic

Key Herbs: Bayberry, Calendula, **Chastetree (Vitex)**, **Cinnamon**, **Yarrow**, False Unicorn (Helonias), Lady's Mantle, Nettle (Stinging), Rehmannia and Shepherd's Purse

Key Nutrients: Iron

Menstrual Cramps

See *Cramps (menstrual)*

Therapies: Avoid Xenoestrogens

Menstrual Irregularity

See also *PMS (general)*

When a woman's menstrual cycle does not follow the normal 28-day pattern (too long, too short, irregular, etc.) herbs can often be helpful in normalizing periods. The easiest place to start is with a *Female Hormonal Balancing Formula*. There are also specific single herbs that may help more specific problems. For example, chastetree or vitex helps to regulate the menstrual cycle via the pituitary gland and hypothalamus when taken over a period of several months. False unicorn can be helpful when progesterone levels are too low and estrogen levels are too high. Consult with a professional herbalist (*findanherbalist.com*) who can help you select the specific remedies that may be helpful for you.

Therapies: Stress Management

Formulas: Female Hormonal Balancing

Key Herbs: Black Cohosh, **Blessed Thistle**, **Chastetree (Vitex)**, Dong Quai, False Unicorn (Helonias) and Milk Thistle

Key Nutrients: DHEA and Omega-3 Essential Fatty Acids

Menstruation (heavy bleeding)

See *Menorrhagia (Heavy Menstrual Bleeding)*

Menstruation (painful)

See *Dysmenorrhea (Painful Menstruation)*

Mental Illness

See also *Fungal Infections (Yeast Infections, Candida albicans), Heavy Metal Poisoning, Hypoglycemia, Memory and Brain Function* and *Abuse and Trauma*

Mental health problems can be a "touchy" subject because most of us find the idea of "mental illness" disturbing or frightening. These attitudes about mental health problems have been around since ancient times, when the mentally ill were considered to be possessed by devils.

Even though our understanding of mental illness has improved since ancient times, the social stigma attached to these conditions is still negative. Furthermore, modern treatments for "mental" conditions still leave much to be desired. Does drugging the brain or locking up the severely disturbed really solve the problem?

Just like any other disease human beings suffer from, the so-called "mental" illnesses have causes. While the causes of mental illness aren't fully understood, it is highly unlikely that a drug deficiency is one of them. So, while drugs might be of use in stabilizing some situations, they aren't the ultimate cure for mental health problems.

Furthermore, it's not like a person wakes up one morning and thinks, "I'm going to go insane today," so people with mental health problems should be treated with the same compassion and respect we would treat anyone suffering from a "physical" disease. Using criticism, rewards and punishments to try to "correct" the behavior of one suffering from mental health problems is just going to make the situation worse, especially since the underlying cause is often childhood abuse or unresolved emotional trauma.

Likewise, the labels given to mental conditions are often confusing and don't really help. Labels are just names attached to certain patterns of symptoms, and are really of little use in helping to cure anything.

We must get past the stigmas, misunderstanding and symptomatic treatments and start understanding the root causes of mental health issues. Only when we understand the cause can we formulate effective treatments.

Types of Mental Illness

To begin our journey, we need to recognize the difference between three different classes of mental health issues. First, there are mood disorders, such as depression, anxiety, learning disabilities, etc. These are not debilitating issues. People who have them can still function in society. In fact, many are problems from which just about everyone suffers from time to time. Who hasn't felt depressed or anxious once in a while?

Unfortunately, in order to push their wares, drug companies appear to be turning these ordinary issues of mood and mental attitude into diseases. The child who is restless, bored and fidgety at school is suddenly suffering from a disease called ADHD. The person who is socially shy or a little bit anxious is a victim of social anxiety disorder. A person who is exhausted and run down from long-term stress has post traumatic stress disorder. The person who is rightfully "down" because of difficult experiences in life needs medication.

This is not to downplay the idea that mood disorders aren't real; it's just that if a person is basically able to function in their life, they probably don't need drugs to get over these mood problems. Some counseling (or even a listening

ear from a friend), good parenting (for kids), and attention to basic health needs like nutrition, rest and exercise will usually clear up mood disorders. These kinds of problems can often be handled by improving overall nutrition, balancing blood sugar levels, and using the Emotional Healing Work, Flower Essences, Affirmation and Visualization or Stress Management therapies.

A second category of "mental" health problems is those that are caused by actual destruction of the brain. Alzheimer's disease and dementia are examples of physical or chemical damage to the brain tissues, which result in the destruction of brain cells. Much of this damage occurs from oxidative stress and inflammation in the brain. These diseases can be prevented by good nutrition and health practices (detoxification, antioxidants, etc.), but once they occur natural therapies can merely slow deterioration rather than reverse them. For information on how to prevent or slow this physical deterioration of the mind, see Memory and Brain Function.

The third kind of "mental" health problem we want to consider are those problems where there is no actual damage to the brain, but the person has mental problems that are keeping them from being a functional human being. These are the people we usually consider "insane," people who suffer from schizophrenia, severe depression or whatever other labels doctors concoct to describe the person's symptoms.

The following information may help people in this third category, but they will probably need some professional help, too. At a minimum, counseling or some kind of psychotherapy is necessary. But, people with these disorders are not "doomed" to a life of insanity. If root causes are addressed and dealt with, they can become functioning people again. It takes dedication and effort, but it can happen.

Nutrition for the Brain and Nerves

Like any other organ, the brain needs nutrients to function properly. If the brain isn't nourished properly problems will occur. The brain needs water, fats, protein, B-complex vitamins and other nutrients to function properly. It also needs balanced blood sugar. Hypoglycemia or low blood sugar is common in people who have been labeled mentally ill, and stabilizing their blood sugar with the Low Glycemic Diet therapy and appropriate supplements can facilitate big improvements.

For example, Barbara Reed, a parole officer from New York, found that diet contributed to juvenile delinquency. As a parole officer for young offenders, she noticed that most of them were living on a junk food diet. When she was able to persuade these kids to go on a hypoglycemic diet along with a B-complex plus C vitamin supplement, they never got in trouble with the law again. This is not the only case where behavior has been linked to diet; studies have also shown that prisoners have had remarkable improvements in behavior when put on a hypoglycemic diet.

In the documentary "Super Size Me," a school for troubled teens is shown, where the teens are calmer because they are being fed a high quality diet. Research on the link between nutrition and mental ability has been around for a long time. Michael Lesser testified before the Senate Select Committee on Nutrition and Human Needs in the 1970s that 70% of all previously uncontrollable schizophrenics showed improvement when put on a diet to counter hypoglyccmia. Thcy also showcd improvement with vitamin supplements, particularly certain B vitamins.

Toxins and the Brain

The brain is the most chemically sensitive organ in the body, so it is highly susceptible to damage from environmental toxins. So, chemical toxins are another major root cause of "mental" illness.

For example, intestinal inflammation and leaky gut syndrome have been linked with depression, hyperactivity, ADHD and schizophrenia. So, a good cleanse can often help "lighten" a person's mood and clear their thinking.

Yeast infections can also "mess up" one's thought processes. Since yeast feed on sugar, yeast infections can contribute to sugar cravings.

A major contributing factor to mental breakdown is heavy metal poisoning. Mercury, lead, cadmium and aluminum all contribute to the breakdown of brain and nervous system tissue. Obviously, detoxification of heavy metals will help protect the brain and may improve brain function.

Since toxins damage brain tissue by causing inflammation and free radical damage, supplements containing antioxidants, lecithin, lycopene, alpha lipoic acid, ginkgo and other herbs may protect the brain from deterioration due to chemical toxicity and free radical damage.

Unresolved Trauma and Stress

In addition to the issues of nutrition and detoxification, we also have the issue of unresolved trauma and emotional stress. The simple fact is that many of the people who have been labeled "insane" have simply suffered trauma or abuse that overwhelmed their ability to cope. Sexual and physical abuse as a child can set up patterns that contribute to poor mental (and physical) health.

As Peter R. Breggin, M.D., points out in his book *Toxic Psychiatry*, many people who are labeled "mentally ill" are simply in emotional and spiritual crisis. Their language

is metaphoric. It sounds crazy because people can't hear what the person is really trying to communicate. Delusions of grandeur ("I'm God or Napoleon", for example) can indicate a person is struggling with their sense of importance.

Dr. Breggin stresses that locking these people up, drugging them and shocking them doesn't help them work through their inner crises or deal with their repressed emotional pain. He also suggests that drugs (which includes medications, alcohol, tobacco and illegal street drugs) only act to chemically lobotomize the brain, numbing a person to their inner pain.

What people in crisis really need is a good psychologist or counselor who can help them work through their unresolved issues. Flower essences may also be helpful in bringing repressed emotions and issues to the surface. Aromatherapy oils can also be used to help improve mood. Space doesn't permit a full discussion of these tools, but there are plenty of resources for learning more about them.

Many people who do bodywork from massage therapists to rolfers have observed that people seem to store stress and pain in the body. When people experience intense feelings they don't know how to deal with, they hold their breath, suppress them, or disassociate from them in order to avoid feeling them. This creates tension in the body and "stores" the memory of the trauma in the tissues.

Bodywork can release these tense areas and help a person reconnect with pain and emotions they have repressed, promoting release and healing. So, bodywork techniques like chiropractic care, rolfing, deep tissue massage, yoga and other bodywork techniques can be very helpful in improving mental health. A number of innovative psychologists have used movement and bodywork to improve mental health.

Obviously, this is an area where it is best to seek professional help, but these general guidelines and some of the supplements and basic therapies we've listed here are avenues to consider.

Therapies: Affirmation and Visualization, Aromatherapy, Emotional Healing Work, Flower Essences, Fresh Fruits and Vegetables, Healthy Fats, Heavy Metal Cleanse, Low Glycemic Diet, Mineralization and Stress Management

Formulas: Brain and Memory Tonic, Heavy Metal Cleansing and **Adaptogen**

Key Herbs: Bacopa (Water Hyssop), Barberry, **Schisandra (Schizandra)**, **Scullcap (Skullcap)**, Ginkgo, Licorice and Oat seed (milky)

Key Nutrients: Calcium, Omega-3 Essential Fatty Acids, Magnesium, DHA, Chromium, Colloidal Minerals, **Vitamin B-Complex**, Vitamin C and Alpha Lipoic Acid

Mercury Poisoning

See also *Heavy Metal Poisoning* and *Multiple Sclerosis (MS)*

Mercury is one of the most toxic substances we can be exposed to and we are exposed to it on a fairly regular basis. It is found in fungicides, pesticides, dental fillings, contaminated seafood, thermometers and a host of products, including cosmetics, fabric softeners, inks, tattoo ink, latex, medications, paints, plastics, polishes, solvents and wood preservatives.

Mercury can be absorbed through the skin or inhaled. It passes through the blood-brain barrier and is attracted to and absorbed by nerve endings. This neurotoxin lodges inside neuron cells disrupting cellular communication. It can cause autoimmune disorders, arthritis, blindness, candidiasis, depression, dizziness, fatigue, gum disease, hair loss, insomnia, memory loss, muscle weakness, multiple sclerosis, lateral sclerosis (ALS), Alzheimer's, Parkinson's, paralysis, lupus, food and environmental allergies, menstrual disorders, miscarriages, behavioral changes, depression, irritability, hyperactivity, allergic reactions, asthma, metallic taste in the mouth, loose teeth and more.

Remember those silver fillings that dentists put into your mouth? Well, they are really 50% mercury! Although the American Dentists Association will do everything they can to deny that amalgam fillings can affect health, many European countries now completely outlaw the use of silver/mercury amalgam fillings! According to the World Health Organization, amalgam dental fillings are a major source of mercury exposure. Mercury fillings may be a contributing factor to many chronic, degenerative and autoimmune conditions, because many people with these conditions have had significant improvement to their health when they have been removed. It is important to note that a mercury detox program is usually needed after fillings have been removed.

Mercury damages the nervous system and the immune system, and it can be a contributing factor in a wide variety of ailments, including autoimmune disorders.

A number of nutrients and herbs may be helpful in helping get mercury out of the body. These include cilantro, milk thistle, alpha lipoic acid, vitamin C and n-acetyl cysteine. Some of these ingredients can be found in *Heavy Metal Cleansing Formulas*. Full directions for doing a Heavy Metal Cleanse are found in the Therapies section.

Therapies: Dietary Fiber, Drawing Bath, Healthy Fats and Heavy Metal Cleanse

Formulas: Heavy Metal Cleansing and Fiber Blend

Key Herbs: Bee Pollen, **Cilantro/Coriander**, Echinacea, Eleuthero (Siberian ginseng), Garlic, Lobelia, Milk Thistle, Red Clover and Sarsaparilla

Key Nutrients: N-Acetyl Cysteine, **Alpha Lipoic Acid**, Sodium Alginate (Algin), Omega-3 Essential Fatty Acids, DHA and Vitamin C

Metabolic Syndrome

See *Hyperinsulinemia (Metabolic Syndrome, Syndrome X)*

Migraine

See also *Headache (general)*

A migraine is a recurrent, moderate to severe headache often accompanied by visual symptoms, nausea and vomiting. Migraines affect about 28 million Americans. People experiencing a migraine typically have an intense unilateral headache, with one half of their head in pain of a pulsating nature. Migraines can last from 2-72 hours and can cause nausea, vomiting, increased sensitivity to light and/or sound with pain normally exacerbated by physical activity.

Migraines are typically associated with a dilation of the cranial blood vessels, as opposed to the constriction of cranial vessels with common tension headaches. Migraines are also associated with the release of the neurotransmitter serotonin from affected nerve endings. These kinds of headaches can be much more difficult to relieve than simple tension headaches.

The modern medical treatment of migraines is woefully inadequate because, as with many diseases, treatment is based on correlation, not causation. Simply put, the use of calcium channel blockers, beta-blockers, anti-seizure medications, antidepressants, and even Botox injections for the prevention of migraines is based on a superficial understanding of the body processes involved.

While some people find relief from these medicines, they do not address the underlying causes of the headaches and run the risk side effects. The most used class of migraine medications are triptans (i.e. Imitrex, Maxalt, and Zomig), which carry an increased risk of stroke, and can cause high blood pressure, vascular spasms and birth defects. Triptans and common OTC analgesics like Tylenol, aspirin and ergotamine are all associated with rebound migraines, thus perpetuating the pain.

The root causes of migraines are more difficult to figure out than some diseases because there are so many. It's speculated that there are over 20 different processes that individually or in concert can cause a migraine. Here are some of the most common causes and natural therapies that can help.

1. GI Imbalances/Food Allergies/Autoimmunity

Migraines often have food allergy triggers, including chocolate, citrus, alcohol, or aged or cured foods. An exaggerated immune response is correlated with migraines. For example, people with celiac disease, an immune attack on the intestinal tract from a gluten allergy, are 10 times more likely to have migraines! People with any autoimmune disorder including rheumatoid arthritis, lupus, Hashimoto's thyroiditis and multiple sclerosis are also much more prone to migraines.

In people with healthy GI tracts, food is completely digested, the nutrients absorbed and the non-nutritive components eliminated. However, in people with impaired digestion and intestinal irritation, undigested food proteins are absorbed into the blood stream, causing an inflammatory immune response that can manifest as a migraine or a host of other disorders including autoimmune diseases. So, Leaky Gut Syndrome and Small Intestinal Bacterial Overgrowth (SIBO) are major underlying causes of migraines.

Symptoms of gut problems that may be triggering migraines include: fatigue after meals, bloating and gas normally occurring within an hour of eating, brain fog after the consumption of certain foods, joint and muscle pain or other signs of systemic inflammation like IBS, chronic sinus congestion, post nasal drip, and chronic skin disorders (eczema, psoriasis etc.). Having any of the above symptoms would make a trial elimination diet and therapies to heal the gut worth trying. If you feel the need to confirm food allergies and intestinal permeability with medical testing find a qualified, natural minded practitioner to order a comprehensive digestive stool analysis and IgG food allergy panel.

Follow the suggestions for the Gut Healing Diet therapy and the recommendations under Leaky Gut Syndrome and Small Intestinal Bacterial Overgrowth. You may also wish to consult a qualified herbalist (*findanherbalist.com*) to determine the need for herbal therapies to heal the gut. Possibilities include: cats claw, St. John's wort, calendula, chamomile, catnip, kudzu, aloe vera, artemesia, yellow root, wild yam, peach, marshmallow and astragalus.

2. Chemical Triggers

Certain chemicals, both manmade and some found in nature are known to trigger migraines. So, you want to minimize chemical exposure by avoiding aspartame, MSG (monosodium glutamate), nitrates (in deli meats), sulfites (found in wine, dried fruit, and some foods in salad bars). In addition, avoid the following foods that are high in histamine, arginine and tyramine for 60 days. You can then slowly reintroduce them one at a time to see if they are problematic for you.

Strong smelly cheeses (e.g. Camembert, Brie, Gruyere, Cheddar, Roquefort, Parmesan)

Canned fish, deli chicken, chicken sausage, pork sausage, beef sausage, ham

Beverages: Coffee, Tea, Wine, Beer, Milk

Fermented foods including: soy products, and all fermented vegetables, such as sauerkraut, kimchi etc.

Vegetables: eggplant, pumpkin, spinach, tomatoes

Fruits: apricots, cherries, cranberry, currants, dates, loganberries, nectarines, oranges, papaya, peach, pineapple, prunes, plums, raisins, raspberries, red grapes (white are OK), strawberries

Chocolate

Beans: soy beans, red beans, fava beans, lima beans, romano and Italian beans

All nuts and seeds

Spices: anise, cinnamon, cloves, curry powder, hot paprika, nutmeg, seasoning packets and foods labeled "with spices"

Commercial ketchup

Brewers yeast

3. Magnesium Deficiency

Many people have magnesium deficiencies. If your migraines are accompanied by muscular tension or cramping (anything that feels too tight), constipation, heart palpitations, anxiety, insomnia or fatigue, this may be a factor. Blood tests are an inaccurate reflection of cellular magnesium levels. So, go by symptoms not blood tests.

Take magnesium glycinate, citrate, or aspartate in slowly increasing doses until your symptoms disappear or you get loose bowels. Then back off to a slightly lower dose. If you have kidney disease of any kind, do this only with a doctor's supervision. Because magnesium is poorly absorbed when taken orally, many people find that topical application of magnesium chloride oil or regular Epsom salts baths are a faster way to treat the symptoms of deficiency.

4. Anemia

There are about 400 types of anemia from a variety of causes. Anemia from an iron deficiency results in a lack of red blood cells, and a deficiency of folate or B12 causes the formation of damaged red blood cells that can't hold onto oxygen properly. The end result of anemia, no matter the cause, is reduced oxygen to the brain. Insufficient oxygen to the brain means headaches; think of a high altitude headache but without the nice scenery.

The migraine-related symptoms of anemia include general weakness, fatigue even when rested, malaise, poor concentration, pale tongue and gums, the compulsive consumption of non-food items like ice, soil, paper, wax and grass (pica), restless legs, and twitching muscles. Anemia is easy to test for because it causes lowered hemoglobin and hematocrit on a CBC panel. Additionally, testing for ferretin and iron saturation can be useful. If anemia is an issue, see the suggestions under Anemia.

5. Hypothyroidism

90% of low thyroid in America is from Hashimoto's thyroiditis, an autoimmune condition. Since autoimmune diseases and migraines likely have many of the same causes, addressing step 1 is essential. In addition fluctuations in thyroid hormone levels can stimulate migraines. Often with hypothyroidism prescription medication is necessary, especially in the beginning of treatment.

Symptoms that low thyroid may be a factor in migraines include depression, weight gain, cold intolerance, fatigue, anxiety, cold hands and feet, chronic muscle pain (fibromyalgia), constipation and dry skin. If these symptoms accompany migraines, see the suggestions under Hashimoto's Disease and Hypothyroid.

6. Hormonal Imbalances

If migraines are accompanied by PMS with bloating, fluid retention, breast tenderness, menstrual cramps and/or heavy or irregular menstrual cycles, hormonal imbalances may be a factor. Birth control pills can also be an issue. If symptoms or hormone saliva testing indicates imbalances in progesterone and estrogen levels, supplements to balance estrogen or progesterone may be helpful. See Estrogen (low) or Progesterone (low) for suggestions.

Other Tips

Migraines are often liver related and respond well to bitter herbs that help to detoxify the liver. In most migraines it seems like too much blood and energy is flowing upward into the head. Bitters draw blood and energy downward into the digestive tract and eliminative organs. So, it may also be helpful to take a *Digestive Bitter Tonic Formula* prior to meals and when one is having a migraine.

One of the most popular bitter herbs used to relieve migraines is feverfew. Studies have shown that feverfew can reduce both the symptoms and the severity of migraines in many people when taken regularly. It is important to understand that feverfew is not very effective at easing a migraine once it has started. It needs to be taken regularly to help prevent migraines. The active constituent is believed to be parthenolide, but there are other constituents that appear to be important as well.

Feverfew is a bitter and is often a key ingredient in *Migraine/Headache Formulas*. Another single herb that has proven helpful for some migraine sufferers (and may be found in some *Migraine/Headache Formulas*) is butterbur.

Because migraines are often liver related, it is sometimes helpful to use a *Hepatoprotective Formula* to support the liver. It may also be helpful to do some colon cleansing. Staying well hydrated can also reduce the frequency and severity of migraines.

Finally, if you suffer from migraines, in addition to finding and treating the root cause, try the following to boost mitochondrial function and reduce the inflammatory response:

400 mg of riboflavin (B2) twice a day

200 mg a day of Co-Q10

Butterbur 75 mg standardized extract twice a day

Finally, most migraines are vasodilative and feel like the head is pounding or exploding. In some cases, people may have migraine-like headaches that are vasoconstrictive in nature. In vasoconstrictive headaches, the head feels like it is in a vice or being squeezed. There is too little blood flow to the brain so remedies that enhance circulation to the brain and relax muscles such as periwinkle, ginkgo, lobelia or ginger may help.

Muscle tension is involved in vasoconstrictive headaches. So, also find ways to reduce your stress and relax. If you work at a computer, take a break periodically to stretch and do some self-massage on your neck and shoulders. Rub a small amount of *Topical Analgesic Formula* along with some lobelia extract or tincture into your neck and shoulders while doing the massage to ease the tension. You may find that the services of a massage therapist or chiropractor will be helpful, too. Having a massage is a great way to reduce stress and tension and can help reduce the frequency of headaches. Chiropractors often relieve headaches by adjusting the vertebrae in the upper back and neck to release pressure on nerves.

Therapies: Colon Cleanse, Eliminate Allergy-Causing Foods, Gut Healing Diet and Hydration

Formulas: Topical Analgesic, Digestive Bitter Tonic and Hepatoprotective

Key Herbs: Butterbur Root, **Feverfew**, Dong Quai, Ginger, Ginkgo, Linden, Lobelia, Periwinkle (Lesser) and Wood Betony

Key Nutrients: Co-Q10, **Vitamin B-2 (Riboflavin)**, Vitamin B-3 (Niacin), **Magnesium**, L-Arginine and SAM-e

Miscarriage (prevention)

The body has to maintain a higher level of progesterone than estrogen during pregnancy. If this balance is upset, bleeding can occur and miscarriage will eventually result. This is not the only cause of miscarriage, but one of the more common ones. Taking red raspberry during pregnancy can help to prevent miscarriages. If a woman starts spotting during pregnancy, the miscarriage can sometimes be prevented by taking 2 capsules (or about 60 drops of the tincture) of false unicorn (Helonias) every 2-4 hours along with black haw or cramp bark. Follow the therapy Avoid Xenoestrogens to reduce the chance of miscarriage. Using a *Uterine Tonic Formula* prior to pregnancy may also be helpful.

Therapies: Avoid Xenoestrogens

Formulas: Uterine Tonic and Pregnancy Tonic

Key Herbs: Capsicum (Cayenne), **Black Haw**, **Cramp Bark**, **False Unicorn (Helonias)**, Lobelia, Red Raspberry and Wild Yam

Key Nutrients: Vitamin E and **Magnesium**

Mononucleosis

See also *Epstein Barr Virus*

Mononucleosis ("mono") is an infectious viral disease that causes an increase in a specific type of white blood cell. Mono is usually linked to the Epstein-Barr virus (EBV), but can also be caused by other viruses, such as cytomegalovirus (CMV). It is passed via saliva and has been called the "kissing disease." Mono causes fever, sore throat, and swollen lymph glands—especially in the neck.

Use an *Antiviral Formula* along with a *Lymphatic Drainage Formula* to reduce swelling in the lymph glands.

Therapies: Hydration

Formulas: Antiviral and **Lymphatic Drainage**

Key Herbs: Astragalus, **Andrographis**, **Echinacea**, **Red Root**, Elder berry, Isatis, Lomatium, Red Clover and Wild Indigo (Baptista)

Key Nutrients: L-Lysine and Probiotics

Mood Swings

See also *Adrenals (exhaustion, weakness or burnout)*, *Hypoglycemia* and *Liver Detoxification*

Mood swings are abnormal and often rapid changes in one's state of mind or predominant emotions. They may be caused by hypoglycemia, liver issues or hormonal imbalances. They may also be caused by unresolved emotional wounds. Start by adopting the Low Glycemic Diet therapy to balance blood sugar levels. Licorice root can help to stabilize blood sugar levels.

Practice the techniques found in the Stress Management therapy and use an *Adaptogen Formula* to help reduce the output of stress hormones. Eleuthero root can also be helpful.

Good fats are especially important for the nervous system in helping to keep moods stable. Include good fats in the diet and consider taking some fatty acid supplements such as DHA or omega-3 essential fatty acids.

If mood swings include periods of depression, try using SAM-e to support the liver function. *Hepatoprotective Formulas* or St. John's wort may also be of benefit.

If mood swings are accompanied by severe fatigue, they could be caused by exhausted adrenal glands. An *Adrenal Tonic Formula* would be helpful in this case. *Energy-Boosting Formulas* might also be of help.

Therapies: Emotional Healing Work, Flower Essences, Healthy Fats, Low Glycemic Diet and Stress Management

Formulas: **Adaptogen**, Hepatoprotective, Relaxing Nervine, Energy-Boosting and **Adrenal Tonic**

Key Herbs: **Mimosa (Albizia, Silk Tree)**, **Scullcap (Skullcap)**, Eleuthero (Siberian ginseng), Licorice and St. John's wort

Key Nutrients: SAM-e, DHA and Omega-3 Essential Fatty Acids

Morning Sickness

See also *Pregnancy (herbs and supplements for)*

Morning sickness is mild to severe nausea, often accompanied by vomiting, that occurs in pregnancy, usually only in the early stages, but in some cases throughout pregnancy. Although common upon rising in the morning, hence the name, it can occur during any part of the day or night.

Some of the simplest remedies to try include ginger, peppermint or red raspberry, taken as a tea. Alfalfa and peppermint tea may also be helpful. Another option is a tea of peach leaf. A *Carminative Formula* that contains any of these herbs could also be helpful.

Many women also find morning sickness is reduced by taking B-complex vitamins.

Morning sickness is often related to liver function. A small dose of a *Blood Purifier* or *Liver Tonic Formula* may help.

Formulas: Carminative, Blood Purifier and Liver Tonic

Key Herbs: Alfalfa, **Peppermint**, **Red Raspberry** and Ginger

Key Nutrients: Vitamin B-6 (Pyridoxine) and Vitamin B-Complex

Motion Sickness

See also *Nausea and Vomiting* and *Vertigo*

Nausea usually caused by traveling in a vehicle such as a car, ship or plane is called motion sickness. Studies have suggested that ginger can be very effective in preventing motion sickness when taken prior to travel. A drop of peppermint oil on the back of the tongue may also be helpful.

Key Herbs: Ginger and Peppermint

Key Nutrients: L-Glutamine and Vitamin B-6 (Pyridoxine)

Mouth Ulcers or Sores

See *Canker Sores (Mouth Ulcers, Stomatitis)*

Mucus

See *Congestion (general)*

Multiple Personal Disorder

See *Mental Illness*

Multiple Sclerosis (MS)

See also *Autoimmune Disorders*

Multiple Sclerosis is an autoimmune disease that attacks the insulating coverings (myelin sheath) of the nerves and brain cells. Symptoms often include weakness, fatigue, debility and numbness and occur in varied regions of the body depending on the nerves affected. This is not an easy condition to treat and there are not quick fixes, so professional assistance should be sought. There are, however, some basic natural remedies to consider.

Fats are very important for the myelin sheath. So, make sure to include plenty of healthy fats in the diet. It may be helpful to supplement with omega-3 essential fatty acids or DHA and fat soluble vitamins (which help protect fatty tissues) such as Vitamins A, D and E.

Another important component of the myelin sheath is silica. Horsetail is rich in this nutrient and herbal *Mineral Formulas* high in horsetail should also be considered.

Antioxidant nutrients in general can help to protect the myelin sheath from damage. Rosemary is a good antioxidant herb that helps protect the nerves, so look for an *Antioxidant Formula* high in rosemary.

One possible cause of MS is mercury poisoning. Some MS patients have improved after having all metal fillings removed from their mouth, followed by a mercury detoxification program. N-acetyl cysteine, cilantro and *Heavy Metal Cleansing Formulas* may all be helpful.

General therapy for autoimmune disorders can be helpful. This includes using digestive enzyme supplements, supporting the adrenal function and reducing stress.

Therapies: Affirmation and Visualization, Dietary Fiber, Fresh Fruits and Vegetables, Gut Healing Diet, Healthy Fats, Heavy Metal Cleanse and Mineralization

Formulas: Antioxidant, Mineral, **Heavy Metal Cleansing**, Mushroom Blend and Immune Balancing

Key Herbs: Astragalus, Cilantro/Coriander leaf, Codonopsis, **Ashwaganda**, **Rosemary**, Ginkgo, Horsetail and Reishi (Ganoderma)

Key Nutrients: N-Acetyl Cysteine, **Vitamin D**, Omega-3 Essential Fatty Acids, DHA, Colloidal Minerals, Vitamin A, Vitamin E, Digestive Enzymes, **Vitamin B-Complex**, **Vitamin B-12** and Vitamin B-1 (Thiamine)

Mumps

See also *Contagious Diseases*

Mumps is an acute contagious viral disease marked by fever and the swelling of lymph nodes, causing a swollen, puffy, full appearance to the cheeks. Herbs that enhance lymphatic drainage such as burdock, lobelia, mullein and red root can be helpful for the mumps. Consider using a *Lymphatic Drainage Formula* containing these herbs. Infection-fighting herbs like echinacea, garlic and yarrow can also be helpful. Drink plenty of water and use the Sweat Bath therapy to help flush out the system.

Therapies: Hydration and Sweat Bath

Formulas: Lymphatic Drainage

Key Herbs: Burdock, Catnip, Clove, **Echinacea**, **Red Root**, Garlic, Isatis, Lobelia, Mullein, Peppermint and Yarrow

Key Nutrients: Vitamin A and **Vitamin D**

Muscle Spasms or Cramps

See *Cramps and Spasms (general)*

Key Nutrients: Zinc

Muscle Twitch

See *Twitching*

Myasthenia Gravis

See also *Autoimmune Disorders*

Myasthenia gravis is a disease of progressive weakness and exhaustion of the voluntary muscles of the body without any wasting. It is caused by a defect at nerve and muscle junctions, and is considered an autoimmune disease. Improve general health habits, such as increasing antioxidants, using good fats and supplementing with minerals and digestive enzymes. You can also follow the general guidelines for Autoimmune Disorders. Seek professional assistance.

Therapies: Fresh Fruits and Vegetables, Healthy Fats, Heavy Metal Cleanse and Mineralization

Formulas: Digestive Enzyme and Antioxidant

Key Herbs: Blue Vervain, **Scullcap (Skullcap)**, Licorice, St. John's wort and Yucca

Key Nutrients: Magnesium, Colloidal Minerals, **Digestive Enzymes**, **Omega-3 Essential Fatty Acids**, Vitamin B-Complex, Vitamin C, Vitamin E, Vitamin B-2 (Riboflavin) and Vitamin B-1 (Thiamine)

Narcolepsy

See also *Adrenals (exhaustion, weakness or burnout)*, *Fatigue* and *Hypoglycemia*

Narcolepsy is a sleeping disorder that causes an overwhelming need to sleep during the day. This can happen very suddenly and attempts to stay awake will fail. It is caused by damage to the nerves that control sleep and wakefulness. Strengthening the nerves using *Nerve Tonic Formulas* may help. Also consider the possibility of Adrenal Exhaustion and use remedies like *Adrenal Tonic* or *Adaptogen Formulas* to increase stamina and energy. Eliminating food allergens has helped in some cases. Very low blood sugar has also been known to cause people to pass out, so make sure the blood sugar stays balanced with the Low Glycemic Diet therapy and use B-complex vitamins, chromium and magnesium to aid cellular energy production.

Since there is no simple answer to this problem, professional help should be sought.

Therapies: Eliminate Allergy-Causing Foods and Low Glycemic Diet

Formulas: Adrenal Tonic, Adrenal Tonic and Adaptogen

Key Herbs: Ashwaganda, **Oat seed (milky)**, **Prickly Ash**, Damiana, Sage and St. John's wort

Key Nutrients: Chromium, L-Glutamine, Calcium, Omega-3 Essential Fatty Acids, Magnesium, Co-Q10, **Vitamin B-Complex** and Vitamin E

Nausea and Vomiting

See also *Morning Sickness*

Nausea is a queasiness in the stomach that makes one resist food and have the urge to vomit. Vomiting is disgorging the contents of the stomach through the mouth. Carminative herbs like anise, cinnamon, clove, ginger, lavender, lemon balm and peppermint have all been used to settle the stomach and ease nausea and vomiting. They are best taken as warm teas and sipped slowly. There are many *Carminative Formulas* available in tea form that could be used for this purpose.

Essential oils can also be used. Simply add a drop of an essential oil like peppermint or clove to a glass of hot water sip it slowly.

Therapies: Aromatherapy

Formulas: Carminative

Key Herbs: Aloe vera, Anise, Cinnamon, Clove, **Ginger**, **Peppermint**, Lavender, Lemon Balm and Red Raspberry

Key Nutrients: Vitamin B-Complex and Vitamin B-6 (Pyridoxine)

Nephritis

See also *Inflammation*

Nephritis is inflammation of the kidney. Juniper berry and other kidney stimulants should be avoided. *Diuretic* and *Urinary Infection Fighting Formulas* that are based primarily on herbs like cornsilk, marshmallow, dandelion leaf, goldenrod, horsetail and cleavers should be used. These herbs have a more soothing and cooling action on the kidneys. Hydration therapy is essential to working with any kidney disorder.

Therapies: Fresh Fruits and Vegetables, Healthy Fats and Hydration

Formulas: Diuretic and Urinary Infection Fighting

Key Herbs: Astragalus, **Cleavers (Bedstraw)**, **Cordyceps**, **Cornsilk**, Dandelion, Echinacea, Goldenseal, Horsetail and Marshmallow

Key Nutrients: Omega-3 Essential Fatty Acids and Magnesium

Nerve Damage

When nerves have been damaged, there are a number of nutrients that can maximize their ability to repair. Those include good fats (DHA, omega-3 EFA), magnesium, potassium, silicon and B-complex. St. John's wort is particularly helpful for stimulating nerve repair. It can be used internally, topically or as a homeopathic. In homeopathic form, it has been called the "arnica of the nervous system," because of its ability to stimulate nerve healing after injuries.

Horsetail, prickly ash and wood betony are other herbal remedies to consider where there is nerve damage. A *Nerve Tonic Formula* may be helpful, too.

Therapies: Epsom Salt Bath and Healthy Fats

Key Herbs: St. John's wort, Horsetail, Prickly Ash, Scullcap (Skullcap) and Wood Betony

Key Nutrients: Omega-3 Essential Fatty Acids, DHA, Magnesium, Potassium, Silicon and **Vitamin B-Complex**

Nervous Disorders

See *Nervousness*, *Restlessness* and *Anxiety Disorders*

Nervous Exhaustion (Enervation)

See also *Adrenals (exhaustion, weakness or burnout)*

Closely related to adrenal exhaustion, enervation occurs after long periods of stress where the nervous system becomes depleted. The person feels shaky, tired and "on edge." They have a hard time holding their hands steady.

It is usually important to support the adrenal glands when treating nervous exhaustion. This is done using *Adaptogen Formulas* and other therapies discussed under Adrenals (exhaustion, weakness or burnout).

To support the nerves B-complex vitamins are usually necessary along with a good *Nerve Tonic Formula*. Milky oat seed, blue vervain, scullcap, damiana and sage are all good single herbs to consider. Potassium and magnesium may also be helpful.

The Epsom Salt Bath Therapy with essential oils like lavender or rose can also do wonders for helping relaxed nerves that feel "frayed." So can staying well hydrated and using healthy fats.

In the long run, following the techniques listed in the Stress Management therapy, getting a good night's sleep and practicing Deep Breathing therapy will all help. Emotional Healing Work may be needed in some cases. Flower Essences therapy using olive, oak and elm can be helpful, too.

Therapies: Affirmation and Visualization, Aromatherapy, Avoid Caffeine, Deep Breathing, Emotional Healing Work, Epsom Salt Bath, Healthy Fats, Hydration and Stress Management

Formulas: Adaptogen

Key Herbs: Ashwaganda, Blue Vervain, **Cordyceps**, **Damiana**, **Oat seed (milky)**, **Olive flower essence**, **Scullcap (Skullcap)**, Kava-kava, Lavender, Muira Puama, Reishi (Ganoderma), Rose essential oil, Rosemary flower essence, Sage, Schisandra (Schizandra), Shatavari and White Oak flower essence

Key Nutrients: Pantothenic Acid (Vitamin B5), Omega-3 Essential Fatty Acids, **Vitamin B-Complex**, **Magnesium** and Potassium

Nervousness, Restlessness

See also *Stress* and *Anxiety Disorders*

When a person feels on edge all the time and suffers from an excessive sense of nervousness and restlessness, they are in a hypervigilant mode. This means that the hormones and neurotransmitters that trigger their fight or flight response are over stimulated and they are having a hard time returning to a state of relaxation. On a physical level, they need to calm down their sympathetic nervous system and activate their parasympathetic nervous system. They also need to calm down the release of stress hormones from the adrenal glands. On an emotional level, they often need to heal from previous traumas and stressful experiences using Emotional Healing Work.

To calm down the sympathetic nervous system, use nervines such as California poppy, chamomile, kava kava and lavender. These are common ingredients in *Relaxing Nervine Formulas*.

If one's hands are shaky, one may also need some milky oat seed or a *Nerve Tonic Formula*. Using the Epsom Salt Bath therapy and/or supplementing with magnesium will also be helpful.

.To calm down the adrenal glands, one can use adaptogens like eleuthero, ashwaganda and schisandra berries. These are key ingredients in a good *Adaptogen Formula*, which can be very helpful for reducing nervousness.

It is also important to avoid stimulants like caffeine and to stay well hydrated. Good fats and B-complex vitamins are also helpful in calming down the nerves.

Therapies: Aromatherapy, Avoid Caffeine, Deep Breathing, Emotional Healing Work, Epsom Salt Bath, Flower Essences, Healthy Fats, Hydration and Stress Management

Formulas: Relaxing Nervine and **Adaptogen**

Key Herbs: California Poppy, Chamomile (English and Roman), **Ashwaganda**, **Eleuthero (Siberian ginseng)**, **Motherwort**, **Oat seed (milky)**, Kava-kava, Lavender, Schisandra (Schizandra) and Skunk Cabbage

Key Nutrients: Omega-3 Essential Fatty Acids, **Vitamin B-Complex**, Vitamin B-12, Vitamin D and **Magnesium**

Neuralgia and Neuritis

See also *Diabetes*

Neuralgia is a pain that radiates along the course of one or more nerves. In neuralgia, irritated nerves cause severe pain in the body. Neuritis is inflammation of the nerves, similar to neuralgia, except there may not be any pain. There may also be degeneration of the nerves.

There are many reasons why nerves can become irritated or inflamed, so it is important to search for and deal with the cause. Pressure on the nerve from mechanical misalignment of body structures may be a factor, so some type of bodywork (massage, Chiropractic, etc.) may be helpful.

Diabetes is often involved in nerve inflammation and should be brought under control. Infection, a lack of good fats in the diet, heavy metals and environmental toxins, and unresolved emotional issues are additional factors to consider.

Start by feeding the nerves with good fats and B-complex vitamins. Try using nervines like blue vervain, St. John's wort or wood betony. Look for an herbal *Analgesic* or a *Relaxing Nervine Formula* containing these ingredients.

If the person has been exposed to a lot of chemicals or metals, some cleansing therapies may be helpful. Try using a *General Detoxifying* or a *Heavy Metal Cleansing Formula* along with a fiber supplement to eliminate toxins that may be irritating the nerves.

Herbs that may help reduce inflammation in the nerves include yucca, wild yam and Devil's claw. These can be helpful in neuritis. Nerves can become inflamed from deficiencies of vitamins B12, B1 (thiamine) and B3. High doses of coenzymated B vitamins are essential to heal damaged or inflamed nerves.

Therapies: Colon Cleanse, Emotional Healing Work, Fresh Fruits and Vegetables, Healthy Fats and Heavy Metal Cleanse

Formulas: Analgesic, Relaxing Nervine, General Detoxifying and Heavy Metal Cleansing

Key Herbs: Black Cohosh, **Blue Vervain**, **St. John's wort**, Devil's Claw, Jamaican Dogwood, Lavender, Linden, Passionflower, Stillingia, Wood Betony and Yucca

Key Nutrients: Vitamin B-12, Pantothenic Acid (Vitamin B5), **Omega-3 Essential Fatty Acids**, DHA, **Vitamin B-Complex** and Fiber

Neurosis

See also *Mental Illness* and *Abuse and Trauma*

Neurosis is a mental and emotional disorder that affects only part of the personality. It usually involves a less distorted image of reality than a psychosis and does not result in a disturbance of language. It is accompanied by various physical, physiological and mental disturbances such as anxieties and phobias.

On a physical level, nutrients that support the nerves such as B-complex vitamins, calcium and magnesium may be helpful. Nervines like kava kava, St. John's wort, valerian and passion flower may also be beneficial. Consider using a *Relaxing Nervine Formula*.

Heavy metals like mercury and lead can damage the nerves and create neurological symptoms. If heavy metals are involved, do some Heavy Metal Detoxification.

For many people, neurological problems like neurosis are the result of abuse and trauma and require counseling or Emotional Healing Work.

Therapies: Emotional Healing Work, Flower Essences, Heavy Metal Cleanse and Low Glycemic Diet

Formulas: Relaxing Nervine

Key Herbs: Ginseng (American), Ginseng (Asian, Korean), Kava-kava, Passionflower, St. John's wort and Valerian

Key Nutrients: Calcium, **Magnesium** and **Vitamin B-Complex**

Night Blindness (Night Vision)

Night blindness is a difficulty in seeing at night. Bilberry and vitamin A may be helpful for improving night vision. Also consider using a *Vision Supporting Formula*.

Formulas: Vision Supporting

Key Herbs: Bilberry (Blueberry, Huckleberry)

Key Nutrients: Vitamin A and Proanthocyanidins

Night Sweating

See also *Perspiration (excessive)*

When there is profuse perspiration during sleep, the problem is often due to an imbalance in the hypothalamus or adrenals. Remedies that have been helpful for reducing night sweats include sage (drunk as a cold tea), astragalus and schisandra.

Key Herbs: Astragalus, **Sage** and **Schisandra (Schizandra)**

Nightmares

See also *Restless Dreams*

Nightmares are often a sign of a toxic liver, blood sugar problems or adrenal fatigue. Use the Low Glycemic Diet therapy and have a protein snack (nut butter, cheese, etc.) at bedtime. Take an *Adaptogen Formula* if stressed, or an *Adrenal Tonic Formula* if suffering from fatigue. Try cleansing and supporting the liver using a *General Detoxifying* or a *Liver Tonic Formula*. Chaparral or St. John's wort flower essences may be helpful for nightmares, especially in children.

Therapies: Flower Essences, Healthy Fats and Low Glycemic Diet

Formulas: Liver Tonic, General Detoxifying, Adaptogen and Adrenal Tonic

Key Herbs: Chaparral flower essence, **St. John's wort flower essence**, **St. John's wort herb** and Milk Thistle

Key Nutrients: Omega-3 Essential Fatty Acids

Nocturnal Emission (Wet Dreams)

Nocturnal emissions, also known as wet dreams, are the involuntary release of semen by the male during sleep. This is often accompanied by erotic dreams. There is nothing harmful about this unless it occurs excessively. Chaste tree, false unicorn, tribulus and wild yam have all been used to help reduce nocturnal emissions. Look for a *Male Glandular Tonic Formula* with these herbs as key ingredients.

Formulas: Male Glandular Tonic

Key Herbs: Chastetree (Vitex), False Unicorn (Helonias), Tribulus and Wild Yam

Nose Bleeds

The following may help stop or reduce nose bleeds. Yarrow and bayberry may be snuffed directly into the sinuses to arrest bleeding. Bayberry, capsicum, yarrow and shepherd's purse can all be taken internally to help stop nose bleeds. Horsetail, vitamin C, bioflavonoids and rose hips may help strengthen capillaries to prevent nose bleeds. Hydration therapy is important in preventing nose bleeds.

Therapies: Hydration

Key Herbs: Bayberry, Capsicum (Cayenne), Coptis (Chinese Goldenthread), **Yarrow**, Horsetail, Rose, Shepherd's Purse and Wood Betony

Key Nutrients: Vitamin C and Bioflavonoids

Numbness

See also *Nerve Damage*

Sensations of numbness and tingling in the extremities are often helped by enhancing circulation to the extremities with remedies like capsicum, ginkgo, hawthorn and prickly ash. A *Cardiovascular Stimulant* may also be used. Numbness and tingling in the extremities are also signs of B12, folate and B1 deficiency.

Numbness and tingling may also involve irritation or pressure on nerves which may be corrected by chiropractic care or bodywork. St. John's wort stimulates nerve regeneration and repair where the problem is caused by bruised or damaged nerves. It can be taken internally or used topically as an oil. When the numbness is due to an injury, a topical application of arnica and St. John's wort in oil form can be helpful in reducing swelling and promoting healing and sensation.

Formulas: Cardiovascular Stimulant

Key Herbs: Arnica, Capsicum (Cayenne), **St. John's wort**, Ginkgo, Hawthorn and Prickly Ash

Key Nutrients: Vitamin B-12, Vitamin B-1 (Thiamine), **Folate (Folic Acid, Vitamin B9)** and Vitamin B-Complex

Nursing

Nursing is one of the best ways to build a healthy immune system in an infant. Ideally, mothers should nurse their children for one year and longer, if possible. Breast milk not only contains the right ratios of nutrients needed for healthy children, it also passes immune factors from mother to child and enhances mother-infant bonding.

Women who are pregnant or nursing need extra nutrition to provide for their own needs and the needs of their offspring. Just as in pregnancy, a good multivitamin or whole food supplement, along with a good diet are very important while nursing.

Nursing also helps to develop a healthy gut flora in an infant, which contributes to lifelong immunity in the child. However, mom has to have the friendly bacteria in her own body before she can pass them on to her offspring, so probiotic supplements or eating cultured foods may also be helpful while nursing, particularly if mom has a history of bowel disorders or yeast infections.

Nursing mothers also need extra water and should pay attention to their stress levels. Staying calm and relaxed while nursing aids baby's digestion and helps the child develop a sense of well-being.

There are a number of herbs that can increase the flow of and/or enrich breast milk. These include blessed thistle, marshmallow, nettles and milk thistle. There are *Nursing Aid Formulas* that contain these herbs to enhance breast milk. herbal *Mineral Formulas* can also help to enrich breast milk and develop healthy bones, teeth and nerves in developing infants.

When it comes time to stop nursing, parsley and sage can be used to help dry up breast milk.

Therapies: Healthy Fats, Hydration and Stress Management

Formulas: Nursing Aid and Mineral

Key Herbs: Alfalfa, Anise, **Blessed Thistle**, **Fenugreek**, **Marshmallow**, **Milk Thistle**, Nettle (Stinging) and Shatavari

Key Nutrients: Probiotics

Obesity

See *Weight Loss (aids for)*

Obsessive Compulsive Disorder

See also *Mental Illness, Anxiety Disorders* and *Abuse and Trauma*

Obsessive-compulsive disorder (OCD) is one of a number of Anxiety Disorders. It is characterized by involuntary thoughts that cause the sufferer to develop a dread that something bad will happen. This makes them feel compelled to perform involuntary, irrational and time-consuming behaviors. Symptoms range from repetitive hand-washing to preoccupation with sexual, religious, or aggressive impulses.

This condition requires counseling and/or Emotional Healing Work. It is often rooted in unhealed abuse and trauma. Healing can be aided, however, by using the general principles for working with anxiety disorders. Here are a few basic pointers:

Adaptogen Formulas can calm down the production of stress hormones, which can be helpful in reducing underlying feelings of anxiety. If the person is chronically tired or has been diagnosed with post traumatic stress disorder an *Adrenal Tonic Formula* will be helpful.

General remedies to support the nerves, including good fats, like omega-3 EFA, B-complex vitamins and magnesium, will also be helpful. Kava kava will help the person to relax and can also be helpful in reducing anxiety. Zinc and vitamin B-6 are often helpful for balancing brain chemistry.

For more information, see Anxiety Disorders and Abuse and Trauma.

Therapies: Affirmation and Visualization, Emotional Healing Work, Flower Essences, Healthy Fats and Low Glycemic Diet

Formulas: Adaptogen and **Adrenal Tonic**

Key Herbs: Bacopa (Water Hyssop), Blue Vervain flower essence, Blue Vervain herb, **Ashwaganda, Eleuthero (Siberian ginseng), Schisandra (Schizandra)** and Kava-kava

Key Nutrients: Omega-3 Essential Fatty Acids, Vitamin B-Complex, **Magnesium, Vitamin B-6 (Pyridoxine)** and **Zinc**

Oral Surgery

See also *Surgery (healing from)*

Goldenseal, myrrh, oak and plantain may help the mouth to heal after oral surgery. These can be used as mouth rinses or applied topically to damaged areas. An herbal *Analgesic Formula* can be used to reduce pain and swelling.

Formulas: Analgesic

Key Herbs: Goldenseal, **Plantain**, Myrrh and White Oak

Key Nutrients: Colloidal Minerals

Osteoarthritis

See *Arthritis*

Osteoporosis

See also *Menopause*

Osteoporosis is a decrease in bone density that causes skeletal weakness. Prior to the 1970s, osteoporosis was considered rare and was only diagnosed in the elderly after a fracture. Today, this problem has become epidemic in both the United States and many European countries.

Studies by the National Osteoporosis Foundation show that one in two females and one in four males over 50 years old will have an osteoporosis-related fracture. This means that 50% of older women and 25% of older men are at risk for fractures due to weakened bones. Recent estimates suggest that at least ten million people in the U.S. have osteoporosis.

The numbers show no signs of improving despite the millions of dollars spent on pharmaceutical research, as well as increased bone mineral density screening. Christine Northrup, M.D, a specialist in women's health, states that bone density scans do not measure bone strength or quality. In fact, 50% of people with thin osteoporotic bones never fracture. Also, older folks in France, Germany, China and Japan have lower bone density than Americans, yet suffer fewer osteoporosis-related fractures.

Osteoporosis didn't exist in native cultures and according to Dr. Susan E. Brown, director of the Osteoporosis Education Project, hip-fracture rates vary worldwide by as much as 40-fold. The greatest problems exist in the U.S. and Europe. Osteoporosis is not a major problem in underdeveloped countries and Asia. (Interestingly, the Chinese have a very low incidence of osteoporosis and they don't consume dairy products, take calcium supplements or use hormone replacement therapy.) Like so many health prob-

lems we experience in modern civilization, bone weakness is a result of our modern lifestyle and is not going to be solved by magic "pills" or quick fixes.

Bones are neither solid nor static; they are living tissue that is continually being renewed. A normally functioning body builds and maintains lifelong healthy bones that are strong and resistant, yet flexible enough to tolerate twisting and bending without breaking. Bone building consists of an array of complex biochemical reactions that maintain a balance between breaking down old and injured bone and building new strong but flexible bone. Old bone is constantly being dissolved and reabsorbed, and new bone is constantly being laid down in its place. Because of this, bones, like every other tissue in the body, need a constant supply of nutrients to keep them healthy. Bones weaken when the breaking down process occurs more rapidly than the building up process.

The common belief is that we aren't getting enough calcium in our diets. However, if that were actually the case, then all the dairy products, calcium-fortified foods, calcium-based antacids and calcium supplements we consume would be fixing the problem. The fact is, that this increased calcium intake doesn't make the problem better. It is true that calcium is both the most abundant mineral in the body and the most abundant mineral in bones, but bones are made of much more than calcium. Bones contain other macro minerals such as magnesium, phosphorus, sodium, chloride, potassium and sulfur. They also need trace minerals such as silica, iron, molybdenum, copper, zinc, fluoride, selenium, chromium, manganese, iodine, and cobalt. In addition, vitamins like C and D, protein and other nutrients are also required for bone health.

This explains why calcium supplements alone will not build strong bones, especially since few Americans are, in fact, deficient in calcium. What they are actually deficient in are the other trace nutrients that are needed to make proper use of the calcium already in their diets. So, the biggest problem contributing to osteoporosis is a lack of nutritional density in our diets.

This problem starts with modern agricultural methods. Plants absorb minerals via bacteria and other microbes which are present in "living" soil that is rich in natural organic material. Modern agricultural practices not only fail to replenish trace minerals in the soil, they also kills the microbes through the use of agricultural chemicals. This has caused dramatic drops in the mineral levels of modern foods. This loss of minerals (and general nutrient value) is further compounded by processing methods, which further depletes nutrients from foods.

A lack of trace minerals and nutritional density is the primary reason our bones are weaker, but there is another contributing factor. Remember that building up bone (which requires all these nutrients) is balancing a constant break down of bone from wear and tear.

When astronauts spend long periods in outer space, they suffer a loss of bone mass. This is because their bodies are not having to work against gravity. Bone is built in response to the body's need for structural support. This is why weight-bearing exercise helps keep bones healthy.

There are also a number of hormones involved with the breakdown and rebuilding of bone. So, health of the glandular system is important to bone health. However, it's not as simple as just using estrogen or progesterone supplements, because many other glands are involved in bone health.

Parathyroid hormone stimulates the kidneys to convert vitamin D to its active form. It also acts to dissolve calcium and other alkaline minerals out of the bone into the blood stream to neutralize excess acid in the body. Glucocortical adrenal hormones and the sex hormones estrogen and androgen play a role in remodeling bone as well as calcitonin and thyrosin from the thyroid, insulin from the pancreas, and growth hormone from the pituitary.

The bottom line is that bone health is connected to overall health. So, you can't have healthy bones without working on your health in general.

Your bones support you, but as you can see, you also need to support your bones with good nutrition. Fortunately, there are numerous herbs and nutritional supplements that can help support the health of bones and joints. Calcium, of course, is an essential element for the health of bones, but it needs to be combined with other nutrients in order to be effective.

Calcium requires vitamin D for proper absorption and utilization. In concert with the parathyroid hormone, vitamin D is essential for absorbing calcium in the small intestines and for maintaining adequate serum calcium and phosphate concentration that enable normal mineralization of bones. The best form of vitamin D is vitamin D3 (cholecalciferol). This fat-soluble vitamin is produced in the skin when it is exposed to sunlight, specifically ultraviolet B radiation. Many studies have shown that vitamin D3 supports bone health, organ health and even helps fight cancer. Vitamin K-2 works with D3 to get calcium into the bones.

Phosphorus is the second most abundant mineral in the body and is necessary for strong bones and teeth, which are composed primarily of calcium phosphate. Diets high in fructose (including high fructose corn syrup) increase urinary loss of phosphorus.

Magnesium is another mineral that works in concert with calcium and is involved in the structure of bones, cell membranes and chromosomes. Sixty percent of magnesium is found in the skeleton, and 27% is found in muscle. The ratio of calcium to magnesium for humans should be 2:1, and it has been established that more people are deficient in magnesium than calcium.

The third most abundant mineral in the body is potassium. Potassium also plays a role in bone density. It helps prevent osteoporosis by counteracting increased urinary calcium loss due to high dietary salt intake. Potassium is abundant in green leafy vegetables.

Trace minerals, such as boron, vanadium, zinc and copper are all important for bone health. Bone Broth therapy is one of the best ways to get all of these minerals (and other key nutrients for healthy bones). Colloidal mineral supplements or, better yet, herbal *Mineral Formulas* can also be helpful.

In women, remedies that help to balance hormones, like those found in *Menopause Balancing* or *Female Hormonal Balancing Formulas*, can also be helpful. See Menopause for more information.

Therapies: Bone Broth, Healthy Fats and Mineralization

Formulas: Mineral, Female Hormonal Balancing and Menopause Balancing

Key Herbs: Alfalfa, Ashwaganda, Horsetail, Nettle (Stinging) and Oat straw

Key Nutrients: Calcium, Copper, DHEA, Zinc, **Vitamin K**, **Vitamin D**, Vitamin B-3 (Niacin), Silicon, Magnesium, Omega-3 Essential Fatty Acids, Colloidal Minerals, **Betaine Hydrochloric Acid (HCl)** and Bromelain

Ovarian Cysts

See *Cysts*

Ovarian Pain

See also *Cysts, Endometriosis* and *Pain (general remedies for)*

Ovarian pain should be checked out by a doctor to determine the cause. It could be due to cysts, endometriosis, or other causes. Helpful herbs include chastetree, false unicorn and black cohosh. You could try a *Female Hormonal Balancing Formula* with these herbs as key ingredients.

Formulas: Female Hormonal Balancing

Key Herbs: Chastetree (Vitex), **Black Cohosh** and False Unicorn (Helonias)

Key Nutrients: Magnesium

Pain (general remedies for)

See also *Arthritis*, *Migraine* and *Headache (general)*

Pain is the primary and nearly universal symptom of all our human afflictions, whether it be physical or emotional. Pain is why we seek help when we are sick. If illness didn't cause "dis-ease" ("lack of ease" or pain), we would not be motivated to avoid doing things that damage the body.

So, no matter how much we dislike it and want to make it go away, pain is not an enemy. Pain is a form of communication. It is how the body tells us it is having a problem. It is the "911 system" that the cells of our body use to call for help. Pain is also the teacher that motivates us, if we let it, to take care of our bodies and pursue a healthy lifestyle.

Modern pain-relieving drugs are wonderful things. They enable us to undergo necessary surgery or dental work without pain. They can also be of great relief to the person who is suffering because of a serious accident or illness.

Unfortunately, pain-relieving medications allow people to disconnect from taking responsibility for their health. Instead of asking "why" they are getting headaches, upset stomachs, muscle aches or other pain, they simply pop a painkiller. Thus, they never make the connection that their pain is originating from their diet, lifestyle and stress, and they usually don't make the changes they need to make to be healthy.

We need to stop seeing pain as an "enemy" that needs to be killed. We need to see pain as a teacher giving us a "wake-up call" and reminding us that we need to take better care of our bodies.

Let's take headaches for example. Headaches have causes. The cause may be as simple as dehydration. Drinking more water has greatly reduced the number of headaches some people have. A headache can also be a sign of poor bowel elimination or of excess stress and tension.

Taking pain killers may relieve today's headache, but it won't stop us from having another one tomorrow. When we start "listening" to the headache's message, we can actually learn to stop having headaches altogether. Headaches are a normal part of most people's lives only because the average person has bad health habits.

When we just keep taking painkillers without changing bad health habits, we keep doing small things that damage our health. After twenty years of failing to heed these little warnings that something is wrong, we get a bigger "wake up call" in the form of a heart attack, cancer, diabetes or some other serious illness. Then we wonder, "How could this happen to me?"

Besides, painkillers themselves are toxic drugs. Sure, they're okay for occasional relief of pain, but when used frequently, they can damage the liver, kidneys, nerves and other organs. They can even increase the risk of heart disease and other serious health problems.

Since pain has a cause, we need to try to identify the source of our pain. When we suffer an acute injury such as a burn, cut or bruise, it's usually pretty easy to see what caused it. When we experience more long-lasting, chronic pain, it's often more difficult to see what is causing the damage. In fact, you may have to search and experiment a little to discover what is causing your pain, but the reward will be worth it. Here are some places to start.

At a cellular level, one cause of pain is lack of oxygenation to the tissues. The sharp pain of acute injuries is caused by the inflammatory process that both deprives cells of oxygen and activates pain receptors. When cells are chronically deprived of oxygen, you'll get chronic dull pain. Many people have experienced a great deal of relief from chronic pain just by practicing Deep Breathing therapy. So, if you are in chronic pain, start practicing deep abdominal breathing for 5-10 minutes twice daily. The results may amaze you.

Accumulation of toxins in the tissues is another underlying cause of pain. Dehydration inhibits oxygen transport and allows toxins to accumulate. Another simple but highly effective strategy for reducing chronic pain is to increase your water intake. This simple practice can greatly reduce the frequency of headaches, constipation, indigestion and muscle aches.

When tissues become congested due to poor lymphatic drainage, cells experience accumulation of toxic acid waste and low oxygenation. Ear aches, sore throats, menstrual pain and headaches can all occur because of swelling in the lymph nodes and congestion of the lymphatic system. Drinking lots of water and taking a *Lymphatic Drainage Formula* will help when pain is associated with congestion.

Massage can also relieve stagnant lymph, especially if you use a *Topical Analgesic Formula* when you do the massage. Lobelia and capsicum extracts mixed in equal parts can also be massaged into painful areas of the body. The secret is to massage the painful areas 6-8 times per day or more to keep the lymph flowing.

Moderate physical activity such as walking or swimming helps increase lymphatic drainage. Gentle bouncing on a mini-trampoline while doing Deep Breathing therapy is an excellent way to move lymph and has proven very effective in reducing many kinds of chronic pain.

Cells produce waste in the process of metabolism. If this waste isn't flushed properly from the system it can contribute to chronic pain. Drinking more water helps to flush this acid waste. Many people have also found that a short fast using lemon water or fresh vegetable juices is also helpful.

Muscle tension is a frequent cause of pain. This may be due to stress, but it can also be due to repetitive movements or bad posture that stress the structural alignment of the body. For example, sitting at a computer and typing all day can cause chronic tension in the neck, shoulders and upper back. This can lead to sore throats, headaches and back pain.

Periodic stretching and better posture will often correct this type of pain. Chiropractic adjustments, massage therapy or other forms of body work can help a person have better structural alignment, thereby easing pain.

Antispasmodic Formulas can help ease tension, especially when taken with plenty of water. Lobelia and kava kava are two great herbs for easing muscle tension to relieve pain. Muscle tension can also be eased by taking a magnesium supplement.

All of these causes of pain are linked with chronic inflammation. Antioxidants and anti-inflammatories will help to reduce this inflammation and relieve chronic pain. An *Anti-Inflammatory Formula* will often be very helpful for easing chronic pain. Eating fresh fruits and vegetables (which are loaded with antioxidants) will greatly reduce chronic inflammation.

Besides these changes in diet, consider taking an antioxidant supplement.

Omega-3 essential fatty acids have also proven helpful in easing chronic inflammation and pain. They help with the production of anti-inflammatory and pain-relieving prostaglandins in the tissues. It also helps to avoid bad fats (margarine, shortening and processed vegetable oils) and refined carbohydrates.

Of course, one can always take an herbal *Analgesic Formula* for relief of minor pain. Most of these formulas are based on herbs like willow bark, which contain salycilates (compounds similar to aspirin). For headaches, a *Migraine/Headache Formula* may be in order. These formulas are usually milder acting than their drug counterparts, but are also safer. When used in combination with some of the aforementioned pain relief techniques, however, they can be very effective. You can also look up some of the specific herbs mentioned for pain and see if they work on your particular type of pain.

Therapies: Aromatherapy, Colon Cleanse, Colon Hydrotherapy, Deep Breathing, Drawing Bath, Fast or Juice Fast, Healthy Fats, Hydration and Poultice

Formulas: Lymphatic Drainage, **Topical Analgesic**, Antispasmodic, Anti-Inflammatory and **Analgesic**

Key Herbs: Arnica, Boswellia, California Poppy, Camphor, Capsicum (Cayenne), **Corydalis**, **Jamaican Dogwood**, **Willow**, Hops, Indian Pipe, Kava-kava, Lobelia, Prickly Ash, Safflowers, St. John's wort, Stillingia, Turmeric and Valerian

Key Nutrients: Omega-3 Essential Fatty Acids, Magnesium and Digestive Enzymes

Pancreatitis

See also *Inflammation*

Pancreatitis is an inflammation of the pancreas. This can be a serious, life-threatening condition requiring medical attention. Seek professional assistance. An Anti-inflammatory Formula may help reduce inflammation.

Therapies: Hydration and Low Glycemic Diet

Formulas: Anti-Inflammatory

Key Herbs: Black Walnut, **Bilberry (Blueberry, Huckleberry) leaf**, **Juniper Berry**, Goldenseal, Horsetail, Licorice and Uva ursi

Key Nutrients: Chlorophyll, Probiotics, Digestive Enzymes and Vitamin B-Complex

Panic Attack

See *Anxiety or Panic Attack*

Pap Smear (abnormal)

See also *Cervical Dysplasia*

An abnormal Pap smear is caused by cervical dysplasia.

Paralysis

See also *Nerve Damage*

Paralysis is a complete or partial loss of motor function usually involving loss of motion with or without loss of sensation in any part of the body. This is usually due to damage to the nervous system, especially the spinal cord. Obviously, this is a condition that requires medical attention, but there are some remedies that may help nerves to heal. The extent of their ability to heal depends on the amount of damage. St. John's wort has been called the "arnica of the nervous system" because of its ability to stimulate nerve repair. It can be used internally (as an herb or homeopathic remedy) or topically (as an oil). Good fats are essential for the nerves as nerves are 50% fat by dry weight and magnesium and B-complex vitamins are also helpful for nutritionally supporting nerve function. Lobelia and capsicum applied topically over injured areas can stimulate healing and improving circulation by using prickly ash internally may also be helpful.

Therapies: Fresh Fruits and Vegetables and Healthy Fats

Key Herbs: Capsicum (Cayenne), **St. John's wort**, Lobelia, Muira Puama and Prickly Ash

Key Nutrients: Vitamin B-12, Omega-3 Essential Fatty Acids, **Magnesium** and Vitamin B-Complex

Parasites (general)

See also *Giardia*, *Parasites (tapeworm)*, *Parasites (nematodes* and *worms)*

When most of us think of parasites hideous images come to mind, such as ten foot tape worms being coaxed out of human hosts—or starving children in developing countries with swollen bellies. But, not all parasites are giant worms; many are microscopic, single-celled organisms. Furthermore, parasites aren't limited to people living in developing countries. Many people in North American also have problems with parasites and don't realize it.

People can pick up parasites from food, water or pets, or through the skin or mucus membranes. Fortunately, where clean food and water are the norm, odds are very small that people will have a serious parasite problem. However, as more and more food is coming out of developing countries, parasite problems are on the rise.

Furthermore, if you have pets or animals with parasites, there is a high probability that you have them, too. It's also easy to pick up parasites while traveling in foreign countries. So, if you've experienced a change in your health after traveling, parasites may be the reason.

Once parasites are in the body, they can be very hard to diagnose. A standard stool analysis may or may not reveal their presence because a particular sample may not contain them. In fact, parasite problems are often so evasive to standard medical investigation that no one can accurately estimate how much of the population may be afflicted. Fortunately, stool tests that not only check with a microscope but check for parasite antibodies have recently increased the reliability of diagnosis.

Parasites leave telltale signs, including chronic fatigue, anemia, an illness that won't go away, nervousness, teeth grinding, diarrhea, ulcers or digestive pain, nausea or diarrhea, extremes of appetite, weight loss or gain, itching (especially in the rectal area), aches and pains that move from place to place, chronic foul breath, furred tongue, liver jaundice, wide mood swings, fever, colitis, insomnia, and lowered immune response. Just because you have these symptoms doesn't mean that you have parasites, but if you do have a lot of these symptoms and other therapies you've tried aren't working, a parasite cleanse may be useful.

The core of a parasite cleanse is an *Antiparasitic Formula*. This should be taken along with herbs to help cleanse the colon, such as a good *General Detoxifying Formula*. In some cases, a *Fiber Blend Formula* and a *Stimulant Laxative* may also be a helpful part of the cleanse. Take these products as directed on the label.

Enzymes can be taken between meals to help destroy parasites. Protease enzyme supplements are particularly helpful. One can also use foods that tend to be antiparasitic. One of the best is raw garlic. It has been used for worms (pinworms, roundworms, hookworms, tapeworms), giardia, amoebic dysentery and yeast. A garlic enema is an effective way to get rid of worms. Other antiparasitic foods and herbs include cloves, pumpkin seeds, watermelon seeds and horsetail, raw almonds (with skins), raw carrots, raw onions, raw papaya, figs, cucumbers and lemon water. Food-based remedies can be especially helpful for parasites in children.

During the cleanse it is helpful to avoid simple sugars, starchy foods, alcohol and caffeine. In fact, fasting on water for several days while taking the antiparasitic herbs will greatly intensify the effectiveness of the program as it starves the parasites.

Always drink plenty of water when doing any cleanse. Follow up a parasite cleanse with probiotics to help restore normal gut flora.

Therapies: Aromatherapy, Colon Hydrotherapy, Fast or Juice Fast, Friendly Flora, Gut Healing Diet and Hydration

Formulas: Antiparasitic, General Detoxifying, Fiber Blend and Stimulant Laxative

Key Herbs: Bitter Melon, Chaparral, Clove, **Andrographis**, **Black Walnut**, **Garlic**, **Sweet Annie (Ching-Hao)**, **Wormwood**, Elecampane, Goldenseal, Horsetail, Oregano, Pau d' Arco and Quassia

Key Nutrients: Digestive Enzymes, Probiotics and **Protease Enzymes**

Parasites (nematodes, worms)

See also *Parasites (general)*

Nematodes are tiny worms such a pinworms (*Enterobius vermicularis*), whipworms (*Trichuris trichiura*) and hookworms (*Ancylostoma duodenale* and *Necator americanus*). The most prevalent of these are pinworms, which are common in school children. They are highly contagious and easily passed around the family.

Pinworm eggs can contaminate clothing, bed linens and toilet seats. When the eggs are ingested, the worms hatch in the intestines and their eggs are passed from the rectum. Pinworms can also infect the vulva, uterus and fallopian tubes in women.

Fortunately, pinworms are one of the easier parasites to detect because they cause rectal itching. If one examines the rectal area at night with a flashlight, the worms appear as white threads at the anal opening. Other symptoms include: nervousness, inability to concentrate, lack of appetite and unusual dark circles around the eyes.

Take precautions to prevent pinworms from spreading by washing bed linens, bed clothes and underwear of the entire family, having the infected child take daily morning showers to remove eggs deposited in the rectal region during the night, disinfecting toilet seats, bathtubs, sinks and door handles daily, and being sure everybody washes their hands (and fingernails) before meals. Clean cat litter boxes daily. Also, avoid a diet high in sugar and other junk food, which gives parasites more to feed on.

Whipworms and hookworms are less common, but pose a more serious threat to human health. Whipworms inject a fluid that liquefies colon tissue so the worms can ingest it. This creates severe nutritional deficiencies and infections.

Hookworms bite and suck on the intestinal wall, causing bleeding and destroying tissue. This can be severe enough to cause death. Since they consume iron, they cause severe anemia, which can help in detecting them.

Natural therapies for nematodes include garlic enemas or suppositories, wormwood, black walnut and pumpkin seeds. Use an *Antiparasitic Formula* and take protease enzyme supplements between meals. For serious parasite infections seek medical assistance.

Therapies: Colon Cleanse and Colon Hydrotherapy

Formulas: Antiparasitic and General Detoxifying

Key Herbs: Butternut bark, Cascara Sagrada, **Black Walnut**, **Sweet Annie (Ching-Hao)**, Garlic, Horseradish, Horsetail, Male Fern, Papaya, Pumpkin Seed, Thuja, Thyme and Wormwood

Key Nutrients: Protease Enzymes and Digestive Enzymes

Parasites (tapeworm)

See also *Parasites (general)*

Other parasites may actually be more dangerous to one's health, but tapeworms (*Taenia saginata*—beef tapeworm and *T. solium*—pork tapeworm) are emotionally disturbing because of their size. Tapeworms require an intermediate host, so they are usually ingested by eating improperly cooked beef, pork or fish.

Tapeworms are composed of 3,000 to 4,000 segments per worm. New segments are formed near the head, and the ones on the end are cast off with egg packets. When passed, these segments look like grains of uncooked rice or cucumber seeds. This is one of the ways they can be diagnosed. Other symptoms of tapeworms include diarrhea or constipation—or alternating diarrhea and constipation. Some people lose weight with tapeworms, but it is more common for the host to be overweight and retaining water. Tapeworms raise blood sugar levels, cause anemia, and interfere with vitamin B12 uptake.

Natural therapies for tapeworms include *Antiparasitic Formulas* and protease enzyme supplements. Fasting on raw pineapple has helped in destroying them. Raw fig juice and pumpkin seeds have also proven helpful. See Parasites (general) for more information.

Therapies: Colon Cleanse

Formulas: Antiparasitic

Key Herbs: Black Walnut, Male Fern and Wormwood

Key Nutrients: Protease Enzymes

Parkinson's Disease

Parkinson's disease is a chronic, progressive disease of the nervous system, usually occurring later in life. It involves the destruction of neurotransmitters that produce acetylcholine and dopamine and is marked by tremor and weakness in resting muscles and a gradual loss of muscle control. Seek appropriate medical assistance, because this disease is not easy to treat naturally once it has begun.

To prevent this disease, protect the brain by making sure your diet contains good fats and fat soluble vitamins. Also make sure you get adequate amounts of antioxidant foods and nutrients and stay well hydrated. Avoid heavy metals and other evironmental toxins.

Once the disease has started, natural remedies can be helpful in slowing its progress. *Antioxidant* and *Brain and Memory Tonic Formulas* may be helpful in protecting neurons from damage. Since the brain is 50% fat by dry weight, it is essential to use healthy fats in the diet and possibly supplement with omega-3 fatty acids or DHA (the most prominent fatty acid in the brain). *Antispasmodic Formulas* and nervine herbs like scullcap, valerian and wood betony may help to ease tremors.

Therapies: Fresh Fruits and Vegetables, Gut Healing Diet, Healthy Fats, Heavy Metal Cleanse and Hydration

Formulas: Antioxidant, Antispasmodic and Brain and Memory Tonic

Key Herbs: Blue Vervain, Licorice, Milk Thistle, Passionflower, Schisandra (Schizandra), Scullcap (Skullcap), Valerian and Wood Betony

Key Nutrients: Alpha Lipoic Acid, Co-Q10, GABA, **N-Acetyl Cysteine**, **Omega-3 Essential Fatty Acids**, Vitamin C, Vitamin E, DHA and Pantothenic Acid (Vitamin B5)

Peptic Ulcer

See *Ulcers*

Periods (lack of)

See *Amenorrhea*

Peripheral Neuropathy

See also *Diabetes*

Peripheral neuropathy is a disorder where the peripheral nerves that carry signals to and from the spinal cord to the rest of the body aren't working properly. It can involve damage to just one nerve or damage to the nerves in general.

Diabetes is the most common cause of peripheral neuropathy, but it can be caused by autoimmune conditions, chronic kidney disease, infections, nutritional deficiencies, poor blood flow and low thyroid. Drugs and toxins can also damage nerves. In some cases mechanical pressure may be the cause (as in carpal tunnel syndrome) or a physical injury may damage a nerve.

Symptoms of neuropathy include pain, numbness, tingling or burning sensations. You may also start to lose feeling in your arms or legs. Nerve damage can also make it harder to control your muscles.

Damage to nerves can also affect internal organs. It can cause digestive problems and heart problems, for example. It can cause problems with the bladder and sweat glands. It can also affect reproductive function, causing erectile dysfunction in men or vaginal dryness in women.

In treating peripheral neuropathy it is essential that you work with a medical doctor or other qualified health care practitioner to help you determine and correct the cause. You may need to control your blood sugar, stop taking certain medications or get bodywork to take pressure off of nerves.

Natural remedies may be of help. Start by eating a whole food diet (preferably a low glycemic one). Use fresh fruits and vegetables. Avoid caffeine, sugar and artificial sweeteners, particularly Aspartame.

Since nerves are composed of fat, eating healthy fats like omega-3 fatty acids or DHA can be very helpful. The fat soluble vitamins, particularly D and E, can be very helpful in protecting the nerves from damage.

Nerve Tonic Formulas may also be helpful. In particular milky oat seed and St. John's wort can help damaged nerves to heal. B-complex vitamins are also helpful for nerve function and repair.

Alpha lipoic acid can be helpful when the neuropathy is due to blood sugar problems. In this case, it will also be helpful to take a *Blood Sugar Reducing Formula*.

Sometimes using herbs which improve peripheral circulation will help, too. These include prickly ash and capsicum. An herbal *Analgesic Formula* may help with pain.

Because this situation is complex, it is wise to seek professional help so you can design a program customized to your needs.

Therapies: Affirmation and Visualization, Healthy Fats, Hydration and Stress Management

Formulas: Analgesic and Blood Sugar Reducing

Key Herbs: Capsicum (Cayenne), **Prickly Ash**, Oat seed (milky), Scullcap (Skullcap), St. John's wort and Wood Betony

Key Nutrients: Alpha Lipoic Acid, Omega-3 Essential Fatty Acids, Vitamin B-Complex, Vitamin E, Vitamin D, **Vitamin B-12**, Vitamin C, DHA, **Vitamin B-1 (Thiamine)**, Vitamin B-6 (Pyridoxine), **Folate (Folic Acid and Vitamin B9)**

Pernicious Anemia

See also *Anemia*

Pernicious anemia is one form of megaloblastic anemia, and is marked by a progressive decrease in number and increase in size and hemoglobin content of red blood cells. Pernicious anemia is caused by an immune attack on the gastric parietal cells in the stomach that produce intrinsic factor. This causes a deficiency in B12. The condition is characterized by paleness, weakness, and gastrointestinal and nervous disturbances. B-12 shots may be needed, although B-12 can also be taken sublingually in some cases.

Formulas: Immune Balancing

Key Herbs: Astragalus, Licorice and Reishi (Ganoderma)

Key Nutrients: Vitamin B-12, Vitamin B-Complex, Folate (Folic Acid and Vitamin B9)

Perspiration (excessive)

See also *Night Sweating*

Sage is a good remedy for reducing excessive perspiration. It needs to be taken as a cold decoction or a capsule because a hot tea of sage increases perspiration. Excessive perspiration can be caused by imbalances in the hypothalamus and the adrenal glands. *Adaptogen Formulas* or herbs like atractylodes or lycium may also be helpful. Chlorophyll, while not reducing perspiration, can be helpful in reducing odor associated with perspiration.

Formulas: Adaptogen

Key Herbs: Atractylodes, **Sage**, Lycium (Wolfberry, Gogi) and Schisandra (Schizandra)

Key Nutrients: Chlorophyll

Perspiration (deficient)

When a person has a difficult time sweating, the skin does not detoxify the body properly. Sudorifics (or diaphoretics) are herbs used to induce perspiration. They are taken as a hot tea or infusion for this purpose. Sudorifics can also be used to encourage sweating to help throw off acute illnesses like colds and flu. Yarrow is one of the best diaphoretic herbs. It can be mixed with peppermint to make the tea palatable. Catnip is a good diaphoretic for children and can be mixed with elderflowers and/or peppermint. *Sudorific Formulas* can be used to induce perspiration when taken with warm liquids, an excellent therapy for colds and flu.

Therapies: Sweat Bath

Formulas: Sudorific

Key Herbs: Boneset, Catnip, **Blue Vervain**, **Yarrow**, Elder flowers, Ginger, Lemon Balm, Peppermint and Pleurisy Root

Pertussis (Whooping Cough)

See also *Cough (spastic)*

Pertussis is a contagious bacterial infection, usually seen in children, marked by a spasmodic cough. It is also called whooping cough. Herbs used traditionally to treat this condition include garlic, wild cherry, elecampane, thyme and rosemary. Look for *Cough Remedy* or *Expectorant Formulas* with these ingredients. Because the cough associated with this disease is often spastic, *Antispasmodic* or *Bronchialdilator Formulas* containing herbs like lobelia, khella or blue vervain can also be helpful. Colon Hydrotherapy and the Sweat Bath therapy will also be helpful in promoting rapid recovery.

Therapies: Colon Hydrotherapy and Sweat Bath

Formulas: Antispasmodic, **Bronchialdilator**, Cough Remedy and Expectorant

Key Herbs: Black Cohosh, Blue Vervain, **Cherry (Wild)**, **Lobelia**, **Red Clover**, **Skunk Cabbage**, Elecampane, Garlic, Grindelia (Gumweed), Khella, Licorice, Oregano, Pleurisy Root, Rosemary and Thyme

Key Nutrients: Vitamin A, Vitamin C and **Vitamin D**

Pets (supplements for)

Pets can benefit from herbs and nutritional supplements, too. Here are some basic suggestions.

Many pet owners add liquid chlorophyll to the drinking water of their pets. Chlorophyll is found in green plants and is nature's blood-cleanser for animals. It helps red blood cells take up oxygen and supports the immune system. It also aids digestion and deodorizes the body. Taken daily it will help prevent halitosis, reduce body odors and dispel gas.

Animals also need good fats in their diet, so omega-3 fatty acids can be a good supplement for your pet. Good fats will help maintain healthy skin and bones and protects cell membranes form oxidative damage. They also support the immune system, helping your pet resist inflammation and arthritis.

A good supplement for your pet's immune system is a mixture of goldenseal, echinacea and garlic powders in equal parts. Just mix the powders with their food. This strengthens the immune system, promotes gastrointestinal health and prevents parasites and infections.

One of the big problems pets often have is parasites. Pets can have both external and internal parasites, the most common being fleas, lice, ear mites, fly larvae, ticks and Giardia.

Prevention is the best treatment. To avoid topical parasites, treat injuries as described above. Regular grooming will reveal the occasional hitchhiker, especially ticks. Keeping a clean environment for your pet and providing fresh drinking water everyday and good food will help prevent internal parasites.

Antiparasitic Formulas can be used for pets as well as people to get rid of internal parasites in dogs and cats. Artemesia or wormwood has been used for centuries for the purpose of riding the body of amoebas, tapeworm and other parasites of the respiratory, digestive and intestinal system. It can be mixed with the animal's food. Garlic is another herb that can help get rid of internal parasites.

If you have pets in your household, it is probably a good idea not only to give *Antiparasitic Formulas* to your pets, but to everyone in the family.

Generally speaking, most dogs and cats will respond to the same remedies you use for human beings.

Therapies: Friendly Flora, Healthy Fats and Mineralization

Formulas: Mineral, Goldenseal & Echinacea and **Antiparasitic**

Key Herbs: Echinacea, Garlic, Goldenseal and Wormwood

Key Nutrients: Omega-3 Essential Fatty Acids, Colloidal Minerals and Chlorophyll

Phlebitis

See also *Varicose Veins*

Phlebitis is inflammation of a vein, usually in the legs. A *Vascular Tonic Formula* containing butcher's broom and/or horse chestnut can be very helpful. It is also important to use fat soluble vitamins like vitamin E. A decoction of oak bark can be applied topically using the Compress therapy to reduce the inflammation.

Therapies: Compress, Healthy Fats and Mineralization

Formulas: Vascular Tonic

Key Herbs: Capsicum (Cayenne), **Butchers Broom**, **Horse Chestnut** and White Oak

Key Nutrients: Vitamin E

Phobias

See also *Anxiety Disorders*

A phobia is an excessive, unreasonable desire to avoid something because of fear. When this fear is beyond control and interferes with daily life, the phobia becomes an anxiety disorder. Counseling and Emotional Healing Work will be necessary, but supplements that help anxiety disorders may also be useful.

Therapies: Emotional Healing Work and Flower Essences

Formulas: Adrenal Tonic

Key Herbs: Blue Vervain, **Pulsatilla** and Licorice

Key Nutrients: Vitamin B-Complex and Vitamin C

Piles

See *Hemorrhoids*

Pimples

See *Acne (Pimples, Blackheads)*

Pin Worms

See *Parasites (nematodes, worms)*

Pink Eye

See *Conjunctivitis (Pink Eye)*

Pleurisy

Pleurisy is inflammation of the tissues that cover the lungs and line the thoracic cavity, creating painful and difficult breathing, cough, and collection of fluid or fibrous tissue in the thoracic cavity. The herb pleurisy root is a specific for this problem. Lobelia and various *Expectorant* and *Decongestant Formulas* may also be helpful. Since this is a very painful condition, an herbal *Analgesic Formula* may also be helpful.

Formulas: Analgesic, Decongestant and Expectorant

Key Herbs: Cherry (Wild), Coltsfoot, **Lobelia**, **Pleurisy Root**, Fenugreek, Marshmallow, Ocotillo, Sarsaparilla and Yarrow

Key Nutrients: Vitamin C and MSM

PMS (general)

See also *Dysmenorrhea (Painful Menstruation)*, *Menstrual Cramps* and *Menorrhagia (Heavy Menstrual Bleeding)*

PMS is an abbreviation for premenstrual syndrome and is not a specific ailment. A syndrome is a collection of symptoms with multiple causes. Pre-Menstrual Syndrome includes over 150 signs and symptoms which have been classified into four major types. Therapy for PMS will depend largely on which type of PMS you have. Please check out the four PMS types listed next to see which type or types match your symptoms best. The remedies listed here are general remedies for PMS, which can be helpful for most, if not all, types.

Therapies: Avoid Xenoestrogens, Colon Cleanse and Healthy Fats

Formulas: PMS Relieving

Key Herbs: Black Cohosh, Blue Cohosh, **Chastetree (Vitex)** and Peony

Key Nutrients: Vitamin B-6 (Pyridoxine), **Magnesium**, **Omega-3 Essential Fatty Acids** and Vitamin E

PMS Type A

See also *PMS (general)* and *Anger (excessive)*

A stands for anxiety. This PMS type is characterized by high levels of estrogen and low levels of progesterone, and is the most common type of PMS. In fact, 80% of the cases of PMS usually involve too much estrogen and a deficiency of progesterone. Since symptoms include a tendency to anxiety, irritability, mood swings, moodiness and nervous tension, this is the type that is commonly joked about.

The main therapy is to decrease estrogen levels and increase progesterone. Too much estrogen increases levels of adrenaline, noradrenaline, and serotonin, while the levels of dopamine and phenylethlamine drop. Estrogen also seems to block vitamin B6, which is instrumental in many important functions of the body, including maintaining normal blood sugar levels and stabilizing one's moods.

Herbs that enhance progesterone are helpful, of course, since estrogen and progesterone compete for receptor sites. Higher levels of progesterone, therefore, neutralize the excess estrogens.

It is also important, however, to minimize exposure to xenoestrogens and reduce estrogen levels in the body by improving the liver's ability to detoxify excess estrogens. Indole-3 carbinol and *Liver Tonic Formulas* are good possibilities for reducing estrogens.

Poor nutrition really aggravates this condition. Generally, women suffering from PMS A have a high consumption of animal fats, which often contain xenoestrogens and interfere with progesterone production. All these symptoms of type A PMS are further heightened by stress, too much sugar, refined carbohydrates, alcohol and caffeine.

To treat PMS A, reduce fats in the diet, especially animal fats of dairy and meat. Use organic meat and dairy products. Cleansing the liver, especially in the first half of the cycle, is also helpful. Anxiety-relieving supplements such as magnesium and vitamin B6 are helpful for this type of PMS.

Therapies: Avoid Xenoestrogens and Stress Management

Formulas: PMS Relieving and Liver Tonic

Key Herbs: Angelica, Chamomile (English and Roman), **Chastetree (Vitex)**, False Unicorn (Helonias) and Lavender

Key Nutrients: Magnesium, Indole-3 Carbinol (DIM) and **Vitamin B-6 (Pyridoxine)**

PMS Type C

See also *Hypoglycemia* and *PMS (general)*

C stands for cravings. These cravings are generated by a hypoglycemic type of reaction. Blood sugar levels actually do drop significantly, but only between ovulation and the onset of menses. At this time there are strong desires for refined carbohydrates, chocolate, and pretty much anything that is sweet. Unfortunately, because the body's insulin balance is even more sensitive than it would normally be, the drop in blood sugar is faster and more dramatic, causing greater fatigue. It's the fatigue that prompts one to crave those sugars, thus starting the cycle again.

If magnesium levels are low, the pancreas will produce more insulin. Too much salt will also increase insulin production upon ingestion of sugar. In PMS C it seems that prostaglandin 1 (PGE1) is deficient, and this is known to contribute to insulin production.

To treat PMS C, following a diet similar to that of a hypoglycemic diet can minimize the discomforts of PMS C. Stay off of refined sugars. Magnesium supplements with good fats will help keep the hormonal balance in check. Vitamin B6, zinc and chromium help serotonin levels and balance blood sugars and insulin. Reduce dairy, eat nuts, sesame seeds, millet and cashews. Licorice root also helps balance blood sugars.

Therapies: Low Glycemic Diet

Key Herbs: Licorice

Key Nutrients: Chromium, Omega-3 Essential Fatty Acids, **Magnesium**, Vitamin B-6 (Pyridoxine), Zinc and **L-Glutamine**

PMS Type D

See also *Depression*, *Lead Poisoning* and *PMS (general)*

D is for Depression. This type of PMS is associated with depression, anxiety and rage—coupled with confusion, forgetfulness, crying easily and being accident-prone. These women often feel suicidal.

PMS D is due to too much progesterone and not enough estrogen. It is exactly the opposite problem of PMS Type A. In balance, progesterone has a calming effect. When progesterone is in excess, it becomes a depressant to the brain.

An interesting feature to this type of PMS is the high levels of lead found in hair samples. When a deficiency of magnesium occurs, the body seems to be more susceptible to taking in lead. High levels of lead are known to be the cause of some types of chronic depression. Heavy Metal Detoxification may be helpful.

A diet of fresh fruits, raw or steamed vegetables of all types, leafy greens, whole grains, seeds, nuts, olive oil, essential fatty acids, sea salt, and herbal salts along with the right supplements will work wonders in alleviating PMS depression. St. John's wort is good for depression in general, but black cohosh is one of the best remedies for this type of depression. Vitamin B6 and magnesium are absolutely required for this type. Essential oils of clary sage, rose, lavender and bergamot can also bring relief.

Therapies: Aromatherapy and Heavy Metal Cleanse

Formulas: PMS Relieving and Antidepressant

Key Herbs: Black Cohosh, **Rose essential oil**, Lavender essential oil and St. John's wort

Key Nutrients: Magnesium and **Vitamin B-6 (Pyridoxine)**

PMS Type H

See also *Edema (Dropsy, Water Retention, Swelling)* and *PMS (general)*

H is for Hyperhydration, which brings on that uncomfortable feeling caused by water retention. Water retention during times of PMS can be due to too much aldosterone, a hormone made by the adrenal glands, high levels of estrogen, or low levels of magnesium. A *Diuretic Formula* is helpful for this PMS type.

Again, when the levels of magnesium are low, it seems to upset the balance of the hormones in many different ways. Vitamin B6 depends upon magnesium in order to convert into its active form, so a B6 deficiency is also indicated here with PMS H.

Diuretics are needed in PMS Type H. Other supplements that can help include: magnesium, vitamin B6, vitamin E and evening primrose oil. Adding beans, whole grains and leafy vegetables to the diet can be helpful, too. The essential oils of frankincense, juniper and lemon can also help.

Therapies: Aromatherapy

Formulas: Diuretic

Key Herbs: Nettle (Stinging) leaf, Dandelion leaf and Juniper Berry

Key Nutrients: Vitamin B-6 (Pyridoxine), **Magnesium** and Vitamin E

PMS Type P

See also *Dysmenorrhea (Painful Menstruation)*

P is for Pain. Pain associated with menstruation is called dysmenorrhea. Try using a *Menstrual Cramp Formula* and/or magnesium supplements. Ginger can be used to enhance pelvic circulation when the pain is congestive. See *Dysmenorrhea* for more options.

Formulas: Menstrual Cramp

Key Herbs: Ginger, **Kava-kava** and Lobelia

Key Nutrients: Magnesium

PMS Type S

See also *Acne (Pimples, Blackheads)*, *Adrenals (exhaustion* and *weakness or burnout)*

S is for Skin. Some women get outbreaks of acne due to high levels of androgens, which are a side effect of stress. Chronic stress will eventually fatigue the adrenal glands. Exhausted adrenal glands are aggravated by non-organic, non-pastured animal fats and dairy products. Eat more green leafy vegetables, vegetable proteins, and fruit. A colon and liver cleanse would add vital energy to the body and clear the skin. *Blood Purifier Formulas* are good for helping to clear skin conditions. Decrease nicotine, caffeine, sugar and salt consumption.

Therapies: Colon Cleanse

Formulas: Blood Purifier and **Skin Healing**

Key Herbs: Burdock, **Dandelion** and **Red Clover**

Key Nutrients: Vitamin C and Vitamin B-Complex

Pneumonia

Pneumonia is a disease of the lungs characterized by inflammation and fluid accumulation; usually caused by infection. It may be caused by a viral or a bacterial infection, so use an *Antibacterial* or *Antiviral Formula* as needed. *Expectorant Formulas* can help clear the lungs of fluid and mucus. Raw garlic is particularly helpful for pneumonia, especially when combined with an *Expectorant Formula*. Seek appropriate medical assistance.

Therapies: Colon Hydrotherapy

Formulas: Expectorant, Antibacterial and Antiviral

Key Herbs: Andrographis, **Cherry (Wild)**, **Garlic**, **Osha**, Licorice, Lobelia, Lomatium, Pleurisy Root, Usnea and Yarrow

Key Nutrients: Zinc, Omega-3 Essential Fatty Acids and Vitamin C

Poison Ivy or Oak

See also *Rashes and Hives*

Certain plants cause a mild to severe contact allergic reaction when touched, such as poison ivy or poison oak. Symptoms of this allergic reaction may include mild to severe redness, rash, itching, burning and/or oozing blisters. Wash the skin immediately with plenty of soap and water after contact with these plants. Then apply herbs topically to reduce swelling and inflammation such as aloe vera, plantain, uva ursi, jewelweed, etc. Make these herbs into a liquid form (infusion or decoction) for application.

Internally, vitamin C and *Blood Purifier Formulas* containing burdock, yellow dock or red clover may be helpful. If you are hypersensitive to these plants, try using homeopathic poison ivy (Rhus tox) to desensitize the body.

Therapies: Compress and Poultice

Formulas: Topical Vulnerary and Blood Purifier

Key Herbs: Aloe vera, Burdock, Collinsonia (Stoneroot), **Grindelia (Gumweed)**, **Plantain**, **Uva ursi**, Red Clover, White Oak, Yellow Dock and Yerba Santa

Key Nutrients: Vitamin A, Vitamin C and Vitamin D

Poisoning (general)

There are numerous toxic substances that can accidentally be inhaled, ingested or absorbed through the skin. Call a poison control center near you for help with any kind of acute poisoning. Activated charcoal absorbs many toxins, and milk thistle helps protect the liver against toxins. For some toxins, lobelia or ipecac can be taken to induce vomiting. Always contact a poison control center for advice before administering any remedy.

Key Herbs: Milk Thistle and Lobelia

Key Nutrients: Charcoal (Activated), Chlorophyll and Vitamin C

Poisoning (food)

Consuming contaminated food can create severe symptoms of food poisoning, which include nausea, vomiting and diarrhea. In severe cases, medical attention should be sought.

Lobelia can be used to induce vomiting to expel the toxic material more quickly from the body. If lobelia isn't available, ipecac, available at most drug stores, is an alternative. Other herbs that may help induce vomiting include boneset, blue vervain and mustard.

To absorb irritants in the digestive tract and ease diarrhea, activated charcoal is the very best. Alternatives include slippery elm and psyllium. Taking probiotics can also help prevent food poisoning.

Therapies: Dietary Fiber and Friendly Flora

Key Herbs: Aloe vera, Blue Vervain, **Lobelia**, Echinacea, Garlic, Goldenseal, Milk Thistle, Psyllium and Slippery Elm

Key Nutrients: Probiotics and **Charcoal (Activated)**

Polyps

A polyp is a projecting mass of swollen, overgrown or tumorous tissue, usually found in the nasal cavity or intestine. They are benign (non-cancerous) growths. Natural healers typically view polyps as a toxic condition in the body and use blood purifiers to clean up the system. Internally, consider using a *Blood Purifier Formula* containing herbs like burdock, pau d'arco and red clover. Also consider doing the Colon Cleanse therapy.

Bayberry is an astringent and can be used to shrink polyps. For nasal polyps make a mixture of equal parts powdered bayberry and goldenseal and snuff it up the nose once or twice daily.

Therapies: Colon Cleanse

Formulas: Blood Purifier

Key Herbs: Aloe vera, Burdock, **Bayberry**, **Goldenseal**, Pau d' Arco and Red Clover

Key Nutrients: Vitamin A, Vitamin D, Vitamin C, Folate (Folic Acid and Vitamin B9)

Post Partum Depression

See also *Depression*

Depression after having a baby is caused by low levels of hormones. Black cohosh or an *Antidepressant Formula* containing black cohosh can be helpful.

Therapies: Flower Essences

Formulas: Antidepressant

Key Herbs: Black Cohosh, **Blessed Thistle** and Partridge Berry (Squaw Vine)

Key Nutrients: 5-HTP and Vitamin B-3 (Niacin)

Post Traumatic Stress Disorder (PTSD)

See also *Adrenals (exhaustion, weakness or burnout), Stress, Anxiety Disorders* and *Abuse and Trauma*

Post Traumatic Stress Disorder (PTSD) used to be called "shell shock" or "battle fatigue." It was identified as a condition affecting soldiers who had undergone so much stress that they simply couldn't cope anymore. You don't have to have gone to war to suffer post traumatic stress disorder. Anytime you've had a series of extremely stressful situations that overwhelmed your ability to cope and left you in a chronic state of stress and anxiety, you may experience PTSD to one degree or another.

The name PTSD "sanitizes" the condition, which is actually a result of severe trauma or abuse. This results in adrenal burnout and enervation. So, *Adrenal Tonic* and *Relaxing Nervine Formulas* are physically helpful. Kava kava, blue vervain or motherwort can be used to reduce anxiety and adaptogens like eleuthero or schisandra can be used to reduce the output of stress hormones. Sleep is essential, so using a *Sleep Formula* to help the person get a good night's sleep can be important.

Physical remedies can be helpful, but ultimately counseling and/or Emotional Healing Work is essential to allow the system to discharge the emotional energy and reset the nervous system. PTSD is considered an Anxiety Disorder, so see that heading for more ideas on what to do for it.

Therapies: Emotional Healing Work, Flower Essences, Hiatal Hernia Correction, Hydration, Low Glycemic Diet and Stress Management

Formulas: Adrenal Tonic, Relaxing Nervine, **Adaptogen** and Sleep

Key Herbs: Eleuthero (Siberian ginseng), **Kava-kava**, **Scullcap (Skullcap)**, Motherwort, Passionflower, Pulsatilla and Schisandra (Schizandra)

Key Nutrients: Pantothenic Acid (Vitamin B5), GABA, **Magnesium** and Vitamin B-Complex

Pregnancy (herbs and supplements for)

See also *Labor and Delivery*

During pregnancy, a woman needs the nutrients necessary to form two extra pounds of uterine muscle, several pounds of amniotic fluid and the placenta. She also experiences a 50% increase in blood volume, and her liver and kidney cells need to process the waste from two living beings—all in addition to forming the bones, muscles, skin, glands, nervous system and other vital organs of her developing child.

This means her body will require larger than normal amounts of protein, good fats, vitamins and minerals-nutrients she isn't going to get from eating a diet of refined and processed foods. A pregnant woman needs to take extra good care of her body by consuming fresh fruits and vegetables, whole grains and organically raised meat and dairy products. She should also avoid alcohol, coffee, tobacco, refined sugar, white flour, shortening, margarine, commercially fried foods and hydrogenated oils. Ideally, all these dietary changes should take place several months before conception in order to prepare the body for a healthy pregnancy. A good prenatal vitamin can be very helpful.

Chemicals are a major cause of birth defects and health problems in infants, so a pregnant woman should be very careful to minimize her exposure to toxic chemicals of all kinds, particularly pesticides. Many pesticides will cause a miscarriage because of their xenoestrogenic nature. A pregnant woman should also be careful to use only natural, non-toxic household cleaning and personal care products. It is also a good idea to do a cleanse prior to conception. This will minimize a woman's risk of morning sickness, toxemia and other health problems during pregnancy.

Traditional cultures used special foods for pregnant women to ensure healthy babies. Supplements can do the same for modern pregnant women. Megadoses of vitamins and minerals aren't wise, but a good prenatal vitamin can be beneficial. These contain essential nutrients for energy and basic health during pregnancy, such as 800 mg of folic acid (as 5MTHF or l-methylfolate), which is essential in the prevention of neural tube defects.

Many women, however, find that using whole foods and herbs are even more important than taking a prenatal in maintaining good health during pregnancy.

Good fats are a must for pregnancy, as a developing child's brain and nervous system need good fats. Supplementing with omega-3 fatty acids has been shown to reduce the risk of developing pre-eclampsia, postpartum depression and pre-term labor. Deep ocean fish (especially sardines), walnuts, flax seeds, hemp seed, avocados, coconut oil and organic butter from grass-fed cows are also great sources of good fats for pregnancy.

Due to modern agricultural practices, the population as a whole is deficient in minerals. Even when consuming a wholesome organic diet, pregnant women usually need extra amounts of trace minerals. Many problems in pregnancy have been attributed to trace mineral deficiencies because the developing infant pulls minerals from the mother's bloodstream.

Drinking a pregnancy tea with equal parts red raspberry leaf, alfalfa and peppermint is an easy way to get the needed trace minerals. Expectant mothers should steep 3-4 heaping tablespoons of this mixture in a quart of boiling water and drink at least a quart of this tea every day. Other mineral-rich herbs like nettles, oat straw and horsetail can be added to the tea for an even better effect. This tea helps prevent morning sickness and strengthens a woman's body during pregnancy and delivery.

Red raspberry leaf is especially valuable to pregnant women as it tones the uterus and prepares the body for childbirth, making labor and delivery easier. It also reduces morning sickness, lowers the risk of miscarriage and decreases the risk of postpartum hemorrhage. Women who don't have time to make the pregnancy tea described above, can take red raspberry in capsule or liquid form.

Other great ways to get minerals include adding sea weeds or sea vegetables to the diet, drinking bone broth, and taking colloidal mineral supplements or mineral-rich herbs (herbal *Mineral Formulas*). Adequate mineral intake prevents many of the problems women experience in pregnancy, creates healthier babies and makes delivery easier.

Pregnant women especially need more iron. Eating dark, green leafy vegetables, organic red meat and iron-rich herbs can keep iron levels normal during pregnancy. Consider supplementing with red beets and yellow dock in addition to adding nettles to your pregnancy tea. Drinking liquid chlorophyll will increase utilization of iron. Taken after childbirth, chlorophyll also increases the quality of the mother's breast milk

Therapies: Affirmation and Visualization, Bone Broth, Dietary Fiber, Fresh Fruits and Vegetables, Healthy Fats and Mineralization

Formulas: Mineral, Iron and **Pregnancy Tonic**

Key Herbs: Alfalfa, Bee Pollen, **Nettle (Stinging)**, **Red Raspberry**, Kelp and Yellow Dock

Key Nutrients: Calcium, 5-HTP, Omega-3 Essential Fatty Acids, Melatonin, **Magnesium**, Iron, **Folate (Folic Acid, Vitamin B9)**, Colloidal Minerals, Chlorophyll, Vitamin E, Vitamin B-6 (Pyridoxine), Vitamin B-Complex, Vitamin C and **Vitamin D**

Pregnancy (herbs and supplements to avoid during)

The following supplements and herbs should be avoided during pregnancy: Black cohosh, partridge berry, dong quai and butcher's broom. These should only be used during the last five weeks of pregnancy. Black and blue cohosh can be used after the due date. Women should not do cleanses during pregnancy or use antiparasitic herbs, unless guided to do so under professional supervision. Herbs and supplements that potentially increase estrogen levels, such as black cohosh, may contribute to miscarriage. Glandular herbs that increase progesterone are fine, as progesterone helps a woman stay pregnant. Blue cohosh and anamu are potentially abortive and should be avoided if a woman is trying to get pregnant. They are especially dangerous during the first trimester. While many of the herbs and formulas in the following lists have been used safely during pregnancy, they all have the potential for issues and should be used during pregnancy only under the guidance of a professional herbalist (*findanherbalist.com*).

Formulas to avoid: General Detoxifying, Blood Purifier, Cholagogue, Antiparasitic, Stimulant Laxative, Female Aphrodisiac, Female Hormonal Balancing, PMS Relieving and Drawing Salve

Herbs to avoid: Angelica, Arnica, Barberry, Black Cohosh, Black Walnut, Blessed Thistle, Blue Cohosh, Borage, Buchu, Buckthorn, Butternut bark, Cascara Sagrada, Cats Claw (Uña de Gato, Gambier), Chaparral, Comfrey, Cramp Bark, Damiana, Dong Quai, Elecampane, Eleuthero (Siberian ginseng), Fenugreek, Feverfew, Gentian, Goldenseal, Guggul, Horehound, Hyssop, Licorice, Mistletoe, Motherwort, Myrrh, Ocotillo, Osha, Pennyroyal, Poke Root, Rosemary, Sage, Sarsaparilla, Tea (Green or Black), Thuja, Thuja, Thyme, Wood Betony and Wormwood

Nutrients to avoid: GABA and DHEA

Premature Ejaculation

See also *Erectile Dysfunction*

Men who experience problems with premature ejaculation may benefit from taking herbs to balance male reproductive hormones, such as a *Male Aphrodisiac* or a *Male Glandular Tonic Formula*. It's also wise to follow the Avoid Xenoestrogens therapy. This problem is often due to stress and tension and the inability to relax. *Adaptogen* and *Nerve Tonic Formulas* may be helpful. Emotional Healing Work may also be needed and counseling may also be helpful, as the problem is often an expression of relationship problems.

Therapies: Avoid Xenoestrogens, Emotional Healing Work and Stress Management

Formulas: Male Aphrodisiac, **Male Glandular Tonic** and Adaptogen

Key Herbs: Maca, **Schisandra (Schizandra)**, Damiana, Ginseng (Asian and Korean)

Key Nutrients: Zinc

Progesterone (low)

See also *PMS Type A*

With exposure to xenoestrogens and an excess burden on the liver, many women have too much estrogen and not enough progesterone. Good reproductive health requires a balance between these two hormones. Since the scale in many women is tipped towards estrogen, a natural progesterone supplement is helpful for many women.

Don't overdo it with progesterone creams, however, because you can also get too much progesterone. Symptoms of progesterone overdose include headache, weight gain, fatigue, water retention and depression. Consider getting a test to see where your current hormone balance lies.

Herbs such as sarsaparilla and false unicorn can also be used to counteract excess estrogen by enhancing progesterone. These herbs have been used to help sustain pregnancy and prevent miscarriage and to relieve heavy menstrual bleeding and cramps. Chaste tree, taken regularly for several months, can also balance out estrogen and progesterone.

Therapies: Avoid Xenoestrogens and Healthy Fats

Formulas: Female Hormonal Balancing

Key Herbs: Blue Cohosh, Chastetree (Vitex), **False Unicorn (Helonias)** and Sarsaparilla

Key Nutrients: Magnesium

Prolapsed Colon

A falling down or sagging of the colon from its usual position is called a prolapsed colon. This condition often involves the transverse or horizontal portion of the colon. Laying on a slant board with one's feet elevated and massaging the colon can help. Taking a *Fiber Blend Formula* and a *Stimulant Laxative Formula* to keep the colon working properly can help to tone the colon. A *Tissue Healing Formula* may also be helpful. Vitamin C and calcium help to build structural integrity in tissues.

Formulas: Tissue Healing, Stimulant Laxative and Fiber Blend

Key Herbs: Bayberry, **Yellow Dock**, Red Raspberry and Solomon's Seal

Key Nutrients: Calcium and Vitamin C

Prolapsed Uterus

See also *Prolapsed Colon*

A falling down or sagging of the uterus from its usual position is called a prolapsed uterus. It is more common after pregnancies. It may prevent conception and often puts pressure on the bladder, which may lead to incontinence. A *Uterine Tonic Formula* may be helpful, as well as increased intake of minerals. Laying on a slant board with one's feet elevated and massaging the uterus can help. Good posture (standing and sitting erect) is also helpful. This condition may be caused by a prolapsed colon.

Therapies: Mineralization

Formulas: Uterine Tonic

Key Herbs: Astragalus, Bayberry, Cranberry, **Red Raspberry**, **White Pond Lily**, **Yellow Dock**, Dong Quai and White Oak bark

Key Nutrients: Calcium, Magnesium and Vitamin C

Prostate Problems

See *Benign Prostate Hyperplasia (BPH)* and *Prostatitis*

Prostatitis

See also *Benign Prostate Hyperplasia (BPH)*

Prostatitis is inflammation of the prostate gland that causes painful urination, frequent trips to the men's room, miss-aim, and dribbling because the weak stream of urine is insufficient to fully open the flaps at the tip of the penis. It is sometimes due to infection, but is more often due to other unknown causes.

One reason why the prostate may become inflamed involves its proximity to both the bladder and the rectum. If the body is toxic, the irritants being eliminated from the colon and urinary passages may be irritating the prostate gland, causing it to swell.

If the problem is due to an acute or chronic infection, consider some herbs with natural antibacterial action, such as goldenseal or uva ursi. One can also use a *Urinary Infection Formula*. Daily exercise to increase circulation is also beneficial for prostatitis because it increases circulation to the prostate and reduces swelling. To relieve inflammation, use an *Anti-Inflammatory Formula*.

Omega-3 essential fatty acids can also reduce prostate inflammation. Eskimo men who have a fish-rich diet have significantly lower rates of prostatitis and prostate cancer than other men. Omega-3 fatty acids have also been shown to inhibit prostate cell growth and reduce prostate enlargement. They help decrease pain and fatigue, reduce night-time urination, increase elimination (stream) and increase libido.

Zinc and/or a *Prostate Formula* may also be beneficial at reducing inflammation and prostate swelling. Also avoid xenoestrogens, clean out the colon, and maintain healthy intestinal flora with probiotics.

Therapies: Avoid Xenoestrogens, Colon Cleanse, Fresh Fruits and Vegetables, Friendly Flora, Gut Healing Diet, Healthy Fats and Hydration

Formulas: Prostate, Urinary Infection Fighting and Anti-Inflammatory

Key Herbs: Barberry, Buchu, **Goldenseal**, **Gravel root**, **Hydrangea**, **White Sage**, Pumpkin Seed, Pygeum Bark, Saw Palmetto and Uva ursi

Key Nutrients: Quercitin, **Omega-3 Essential Fatty Acids**, Probiotics, Zinc, Bromelain and Chondroitin

Psoriasis

See also *Eczema* and *Leaky Gut Syndrome*

Psoriasis differs from eczema because it involves rapid skin growth and appears to be an autoimmune disorder, like multiple sclerosis or lupus. Psoriasis primarily affects the skin, but in about 10% of the cases the joints are also affected. Research suggests that psoriasis is triggered when certain T-cells reproduce very rapidly, which starts an inflammatory reaction that causes skin cells to multiply seven to twelve times faster than normal. In natural medicine this may be taking place because the skin is malnourished and weak or because of allergic reactions to food.

Because this hyperactivity of the immune system also creates a form of inflammation, psoriasis has symptoms similar to eczema. The skin is often itchy and dry, and frequently cracking or blistering. Oils are needed to keep the skin moist. In particular, omega-3 essential fatty acids may be helpful.

Diet is important in the effective treatment of psoriasis. Using the Eliminate Gluten therapy has also benefited some sufferers. Since food allergies are a contributing factor in psoriasis, it would be a good idea to follow the Eliminate Allergy-Causing Foods therapy.

Incomplete protein digestion and bowel toxemia may be underlying factors in psoriasis. Digestive enzyme supplements, taken between meals, will help break down un-digested protein and detoxify the colon. Psoriasis is often linked to Leaky Gut Syndrome, so healing the gut can help.

Detoxifying the liver is also important. Products containing liver protecting herbs like milk thistle and nutrients that enhance liver detoxification like N-acetyl-cysteine and detoxifying herbs can accomplish this. Use a good *Liver Tonic* or *Blood Purifier Formula*. Combined with a *Fiber Blend* formula and plenty of water, these formulas will also help to gently cleanse the bowel to get rid of the gut-derived toxins that may be involved in this disease.

Nutrients that have been reported helpful for psoriasis include vitamin A (in large doses of about 50,000 to 75,000 IU per day for a short time), vitamin E (400 to 800 IU per day), B-complex vitamins and vitamin B6 in particular, vitamin C, zinc and chromium. Feverfew can be used both internally and topically to ease psoriasis. Finally, the polyphenols in green tea can also help to reduce irritation of the skin and ease psoriasis.

Therapies: Colon Cleanse, Eliminate Allergy-Causing Foods and Healthy Fats

Formulas: Liver Tonic, **Blood Purifier** and Fiber Blend

Key Herbs: Chamomile (English and Roman), **Burdock**, **Red Clover**, **Turmeric**, Gotu kola, Licorice, Milk Thistle, Psyllium, Sarsaparilla and Tea (Green or Black)

Key Nutrients: Vitamin D, Vitamin B-6 (Pyridoxine), Protease Enzymes, Omega-3 Essential Fatty Acids, MSM, Vitamin B-Complex, Vitamin A, Vitamin E, Zinc, Digestive Enzymes, N-Acetyl Cysteine, **Betaine Hydrochloric Acid (HCl)** and DHA

Puberty (hormone balancer)

It's no great secret that teenagers experience major hormonal changes. These changes affect not only a teen's body, but also their thoughts and emotions, so it is important to talk with kids about these changes and help them through this critical time in their lives. Appropriate herbs and supplements can also help.

For young women who are just starting their periods, a *Female Hormonal Balancing Formula* can help. It cleanses the genito-urinary system, makes periods easier, and reduces the risk of urinary tract infections while counteracting environmental estrogens. It can also help reduce androgens in teenage boys to lessen acne.

Another good hormone balancer is chaste tree. It regulates the pituitary gland to balance hormone levels. It is a useful remedy for teenage acne but can also help with excessive aggression in boys and menstrual cramps in girls.

If young women are having problems with painful periods, irregular periods and other menstrual problems, a

Female Hormonal Balancer can counteract PMS and normalize the reproductive cycle.

Therapies: Avoid Xenoestrogens, Healthy Fats, Low Glycemic Diet, Mineralization and Stress Management

Formulas: Female Hormonal Balancing

Key Herbs: Chastetree (Vitex) and Red Raspberry

Key Nutrients: Colloidal Minerals, **Omega-3 Essential Fatty Acids**, Vitamin B-6 (Pyridoxine) and **Magnesium**

Puncture Wounds

See *Tetanus* and *Wounds and Sores*

Pyorrhea

See *Gingivitis (Bleeding Gums, Gum Disease, Pyorrhea)*

Radiation Sickness

When the body is exposed to radiation, cellular DNA is damaged and a toxic condition is created in the body. X-rays, radon, microwave ovens, radar and radiation treatments for cancer are among the ways the body can be exposed to radiation. One of the most important supplements to take when one has been or will be exposed to radiation is iodine, as it protects the thyroid against radioactive iodine. Radiation also causes free radical damage, so antioxidants are helpful.

Therapies: Fresh Fruits and Vegetables

Formulas: Antioxidant

Key Herbs: Aloe vera, **Barley grass**, **Codonopsis**, **Reishi (Ganoderma)**, Eleuthero (Siberian ginseng), Ginseng (American), Ginseng (Asian, Korean), Kelp and Rhodiola

Key Nutrients: Iodine, **Sodium Alginate (Algin)**, Vitamin A and Vitamin D

Rapid Heart Beat

See *Tachycardia*

Rashes and Hives

See also *Itching* and *Dermatitis*

A rash is a skin eruption, which can be local or general. It is an inflammatory process and may involve allergic reactions or toxicity. Symptoms include redness, swelling, itching, burning and sometimes blisters.

The Drawing Bath therapy is very helpful in easing rashes and hives. It can soothe the irritated skin and reduce itching. Any of the following could be used in the bath: chickweed (good for itching), comfrey (healing and soothing to the skin), marshmallow (soothing) or seaweeds like kelp (nourishing to the skin). Also consider topical applications of *Topical Vulnerary Formulas* containing aloe vera, chickweed and other herbs that soothe irritated skin. Internally, consider *Blood Purifier Formulas*, as blood purifiers like burdock, Oregon grape, pau d'arco and yellow dock have been historically used to clear up skin conditions.

Therapies: Drawing Bath and Hydration

Formulas: Blood Purifier, Topical Vulnerary and **Skin Healing**

Key Herbs: Aloe vera, Chamomile (English and Roman), Chickweed, **Burdock**, **Yellow Dock**, Dandelion, Marshmallow, Mullein, Oregon Grape, Pau d' Arco, Tea Tree essential oil and Turmeric

Key Nutrients: MSM, Vitamin A and Vitamin D

Raynaud's Disease

Raynaud's disease is a vascular disorder marked by recurrent spasm of the capillaries (especially those of the fingers and toes upon exposure to cold), skin changes from white to blue to red in succession, and pain. Remedies that enhance peripheral circulation, such as capsicum, ginkgo and prickly ash, can be helpful. Look for *Cardiovascular Stimulant Formulas* based on these herbs.

Formulas: Cardiovascular Stimulant

Key Herbs: Capsicum (Cayenne), **Prickly Ash**, **Turmeric**, Ginger, Ginkgo, Hawthorn and Lobelia

Key Nutrients: Co-Q10, Chlorophyll, **Magnesium**, Vitamin B-Complex and **Vitamin B-12**

Recuperation

See *Convalescence*

Respiratory Congestion

See *Congestion (lungs)*

Respiratory Infections

See *Congestion (lungs)*, *Infection (bacterial)*, *Infection (viral)*, *Pleurisy* and *Pneumonia*

Restless Dreams

See also *Adrenals (exhaustion, weakness or burnout)*

Restless and disturbing dreams are often one of the first indications that a person is under too much stress and in danger of developing enervation and adrenal burnout. Practice some the skills listed under Stress Management in the *Therapies Section* and take an *Adaptogen Formula*. It also helps to balance blood sugar using the Low Glycemic Diet and to Avoid Caffeine therapies.

Therapies: Aromatherapy, Avoid Caffeine, Emotional Healing Work, Flower Essences, Low Glycemic Diet and Stress Management

Formulas: Adaptogen

Key Herbs: Chamomile (English and Roman), Chaparral flower essence and **Passionflower**

Key Nutrients: GABA

Restless Leg Syndrome

See also *Anemia*

Restless leg syndrome is a condition where the legs itch, tickle or burn, often at night. Moving them brings temporary relief, but the urge to move them returns seconds or minutes later. It can hinder sleep. Food allergies, mineral deficiencies, anemia and stress could be underlying problems. Start by taking magnesium, B-complex vitamins and a *Relaxing Nervine Formula*. If there are signs of anemia, build up the blood. Seek professional help to determine the underlying cause if symptoms persist.

Therapies: Mineralization and Stress Management

Formulas: Relaxing Nervine, Iron and Antiparasitic

Key Herbs: Scullcap (Skullcap), Kava-kava, Lobelia and St. John's wort

Key Nutrients: Magnesium, **Folate (Folic Acid, Vitamin B9)**, Colloidal Minerals, **Vitamin B-Complex** and **Iron**

Reye's Syndrome

Reye's Syndrome is a serious illness that occurs after a viral infection such as a cold, flu or chicken pox. Research has linked the development of this disease to the use of aspirin and other salicylates to treat symptoms. In Reye's Syndrome, abnormal accumulations of fat begin to develop in the liver and other organs of the body. Pressure in the brain also increases. Early diagnosis and treatment is essential, as death can occur rapidly. This disorder requires immediate medical attention. Supplements listed may be beneficial as adjuncts to medical treatment. It is important to know that natural sources of salycilates, such as willow bark, can also trigger Reye's syndrome. We do not recommend the use of herbal *Analgesic Formulas* or *Topical Analgesic Formulas* containing salycilate-bearing herbs to treat symptoms of viral diseases.

Key Herbs: Cats Claw (Uña de Gato, Gambier)

Key Nutrients: L-Carnitine

Rheumatic Fever

Rheumatic fever is an acute, often recurrent, disease found mainly in children and young adults. It is characterized by fever, inflammation, pain and swelling in and around the joints. The inflammation also affects the surface and valves of the heart and may involve the formation of small nodules in the heart or other tissues. Appropriate medical assistance should be sought. Garlic and Oregon grape are good remedies to help with infection. Co-Q10 and l-carnitine can help protect the heart.

Formulas: Antibacterial and Cardiac Tonic

Key Herbs: Garlic, **Hawthorn** and **Oregon Grape**

Key Nutrients: L-Carnitine and Co-Q10

Rheumatoid Arthritis (Rheumatism)

See also *Allergies (food)*, *Arthritis*, *Autoimmune Disorders* and *Leaky Gut Syndrome*

Rheumatoid arthritis is a type of arthritis that has an autoimmune component. It is characterized by inflammation and pain in muscles, joints or fibrous tissues. Juice Fasting and using remedies that modulate immune responses can be very helpful for rheumatoid arthritis. See Arthritis for a complete discussion of how to work with arthritis naturally.

Therapies: Colon Cleanse, Eliminate Allergy-Causing Foods, Eliminate Gluten, Fast or Juice Fast, Gut Healing Diet, Healthy Fats and Hydration

Formulas: Joint Healing, Immune Balancing and Mushroom Blend

Key Herbs: Alfalfa, Ashwaganda, Blue Cohosh, Boswellia, Celery, **Cats Claw (Uña de Gato, Gambier)**, **Devil's Claw**, **Solomon's Seal**, **Turmeric**, Eucalyptus, Gravel root, Meadowsweet, Nettle (Stinging), Prickly Ash, Sarsaparilla, Stillingia and Yucca

Key Nutrients: Glucosamine, **Omega-3 Essential Fatty Acids**, **MSM**, Vitamin B-3 (Niacin), **Vitamin D** and Bromelain

Rhinitis

See also *Rhinitis, Allergic*

Rhinitis as an inflammatory condition that affects the sensitive membranes of the nasal and sinus passages, the eyes and the throat. In allergic rhinitis the inflammation is caused by allergic reactions, but any irritation to the sensitive membranes of the upper respiratory passages and eyes can cause rhinitis. Whatever the cause, having congested nasal passages, a runny nose, itchy, watery eyes and an irritated throat can make life miserable.

Here's what's happening—anytime the sensitive membranes in your upper respiratory tract are exposed to irritants, inflammation can occur. Tissues swell and mucus is secreted to try to flush the irritation away.

In most people, these symptoms include sneezing, wheezing, stuffiness, itchy, runny nose and throat, post-nasal drip, itchy, watery eyes, conjunctivitis, earaches, and insomnia. Many feel a reduced sense of taste or smell and even difficulty hearing. Other suffers have a nasal voice, breathe noisily or snore. Still others complain of frequent headaches and feeling chronically tired. Some people are more sensitive and will experience nasal and respiratory congestion, pain and pressure in the face. In more severe cases, rhinitis can produce yellow or greenish discharge from the nose, a chronic cough that produces mucus, poor appetite, nausea and sometimes a fever.

To deal with this problem, you need to identify, if possible, the source of the irritation. In the case of non-allergic rhinitis, this is usually chemical in nature. Avoid household cleaning products or other chemicals that cause respiratory irritation. People have found permanent relief just by switching to non-toxic household cleaning products.

For symptomatic relief try using an *Anti-Inflammatory* and a *Decongestant Formula*. Eyebright and osha are two ingredients to look for as both are very good at reducing the symptoms of rhinitis. Vitamin C can block the histamine involved in the immune reactions and reduce symptoms. It can also be helpful to use the Colon Cleansing and Eliminate Allergy-Causing Foods therapies.

A very simple way to ease rhinitis is to drink lots of water and take a small amount of natural salt with it. The salt and water increase secretions of tears and mucus, which helps the body flush away irritants faster. By staying well hydrated, the body is able to keep irritants flushed away, which prevents the inflammatory reactions.

Therapies: Colon Cleanse, Eliminate Allergy-Causing Foods and Hydration

Formulas: Allergy-Reducing, Decongestant and Anti-Inflammatory

Key Herbs: Eyebright, **Nettle (Stinging)** and Osha

Key Nutrients: Digestive Enzymes, **Vitamin C** and **Quercitin**

Rhinitis, Allergic

See *Allergies (respiratory)*

Ringing In Ears

See *Tinnitus (Ringing in the Ears)*

Ringworm

See *Parasites (nematodes, worms)*

Rosacea

See also *Allergies (food)*, *Leaky Gut Syndrome* and *Small Intestinal Bacterial Overgrowth (SIBO)*

Rosacea is a chronic inflammatory skin condition. It is very similar to facial acne, except that it typically appears after the age of thirty. Rosacea is usually restricted to the face, but occasionally spreads to other parts of the body. It is more commonly experienced by people with deficient amounts of hydrochloric acid and poor digestion and is directly linked to Small Intestinal Bacterial Overgrowth and Leaky Gut. Red raspberry or feverfew can help when applied topically as a facial mask. Healthy fats, especially omega-3 fatty acids and fat soluble vitamins A, D and E may be helpful.

Therapies: Bone Broth, Eliminate Allergy-Causing Foods, Fresh Fruits and Vegetables, Gut Healing Diet and Healthy Fats

Formulas: Digestive Bitter Tonic and Adrenal Tonic

Key Herbs: Chamomile (English and Roman), **Feverfew**, **Goldenseal**, Hawthorn and Red Raspberry

Key Nutrients: Omega-3 Essential Fatty Acids, **Vitamin A**, **Vitamin D**, Vitamin E, **Zinc**, **Digestive Enzymes**, **L-Glutamine** and **Betaine Hydrochloric Acid (HCl)**

Runny Nose

See *Congestion (sinus)*

Scabies

Scabies is a parasitic mite that lives in the skin causing severe itching. Paw Paw, lemon oil, tea tree oil or thyme oil can be added to a shampoo or soap and used as a wash.

Key Herbs: Garlic, Goldenseal, Paw Paw, Tea Tree and Thyme

Scars / Scar Tissue

A scar is a mark left in the skin by the healing of injured tissue. Scarring can be prevented by proper treatment of injuries. Applying herbs or essential oils that speed tissue healing, such as lavender essential oil, helichrysum essential oil, yarrow or calendula can help wounds heal without scarring. Helichrysum essential oil is especially effective, both at preventing scars and also helping to heal them. It can be mixed with vitamin E and applied to scar tissue to help dissolve it.

Therapies: Compress

Key Herbs: Aloe vera, **Calendula**, Lavender essential oil and Yarrow

Key Nutrients: MSM and **Vitamin E**

Schizophrenia

See also *Mental Illness* and *Abuse and Trauma*

Schizophrenia is a psychotic disorder characterized by loss of contact with the environment, and by noticeable deterioration in the level of functioning in everyday life. There is a disintegration of personality expressed as disorder of feeling, thought and conduct.

This condition may be associated with high copper levels that depress levels of vitamin C and zinc. Prenatal zinc deficiency has been linked with development of this disorder later in life. Possible damage to the pineal gland, which contains high levels of zinc, is another possible cause.

Schizophrenia may be related to excess dopamine in the brain. Magnesium deficiencies and hypoglycemia are very common in schizophrenia. Avoiding refined carbohydrates, stimulants like caffeine and consuming adequate protein often helps to stabilize this condition. It is also helpful to support the nerves with B-complex vitamins.

Supplementing with high doses of niacin can be curative in some people.

Emotional Healing Work is essential. Professional assistance should also be sought. See Mental Illness for more ideas.

Therapies: Avoid Caffeine, Emotional Healing Work and Low Glycemic Diet

Key Herbs: Scullcap (Skullcap) and Licorice

Key Nutrients: Folate (Folic Acid, Vitamin B9), **GABA**, **L-Glutamine**, **Zinc**, **Vitamin D**, **Vitamin B-12**, **Vitamin B-3 (Niacin)**, **Omega-3 Essential Fatty Acids**, **Magnesium**, **Vitamin C** and **Vitamin B-Complex**

Sciatica

See also *Backache (Back Pain, Lumbago)*

Sciatica is a pain along the course of the sciatic nerve, making pain common in the lower back, buttocks, hips and back of the thighs. This usually is isolated to one side of the body. It may involve pressure on the nerve from the hips being out of alignment. Chiropractic care can be very helpful. In Traditional Chinese medicine, the kidney energy (qi) builds the bones and structural misalignment may indicate poor kidney function. Hence, in addition to bodywork, Hydration therapy and a *Kidney Tonic Formula* may be of help. An herbal *Analgesic Formula* or MSM may help with pain.

Therapies: Hydration

Formulas: Kidney Tonic and Analgesic

Key Herbs: Black Cohosh, Corydalis, **St. John's wort**, Jamaican Dogwood and Prickly Ash

Key Nutrients: MSM

Scratches and Abrasions

See also *Wounds and Sores*

Wounds to the skin from sliding contact with sharp or rough objects or surfaces may benefit from various tissue healing herbs, including aloe vera, tea tree oil, yarrow and calendula. Topical application of plantain has helped to draw dirt out of abrasions.

Formulas: Topical Vulnerary

Key Herbs: Aloe vera, **Calendula**, **Plantain**, **Tea Tree essential oil**, Goldenseal and Yarrow

Scrofula

See *Tuberculosis (Consumption, Scrofula)*

Scurvy

Scurvy is a deficiency of vitamin C.

Key Herbs: Rose hips

Key Nutrients: Vitamin C

Seasonal Affective Disorder

See also *Depression*

Seasonal affective disorder (SAD) is a form of depression that occurs in the dark and dreary fall and winter months. It is believed to be due to a lack of exposure to natural sunlight. Full spectrum lighting is very helpful in preventing this condition, as is taking the "sunshine vitamin," vitamin D3. An *Antidepressant Formula* that uses lemon balm and St. John's wort as key ingredients may also be helpful.

Therapies: Affirmation and Visualization, Healthy Fats and Stress Management

Formulas: Antidepressant

Key Herbs: Lemon Balm and St. John's wort

Key Nutrients: Vitamin D and Omega-3 Essential Fatty Acids

Seborrhea

Seborrhea is characterized by scaly patches of skin. It is caused by a disorder of the oil producing glands. Good fats and fat soluble vitamins may be helpful, as well as topical applications of aloe vera gel with lemon or tea tree oils.

Therapies: Healthy Fats

Key Herbs: Aloe vera, Burdock and **Tea Tree essential oil**

Key Nutrients: Omega-3 Essential Fatty Acids, **Vitamin A** and Vitamin D

Seizures

See also *Epilepsy*

A seizure is a sudden convulsive attack. There is usually a clouding of consciousness involved. These are often a result of epilepsy. Seizures should be treated medically, but there are some herbs and nutrients that may be helpful as well. GABA is a calming neurotransmitter in the brain that keeps the brain from over firing, It may be helpful for seizures. Passionflower and valerian affect GABA receptors. Scullcap, lobelia, blue vervain and mistletoe are single herbs that have been historically used for seizures. A high fat diet may be helpful in controlling seizures. Seek appropriate medical attention.

Therapies: Healthy Fats

Formulas: Relaxing Nervine and Brain Calming

Key Herbs: Lobelia, **Scullcap (Skullcap)**, Hyssop, Mistletoe, Passionflower and Valerian

Key Nutrients: GABA and DHA

Senility

See also *Alzheimer's Disease*, *Memory and Brain Function* and *Dementia*

One of the potential physical and mental infirmities of old age is senility, an increasing loss of brain function. It is often a sign of poor circulation to the brain, a high carbohydrate and low fat diet, or a general lack of good nutrition for brain function. Staying physically and mentally active helps prevent senility. Antioxidants protect the brain from damage that lead to memory loss. *Brain and Memory Tonic Formulas* containing ginkgo, gotu kola, rosemary and/or sage may be helpful in maintaining healthy brain function as one ages. See related conditions for more suggestions.

Therapies: Fresh Fruits and Vegetables, Heavy Metal Cleanse and Low Glycemic Diet

Formulas: Brain and Memory Tonic

Key Herbs: Capsicum (Cayenne), **Ginkgo**, **Gotu kola**, **Rosemary**, Sage and Wood Betony

Key Nutrients: Omega-3 Essential Fatty Acids, **L-Glutamine**, GABA and **Vitamin B-12**

Sepsis

See *Blood Poisoning (Sepsis)*

Sex Drive (excessive)

See also *Abuse and Trauma*

When sex drive is excessive, resulting in promiscuous behavior, it is often a sign of emotional trauma and abuse. Emotional Healing Work and Flower Essences therapies can be helpful in working through these issues. Hops and chastetree can also be used to balance hormone function in males with excessive sex drive. Oat seed can be helpful in balancing hormones and stress in women.

Therapies: Emotional Healing Work, Fast or Juice Fast and Flower Essences

Formulas: Adaptogen

Key Herbs: Chastetree (Vitex), **White Pond Lily**, Hops and Oat seed (milky)

Sex Drive (low)

See also *Adrenals (exhaustion, weakness or burnout), Endometriosis, Fibroids (uterine), Hypothyroid, Erectile Dysfunction* and *Abuse and Trauma*

Health problems that interfere with sexual intimacy may not be life-threatening, but they can threaten the health of a marriage or relationship. Intimacy helps to forge a loving bond between a man and a woman, while the lack of intimacy can cause increased tension and friction in a relationship.

No two people are going to have the exact same needs when it comes to intimacy, so negotiation is always necessary in a relationship. But when one party loses interest completely or has health problems that make intimacy undesirable, it's time to seek some help.

While loss of desire is often due to unresolved conflicts in a relationship, it can also be an early warning sign of other health problems such as low thyroid, hormonal imbalances, depression or excess stress. These problems should be identified and corrected.

When there is no physical reason for loss of desire, honest communication and perhaps even counseling may be necessary. Touch and intimacy are forms of non-verbal communication, and according to David Schnarch, author of *Passionate Marriage: Keeping Love and Intimacy Alive in Committed Relationships*, what is happening in the bedroom is communicating very clearly what is happening in the marriage.

Sex and Nutrition

Healthy sexual desire and function starts with a healthy glandular system, and it's not just the reproductive glands we're talking about. The endocrine system is highly interconnected, so the thyroid, adrenals, pancreas and pituitary glands all play a role in reproductive health. The general poor nutrition of most modern Americans, coupled with exposure to xenoestrogens and other environmental toxins, is taking a huge toll on the endocrine system, which, in turn, is having an effect on our reproductive health (and our ability to be attractive to a partner).

For starters, let's look at the whole issue of attraction. The common saying is that beauty is only skin deep, but this isn't exactly true. General physical and emotional health increases our attractiveness to the opposite sex. This is because attraction is primarily based on instinctive programming in our lower (or reptilian) brain. Researchers have found that certain clues that trigger attraction are actually linked to signs of good health in a prospective partner.

For example, most of us are instinctively drawn to healthy skin. Skin problems, such as acne, aren't just cosmetic problems, they are usually signs of deeper health issues, such as a toxic condition of the liver and colon, overburdened kidneys and hormonal imbalances. So, taking care of your skin is an inside job that starts with good nutrition and detoxification.

Another piece of information research has uncovered about attraction has to do with waist-to-hip ratios. Both sexes find a slimmer waistline more naturally attractive. Again, excess weight around the abdomen is a sign of internal health problems such as blood sugar imbalances, stressed adrenals, low thyroid and so forth.

So, if we improve our general health, we improve our attractiveness. We should start by getting refined carbohydrates like sugar and white flour out of our diet as much as we can. We should also eliminate bad fats like margarine, shortening, processed vegetable oils and deep fried foods.

On the positive side, we should increase our consumption of fresh fruits and vegetables and select high-quality proteins and fats. Ideally, our proteins should be organic and from grass-fed animals or deep ocean fish. Good fats, such as wild salmon, sardines, avocados, olive oil and omega-3 essential fatty acids are also important.

Feeding our body right will not only help us look and feel our best, it will also give us more energy. This is important, since fatigue is a major reason for low sex drive.

Supporting Glandular Health

Although our sex drive is a complicated thing, it is largely the result of our hormones, so keeping our glandular system balanced is important. Xenoestrogens are disrupting hormonal balance in both men and women and should be avoided, but they aren't the only hormonal imbalance that results in reduced sex drive and health.

Low Thyroid

Low thyroid is a major cause of loss of desire in women. In fact, the thyroid plays such a critical role in reproductive health that naturopathic doctor Jack Ritchason has referred to it as the "third ovary." In addition to reduced sexual desire, low thyroid can cause weight gain, dry and lackluster skin, hair thinning, fatigue and depression. So, it's easy to see why thyroid health is important to feeling attractive and having energy for intimacy. A *Hypothyroid Formula* may help. See Hypothyroid for more suggestions.

Low Testosterone

Male testosterone levels have been falling in recent decades. This could be due to the combination of xenoestrogens, poor diet and lack of exercise. Testosterone isn't just important for a man's reproductive health, it's absolutely vital to his general health. Testosterone reduces fat, builds muscle and improves a man's mood and confidence.

While testosterone is the hormone that makes a man, a man, women also need it, only in lesser amounts. A certain amount of testosterone combined with estrogen is essential for a woman's sex drive. Progesterone, on the other hand, tends to lower sex drive in women.

One supplement for enhancing testosterone levels is DHEA. DHEA is the basic building block for all reproductive hormones, including testosterone, estrogen and progesterone. Herbs that enhance testosterone, such as ginseng, horny goat weed, maca and muira puama will also be helpful. Look for a *Male Aphrodisiac Formula* that contains these herbs.

Low Estrogen

Estrogen is a hormone that enhances female sex drive. If a woman's estrogen levels are low, she may experience a loss of sex drive along with vaginal dryness. Remedies that can balance estrogen in women include chaste tree berries and maca. These are often used in *Female Aphrodisiac Formulas*.

Adrenal Fatigue

DHEA is produced in the adrenal glands, along with numerous other hormones that affect metabolism, stress levels and fluid retention. The adrenal glands even produce sex hormones.

High stress levels deplete the adrenal glands, which can result in severe fatigue, excessive emotional sensitivity, poor sleep and a loss of interest in sex. It's only natural that our sex drive would diminish when we're in stressful times, as this isn't the best time to be bringing children into the world.

Adaptogen Formulas will often help restore sex drive when a person is under stress. When a person is exhausted from long term stress they may need an *Adrenal Tonic Formula* or DHEA.

Other Barriers to Intimacy

For some women vaginal dryness may interfere with the pleasure of intimacy. This may be due to low hormone levels, but using a natural lubricant can help.

Uterine fibroids or endometriosis can make intimacy painful for women. If intercourse is painful, seek medical help to determine the cause before determining an approach to treatment. Suggestions for dealing with these conditions are found in this book.

Unresolved sexual or emotional abuse can also adversely affect a person's sex drive. Emotional Healing Work may be necessary to overcome these problems.

Most barriers to intimacy can be overcome with patience, love, good communication and appropriate natural remedies. Seek professional assistance if necessary.

Therapies: Affirmation and Visualization, Avoid Xenoestrogens, Emotional Healing Work, Healthy Fats, Low Glycemic Diet and Stress Management

Formulas: Hypothyroid, **Male Aphrodisiac**, **Female Aphrodisiac**, Adrenal Tonic and Adaptogen

Key Herbs: Black Cohosh, **Damiana**, **Shatavari**, Eleuthero (Siberian ginseng), Ginseng (American), Ginseng (Asian, Korean), Horny Goat Weed (Epimedium), Kava-kava, Licorice, Maca, Muira Puama, Oat seed (milky) and Sarsaparilla

Key Nutrients: Omega-3 Essential Fatty Acids, Vitamin E, DHEA and **L-Arginine**

Shame and Guilt

See also *Abuse and Trauma*

The concept of guilt is associated with committing a trespass or "crime" against another person. When I injure someone by harming them, stealing from them or otherwise violating their inalienable rights I am guilty. When we are guilty of a trespass against others, it is natural and healthy to experience shame. Shame allows us to recognize that we have done something wrong and change our behavior. To be without shame, or "shameless," is to be without conscience and to be capable of harming others without remorse.

Shame is not healthy, however, when that shame is a result of being abused. Many times abusers try to make their victims feel like they were deserving of the abuse. The person internalizes this sense of guilt and feels ashamed of being who they are, even when they are not actually harming others. This toxic shame and guilt is unhealthy and needs healing.

Toxic shame not only creates poor self-esteem, which causes a person to tolerate abuse, it can actually cause a person's immune system to weaken. Because they have a hard time standing up for themselves, they lack the "fight" necessary to defend themselves and their body against harm.

Emotional Healing Work and Flower Essences therapy can be very helpful in healing this toxic shame.

Therapies: Affirmation and Visualization, Emotional Healing Work and Flower Essences

Formulas: Immune Stimulating

Key Herbs: Pine (White) flower essence

Shingles

See also *Chicken Pox*

Shingles is an infection by the *Herpes zoster* virus that causes chicken pox. It is theorized that by suppressing the fever in chicken pox, it inhibits the immune system from expelling the virus, which allows it to lie dormant until it flares up. Then, it causes acute inflammation and severe pain along the path of a specific nerve or nerves.

Antiviral Formulas may be helpful. St. John's wort can be particularly helpful, since it is anti-inflammatory, antiviral and helps ease nerve pain. Since flare-ups tend to occur when a person is under stress, *Relaxing Nervine* and *Adaptogen Formulas* may be helpful.

Therapies: Stress Management

Formulas: Antiviral, Relaxing Nervine, Adaptogen and Immune Stimulating

Key Herbs: Lemon Balm, **St. John's wort**, **Yarrow**, Isatis and Licorice

Key Nutrients: L-Lysine and **Vitamin A**

Shock

A sudden or violent disturbance in the mental or emotional faculties can put a person into a state of shock. Shock is characterized by paleness, rapid but weak pulse, rapid and shallow respiration, restlessness, anxiety or mental dullness, nausea or vomiting associated with reduced blood volume and low blood pressure and subnormal temperature. It usually results from severe injuries, hemorrhage, burns or major surgery.

Capsicum powder on the tongue can help relieve shock. Other aromatic herbs may have a similar effect. The Bach flower essence blend, Rescue Remedy®, is often helpful taken under the tongue. Have the person lie down and cover them with a blanket. If there is no sign of a spinal injury, attempt to elevate their feet above the level of their heart. Have them sip fluids to stay hydrated. Shock can be severe and medical attention is sometimes needed.

Therapies: Hydration

Key Herbs: Cinnamon, **Capsicum (Cayenne)**, Ginger, Hawthorn, Hops and Peppermint

Sickle Cell Anemia

See also *Anemia*

Sickle Cell Anemia is a hereditary form of anemia that causes abnormally shaped red blood cells. Although natural remedies may not cure the condition, some can be helpful in easing symptoms. Chlorophyll and zinc have helped some people. Herbs that help to build the blood such as *Iron Formulas* can be helpful.

Therapies: Mineralization

Formulas: Iron

Key Herbs: Alfalfa and Nettle (Stinging) leaf

Key Nutrients: Chlorophyll and Zinc

Sinus Infection

See also *Congestion (sinus)* and *Rhinitis*

Although antibiotics are commonly recommended for sinus infections, they rarely have a positive effect. Chronic sinus infections are typically the result of problems in the digestive tract and may be related to food allergies, food sensitivities and/or leaky gut syndrome. Using the Colon Cleansing and Eliminate Allergy-Causing Foods therapies is often the best long-term solution.

A number of companies sell *Sinus Decongestant Formulas*. Two very effective ingredients to look for in these formulas are fenugreek and thyme. Osha, Mormon or Brigham tea and horseradish can also help clear the sinuses.

Drink plenty of water and take a small pinch of salt with it. This helps increase mucus flow and helps the sinuses to drain properly.

For rapid relief, make a solution of sea salt and water, add a little xylitol to it, and use it as a nasal wash (neti pots are the perfect tool to use). Snuffing a mixture of equal parts goldenseal and bayberry into the sinuses may also bring rapid relief, but this can be uncomfortable.

Therapies: Colon Cleanse, Dietary Fiber, Eliminate Allergy-Causing Foods, Friendly Flora and Hydration

Formulas: Sinus Decongestant and Goldenseal & Echinacea

Key Herbs: Andrographis, Bayberry, **Thyme**, **Yerba Santa**, Echinacea, Fenugreek, Goldenseal, Lomatium and Osha

Key Nutrients: Digestive Enzymes, Probiotics, **Vitamin A**, **Vitamin C**, Bromelain and Colloidal Silver

Sinusitis (Sinus Problems)

See *Congestion (sinus)*, *Sinus Infection* and *Rhinitis*

Therapies: Aromatherapy and Fast or Juice Fast

Skin (acne)

See *Acne (Pimples, Blackheads)*

Therapies: Aromatherapy

Skin (dry and/or flaky)

See also *Fat Metabolism (poor)*, *Gall Bladder (sluggish or removed)*, *Hashimoto's Disease (Thyroiditis)* and *Hypothyroid*

The skin is kept moist by the secretion of sebum, a waxy-oily substance secreted by the sebaceous glands in the skin. This substance holds moisture in the skin, helping to keep it soft and moist. Dry skin is typically due to a lack of this secretion. A lack of healthy fats in the diet, poor fat digestion and metabolism, and low thyroid function are all possible causes of dry and flaky skin.

If you have problems with dry skin make sure you are eating healthy fats and avoiding processed fats like margarine, shortening and refined vegetable oils. Make sure you are able to properly digest fats by taking lipase enzyme or digestive enzyme supplements. Also make sure your liver and gallbladder are secreting bile to emulsify and digest the fats. A *Cholagogue Formula* can help with this. Skin problems often trace back to the liver, so a *Liver Tonic Formula* may also help.

Most frequently, however, dry skin is a sign of poor thyroid function. If your dry skin is accompanied by feeling easily chilled and tired, you may have a thyroid problem. The thyroid hormone regulates the combustion of fats and is essential for soft, moist skin. A *Hypothyroid Formula* may help, but be sure to look up additional suggestions under Hypothyroid and *Hashimoto's Disease*.

Therapies: Healthy Fats

Formulas: Hypothyroid, Cholagogue and Liver Tonic

Key Herbs: Burdock, Irish moss and Kelp

Key Nutrients: Omega-3 Essential Fatty Acids and MSM

Skin (infections)

See also *Fungal Infections (Yeast Infections, Candida albicans)*, *Infection (bacterial)* and *Infection (viral)*

When there is an infection in the skin, you can apply a *Topical Antiseptic Formula* directly to the affected areas or use the Compress therapy with extracts of infection-fighting herbs such as a *Goldenseal & Echinacea Formula*. You can also dilute essential oils like rosemary, tea tree and/or thyme with a fixed oil (such as olive oil) and apply this to affected areas. Dilution should be one part essential oil to ten parts fixed oil for normal situations or one part essential oil to twenty parts essential oil for sensitive skin or children. Internally, *Blood Purifier Formulas* have been used traditionally to help clear up skin infections. Gotu kola is a good single herb to take internally for fighting infections in the skin. If you know whether the infection is viral, fungal or bacterial, you can look up additional remedies under those related conditions.

Therapies: Aromatherapy and Compress

Formulas: Topical Antiseptic, Goldenseal & Echinacea, Blood Purifier and Skin Healing

Key Herbs: Burdock, **Echinacea**, **Tea Tree essential oil**, Goldenseal, Gotu kola, Pau d' Arco, Rosemary essential oil, Thyme essential oil and Yarrow

Key Nutrients: Vitamin A, Vitamin D, Vitamin C and **Colloidal Silver**

Skin (oily)

Oily skin can be a sign of problems with fat metabolism. Lipase enzyme supplements and *Cholagogue Formulas* can help the body process fats more effectively. The Drawing Bath therapy can be used to pull excess oil from the skin. A fine clay (such as Redmond clay) can be moistened and applied to the skin as a mask to draw out excess oils. Adding a drop or two of rosemary or rose essential oils to the mask will also be helpful.

Therapies: Colon Cleanse and Drawing Bath

Formulas: Blood Purifier and Cholagogue

Key Herbs: Burdock, Rose essential oil and Rosemary

Key Nutrients: Lipase Enzymes

Skin Care (general)

See also *Hypothyroid* and *Leaky Gut Syndrome*

The skin is the largest sensory organ in the body. Loaded with nerves that allow us to sense heat, cold, texture, pressure and pain, the skin allows us to "touch" the outside world. The fact that the skin is so connected with our nervous system is also revealed by how our skin communicates what is going on inside of us mentally and emotionally.

Through our skin we flush from excitement, we blush when we're embarrassed, we grow pale because of fear and we sweat over the "small stuff" that sometimes makes us feel overwhelmed and nervous. It is why we say that a person who is confident is "comfortable in their own skin." This strong connection to our emotions suggests we shouldn't discount the importance of positive mental attitudes and Emotional Healing Work in keeping the skin healthy.

Unhealed shame can be a big factor in skin diseases because how we look affects our self-esteem. Feeling ashamed of who we are, not wanting to be "seen" or feeling undesirable and unattractive can manifest in our skin. Likewise, skin conditions that arise from physical problems with our skin, can contribute to these emotional issues. The two go hand-in-hand and should always be worked on together.

Physically, the skin needs nutrition to be healthy, just like any other organ of the body. Skin conditions are not just "skin deep." They point to more deep-seated conditions like poor nutrition, toxicity of the liver, poor kidney function and problems with the mucus membranes of the gut. They can also point to imbalances in the glandular system.

Nutrients the skin needs include silica, calcium, trace minerals, good fats, fat soluble vitamins like A, D, E and K and vitamin C. Antioxidants protect the skin from damage from the sun and other environmental influences. Herbs helpful for topical application to the skin include seaweeds (dulse, kelp, etc.), rosemary, sage and chamomile. Internally, horsetail, dulse and gotu kola are helpful.

Traditionally *Blood Purifier Formulas* have been used to clear up skin conditions. Sweat Bath and Drawing Bath therapies are also great ways to detoxify the body and improve skin health.

When using products on your skin such as cosmetics, soaps and beauty care products, remember that your skin absorbs things. Don't put chemicals on your skin that you don't want in your body.

Since the skin reflects our emotions, managing stress is important in maintaining healthy skin. Emotional Healing Work may be needed to clear up emotional issues that are contributing to skin problems.

Therapies: Aromatherapy, Drawing Bath, Emotional Healing Work, Flower Essences, Fresh Fruits and Vegetables, Healthy Fats, Mineralization, Poultice and Sweat Bath

Formulas: Mineral and Blood Purifier

Key Herbs: Aloe vera, Bladderwrack, Chamomile (English and Roman), Chickweed, Comfrey, Elder flowers, Gotu kola, Horsetail, Irish moss, Kelp and Rosemary

Key Nutrients: Omega-3 Essential Fatty Acids, Colloidal Minerals, Vitamin A, Vitamin C, Vitamin D, Vitamin E, Silicon and Calcium

Sleep (restless and disturbed)

See also *Insomnia* and *Restless Dreams*

When a person falls asleep easily, but tosses and turns throughout the night, wakes up frequently and/or has disturbing dreams, this can be a sign of adrenal fatigue, blood sugar problems or liver problems. Start by adopting the Low Glycemic Diet therapy and avoiding stimulants like caffeine and spicy foods (especially in the evening). Make sure you are adequately hydrated.

If you wake up at night with thoughts racing through your head that prevent you from going back to sleep, try taking passionflower and/or GABA or an herbal *Sleep Formula* that contains them. Both GABA and passionflower calm the mind and help reduce mental chatter.

A protein snack (cottage cheese, nut butter, etc.) at bedtime can keep blood sugar levels stable during the night. This can help to prevent you from waking up after four or five hours unable to go back to sleep. An *Adaptogen Formula* may also help with this.

If you are disturbed by small noises and have highly sensitive nerves, you may be deficient in magnesium. Try taking magnesium at bedtime along with the herb scullcap.

For additional suggestions see Insomnia.

Therapies: Avoid Caffeine, Hydration, Low Glycemic Diet and Stress Management

Formulas: Sleep and **Adaptogen**

Key Herbs: Passionflower, **Scullcap (Skullcap)**, Hops, Licorice and Valerian

Key Nutrients: Melatonin, **Magnesium**, Vitamin C, Vitamin B-Complex and GABA

Sleep Apnea

See also *Weight Loss (aids for)*

Sleep apnea occurs when the throat closes down completely making it impossible to breathe while sleeping. This starves your tissues for oxygen, which can cause you to wake up after about a minute of not breathing, shift positions and go back to sleep. The problem is that you are not aware that you are waking up numerous times each night starved for oxygen.

Sleep apnea doesn't just interfere with your sleep; it is dangerous. Not only does it stress your heart and increase your risk of heart disease, you risk dying in your sleep from oxygen starvation. If you snore very loudly, get checked for sleep apnea. If you do have sleep apnea, medical help may be necessary to ensure you get enough oxygen for a sound night's sleep. To protect your heart, trying taking Co-Q10 and four hawthorn capsules at bedtime.

Factors that can contribute to snoring and sleep apnea include excess weight, swollen lymph nodes, sinus congestion, or any inflammation of the mucus membranes. *Allergy-Reducing* and *Decongestant Formulas* may help shrink swelling of inflamed mucus membranes, reduce sinus congestion and swollen lymph nodes and otherwise help to open respiratory passages. Food and respiratory allergies may be a factor, so use the Eliminate Allergy-Causing Foods therapy. High doses of vitamin C with bioflavonoids (2,000-3,000 milligrams per day) can help to counteract histamine reactions if allergies are a factor. Weight loss and colon cleansing are also helpful.

Therapies: Colon Cleanse and Eliminate Allergy-Causing Foods

Formulas: Cardiac Tonic, Allergy-Reducing and Decongestant

Key Herbs: Hawthorn

Key Nutrients: Vitamin C, Bioflavonoids and **Quercitin**

Slivers

Slivers are tiny pieces of wood or other material embedded in the skin. A *Drawing Salve* can help draw slivers out of the skin. Pine gum and crushed leaves of lily of the valley are also good for this. Apply the remedy and cover with a bandage. Tea tree oil can help prevent infection.

Therapies: Poultice

Formulas: Drawing Salve

Key Herbs: Lily of the Valley, Pine (White) gum and Tea Tree

Small Intestinal Bacterial Overgrowth (SIBO)

See also *Belching, Gas and Bloating, Gastritis* and *Leaky Gut Syndrome*

Intestinal microflora, also called friendly flora or probiotics, play a role in regulating the immune system and keeping the colon healthy. However, most of the bacteria in your intestines should be in your colon or large intestines, not your small intestines.

When abnormally large numbers of bacteria (even friendly bacteria) start growing in the small intestines, they actually cause problems with your health. Small Intestinal Bacterial Overgrowth (SIBO) is a condition where abnormally large numbers of bacteria are present in the small intestines.

These bacteria feed off of sugars and starches in the diet (both refined sugars and natural sugars) and produce methane and hydrogen gas. They also inhibit the enzymes in the small intestines that break down starches into simple sugars for absorption. This can result in abdominal bloating, belching and/or flatulence (intestinal gas), especially when you eat grains and other complex carbohydrates. The gases produced by these bacteria can also cause abdominal pain, intestinal cramping, and IBS with constipation and/or diarrhea.

Gas pressure in the small intestines can push upwards against the stomach, contributing to the development of a hiatal hernia and causing heartburn, acid reflux (GERD) and nausea.

SIBO increases a hormone called zonulin, causing an increase in small intestinal permeability (aka leaky gut syndrome), which results in the intestines absorbing large molecules they shouldn't. The bacteria also like to gobble up essential nutrients like fats, iron and vitamin B-12. The nutrient deficiencies from SIBO along with the absorption of large protein molecules can cause problems with the immune system and contribute to allergies, asthma, autoimmune disorders, and a general decline in health.

SIBO has wide ranging implications and may be a cause or a major factor in many diseases. GERD (or acid reflux), gas and bloating, and frequent belching are clues that SIBO may be a problem.

Other clues include having better bowel movements after taking antibiotics and bowel problems getting worse when taking probiotics or fiber. If bowel problems began after using opiates for pain, this is another clue that SIBO may be a factor.

Diagnosing SIBO

Experts in SIBO have estimated that about 35-50% of the general public has this problem. Unfortunately, it is not widely understood and hence, is not properly diagnosed. Many people who have SIBO think they have a candida or yeast infection. However, while yeast overgrowth can occur with or without SIBO, candida is often over diagnosed and SIBO is under diagnosed.

Medical diagnosis of SIBO is difficult because it is hard to get a culture from the small intestines. There are tests involving collecting breath samples from patients that drink either glucose or lactulose. The lactulose test is the most accurate. These tests must be ordered by a physician.

However, you can also assess this condition fairly accurately by symptoms. If you have an autoimmune disorder, pain in multiple joints, chronic allergies, chronic skin conditions, chronic fatigue or depression, or general malaise (just don't feel good) you may have leaky gut. When you have symptoms of leaky gut coupled with chronic diarrhea or constipation, regular abdominal pain, IBS, bloating or belching after meals, GERD and/or regular indigestion, you may have SIBO.

What Causes SIBO?

There are several major factors that contribute to the development of SIBO. The first is a lack of hydrochloric acid (HCl) in the stomach. HCl helps the body digest proteins, but it also helps to kill bacteria in the food we eat and prevent them from colonizing the small intestines.

A second factor is a lack of intestinal motility. In between meals migrating motor complexes (MMCs) sweep down the intestines, helping to flush bacteria. These movements of the small intestine are responsible for what we call hunger pains, the "rumblings" we feel in our gut when we haven't eaten in a while. These MMCs may be damaged by surgery, intestinal scarring, various diseases, intestinal infections, and certain drugs. Medications that can inhibit these intestinal movements include antibiotics, proton pump inhibitors, antacids and opiates (pain killers) like morphine.

Stress can be a factor in both low hydrochloric acid and the lack of intestinal motility, as the sympathetic nervous system (responsible for the fight or flight response) inhibits both digestive secretion and intestinal motility. When we are relaxed, the parasympathetic nervous system is more active and digestion and intestinal motility are enhanced. Unfortunately, many people in our society are eating on the run and do not take time to relax, chew their food thoroughly and enjoy their meals.

A final factor in SIBO is a malfunctioning ileocecal valve. This valve lies between the small and large intestines and is designed to prevent back flow (that is, to keep material in the large intestine from migrating back into the small intestine). When this valve is not shutting properly, intestinal bacteria migrate from the colon into the small intestine, causing gas, bloating and general weakness and malaise.

Natural Therapy for SIBO

Here are seven things you can do to overcome SIBO. Many of these things are also done for leaky gut.

Step One: Remove food and chemical irritants

Dietary adjustments are essential to overcoming both SIBO and leaky gut. It is absolutely essential to eliminate all refined sugars from the diet and most starchy foods. At the least one should eliminate grains containing gluten (wheat, rye, barley), but eliminating all grains may be required.

Dairy may also be problematic because the bacteria love to feast on lactose, the sugar in dairy. Goat milk products and cultured dairy foods can be beneficial for some people, yet other people may have to eliminate all dairy foods.

Fermented foods are generally helpful for SIBO. These are discussed under Step Six: Restore beneficial bacteria.

There are three dietary programs that may be helpful, depending on the severity of the problem. These are the Specific Carbohydrate Diet (SCD), the Gut and Psychology Syndrome (GAPS) diet and the Paleo diet. More information about these diets can be found in a webinar on this topic available at *www.modernherbalmedicine.com*.

Step Two: Stimulate production of and/or supplement stomach acid and enzymes

There are two ways to increase stomach acid and enzymes. One is to take supplements and the other is to take herbs and nutrients that stimulate their production. With SIBO it is normally necessary to do both.

To determine how much Betaine HCl you need, you can do a hydrochloric acid challenge test. Note: do not perform this test if you have an active ulcer or a history of ulcers.

To do the test, take a 400-500 mg capsule of Betaine Hydrochloric Acid (HCl) with pepsin prior to a meal. If you notice no burning, increase to two capsules the next meal. Proceed until you notice a mild burning sensation, then immediately reduce your dose to the number of capsules that preceded the burning or heat sensation. Most people find a comfortable dose between 400 and 1500 mg per meal (2-3 capsules).

If one or two capsules causes burning, you either don't have low stomach acid or your reflux is so severe that you won't be able to take HCL until you get it under control. Also, remember that the more protein you eat with a meal, the greater the need for HCl, so you can vary the dose with the size and content of your meals. Also, if you have severe digestive problems, you may also wish to take a complete food enzyme that has HCl and pancreatic enzymes.

Within 3-6 months most people feel a warmth in their stomach with the same dose they have been taking. When this happens it is time to decrease your dose and start weaning off of Betaine HCl.

You can also use *Digestive Bitter Tonic Formulas* to stimulate digestive secretions. Bitters not only stimulate HCl secretion, they also stimulate pancreatic enzymes and bile from the gallbladder and tend to be mildly antibacterial as well. Bitters should be taken 15-20 minutes prior to meals with one to two large glasses of water. A small pinch of a natural salt can also be taken at the same time, as this also helps stimulate HCl production by providing chloride.

Bitters are contraindicated if you have digestive atrophy. So, if you have dry mucus membranes, as evidenced by a dry and withered (or shriveled) looking tongue, don't take bitters because they dry the mucus membranes.

A lack of HCl may also be due to a lack of the following nutrients: chloride (low serum levels), zinc and thiamine. These are primary nutritional factors required for the synthesis of hydrochloric acid.

Step Three:
Improve intestinal motility (if necessary)

With SIBO it is also important to make certain that there is good intestinal motility between meals to flush the intestines and clear out bacteria. One way to do this is to allow adequate time between meals. Depending on the efficiency of your digestion, you need three to five hours between meals. Ideally, you should wait until you get stomach rumblings indicating your digestive tract is clear before eating the next meal.

If motility is slow there are some supplements that may be helpful. All carminatives increase digestive motility, and many people find that a cup of ginger tea is most helpful. You can also try taking 100 mg of 5-HTP twice daily or MotilPro from Pure Encapsulations (two capsules twice daily). If improvement isn't noted after two weeks, add 6 mg of melatonin before bed and three capsules of Methyl Guard (from Thorne) twice daily.

Step Four: Close the ileocecal valve (if necessary)

If there is severe gas and bloating, you probably need to work on the ileocecal valve. This is done by massaging the valve to reduce swelling and inflammation and get it to close properly. This is demonstrated in Steven's video on techniques for self-correction of a hiatal hernia at *modern-herbalmedicine.com*.

Step Five: Reduce bacteria

If a person has signs of SIBO, they will need to take some supplements to reduce bacterial overgrowth in the small intestines. This can be done with pharmaceutical antibiotics or herbal antibacterial agents.

For starters, one can take a *Digestive Bitter Tonic Formula* containing antibacterial herbs or take a *Digestive Bitter Tonic Formula* along with an herbal *Antibacterial Formula*. Another great remedy is enteric coated peppermint oil. Take one capsule with three meals each day for about 20 days. In clinical trials this was shown to cause a 25-50% reduction in small intestinal bacteria.

Garlic is another possible antimicrobial agent, but if friendly lacto bacteria are overpopulating the small intestines, it won't work. It does kill gram negative bacteria. The best way to take it is to chop up or crush fresh garlic, then mix it with a teaspoon of honey to make it easier to take. Encapsulated garlic products are generally ineffective.

Cinnamon kills both lactic acid bacteria and yeast. It is much more active than peppermint. Use it when you are sensitive to taking probiotics. Take two capsules three times daily with meals.

Goldenseal may also be helpful. It not only reduces intestinal bacteria, it also tones up digestive membranes and reduces irritation. It does lower blood sugar levels, however. Take two capsules three times daily with meals.

Note: It is not necessary to take ALL of the above remedies. That would be overkill. Pick one or two only, depending on your circumstances and what's available to you.

Step Six: Restore beneficial bacteria

All traditional cultures used some kind of cultured foods. Vegetables were commonly cultured, as were fruits and dairy foods. Studies have shown that it takes 10 billion encapsulated bacteria to obtain the same value to the intestines that just 100 million bacteria from food will provide. Furthermore, people with SIBO often do not do well on probiotic supplements, especially if they contain prebiotics which feed the small intestinal bacteria as well as friendly flora.

Cultured vegetables are very valuable in treating SIBO and leaky gut. You can make your own cultured vegetables or you can purchase them from a health food store or some supermarkets. Making your own cultured vegetables is quite easy. Recipes for making cultured vegetables can be found in the materials from our *Leaky Gut and SIBO* webinar (*modernherbalmedicine.com*), online or from the book *Nourishing Traditions* by Sally Fallon.

Step Seven: Repair gut integrity

Since SIBO always causes leaky gut, it is important to rebuild the integrity of the intestinal membranes. One of the best ways to do this is by using the Bone Broth therapy. Bone broth is high in glutamine and glycine, both of which are essential in healing the gut. They are emphasized in both the SCD and GAPS diet. Drink 1-4 cups of bone broth daily. You can also use it to make soups. Recipes for bone broth can be found online or in *Nourishing Traditions*.

If you can't take the bone broth, you can use l-glutamine, which can also be used along with bone broth. The best way to take it is to get l-glutamine powder and take 1 teaspoon three times daily mixed with food. Other remedies that help heal the gut include chamomile tea (one cup three times daily), deglycyrrhizinated licorice (2 capsules three times daily) and colostrum powder, one teaspoon twice daily.

Therapies: Bone Broth, Low Glycemic Diet and Stress Management

Formulas: Antibacterial, **Digestive Bitter Tonic**, Digestive Enzyme and Goldenseal & Echinacea

Key Herbs: Cinnamon, **Goldenseal**, Garlic and Peppermint essential oil

Key Nutrients: Betaine Hydrochloric Acid (HCl), Digestive Enzymes, L-Glutamine, Melatonin, 5-HTP and **Probiotics**

Smell (loss of sense of)

See also *Congestion (sinus)*

A loss of the sense of smell is sometimes due to a zinc deficiency. It can also be due to sinus congestion and nasal polyps, in which case a snuff made of bayberry and goldenseal may be helpful.

Key Herbs: Bayberry, Fenugreek, Goldenseal and Thyme

Key Nutrients: Zinc

Smoking

See *Addictions (tobacco smoking or chewing)*

Snake Bite

Astringent herbs have traditionally been applied topically to snake bites to promote healing and counteract the venom. One of the best astringent herbs for this purpose is plantain. Black cohosh and echinacea are also traditional snake bite remedies. They should be applied topically using the Compress or Poultice therapies, but may also be taken internally. Large doses of vitamin C internally (5,000 milligrams or more) may also be helpful. Seek medical attention if bitten by a poisonous snake and only use these remedies while in route to the hospital.

Therapies: Compress and Poultice

Key Herbs: Black Cohosh, **Echinacea** and **Plantain**

Key Nutrients: Vitamin C

Sneezing

See also *Congestion (sinus)*

Sneezing is a sudden, violent, spasmodic, audible expiration of breath through the nose and mouth, usually as a reflex reaction to an irritant in the nasal mucous membrane. It is often associated with allergies. A *Sinus Decongestant* or an *Allergy-Reducing Formula* may be helpful. Cleaning out the colon with Colon Hydrotherapy and drinking lots of water to stay well hydrated will help the body clear the congestion more quickly. Fenugreek and thyme are two great herbs for clearing congested nasal passages.

Therapies: Colon Hydrotherapy and Hydration

Formulas: Allergy-Reducing and Sinus Decongestant

Key Herbs: Bayberry, **Nettle (Stinging)**, Eyebright, Fenugreek and Thyme

Key Nutrients: Vitamin C and **Quercitin**

Snoring

See also *Allergies (food)*, *Allergies (respiratory)* and *Congestion (sinus)*

Snoring is caused by blockage in the respiratory passages that narrows the airways when sleeping. To clear this congestion use the Colon Cleanse and Eliminate Allergy-Causing Foods therapy. Use a *Sinus Decongestant* or a *Decongestant Formula* to clear the congestion and open up the airways. Hydration therapy also helps.

Therapies: Colon Cleanse, Eliminate Allergy-Causing Foods and Hydration

Formulas: Sinus Decongestant and Decongestant

Key Herbs: Fenugreek and **Thyme**

Key Nutrients: MSM and Co-Q10

Sore Gums

See *Gingivitis (Bleeding Gums, Gum Disease, Pyorrhea)*

Sore or Geographic Tongue

See also *Inflammatory Bowel Disorders (Colitis, IBS)*

A tongue that is covered with bare red patches alternating with heavily coated areas is called a geographic tongue. Both a geographic tongue and a sore tongue can be a sign of a vitamin B12, iron, folate or niacin deficiency. They can also indicate digestive mucosal irritation. Bitter herbs, especially if taken as powders, teas or tinctures can be helpful for cooling down this digestive irritation. Mix some goldenseal or yellow dock powder with powdered marshmallow root or aloe vera juice 15-20 minutes prior to meals. Digestive enzyme supplements may also be helpful.

Therapies: Dietary Fiber, Fresh Fruits and Vegetables and Friendly Flora

Formulas: Digestive Bitter Tonic and Digestive Enzyme

Key Herbs: Goldenseal, **Yellow Dock**, Dandelion and Marshmallow

Key Nutrients: Probiotics, Vitamin B-Complex, Vitamin B-6 (Pyridoxine), **Vitamin B-12**, Vitamin B-3 (Niacin), **Folate (Folic Acid, Vitamin B9)** and Iron

Sore Throat

See also *Strep Throat*

Sore throat is a discomfort in the pharynx due to inflammation. A number of herbs can be used as infusions (teas) and a gargle for sore throats. You can also make the gargle by diluting a tincture or extract in water. Good herbs for gargles include capsicum (stings at first, then numbs the pain), bayberry (great for loosening mucus), goldenseal (fights infection and reduces inflammation), myrrh (antiseptic) and sage (antiseptic).

You can also massage a *Topical Analgesic Formula* to the throat. Lobelia and capsicum extracts mixed in equal parts also make a great topical message for sore throats.

Sucking on slippery elm or licorice powder will ease irritation and dryness. Internally, a *Lymphatic Drainage Formula* can be used to clear swollen lymph nodes, which also helps.

If the problem is a bacterial infection (such as strep throat), then garlic and echinacea are good remedies. They are taken internally, but garlic oil can also be massaged topically into the throat. See Strep Throat for details.

Therapies: Hydration

Formulas: Topical Analgesic and Lymphatic Drainage

Key Herbs: Andrographis, Capsicum (Cayenne), Collinsonia (Stoneroot), **Bayberry**, **Red Root**, **Slippery Elm**, Echinacea, Elder berries, Garlic, Goldenseal, Isatis, Licorice, Lobelia, Lomatium, Myrrh, Osha, Platycodon (Balloon Flower), Sage and Usnea

Key Nutrients: Vitamin A, Vitamin C, Vitamin D and Colloidal Silver

Sores

See *Wounds and Sores*

Spasms

See *Cramps and Spasms (general)*

Spastic Colon

See *Colon (spastic)*

Spider Veins

See also *Cardiovascular Disease (Heart Disease)*

Spider veins can be an early warning sign of cardiovascular inflammation that can lead to cardiovascular disease. *Vascular Tonic Formulas* and *Anti-Inflammatory Formulas* can be helpful. Co-Q10, vitamin C and bioflavonoids will strengthen capillaries and help to reduce these unsightly veins. Spider veins can also indicate a copper deficiency, which should be tested for before supplementing with copper. A compress using an extract of rose hips, butcher's broom or bilberry will also help.

Therapies: Compress, Fresh Fruits and Vegetables and Healthy Fats

Formulas: Vascular Tonic and Anti-Inflammatory

Key Herbs: Bilberry (Blueberry, Huckleberry), **Butchers Broom**, **Horse Chestnut** and Rose

Key Nutrients: Vitamin C, Co-Q10, Omega-3 Essential Fatty Acids and Bioflavonoids

Spinal Meningitis

See *Meningitis*

Sprains

A sprain is caused by a sudden or violent twisting of a joint that causes stretching or tearing of ligaments, resulting in swelling, pain, inflammation, bruising and discoloration. Arnica is a wonderful remedy for sprains and can be applied topically as an oil or ointment and used internally as a homeopathic. Soaking the sprained joint in Epsom salts will help to reduce swelling. You can also make a soak or fomentation using decoctions of herbs like comfrey, willow, white oak bark and/or plantain. Using a *Tissue Healing Formula* internally can also speed healing.

Therapies: Epsom Salt Bath

Formulas: Topical Vulnerary and Tissue Healing

Key Herbs: Camphor, Comfrey, **Arnica**, **Solomon's Seal**, Plantain, White Oak, Willow and Witch Hazel

Key Nutrients: MSM and Vitamin C

Staph Infections

See also *Infection (bacterial)*

Staphylococcus are a particular type of bacteria that can invade the body. Serious infections may require medical attention, but raw garlic, goldenseal, Oregon grape, wild indigo and echinacea can be effective in fighting staph infections when taken internally and applied externally. Choose an *Antibacterial Formula* containing these herbs or use a *Goldenseal & Echinacea* or *Echinacea Blend Formula*. Vitamins A, D, and C can also be helpful. If you take an antibiotic, be sure to supplement with probiotics afterwards.

Therapies: Friendly Flora

Formulas: Antibacterial, **Goldenseal & Echinacea** and Echinacea Blend

Key Herbs: Echinacea, **Goldenseal**, Garlic, Oregon Grape, Tea Tree and Wild Indigo (Baptista)

Key Nutrients: Probiotics, Vitamin A, Vitamin C and **Vitamin D**

Stiff Neck

See also *Cramps and Spasms (general)*

Pain, inflammation and lack of mobility between the head and shoulders can be aided by massaging a *Topical Analgesic Formula* or lobelia extract into the neck and shoulders. Chiropractic care can be helpful. Blue vervain, Jamaica dogwood or wood betony may also be helpful for a stiff neck. Stress and fatigue, especially from working too much at a computer or other desk job can contribute to this problem. Take period breaks to stretch and relax. Make sure to drink plenty of water, too.

Therapies: Colon Cleanse, Hydration and Stress Management

Formulas: Topical Analgesic and Antispasmodic

Key Herbs: Blue Vervain, Jamaican Dogwood, Kava-kava, Kudzu, Lobelia and Wood Betony

Key Nutrients: MSM and **Magnesium**

Stomachache

See *Indigestion*

Strep Throat

See also *Sore Throat*

Strep throat is a sore throat that is caused by a particular type of infectious bacteria. Serious bacterial infections may require medical attention, but there are a few herbs that can be effective against strep. These include garlic (especially when raw), echinacea, usnea and goldenseal. Try making a gargle using a *Goldenseal & Echinacea Formula*. Take an *Antibacterial Formula* internally and drink plenty of water. It also helps to follow some of the general procedures listed under sore throat, such as massaging a *Topical Analgesic* or a *Topical Antiseptic Formula* into the outside of the throat. A type of Strep, specifically Group A Beta hemolytic streptococcal infection, if untreated can lead to rheumatic fever a serious condition. Untreated Strep will lead to rheumatic fever in about 3% of people. We recommend any child younger than 12 years old who tests positive for Strep and is running a fever higher that 102 be treated with antibiotics. For other cases of Strep please consult with a doctor.

Therapies: Hydration

Formulas: Goldenseal & Echinacea, Antibacterial, Topical Analgesic and Topical Antiseptic

Key Herbs: Andrographis, **Echinacea**, Garlic, Goldenseal, Pine (White), Tea Tree, Usnea and Wild Indigo (Baptista)

Key Nutrients: Vitamin C, Vitamin A and Zinc

Stress

See also *Anxiety Disorders*

Stress is a physical, chemical or emotional factor that causes bodily or mental tension and is a contributing factor to disease. Stress Management is discussed as one of the basic therapies in the *Therapies Section* because stress is involved in many different health problems.

Some basic supplements and herbs for stress include the following. Adaptogens help reduce the output of stress hormones, thus lowering baseline stress levels. This increases energy, boosts immunity and helps a person cope better both physically and emotionally with stress. Major adaptogens include ashwaganda, eleuthero, ginseng, gotu kola, holy basil and rhodiola. You can obtain the benefit of a variety of adaptogens by taking an *Adaptogen Formula*.

Nervines help the body relax, which can reduce anxiety and nervousness. They can also promote better sleep, which also helps a person cope with stress. Blue vervain, kava kava, chamomile, passionflower, St. John's wort, scullcap and valerian are all nervines that are helpful for counteracting stress. A *Relaxing Nervine Formula* will contain several of these herbs and have a synergistic effect in helping you to calm down. If sleep is a problem, these herbs also form the basis for *Sleep Formulas*.

Other remedies that help calm the nerves and enable a person to cope with stress better include B-Complex vitamins, vitamin C and magnesium. Avoid caffeine and sugar when under stress, as they cause further depletion of the nerves. Drink plenty of pure water, as hydration also helps the body cope better with stress.

When nerves feel "shot" because of stress, borage, milky oat seed, scullcap and magnesium can all be helpful remedies. You can also look for a *Nerve Tonic Formula*.

Therapies: Avoid Caffeine, Hydration and Stress Management

Formulas: Adaptogen, **Relaxing Nervine** and Sleep

Key Herbs: Borage, Chamomile (English and Roman), **Ashwaganda**, **Blue Vervain**, **Eleuthero (Siberian ginseng)**, **Kava-kava**, **Motherwort**, **Scullcap (Skullcap)**, Ginseng (American), Ginseng (Asian, Korean), Gotu kola, Holy Basil, Oat seed (milky), Passionflower, Pulsatilla, Rhodiola, St. John's wort and Valerian

Key Nutrients: 5-HTP, Vitamin B-3 (Niacin), Pantothenic Acid (Vitamin B5), **Magnesium**, **Vitamin B-Complex**, Vitamin C and Potassium

Stretch Marks

Stretch marks are lines of scarred tissue that form on the surface of the skin when the skin is stressed from rapid growth. For instance, stretch marks are common from pregnancy or rapid weight gain. In pregnancy, they are commonly found on the belly, hips and or thighs. Vitamin E and zinc can help prevent stretch marks. Massaging cocoa butter, coconut, olive or peanut oil into the skin can also help prevent them.

Key Nutrients: Vitamin E and Zinc

Strokes

See also *Blood Clots (prevention of)*, *Hypertension* and *Thrombosis*

A stroke causes temporary or permanent loss of blood flow to an artery of the brain and the part of the brain that artery feeds. It may be caused by an arterial rupture or a blood clot. The type and degree of damage depends on the size and location of the portion of the brain affected. Appropriate medical attention should be sought immediately following a stroke. Capsicum and ginkgo can be administered while waiting for medical assistance.

To reduce one's risk of stroke, *Cardiovascular Stimulant Formulas* can be used to enhance circulation as one gets older. Make sure to keep blood pressure managed, as high blood pressure increases the risk of stroke.

Magnesium, potassium, vitamin C and omega-3 essential fatty acids can all reduce one's risk of stroke. Butcher's broom, horsechestnut, vitamin E and *Vascular Tonic Formulas* can all reduce the risk of blood clots that cause strokes. See related conditions for more information.

Therapies: Fresh Fruits and Vegetables and Healthy Fats

Formulas: Cardiovascular Stimulant

Key Herbs: Capsicum (Cayenne), **Butchers Broom**, **Ginkgo** and Horse Chestnut

Key Nutrients: Potassium, Omega-3 Essential Fatty Acids, Magnesium, Vitamin C and Vitamin E

Stye

See also *Eye Infections*

An inflamed swelling of a sebaceous gland at the margin of the eyelid is called a stye. Eyebright or chamomile, made into a tea and applied to the eyes using the Compress therapy, can be very effective for treating styes. You could also try an herbal *Eye Wash Formula* used as a wash or a compress. Vitamins A and D help eye infections to heal more rapidly.

Therapies: Compress

Formulas: Eye Wash

Key Herbs: Chamomile (English and Roman), Eyebright and Goldenseal

Key Nutrients: Vitamin A and Vitamin D

Sugar Cravings

See *Addictions (sugar and refined carbohydrates)* and *Hypoglycemia*

Sunburn

See also *Burns and Scalds*

Varying degrees of damage to the skin due to overexposure result in sunburn. One of the most effective natural remedies for this problem is aloe vera gel applied topically. Lavender oil is also helpful when applied topically. Keeping the burn moist with pure water in a spray bottle also speeds healing. Large doses of vitamin C taken internally also speeds recovery.

Therapies: Fresh Fruits and Vegetables and Hydration

Key Herbs: Chamomile (English and Roman), **Aloe vera**, **Lavender essential oil** and Tea Tree

Key Nutrients: Vitamin C

Surgery (healing from)

See also *Injuries*

After surgery, the body needs support to complete the healing process. Vulnerary herbs, such as calendula, comfrey, marshmallow, oak bark and plantain, can be used to stimulate tissue repair. You can obtain several of these herbs at once by using a *Tissue Healing Formula* internally. You can also apply a *Topical Vulnerary Formula* to incisions to speed healing.

A number of nutrients also aid the healing process, including vitamin C, vitamin E and zinc. These nutrients help prevent scarring.

Minerals also aid tissue repair when recovering from injury or surgery. Colloidal mineral supplements or an herbal *Mineral Formula* will support more rapid recovery.

The liver has to detoxify any anesthetic drugs used during surgery, so using a *Blood Purifier* or a *Liver Tonic Formula* can aid this process. B-complex vitamins, milk thistle, n-acetyl-cysteine and red clover are also helpful.

Since antibiotics are used to prevent infection during and after surgery, it is very important to restore normal gut flora by using probiotic supplements and/or eating fermented foods following surgery. Taking 2,000 mg of MSM and 2,000 mg of vitamin C twice a day after surgery greatly speeds the healing process. Arnica homeopathic can be taken several times a day to reduce inflammation and pain.

Therapies: Affirmation and Visualization, Friendly Flora, Healthy Fats, Mineralization and Poultice

Formulas: Topical Vulnerary, **Tissue Healing**, Blood Purifier, Liver Tonic and **Mineral**

Key Herbs: Alfalfa, Comfrey, **Calendula**, Milk Thistle, Plantain and Red Clover

Key Nutrients: Bromelain, Pantothenic Acid (Vitamin B5), Colloidal Minerals, Omega-3 Essential Fatty Acids, Vitamin C, Vitamin E, Zinc, Vitamin B-Complex, N-Acetyl Cysteine, Probiotics, **MSM** and L-Arginine

Surgery (preparation for)

Prior to surgery, discontinue any herbs that may have a blood thinning effect, including alfalfa, ginkgo, garlic and willow. It may also be wise to discontinue taking vitamin E. *Hepatoprotective Formulas* containing milk thistle, schisandra and other remedies that aid the liver's ability to cope with chemicals can be taken prior to surgery to help the liver handle the drugs used in the hospital.

Herbal *Iron Formulas*, herbal *Mineral Formulas*, Colloidal Mineral supplements and a good multivitamin might also be helpful in making sure the body is adequately prepared for the surgery. *Mushroom Blend* and *Tissue Healing Formulas* could also be used to strengthen the body prior to surgery.

Since surgery is a stressful event, Stress Management therapy can be practiced before hand to keep stress hormones at a minimum. This will help the body be better prepared to handle the stress of surgery. It also helps to use Affirmation and Visualization therapy, affirming or visualizing that all will go well during the procedure. Prayer has also been documented to improve outcomes during surgery.

Therapies: Affirmation and Visualization, Mineralization and Stress Management

Formulas: Hepatoprotective, Mushroom Blend, Iron, Mineral and Tissue Healing

Key Herbs: Butchers Broom, Capsicum (Cayenne), Milk Thistle and Schisandra (Schizandra)

Key Nutrients: Colloidal Minerals, Vitamin B-Complex and **Vitamin C**

Sweating

See *Perspiration (excessive)*

Swelling

See *Edema (Dropsy, Water Retention, Swelling)*

Syndrome X

See *Hyperinsulinemia (Metabolic Syndrome, Syndrome X)*

Syphilis

Syphilis is a sexually transmitted bacterial infection. It is best treated medically with antibiotics. Echinacea and Goldenseal may be somewhat helpful, but antibiotics are generally needed. After taking antibiotics, be sure to replace friendly flora with probiotic supplements. The disease can be prevented by having sexual relations only within committed relationships or using condoms when having sex with partners who have not been tested for sexually transmitted diseases.

Therapies: Friendly Flora

Formulas: Goldenseal & Echinacea

Key Herbs: Echinacea, Goldenseal and Oregon Grape

Key Nutrients: Probiotics

Tachycardia

See also *Hyperthyroid (Grave's Disease)*

Tachycardia is a rapid beating of the heart. This condition requires medical attention, but can be aided by natural remedies in some cases. Motherwort is one of the safest herbal remedies for this condition. Other remedies that might help include lobelia, which acts as a natural beta blocker, mistletoe (which should be used under professional supervision) and magnesium, which can help calm and strengthen the heart beat. Grave's disease can cause tachycardia. Stress and a lack of mineral electrolytes like magnesium, calcium and potassium can also be causal factors.

Therapies: Hiatal Hernia Correction, Mineralization and Stress Management

Key Herbs: Bugleweed, **Motherwort**, Hawthorn, Lemon Balm, Lobelia and Mistletoe

Key Nutrients: Calcium, Potassium, **Magnesium** and Colloidal Minerals

Teeth (grinding)

See also *Parasites (general)* and *Stress*

The often unconscious habit of gritting the teeth together during sleep or periods of stress is often due to a lack of trace minerals, calcium deficiency, parasites or stress. Look under related conditions for information on how to treat these root causes. Mineral supplements can help relieve this condition.

Therapies: Mineralization and Stress Management

Formulas: Relaxing Nervine

Key Herbs: Bacopa (Water Hyssop), **Blue Vervain** and **Motherwort**

Key Nutrients: Calcium, Pantothenic Acid (Vitamin B5), **Magnesium** and Vitamin B-3 (Niacin)

Teeth (loose)

See also *Gingivitis (Bleeding Gums, Gum Disease, Pyorrhea)*

Teeth which are not properly rooted or firmly attached into the gums of the mouth and thus wiggle back and forth in their sockets may be aided by remedies that strengthen tissue integrity and reduce inflammation. White oak bark tea can be used as a mouthwash. Brushing with a toothpowder made from equal parts white oak bark and black walnut can also be helpful.

Therapies: Fresh Fruits and Vegetables and Mineralization

Key Herbs: Black Walnut and **White Oak**

Key Nutrients: Vitamin C, Co-Q10 and Colloidal Minerals

Teething

In the process of developing the first set of teeth and having them push through the gums, infants often develop pain, irritability, fever and earache. Rubbing clove oil diluted in olive oil can ease gum pain. Lobelia can also be rubbed on the gums. Chamomile tea or homeopathic chamomile is a traditional remedy for this.

Key Herbs: Catnip, Clove essential oil, **Chamomile (English and Roman)**, Lobelia and Passionflower

Tendonitis

Inflammation of a tendon or tendons of the body is often due to injury or overexertion. *Anti-Inflammatory* and *Tissue Healing Formulas* may be helpful in speeding recovery. Use a *Topical Analgesic Formula* to ease pain.

Formulas: Anti-Inflammatory, Tissue Healing and Topical Analgesic

Key Herbs: Boswellia, **Solomon's Seal** and Willow

Key Nutrients: MSM

Tension

See also *Stress* and *Anxiety Disorders*

Uneasiness or stress due to illness or emotional trauma can cause muscles to become tense. *Antispasmodic* herbs are used to relax tense muscles. They may be taken internally or massaged in topically. Kava-kava, lobelia and skunk cabbage are three excellent antispasmodic remedies and can often be found in *Antispasmodic Formulas*. Magnesium is also helpful for reducing muscle tension and can be taken orally or obtained through using the Epsom Salt Bath therapy or magnesium chloride oil topically. When tension is chronic, Emotional Healing Work may be needed.

Therapies: Emotional Healing Work, Epsom Salt Bath and Stress Management

Formulas: Antispasmodic

Key Herbs: Black Cohosh, California Poppy, Chamomile (English and Roman), **Blue Vervain**, **Kava-kava**, **Lobelia**, **Skunk Cabbage**, Jamaican Dogwood, Mimosa (Albizia, Silk Tree) and Wood Betony

Key Nutrients: Magnesium

Testosterone (low)

See also *Erectile Dysfunction* and *Sex Drive (low)*

Testosterone is the principle male hormone. It stimulates sperm production, libido, muscular strength and the physical characteristics of the male. Low testosterone causes a number of symptoms including frustration and anxiety, mild depression, low self-esteem, decreased sex drive, lack of muscle tone and muscle wasting. Men's testosterone levels have fallen sharply; most men have half the levels of testosterone men had 20 years ago, which is bad for their health. Here are some tips for increasing testosterone levels.

Excess estrogens upset the balance between testosterone and estrogen in men, and xenoestrogens are a principle cause of this imbalance. So, follow the therapy Avoid Xenoestrogens to promote better testosterone levels.

Men suffering from any kind of male reproductive problems should also be aware that too many phytoestrogens (estrogenic compounds found in plants) can cause imbalances in testosterone and estrogen levels. One of the principle culprits here is soy. Widely touted as a beneficial health food, according to the Weston Price Foundation, "Numerous animals studies show that soy foods cause infertility in animals ... Japanese housewives feed tofu to their husbands frequently when they want to reduce his virility." So use soy sparingly.

Men should also avoid consuming large amounts of licorice, as it enhances cortisol and decreases testosterone. Hops is another highly estrogenic herb. It contains very potent estrogens that can reduce male sex drive. Since most beer is made with hops, men who are concerned about their fertility or who are suffering from male reproductive health problems should avoid drinking beer made from hops. Finally, grapefruit interferes with estrogen breakdown and should also be consumed sparingly by men who wish to enhance their testosterone levels.

Drugs can also adversely affect testosterone levels. Classes of medications that may interfere with male reproductive function include anti-inflammatories, antibiotics, antifungals, statins (cholesterol-lowering medications), antidepressants, calcium channel blockers, sleeping pills and high blood pressure medications. Carefully read warning labels to discover if any medications you take may be affecting your reproductive health.

Diets that are high in refined carbohydrates and low in good fats and protein will also damage male reproductive health. High carbohydrate diets stress the adrenal glands and pancreas, resulting in increased levels of insulin and reduced levels of DHEA, a building block for male hormones. Also, the current drive to lower cholesterol levels is increasing depression and reproductive health problems in men. DHEA and all reproductive hormones are made from cholesterol, so driving cholesterol levels too low will actually cause reproductive problems in both sexes.

Organic meat, eggs and dairy products are actually good for you, especially if they are from grass-fed animals. Get white bread and refined sugar out of your diet and eat organic fruits and vegetables instead. These foods also protect your body from heart disease and cancer.

Finally, exercise regularly. Regular exercise helps increase testosterone production. It also reduces your risk of cardiovascular disease, diabetes and other degenerative diseases. Resistance training with weights is especially important for men as they grow older.

Herbs that can enhance testosterone levels include ginseng, horny goat weed, maca, muira puama, tribulus and pine pollen. These form the basis for *Male Aphrodisiac*

Formulas. DHEA is a building block for testosterone and supplementing with it can also be helpful. However, we recommend getting your levels tested before using DHEA supplements.

Therapies: Avoid Xenoestrogens, Exercise and Healthy Fats

Formulas: Male Aphrodisiac and Male Glandular Tonic

Key Herbs: Cinnamon, **Ginseng (Asian, Korean)**, **Muira Puama**, Damiana, Eleuthero (Siberian ginseng), Ginseng (American), Horny Goat Weed (Epimedium), Maca, Pine (White) pollen, Sarsaparilla and Tribulus

Key Nutrients: DHEA and Omega-3 Essential Fatty Acids

Tetanus

See also *Wounds and Sores*

Tetanus is an acute infectious disease characterized by tonic spasm of voluntary muscles, especially those of the jaw. It is caused by a toxin from a specific bacteria, which is usually introduced through a wound. Medical advice is to obtain a tetanus shot for any deep puncture wounds. However, if wounds are properly cleansed and topical antiseptics (such as tea tree oil) are applied, the risk of tetanus is very slight. If tetanus does develop, medical attention should be sought, but lobelia has been used in natural treatment.

Therapies: Compress

Formulas: Topical Antiseptic and Topical Analgesic

Key Herbs: Tea Tree essential oil, Lobelia and Thyme

Thinking (cloudy)

See also *Adrenals (exhaustion, weakness or burnout), Hyperinsulinemia (Metabolic Syndrome, Syndrome X), Hypoglycemia* and *Insomnia*

When a person's thinking is "cloudy" or they are having a difficult time concentrating, remembering or thinking clearly, they may be "toxic" and need cleansing, or there may be a deficiency of blood flow to the brain. They may also be dehydrated, not getting enough sleep, have low thyroid or be lacking omega-3 fatty acids. Protein deficiencies and hypoglycemia may also be involved.

Start by adopting the Low Glycemic Diet therapy. Adequate protein intake is necessary for the production of neurotransmitters, which are made from amino acids using B-complex vitamins and minerals. So eat protein foods for breakfast and avoid refined carbohydrates.

Even slight dehydration makes it harder to think clearly, so stay properly hydrated.

You can also use a *Brain and Memory Tonic Formula* to promote better mental alertness. If you are tired and not sleeping well, you may need to build up your adrenal glands (See Adrenals (exhaustion, weakness or burnout). An *Adaptogen Formula* may help if the adrenals and stress are involved. If you aren't getting enough sleep, try an herbal *Sleep Formula* at night and look up other remedies for Insomnia.

Therapies: Colon Cleanse, Heavy Metal Cleanse, Hydration and Low Glycemic Diet

Formulas: Brain and Memory Tonic, Adaptogen and Sleep

Key Herbs: Bacopa (Water Hyssop), **Rosemary**, Ginkgo, Ginseng (American), Gotu kola and Peppermint

Key Nutrients: Digestive Enzymes, Vitamin B-Complex and L-Glutamine

Thrombosis

See also *Blood Clots (prevention of)*

A blood clot within a blood vessel is called thrombosis. The formation of these clots is dangerous because if they break loose they can lodge in the heart or brain, causing a heart attack or stroke. Medical doctors often prescribe blood thinners to avoid thrombosis, but there are many herbs and supplements that can help, too. Butcher's broom, horse chestnut, garlic and ginkgo all help to prevent blood clots from forming in the circulatory system. Vitamin E is also helpful. Keep blood pressure down and stay properly hydrated, as this also helps prevent thrombosis.

Therapies: Hydration

Formulas: Vascular Tonic

Key Herbs: Butchers Broom, Garlic, Ginkgo, Guggul and Horse Chestnut

Key Nutrients: Vitamin E

Thrush

See also *Fungal Infections (Yeast Infections, Candida albicans)*

Thrush is a Candida or yeast infection of the mouth marked by white patches in the oral cavity. It typically occurs in infants and children. For rapid relief mix equal amounts of tea tree oil, thyme oil, and lavender oil and dilute them 20-to-1 in olive oil (20 parts olive oil, 1 part essential oils). Take or administer one drop of this mixture twice daily. You can also use an *Antifungal Formula*. It is also important to supplement with probiotic supplements.

Therapies: Friendly Flora

Formulas: Antifungal

Key Herbs: Lavender essential oil, Pau d' Arco, Tea Tree essential oil and Thyme essential oil

Key Nutrients: Probiotics

Thyroid (high)

See *Grave's Disease*

Thyroid (low)

See *Hypothyroid*

Tick

See also *Lyme Disease*

A tick is a small, blood-sucking insect whose bite can carry diseases such as Lyme's or Rocky Mountain spotted fever. Paw paw may help to kill ticks if applied topically. Ticks should not be crushed when removed. Garlic is a natural tick repellant. If you get bitten by a tick, get checked for infection, as antibiotics can be very helpful in treating tick-born illness if used early on.

Formulas: Antibacterial

Key Herbs: Garlic, Paw Paw and Tea Tree essential oil

Key Nutrients: Vitamin C

Tickle in Throat

See also *Cough (dry)*

An annoying sensation in the pharynx that feels like a tickle can often be relieved by sucking on licorice or slippery elm powder.

Therapies: Hydration

Key Herbs: Licorice, **Slippery Elm** and Marshmallow

Tics

See also *Twitching* and *Tremors*

A tic is a spasmodic muscular contraction. The movement may appear voluntary or purposeful, but is involuntary. These are often due to deficiencies of mineral electrolytes like magnesium, potassium and calcium. *Antispasmodic Formulas* and herbs like lobelia and blue vervain may be helpful for tics.

Therapies: Epsom Salt Bath

Formulas: Antispasmodic

Key Herbs: Blue Vervain and Lobelia

Key Nutrients: Calcium, Potassium, **Magnesium**, Vitamin B-Complex and Vitamin B-12

Tinnitus (Ringing in the Ears)

See also *Ear Infection or Earache*

Tinnitus refers to a sound in the ears when no outside sound is present. Tinnitus can sound like ringing, hissing, roaring, pulsing, whooshing, chirping, humming, whistling or clicking. One third of all adults experience tinnitus at some time in their lives. To see if you have problems with tinnitus, start by answering yes or no to the following questions:

_____ Do you have a problem hearing over the telephone?

_____ Do you hear better through one ear than the other when you are on the telephone?

_____ Do you have trouble following conversation when two or more people are talking at the same time?

_____ Do people complain that you turn the TV volume up too high?

_____ Do you have to strain to understand conversation?

_____ Do you have trouble hearing when there is a lot of background noise?

_____ Do you have trouble hearing in restaurants?

_____ Do you have dizziness, pain or ringing in your ears?

_____ Do you find yourself asking people to repeat themselves?

_____ Do family members or coworkers comment about your missing what has been said?

_____ Do many people you talk to seem to mumble (not speak clearly)?

_____ Do you misunderstand what others are saying and respond inappropriately?

_____ Do you have trouble understanding the speech of women and children?

_____ Do people get annoyed because you misunderstand what they say?

If you answered "yes" to more than two of these questions, you should have your hearing evaluated by a certified audiologist. He or she will perform an audiogram, which shows the results of pure-tone hearing tests. Based on the type, degree and configuration of your hearing loss, the audiologist can make appropriate recommendations.

Tinnitus may be caused by ear infections, circulatory problems or nerve damage. It can also be caused by chronic tension in the muscles holding the bones of the middle ear. These muscles tense to reduce vibration when we hear loud noises and like any other muscle can fatigue from chronic tension.

Lobelia extract warmed to body temperature to use as ear drops may be helpful in treating tinnitus as it will help to relax these tiny muscles. Gingko biloba and *Cardiovascular Stimulant Formulas* may be helpful when the problem is due to circulatory problems. St. Johns wort may be helpful when the problem is due to nerve damage.

For infections, See Ear Infection or Earache

Formulas: Cardiovascular Stimulant

Key Herbs: Black Cohosh, Cordyceps, **Ginkgo**, Garlic, Gotu kola, Hawthorn, Kudzu, Lobelia, Mistletoe, St. John's wort and Wood Betony

Key Nutrients: Vitamin B-12, Vitamin B-Complex and Zinc

TMJ

TMJ stands for temporomandibular joint or the point at which the lower jaw meets the temple region of the skull. Those who suffer from "TMJ" experience headaches and radiating pain from this region. Mechanical work by a massage therapist or chiropractor is often helpful. An *Antispasmodic Formula* to relax muscle tension may also be helpful, both taken internally and applied topically.

Therapies: Stress Management

Formulas: Antispasmodic

Key Herbs: Kava-kava and Lobelia

Key Nutrients: Magnesium and Glucosamine

Tonsillitis (Adenoids)

When there is inflammation and swelling of the tonsils or lymph nodes located at the back of the throat (also known as adenoids), they can obstruct the nasal and ear passages resulting in mouth breathing, snoring and nasal discharge. If chronically inflamed, they can become a site of infection. Some herbs that can be helpful for tonsillitis include echinacea, garlic, red root and wild indigo. Look for an herbal *Antibacterial Formula* containing several of these herbs or try an *Echinacea Blend* or *Goldenseal & Echinacea Formula*.

Therapies: Colon Cleanse and Eliminate Allergy-Causing Foods

Formulas: Antibacterial, Goldenseal & Echinacea and Echinacea Blend

Key Herbs: Blue Vervain, Capsicum (Cayenne), **Andrographis**, **Echinacea**, **Red Root**, Garlic, Goldenseal, Oregano, Slippery Elm and Wild Indigo (Baptista)

Key Nutrients: Vitamin A and Vitamin C

Tooth Decay (prevention)

Helping the teeth to have proper mineralization can help prevent tooth decay. Brushing with a toothpowder made of white oak bark and black walnut hulls can help strengthen enamel. Contrary to popular belief, teeth do remineralize when a person takes fat soluble vitamins (particularly D3 and K2) and minerals.

Therapies: Bone Broth, Healthy Fats and Mineralization

Formulas: Mineral

Key Herbs: Alfalfa, **Black Walnut**, Tea (Green or Black) and White Oak

Key Nutrients: Colloidal Minerals, Omega-3 Essential Fatty Acids, Vitamin B-6 (Pyridoxine), Vitamin B-Complex, **Vitamin D** and Vitamin K

Tooth Extraction

After a tooth has been removed by pulling or surgery goldenseal, oak bark or plantain can be used topically to ease pain and promote more rapid healing. An herbal *Analgesic Formula* can be used to reduce pain.

Formulas: Analgesic

Key Herbs: Goldenseal, Plantain, Valerian and White Oak

Key Nutrients: Vitamin C

Tooth Grinding

See *Teeth (grinding)*

Toothache

Pain in or around a tooth often as a result of a cavity or gum disease can be eased by *Anti-Inflammatory* and herbal *Analgesic Formulas*. Some of the best herbs for easing the pain are Jamaican dogwood, kava-kava and lobelia. Clove oil, diluted in olive oil, can be applied topically to ease pain. You can also slice a piece of garlic, coat it with olive oil and put it in between the cheek and the gum to fight the infection, relieve pain and ease the swelling of dental abscesses until a dentist can repair the tooth. All of these are temporary measures to use while seeking dental assistance.

Formulas: Anti-Inflammatory and Analgesic

Key Herbs: Chamomile (English and Roman), Clove, **Spilanthes**, Garlic, Jamaican Dogwood, Kava-kava, Lobelia, Tea Tree and Thyme

Toxemia

See also *Pregnancy (herbs and supplements for)*

An abnormal condition of toxic substances in the blood is called toxemia. When this occurs in pregnancy it is marked by high blood pressure, protein in the urine, swelling, headache, visual disturbances and possibly even convulsions. Seek appropriate medical assistance. A *Blood Purifier Formula* or a tea of red clover or pau d'arco may be helpful. Proper attention to prenatal care and a healthy diet during pregnancy will reduce the risk of toxemia.

Therapies: Colon Cleanse, Drawing Bath, Fast or Juice Fast and Hydration

Formulas: Blood Purifier and General Detoxifying

Key Herbs: Burdock, **Milk Thistle**, Pau d' Arco and Red Clover

Key Nutrients: MSM, Chlorophyll and **Vitamin C**

Toxic Blood

See *Blood Poisoning (Sepsis)*

Tremors

See also *Adrenals (exhaustion, weakness or burnout)*, *Twitching* and *Tics*

A tremor is an involuntary quivering of a muscle. This can be due to severe depletion of muscle energy or nervous system problems. It often indicates low levels of potassium or magnesium and may also be a sign of exhausted adrenals. Besides these minerals, B-complex vitamins, *Antispasmodic* or *Nerve Tonic Formulas* and herbs like scullcap and wood betony may be helpful.

Formulas: Antispasmodic

Key Herbs: Blue Vervain, **Scullcap (Skullcap)**, Ginkgo and Wood Betony

Key Nutrients: Potassium, **Magnesium**, Vitamin B-1 (Thiamine) and Vitamin B-12

Triglycerides (high)

Triglycerides are blood fats composed of three fatty acids linked together. They travel with cholesterol in the blood stream and are used to produce energy. When triglycerides are high there may be problems with digestion, adrenal function or the hypothalamus. Contrary to popular belief, eating healthy fats is not what elevates triglycerides. Excess consumption of alcohol, sugar, starches and other simple carbohydrates is the primary reason triglycerides are elevated because the excess calories are converted into fats. So, adopt the Low Glycemic Diet and Dietary Fiber therapies as your first steps.

Cholesterol Balancing Formulas may help with the metabolism of excess triglycerides. *Mushroom Blend Formulas* can also be helpful in balancing triglycerides and cholesterol.

Therapies: Dietary Fiber and Low Glycemic Diet

Formulas: Blood Purifier, **Cholesterol Balancing** and Mushroom Blend

Key Herbs: Guggul, Reishi (Ganoderma), Shiitake, Spirulina and Turmeric

Key Nutrients: Alpha Lipoic Acid, Digestive Enzymes, Lipase Enzymes and **Omega-3 Essential Fatty Acids**

Triglycerides (low)

See also *Fatty Liver Disease*

Low triglycerides may be due to a lack of dietary fats, fatty congestion in the liver or digestive problems. If you're on a low fat diet, start including Healthy Fats in your diet. *Cholagogue Formulas* and lipase enzymes can help your body break down fats better. L-carnitine and chickweed can help the body metabolize fats more efficiently.

Therapies: Healthy Fats

Formulas: Liver Tonic and **Cholagogue**

Key Herbs: Barberry, Chickweed, **Dandelion** and Gentian

Key Nutrients: L-Carnitine, Omega-3 Essential Fatty Acids, Digestive Enzymes and **Lipase Enzymes**

Tuberculosis (Consumption, Scrofula)

An infectious disease caused by a bacterial infection, tuberculosis used to be called "Consumption." Scrofula is a particular variety of tuberculosis, involving lymph nodes, especially in the neck. Once very common, the discovery of antibiotics caused this condition to become very rare, but now that antibiotic resistant strains have developed, it is making a comeback. Herbs that have been historically used to treat consumption, such as elecampane, lomatium and usnea may be helpful in antibiotic resistant tuberculosis. *Decongestant Formulas* may also be helpful.

Formulas: Antibacterial and Decongestant

Key Herbs: Cherry (Wild), **Elecampane**, **Usnea**, Devil's Club, Eucalyptus, Lobelia and Lomatium

Key Nutrients: Vitamin D, **Vitamin A** and **Vitamin C**

Tumors

See *Cancer (natural therapy for)*

Tumors (fatty)

See *Fatty Tumors or Deposits*

Twitching

See also *Tics* and *Tremors*

A twitch is a quick spasmodic contraction of a muscle. When repeated in rapid succession this is twitching. Minerals like calcium, magnesium and potassium and *Antispasmodic Formulas* may be helpful for twitching.

Formulas: Antispasmodic

Key Herbs: Lobelia, Hops, Jamaican Dogwood, Valerian and Wood Betony

Key Nutrients: Calcium, Potassium and **Magnesium**

Typhoid

Typhoid is a severe, contagious disease marked by high fever, stupor alternating with delirium, intense headache, diarrhea, intestinal inflammation, and a dark red rash. It is medically treated with antibiotics. herbal *Antibacterial Formulas* may also be helpful.

Formulas: Antibacterial and Goldenseal & Echinacea

Key Herbs: Coptis (Chinese Goldenthread), **Echinacea** and Goldenseal

Key Nutrients: Vitamin A, **Vitamin C** and **Vitamin D**

Ulcerations (external)

See also *Wounds and Sores*

An open sore or break in the skin, often containing pus, can often be healed by topical application of *Topical Vulnerary Formula*, goldenseal, myrrh, propolis or tea tree oil. These remedies may be applied using the Compress or Poultice therapy. Internally, *Cardiovascular Stimulant Formulas* to enhance circulation and *Immune Stimulating Formulas* may be helpful. Vitamin C and zinc helps tissues to heal more rapidly.

Therapies: Compress and Poultice

Formulas: Topical Vulnerary, Cardiovascular Stimulant and Immune Stimulating

Key Herbs: Aloe vera, Calendula, Coptis (Chinese Goldenthread), **Goldenseal**, **Propolis**, **Tea Tree essential oil**, Echinacea, Grindelia (Gumweed) and Myrrh

Key Nutrients: Vitamin C, Digestive Enzymes and Zinc

Ulcerative Colitis

See *Inflammatory Bowel Disorders (Colitis, IBS)*

Ulcers

When most people mention the word "ulcer," or "bleeding ulcer," they usually mean the kind that happens in the stomach. The accurate name for this kind of ulcer is "peptic ulcer," which differentiates it from other kinds of ulcerated tissues. The two major kinds of ulcers are chronic duodenal (found in the first part of the small intestine) and gastric (stomach) ulcers. In both kinds of ulcers, the lining and the tissue underneath have been damaged and eroded by the digestive acids and, in essence, the stomach has begun to digest itself. This leaves an open wound inside of the stomach or duodenum and causes irritation and swelling in the surrounding tissues.

Even though some peptic ulcers are asymptomatic, they are most often experienced as abdominal pain or discomfort about 45 minutes to an hour after eating or during the night. The pain feels like cramping, gnawing, burning, aching, or is described as "heartburn." Relief occurs when the stomach acids are neutralized by antacids or by vomiting or drinking water. Other symptoms can be headaches, low back pain, choking sensations, itching, and nausea.

Contributing factors can be as diverse as food allergies, a poor diet that is too low in fiber, stress, medications and over-the-counter drugs such as aspirin and other pain relievers, cigarette smoking, alcohol consumption and infections. The bacteria *Helicobacter pylori* (*H. pylori*) is believed to be responsible for causing many ulcers, and is reported to be found in 95% of patients with ulcers.

If an ulcer is suspected and symptoms cannot be controlled by natural means, it is important to seek medical help to find out exactly what the problem is. Complications of peptic ulcers can be serious and may need hospitalization.

To deal with peptic ulcers in a natural way, one must first identify and reduce the factors that may have contributed to causing the ulcer. Once the causative factors have been eliminated, the next step is to heal and protect the tissues with proper supplementation and continued lifestyle changes.

Dietary suggestions

Restrict the use of sugar, which increases stomach acid. Restrict salt, as it irritates stomach and intestinal tissues. Eliminate dairy products. Food allergies can cause stomach bleeding, so eliminate suspected foods. Aspirin, alcohol, coffee and tea increase stomach acidity and can interfere with healing.

Drink plenty of water and eat a diet with a variety of whole, unprocessed foods. A high fiber diet is important because fiber slows the movement of food and acidic fluid from the stomach to the intestines and will reduce the frequency of recurrence. Bananas and banana chips have also been proven to help. Fresh cabbage juice has been proven to accelerate the healing of peptic ulcers. Also, exercise regularly.

Supplements that help peptic ulcers include vitamin C (buffered only—take between 500 and 1,000 mg three times daily), vitamin A, zinc and bioflavonoids. Clove, pau d'arco and licorice are believed to inhibit the growth of *H. pylori* bacteria. Licorice root soothes inflamed and injured mucous membranes in the digestive tract. It is the most highly recommended of all single herbs for the treatment of peptic ulcers. Licorice root taken 1/2 hour before meals has been known to be very effective in the healing of ulcers. Myrrh and goldenseal are also antimicrobial and have been helpful for some people with ulcers.

Slippery elm, marshmallow root and aloe vera, highly mucilaginous herbs, have a healing effect on the mucous membranes similar to licorice root.

It's important to obtain adequate fiber and water when trying to heal an ulcer. It may be necessary to use an herbal *Antacid Formula* to calm down acid production in the stomach while the ulcer heals. If you suspect you have an ulcer, going to the doctor for testing or using a home test kit for the bacteria *H. Pylori* is recommended.

Therapies: Dietary Fiber, Fresh Fruits and Vegetables and Hydration

Formulas: Tissue Healing, Antacid and **Ulcer Healing**

Key Herbs: Aloe vera, Bayberry, Calendula, Capsicum (Cayenne), Chamomile (English and Roman), **Licorice**, Elecampane, Goldenseal, Myrrh and Slippery Elm

Key Nutrients: L-Glutamine, Vitamin A, Vitamin C, Bioflavonoids and Zinc

Underweight

See *Weight Gain (aids for)* and *Wasting*

Urethritis

See also *Urination (burning or painful)* and *Urinary Tract Infections*

Inflammation of the urethra or tube that carries urine from the bladder to the outside of the body is called urethritis. Remedies that soothe inflammation in the urinary passages are helpful, such as cornsilk, marshmallow and pipsissewa. If an herbal *Diuretic Formula* is used, look for one that is high in these soothing urinary remedies. Drinking more water helps dilute irritants in the urine, which also soothes irritation and promotes healing. Herbal formulas with irritating diuretics like juniper should be avoided.

Therapies: Hydration

Formulas: Diuretic

Key Herbs: Barberry, Buchu, Cornsilk, **Marshmallow**, **Pipsissewa**, Damiana, Gravel root, Horsetail, Hydrangea, Spilanthes and Uva ursi

Uric Acid Retention

See also *Gout*

The inability of the body to eliminate uric acid results in painful uric acid crystal formation in the joints of the body, which can weaken bones and joints and increase the risk of calcium deposits and kidney stones. When uric acid retention is a problem decrease proteins containing purines and eat more vegetables (especially dark green, leafy vegetables), drink more water and use herbs that help to neutralize the acid. Some of the best herbs to reduce uric acid levels are nettles, celery seed and black cherries.

While most people know that eating foods high in purine raise uric acid levels, what many don't know is that fructose is a bigger culprit! In fact the consumption of fructose from table sugar, high fructose corn syrup and fruits high in fructose, is one of the primary causes of not only elevated uric acid, but the also metabolic syndrome and high blood pressure.

Therapies: Fresh Fruits and Vegetables and Hydration

Key Herbs: Alfalfa, **Celery seed**, **Safflowers**, Devil's Claw, Nettle (Stinging) leaf and Yucca

Key Nutrients: Vitamin B-Complex

Urinary Tract Infections

See also *Bladder Infection*

The following products can help combat urinary tract infections. Cranberry is helpful for preventing them, but is not very effective at treating them once they are active. Some of the best remedies for curing them once they are present are goldenseal, and uva ursi. Take a *Urinary Infection Fighting Formula* and drink lots of water.

Therapies: Hydration

Formulas: Urinary Infection Fighting

Key Herbs: Buchu, Cranberry, **Goldenrod**, **Goldenseal**, **Pipsissewa**, **Uva ursi**, Juniper Berry, Kava-kava, Usnea and Yerba Santa

Urination (burning or painful)

See also *Interstitial Cystitis*

Painful urination is a sign of inflammation and/or infection. Herbs like cornsilk, kava-kava, marshmallow and pipsissewa are useful remedies. Be sure to drink plenty of water to dilute irritants in the urine.

Therapies: Hydration

Formulas: Urinary Infection Fighting

Key Herbs: Cornsilk, **Marshmallow**, Goldenseal, Kava-kava, Pipsissewa and Uva ursi

Urination (frequent)

See also *Adrenals (exhaustion, weakness or burnout)*, *Prolapsed Uterus* and *Stress*

Herbs like cornsilk, marshmallow, schisandra and pipsissewa may help with frequent urination or the frequent urge to urinate. Be sure to drink plenty of water to dilute toxins.

Therapies: Hydration

Formulas: Kidney Tonic

Key Herbs: Cornsilk, **Marshmallow**, **Schisandra** **(Schizandra)**, Erigeron (Fleabane), Jambul, Nettle (Stinging), Pipsissewa and Uva ursi

Urine (scant)

See also *Edema (Dropsy, Water Retention, Swelling)*

When urine production is scant, the kidneys need stimulation and support. In men, this can be a sign of prostate swelling. Diuretic herbs, like those found in herbal *Diuretic Formulas*, can increase output of urine. Make sure you are drinking adequate amounts of water too.

Therapies: Hydration

Formulas: Diuretic

Key Herbs: Buchu, **Juniper Berry**, Goldenrod and Uva ursi

Uterine Fibroids

See *Fibroids (uterine)*

Vaccines (detoxification from)

Vaccines contain chemicals like mercury, aluminum, formaldehyde and other toxic ingredients. These sometimes lodge in the tissues causing irritation, fever and chronic health problems. Vaccines may be an underlying cause of autoimmune disorders. If you choose to be vaccinated, it can be helpful to take a *Blood Purifier* or *Liver Tonic Formula* prior to getting vaccinated and for several weeks thereafter. It is also helpful to do the Heavy Metal Cleanse therapy after getting vaccines. If a child or adult develops a fever or gets cranky or irritable after a vaccine, give them herbs to enhance their immune system, such as an *Immune Stimulating Formula*. You may also want to give them yarrow and/or elderflower (for fever), wild indigo or thuja (to help the immune response), elderberry (for viral vaccines) and lobelia and mullein (if they develop lymphatic swelling).

Therapies: Colon Cleanse, Healthy Fats and Heavy Metal Cleanse

Formulas: Blood Purifier, General Detoxifying, **Heavy Metal Cleansing**, Liver Tonic and Immune Stimulating

Key Herbs: Thuja, **Yarrow**, Elder flower, Lobelia, Mullein, Oregon Grape and Wild Indigo (Baptista)

Key Nutrients: Vitamin C, Sodium Alginate (Algin) and **Omega-3 Essential Fatty Acids**

Vaginal Discharge

See *Leucorrhea (Vaginal Discharge)*

Vaginal Dryness

Vaginal dryness often occurs after menopause when estrogen levels are reduced. Regular sexual activity can help to ease vaginal dryness. When vaginal dryness occurs, use a topical lubricant and try taking a *Menopause Balancing* or Female Hormone Balancing Formula.

Formulas: Menopause Balancing and Female Hormonal Balancing

Key Herbs: Aloe vera, Black Cohosh, **Hops**, **Licorice** and White Pond Lily

Key Nutrients: Omega-3 Essential Fatty Acids

Vaginitis

Inflammation of the vagina is known as vaginitis. It arises from a variety of causes including infection, parasites, or irritation from douches and sprays. Fifty-percent of vaginitis is caused by excessive growth of certain vaginal bacteria. Bacterial vaginitis is characterized by an off-white vaginal discharge (especially after vaginal intercourse) with an unpleasant smell. Discharge occurs without significant irritation, pain, or redness, although mild itching can sometimes occur. A Povidone iodine solution (betadine) 1 oz in a quart of water used as a douche daily for 7 days can relieve most cases of bacterial vaginitis. Follow with application of yoghurt or probiotics.

Vaginitis caused by candida overgrowth causes vulval itching, soreness and irritation, with pain or discomfort during sexual intercourse or urination and vaginal discharge, which is usually odorless. For mild candida infections simply use 2 tsp. cider vinegar mixed in 1 cup warm water as a douche daily for 2 days followed by 1 tbsp. of plain yoghurt (with live cultures) mixed in 1 cup warm purified water as a douche 2 times a day for 7 days.

For severe candida infections mix 1 tablespoon of boric acid powder USP in 1 quart of warm water. Used as a douche 1-2 times per day for 7 days is generally very effective. You should follow this with an application of plain living yoghurt.

If the problem is caused by an infection, use an *Antifungal* or *Antibacterial Formula* internally. Douches with probiotics or an herbal tea or decoction of goldenseal, Oregon grape or red raspberry may also be helpful.

Therapies: Fresh Fruits and Vegetables, Friendly Flora and Stress Management

Formulas: Antibacterial and Antifungal

Key Herbs: Aloe vera, Barberry, **Tea Tree essential oil**, Garlic, Goldenseal, Oregon Grape, Pau d' Arco, Red Raspberry and Usnea

Key Nutrients: Probiotics

Varicose Veins

See also *Hemorrhoids*

Externally visible, prominent veins are called varicose veins. They are common on the legs and are a sign of poor circulation and venous valve collapse. They are not just a cosmetic problem; they may be painful and indicate a lack of tone in the blood vessels. They can also be a sign of congestion in the liver. Eat lots of fresh fruits and vegetables (especially berries) for their antioxidant value. These foods also contain vitamin C, which helps to tone veins.

Vascular Tonic Formulas contain herbs like butcher's broom, ginkgo and horse chestnut, which help to tone up varicose veins and improve venous circulation. Apply the Compress therapy using oak bark, bayberry or yarrow to help veins to shrink more rapidly. Internally, a *Liver Tonic Formula* can also be helpful.

Therapies: Dietary Fiber and Fresh Fruits and Vegetables

Formulas: Vascular Tonic and Liver Tonic

Key Herbs: Aloe vera, Bayberry, Bilberry (Blueberry, Huckleberry), Capsicum (Cayenne), **Butchers Broom**, **Horse Chestnut**, Ginkgo, Milk Thistle, White Oak, Witch Hazel and Yarrow

Key Nutrients: Vitamin C, Copper and Bioflavonoids

Vertigo

See *Dizziness (Vertigo)*

Key Nutrients: Folate (Folic Acid, Vitamin B9)

Viral Infection

See *Infection (viral)*

Vitiligo

Vitiligo is a skin condition where there are white patches of skin surrounded by a dark border. It occurs when menalocytes, the cells responsible for producing pigment, or skin color, die or are unable to function properly. While the exact cause is unknown, treatment with Ultra Violet B (UVB) light, either from the sun or a special UVB lamp, combined with high doses of B12 and folate is a good option. In a study of 100 people with vitiligo, B12, folate and UVB together stopped depigmentation in 65% of people, caused 52% of people to develop new pigment, and totally cured 6% of the people involved in the study.

Key Nutrients: Vitamin B-12, **Folate (Folic Acid, Vitamin B9)**, Vitamin C and Betaine Hydrochloric Acid (HCl)

Vomiting

See *Nausea and Vomiting*

Warts

A wart is a horny projection on the skin usually caused by a virus. A *Drawing Salve Formula* can be applied topically to help get rid of warts. One can also apply the Compress or Poultice therapies using herbs like bloodroot or celandine. These herbs are somewhat caustic, so this should be done with the supervision of a skilled herbalist (*findanherbalist.com*). Raw garlic has also been applied topically to get rid of warts. A banana peel taped over the wart has also been an effective wart remedy.

Formulas: Drawing Salve

Key Herbs: Aloe vera, Bloodroot, **Celandine**, **Paw Paw** and Garlic

Key Nutrients: Vitamin C

Wasting

See also *Weight Gain (aids for)*

Wasting is a condition where a person begins to lose muscle mass and general body weight, usually as a result of aging or a chronic disease. *Digestive Tonic Formulas* can improve appetite and help counteract wasting. Herbalists in the west have used marshmallow or slippery elm as nourishing herbs to rebuild health in people who are wasting. Digestive enzyme supplements improve assimilation of nutrients as well.

Therapies: Eliminate Gluten and Stress Management

Formulas: Digestive Tonic and **Superfood**

Key Herbs: Ashwaganda, **Saw Palmetto**, Ginseng (American), Marshmallow and Slippery Elm

Key Nutrients: Digestive Enzymes

Water Retention

See *Edema (Dropsy, Water Retention, Swelling)*

Weight Gain (aids for)

See also *Hyperthyroid (Grave's Disease)*, *Hiatal Hernia* and *Wasting*

The inability to gain muscle weight is often due to a stress induced hiatal hernia. It can also be due to other digestive problems like malabsorption and occasionally to glandular imbalances like hyperthyroid. Using the Hiatal Hernia Correction therapy will often result in improved muscle tone and healthy weight gain. *Digestive Tonic* and *Digestive Enzyme Formulas* will improve absorption of nutrients. Enzymes, particularly protease enzyme supplements, are also helpful. Digestion relies on water, so a lack of adequate hydration can make protein metabolism difficult. For more suggestions see related conditions.

Therapies: Hiatal Hernia Correction, Hydration and Stress Management

Formulas: Digestive Enzyme and Digestive Tonic

Key Herbs: Saw Palmetto, Ginseng (American), Licorice and Spirulina

Key Nutrients: Protease Enzymes and **Digestive Enzymes**

Weight Loss (aids for)

See also *Hyperinsulinemia (Metabolic Syndrome, Syndrome X)*, *Grave's Disease*, *Hypothyroid* and *Sugar Cravings*

For years, the weight loss mantra has been, "eat less, exercise more." Yet, the research shows that 90% of the people who lose weight in this manner simply gain it back. Why is this so?

Well, for starters, appetite, metabolism and mood are all controlled by messenger chemicals in the body. When you restrict calories, the cells of the body assume that there is a "famine" going on. In response, cells send chemical messengers that elevate cortisol, causing thyroid hormone to become inactive, which reduces metabolism (the rate at which you burn calories). This conserves the body's energy during the "famine."

Because your metabolism is lower, your energy is reduced, so you become less physically active. Your mood also changes because you feel deprived, so your body is attracted to foods that enhance mood—particularly carbohydrates. When food is available, other chemical messengers are released to stimulate appetite and program the body to store energy (fat) in preparation for the next famine. Thus, a vicious cycle of "feast" and "famine" ensues.

In addition, fat itself acts like a gland, secreting its own chemical messengers. One of these is a hormone called leptin. Leptin is supposed to increase your metabolism and reduce your appetite. However, inflammation blocks the action of leptin. Weight can also cause leptin resistance, much like insulin resistance causes type II diabetes.

Inflammation is very common in most Americans because of the large quantity of chemicals in our food, water and air. Inflammation causes fluid retention, and since it is very common for Americans to have intestinal inflammation, it's very common to have excess fluid and fat in the abdominal area. Since a gallon of water weighs eight pounds, it is very easy to have 5-15 pounds of excess water stored in the tissues of the body.

It is evident, then, that unless one changes the type of chemical messages being sent by the cells, one is fighting a losing (or "gaining") battle. Conversely, by getting our cells to send the right chemical messages, we can increase energy, reduce appetite, enhance mood and have a better functioning immune system.

There are four basic keys to achieving this goal:

1. Start with an Attitude Adjustment

There is a simple but powerful principle—whatever we focus our mental energy on, we tend to create. If one is constantly thinking negative things about oneself or one's body, these thoughts will both create and perpetuate health problems, including excess weight. Most people hate certain things about themselves and their bodies. For instance, they may not like their stomach, or their thighs, or their complexion. Even actresses and models who are considered the epitome of beauty have these kinds of issues and often abuse their bodies trying to achieve some unrealistic image of perfection.

Mentally and emotionally, we associate being "wrong" with the need to be "punished." So, negative attitudes about the body make us want to punish the body for being "wrong." This is why many people are driven to unhealthy diet or exercise regimes in trying to achieve the ideal image of weight and beauty. Real beauty comes from health and inner happiness. It radiates from within as a glowing complexion, sparkling clear eyes and a happy countenance.

If you stop and think about it, the biggest reason people "pig out" on junk food (or acquire any other bad habit) is because they are unhappy. Being unhappy sends the wrong chemical messages to your cells. So, "beating yourself up" mentally and emotionally for being overweight is only going to perpetuate the problem.

Conversely, it has been scientifically documented that pleasurable experiences (such as loving relationships, laughter, enjoyable activities, time spent in nature, etc.) cause the body to send out chemical messages that reduce inflammation, enhance immunity, promote healing, improve metabolism and otherwise improve health and well-being. In fact, the biggest single factor in having a long and healthy life isn't your weight, diet or exercise level—it's your attitude. People who experience pleasure in life live longer, healthier lives.

So, instead of being hard on yourself, be gentle with yourself and find ways to experience pleasure in your life. Do things that help you find joy and fulfillment.

Furthermore, enjoy your food! Make a decision to enjoy whatever you decide to eat (even if it isn't the healthiest food). This means taking time to notice the color, aroma, texture and taste of each bite. It also means eating your food slowly and chewing it thoroughly. A good way to train yourself to do this is to put your fork or spoon down after each bite and take some nice deep breaths while chewing. If you just do this, you'll automatically eat less and feel more satisfied.

Remember that all healing, including losing weight, is inherently about love and nurturing, not fear and deprivation. So, if your self-talk is negative, start changing it. A good way to do that is to keep a journal and write down your feelings about yourself and your body. Then, start affirming that you love yourself, that you are loving and caring for your body.

2. Instead of focusing on calories, focus on selecting healthy food

The single biggest reason why so many Americans are overweight and sick is because we are eating refined and processed foods. These foods are lacking in vitamins, minerals, enzymes and other phytonutrients the body is looking to obtain from food. When we eat these foods, we may be getting enough calories, but we still feel hungry because the body is still looking for the nutrition it needs.

Refined sugars (sucrose, high fructose corn syrup, etc.), white flour, polished rice, processed vegetable oils, margarine, shortening and most processed and packaged foods fall into this category. If you want to lose weight and be healthy, you must start eliminating these foods from your diet and replacing them with whole, natural, nutrient-rich, unprocessed foods. When you do so, your body will get the nutrition it needs and stop telling you it is hungry.

Of course, if you focus on the negative (what you shouldn't be eating) you'll never succeed. The way to succeed is to start incorporating more whole, natural foods into your diet. Eat plenty of fresh vegetables and fruits (with a greater emphasis on vegetables that are not starchy). Choose good sources of protein for your blood type and eat high quality protein and vegetables as your primary food source. Go easy on grains (bread, pasta, etc.) and only use whole grains when you do eat them. Eat high quality fats, too. Eat the foods that are good for you first and your body will start craving the good foods while your desire for the "junk" foods will diminish.

3. Eat small but balanced meals on a regular basis

Here is a surefire recipe for gaining weight, even on good food. Skip breakfast and eat a big meal right before going to bed. This puts your blood sugar on a roller-coaster and results in a daily famine-feast cycle. You aren't hungry in the morning, so you don't eat. Your body, thinking it is starving sends messengers to lower your metabolism and energy level throughout the day. By night, your body is starving, and you eat too much. However, since you are inactive (going to sleep), the body stores the excess calories for tomorrow's "famine."

To change this cycle, always "break your fast" by eating something for breakfast. Start the day with some quality fat and protein. For example: avocado, eggs, meat or whole milk yogurt with fruit and nuts. This sets your metabolism to start burning fat instead of storing it. When you eat carbohydrates for breakfast, you raise insulin levels, which prompts the body to store fat. Starting off with a meal that contains fat and protein, not just carbs, kicks a hormone called glucagon into action and mobilizes stored sugars.

Then, whenever you feel a little bit hungry during the day, eat a healthy snack such as nuts, fruit, organic cheese, fresh vegetables, tuna, a salad, etc. By eating small, regular meals your body realizes there's no more famine and will start adjusting your appetite accordingly. You won't be so hungry at night and won't overeat at bedtime. You will feel better and these meals will help you lose weight.

4. Get Physically Active

Forty-eight million Americans are considered sedentary, which contributes directly to obesity. Being sedentary means one doesn't get enough exercise to maintain health.

Almost every system of the body is affected by exercise. Exercise tones the heart, which is a muscle and needs exercise as much as other muscles do. It also increases the body's ability to use oxygen, raises the amount of blood pumping through the body, decreases blood pressure, lubricates the joints and makes the body function better in the use and storing of calories. That means better health and less excess body fat.

Don't worry, this doesn't mean you have to go to the gym. Choose physical activities that you enjoy, such as swimming, riding a bike, playing a sport, gardening or hiking. Just getting out and taking a walk every day is helpful. You can also consider yoga or tai chi, as these exercises also help reduce stress. Resistance exercise (such as weight lifting) helps increase weight loss because muscle tissue burns more calories than fat. So consider doing at least a little bit of weight lifting.

5. Correct Underlying Health Problems

Part of the secret to weight loss is to identify some of the specific health issues that may be inhibiting your ability to lose weight. These can then be corrected with appropriate supplements or lifestyle changes. Consult a natural health professional to help you create a program that is custom-tailored for you, but here are a few of the most important problems to consider.

Low Thyroid

The body burns fat in order to stay warm and the gland that sends the chemical messages to burn that fat is the thyroid. Low thyroid is extremely common, especially among women, and can result in weight gain, fatigue, depression, cold hands and feet, and dry skin. If you have any of these symptoms, consider supporting your thyroid. If lab tests show you have normal levels of thyroid hormones, but you still exhibit symptoms of low thyroid, you may have a problem with conversion of T4 (the inactive form of the thyroid hormone) to T3, the active form.

Toxicity and Inflammation

Toxins contribute to weight gain in two ways. First, toxins cause inflammation, and inflammation causes fluid retention in the tissues. The rapid weight loss most people experience at the beginning of any diet program or cleanse is typically due to a reduction of inflammation and fluid retention.

The second reason toxins contribute to weight gain has to do with the fact that many toxins we're exposed to are fat-soluble. So, if the body can't break them down, it stores them in fat. It may also increase cholesterol levels to transport them. The body won't release the fat if it can't deal with the toxins.

This is why learning to eat natural foods is critical to weight loss. Not only are natural foods free of the chemical additives found in processed foods, they also contain more vitamins and minerals to break down toxins. It also explains why a cleanse can help a person lose weight.

A good herbal cleansing program or *General Detoxifying Formula* can be helpful for anyone trying to lose weight. They not only contain herbs that promote detoxification and reduce fluid retention in the tissues, but they also contain herbs that help balance hormones and metabolism. Be aware that most of the weight lost on a cleanse is not fat, it is simply water retained in the tissues from inflammation. It is not uncommon for people to lose 5-10 pounds after a cleanse, but the loss of fat proceeds more slowly (about one to two pounds per week).

Adding fiber to the diet is another way to increase weight loss. Fiber binds toxins for removal and results in a feeling of fullness that reduces appetite. Be sure to take fiber supplements with plenty of water.

Stress

Stress and unresolved emotional issues can also contribute to weight gain. Many people eat to feed emotional needs. Stress also releases hormones from the adrenals like cortisol, which causes a breakdown of muscle tissue and can contribute to creating fat deposits. Stress can also cause a release of other chemicals which create food cravings and otherwise upset the body's biochemistry.

Keeping an emotional journal where you can write down your feelings when you are having the desire to eat junk food or otherwise fail to take care of your body, can help you identify and fulfill your real emotional needs. Cravings for sugar and sweets often signals a lack of joy or "sweetness" in one's life. Finding ways to bring more joy into your life can help fulfill those emotional needs in more constructive ways.

Supplements that help you deal with stress more effectively, such as *Adaptogen Formulas*, can also be beneficial. These include natural cortisol-reducing formulas to help reduce stress levels and inhibit excess cortisol production. This can be particularly helpful where there is abdominal fat due to stress.

Other options include formulas that support the adrenals and calm the nerves, thereby reducing stress levels and the need for comfort foods.

Depression may also be involved in weight problems and food cravings. 5-hydroxytryptophan (5-HTP) can help increase serotonin levels, which can reduce appetite and improve mood.

Remember that cortisol is also released in response to chronic inflammation, so a supplement with antioxidant and anti-inflammatory properties can also help to reduce cortisol output. Reducing inflammation also increases metabolism and helps leptin, the fat burning hormone, work more efficiently.

Food Cravings

Sometimes it seems that food cravings are our worst enemy when trying to change our diet. Therefore, supplements that reduce appetite or specific food cravings may also be helpful as part of a weight loss program. Cravings for sugar are signs of blood sugar problems and usually indicate that the diet is lacking fat and protein.

Energy-Boosting Formulas containing licorice root, bee pollen, spirulina and/or blue-green algae can control blood sugar levels and reduce cravings for sweets. These formulas also contain herbs that stimulate metabolism. Some herb companies offer *Weight Loss Formulas*, which also increase metabolism and may reduce food cravings.

Therapies: Affirmation and Visualization, Colon Cleanse, Dietary Fiber, Exercise, Fast or Juice Fast, Gut Healing Diet, Healthy Fats, Hydration and Stress Management

Formulas: Fiber Blend, Hypothyroid, General Detoxifying, Adaptogen, Energy-Boosting and **Weight Loss**

Key Herbs: Bee Pollen, Bladderwrack, Chickweed, **Tea (Green or Black)**, Ginseng (American), Guggul, Kelp, Licorice and Psyllium

Key Nutrients: L-Carnitine, 5-HTP, Digestive Enzymes, Omega-3 Essential Fatty Acids and Sodium Alginate (Algin)

Whiplash

Whiplash is an injury to the neck caused by auto accidents or any sudden distortion of the neck. Black cohosh is a good remedy for whiplash. *Antispasmodic Formulas* or single herbs may also be helpful. Magnesium oil or homeopathic arnica can also be applied topically.

Formulas: Antispasmodic

Key Herbs: Arnica homeopathic, **Black Cohosh**, **Skunk Cabbage**, Lobelia and Wood Betony

Key Nutrients: Magnesium

Whooping Cough

See *Pertussis (Whooping Cough)*

Worms

See *Parasites (nematodes, worms)*

Worry

See *Fear (excessive)*

Conditions

Wounds and Sores

See also *Cuts* and *Injuries*

There are many herbs that can help wounds and sores to heal more rapidly. Many of these herbs also prevent infection. Consider applying a *Topical Vulnerary* or *Poultice Formula*. You can also use the Compress or Poultice therapies using herbs like calendula, goldenseal, comfrey and yarrow. Essential oils, such as tea tree or thyme, can also be applied to inhibit infection and promote healing.

Therapies: Aromatherapy, Compress and Poultice

Formulas: Topical Vulnerary and Poultice

Key Herbs: Aloe vera, Bayberry, Capsicum (Cayenne), Chamomile (English and Roman), Comfrey, **Calendula**, **Echinacea**, **Tea Tree essential oil**, Devil's Claw, Eucalyptus, Goldenseal, Grindelia (Gumweed), Lady's Mantle, St. John's wort, Thyme, White Oak, Wild Indigo (Baptista), Yarrow and Yellow Dock

Key Nutrients: Zinc, **MSM**, Vitamin C and Colloidal Silver

Wrinkles

See also *Skin Care (general)*

Avoid cigarette smoke and excessive sun exposure for more youthful, healthy skin. Fat soluble vitamins, good fats and minerals all help to keep skin elastic and moist, which prevents wrinkles.

Therapies: Fresh Fruits and Vegetables, Healthy Fats, Mineralization and Stress Management

Formulas: Mineral

Key Herbs: Witch Hazel and Horsetail

Key Nutrients: Colloidal Minerals, Omega-3 Essential Fatty Acids, Vitamin A, Vitamin C and Vitamin D

Yeast Infections

See *Fungal Infections (Yeast Infections, Candida albicans)*

Therapies Section

Basic Natural Healing Therapies That Work on Root Causes of Illness Or Are Helpful for a Wide Variety of Health Conditions

Consult this section for diet and lifestyle changes you can make to remove the underlying cause of your health problems. This is a critical step in the healing process. Generally speaking, herbs and nutrients work best as part of an overall health program. This section also contains instructions for doing some basic herbal therapies such as compresses and poultices. The suggestions in this section can help a person improve his or her overall health no matter what health challenges he or she may be facing.

Affirmation and Visualization

The discovery that the thoughts we are thinking influence the immune system via the nervous system has given rise to the science of psychoneuroimmunology. Basically, positive thoughts enhance our health and well-being, while negative thoughts detract from it.

What is the difference between a positive thought and a negative one? It's very simple. Positive thinking is focusing our mind on what we want, while negative thinking is focusing our mind on what we don't want. So, when we're focused on thinking about a disease we have and how we want to get rid of it, we're actually thinking negatively. "I'm going to fight this cancer," in other words, is NOT a positive thought because the focus is on the disease.

Positive thinking would entail thinking something like, "I'm getting stronger and healthier every day." This is focused on the goal of what you want, not the elimination of what you don't want.

Affirmation and visualization are two tools that you can employ to help you create positive thoughts that will enhance your health and your ability to heal. Affirmation is auditory and verbal, while visualization is visual and non-verbal. Of the two, visualization is the more powerful, but both can be helpful, so try combining them for the best effect. Here's how to use these mental tools for healing.

An affirmation is a present tense statement that affirms what I want as if I actually had it. Thus, if I had a broken bone and I wanted to speed the healing of that bone

I would affirm "my bone is whole and strong." Notice the present tense statement, "My bone IS." This is a vital key to making affirmations work because it is laying hold of what you desire in the present tense. If you say, "My bone will be whole and strong," this places the fulfillment in the future, not the present and does not convey the same power. If a direct statement like that is difficult to use, a less direct, but equally effective statement would be, "My bone is healing as it should."

Examples of healing affirmations for yourself or others would include statements such as:

My body is healthy and strong.

My body is healing as it should.

You will feel better starting now.

Your body is recovering nicely.

To get the most benefit out of an affirmation, you should write it down and post it somewhere where you will see it every day. A good place is your bathroom mirror. That way, when you brush your teeth in the morning and again in the evening, you can read the affirmations out loud. It is very important to repeat the affirmation aloud, as hearing yourself say it makes it stronger.

During the day, when negative thoughts arise, simply replace them with your affirmation. So, as you start to worry about the disease or problem, simply start saying your affirmation. Since your mind cannot hold two thoughts at the same time, the positive thought crowds out the negative thought.

If you are a person of faith, affirmation can be helpful when combined with prayer. Pray for the outcome you desire and then affirm that the matter is now in God's hands. Always ask in your prayer that God's will be done and that whatever happens will be for the good of all concerned. God may have a better plan for you than you have for yourself. Always be open to guidance.

The main way God answers prayers is by helping us to understand the changes we need to make in our lives to achieve the outcome we desire. So, it doesn't hurt to be prayerful about your choice of herbs, supplements, lifestyle changes, etc.

The second method for helping to create positive thoughts is visualization. Visualization involves getting into a relaxed state and breathing deeply while you picture the final result you desire in your mind. Again, it is important to see what you want, not what you don't want and to picture yourself having it in the present, not in the future.

For instance, cancer patients have practiced visualizing their white blood cells gobbling up the cancer cells and destroying them. If you have an injury, visualize your body healed and whole again. It has been proven in studies that such visualization actually enhances immunity and tissue repair.

Both of these techniques are enhanced by practicing deep breathing and relaxation, as is done in meditation. As one breathes deeply, tissues are oxygenated, which fans the spark of life and increases the flame of life throughout the body. Breath is called the "breath of life" because it is intimately connected with the vital force. To breathe is to connect with feelings, to be alive. Shallow breathing causes a person to stifle his or her feelings by deadening the body.

So, start the healing process by breathing deeply and allowing the body to relax. Then you can pick one of the foregoing methods for "laying hold" on the health you want before you actually have it. Although we've linked these techniques to specific conditions in which they may be particularly helpful, affirmation and visualization can be helpful with any health or non-health related problems.

The therapy *Affirmation and Visualization* helps deal with *Mental and Emotional Stress*, one of the root causes of disease.

Aromatherapy

Aromatherapy is a term coined by the French cosmetic chemist Rene-Maurice Gattefosse in 1937. After an explosion in his laboratory, Gattefosse inserted his painfully burned arm into a nearby vat of lavender oil. He was amazed at the miraculous way the lavender oil instantly relieved the pain and began an immediate process of healing. The arm subsequently healed quickly and without scarring.

Today, aromatherapy is the use of essential oils for mental, emotional and physical healing. Essential oils are volatile compounds found in plants. They are responsible for the aroma or smell of the plant. These non-fatty oils are distilled or expressed from herbs, flowers and trees.

Although individual essential oils have their own qualities, in general essential oils are antibacterial, antiviral and antifungal. They tend stimulate circulation, boost immune responses, increase blood oxygen levels and stimulate cellular growth and repair. They also have strong effects on the nerves and endocrine glands, because the sense of smell directly affects the hypothalamus, which regulates the pituitary and acts as the switching station for the brain. This means that essential oils can also help enhance a person's mood, soothe stress, calm negative emotions, and enhance glandular functions.

Essential oils are potent and highly concentrated remedies. Generally speaking, it is unwise to take most essential oils internally. Those that are safe for internal use should only be used in drop doses that are highly diluted and then only for short periods of time. The best use of aromatherapy oils is topical.

Even then, essential oils should not be used undiluted on the skin for open wounds or burns, except for lavender or tea tree oil. If in doubt, always conduct a patch test to be certain. To do a patch test, double the concentration you plan to use, apply it inside the forearm, and monitor for redness, itching or swelling.

Essential oils should never be used on or around the eyes. If eye contact occurs, the most effective method of flushing is to use a fatty substance that will absorb the oil. Using water will just spread the oil onto the mucous membrane lining of the eye causing additional irritation. Some examples of substances to use include butter, cold milk or vegetable oil. After applying the fatty substance, wash thoroughly with water for five minutes. This also works for spills on the skin.

Overuse and excess dosages can lead to skin irritations, headaches, nausea and a feeling of unease. Always use a more diluted amount with children. And as with any concentrated substance, keep essential oils out of the reach of children and do not leave a bottle of oil, which has no orifice reducer, where a child could take off the cap and consume its contents.

Here are a few of the major ways essential oils can be used:

Inhalation: A simple and easy way to introduce oils to your senses is to take the lid off the bottle and breath deeply. It is very effective and you can use it anytime and anywhere.

Diffuser: This is the best way to disperse oils into the air. This device consists of a glass nebulizer attached to a pump that forces air though creating a fine mist that lingers for a long while. This is an extremely therapeutic use and can kill germs in the air to prevent the spread of infection.

Hydrosol: Create a natural air freshener by adding 40-50 drops of your favorite oil or oil blend to a 2 ounce bottle of pure water with a spray mister. This is great for home, work or car. Shake well before each use. Store in glass container.

Baths: Add 8-15 drops of an essential oil to the tub with a small amount of a natural, odorless soap such as Dr. Bronner's Supermild Baby Soap. Mix the oil in with a capful of soap and hold under the faucet while drawing the bath to emulsify. Baths are very effective for absorbing the oils through the skin as well as for the aromatic effects.

Massage: Create your own massage oil by adding 12-18 drops of an essential oil per one ounce of pure massage oil. For children, reduce by half. Use for a full massage or spot massage at pressure points for a quick effect.

Compress: Add 6 drops of an essential oil to a bowl of hot or cold water. Submerse a cloth in the water, wring it out and place it on the area needing healing. Hot compresses are useful for muscular pain and cramp relief and cold compresses are useful for swelling or headache.

The therapy *Aromatherapy* helps deal with *Mental and Emotional Stress*, one of the root causes of disease.

Avoid Caffeine

Excessive use of caffeine may cause serious damage to the brain and central nervous system. High blood pressure cases are particularly at risk. Caffeine can also be an aggravating factor with breast cysts, hyperthyroidism, irritability and insomnia.

Caffeine stimulates epinephrine production, upping the function of the central nervous system. Habitual use of caffeine causes anxiety, nervousness, insomnia and other nervous symptoms. It depletes the adrenals, causing fatigue. The longer caffeine is used, the more depleted the adrenals become and the more the person craves caffeine.

If you stop using caffeinated beverages you will go through withdrawal symptoms. You may feel tired or get a headache. You may even feel a bit depressed. To help with withdrawal take a caffeine-free Energy-Boosting Formula (read the label carefully as many do contain caffeine-bearing herbs) or an Adaptogen Formula. Also stay well hydrated by drinking lots of water and get plenty of sleep.

It may help to substitute a caffeine-free beverage such as an herbal tea for black tea, an herbal coffee substitute for coffee or sparkling water with a little fruit juice added for sodas. By focusing on healthy substitutes instead of just eliminating the caffeinated beverages, you will ease the transition.

The therapy *Avoid Caffeine* helps deal with *Toxic Overload*, one of the root causes of disease.

Avoid Xenoestrogens

Over 50 years ago it was discovered that chemicals in our environment were having a negative impact on the reproductive capability of wild animals. In spite of this, our society has continued to accept and use these chemicals because they offer "quick fixes" in modern agriculture. Some of these chemicals have now been dubbed as xenoestrogens.

The term estrogen does not refer to a specific hormone. An estrogen is any natural or artificial substance that induces estrus (female fertility and desire to mate). The human body makes three different estrogens—estriol, estrone, and estrodial. Xenoestrogens are chemical compounds from environmental pollutants that bond to estrogen receptor sites. *Xeno* is a Greek word meaning foreigner, stranger or alien. So, xenoestrogens are foreign or alien estrogens.

Xenoestrogens bond to receptor sites within cells to make specific changes to cellular activity. These chemical estrogens can disrupt the function of the endocrine system in two ways. First, they can mimic natural hormones and turn on cellular processes at the wrong time or simply over-stimulate them. A second way they can disrupt the body's hormonal processes is to bond to receptor sites without stimulating them, blocking normal hormonal processes. The results of this bonding can be cellular damage, the inappropriate activation of genes, or the disruption of normal hormonal processes.

Although these chemicals have been "tested" for safety, they have all been tested individually, not collectively. One experiment showed that, when 10 commonly encountered chemicals were mixed at a tenth of their individually active dose, the potency (measured as cell proliferation) was 10 times higher than expected. So, the synergistic effect of these chemicals is dangerous.

Furthermore, they do not readily degrade nor break down in the environment. In fact, they tend to accumulate in the fatty tissues of animals and concentrate the higher up the food chain you go.

Xenoestrogens have been documented as causes in reproductive dysfunction and mutations in wild birds, frogs, reptiles and even mammals. However, the first species of animals to be affected were birds of prey, because they sit at the top of the food chain. The problems these chemicals have caused in wild animals should have clued us into the harm they are causing human beings, but commercial interests have continued to push for their use.

Harmful Effects to Humans

Some of the possible effects these xenoestrogens are having on human beings include:

1. Early onset of puberty in young girls (Precocious puberty).
2. Increases in breast and prostate cancer. These tissues contain estrogen receptor sites and are extremely prone to genetic damage and the stimulation of excess growth by xenoestrogens. Other cancers of the reproductive organs may also be caused by xenoestrogens.
3. Uterine fibroids and other reproductive disorders in women. By over stimulating uterine tissue, excessive tissue growth is encouraged.
4. A worldwide decrease in male fertility.

Some of the chemicals that appear to have serious reproductive and endocrine disruptive effects include:

Pesticides (such as 2,4-D, DDT and many others)

Organochlorides (dioxin, PPBs, PCBs, and others)

Heavy metals (cadmium, lead and mercury)

Plastic ingredients (particularly soft plastics)

Hormones fed to chickens and cows to increase egg and milk production

Both men and women need to become keenly aware of xenoestrogens, avoiding them as much as they possibly can. Organic fruits and vegetables should be purchased whenever available, and commercial produce should be washed in a natural soap like Dr. Bronners to remove pesticide residues. Use only organic meat, dairy and eggs. Use glass or paper cartons instead of plastic containers where possible. Do not microwave food in plastic containers or put hot food in plastic containers. Avoid chemicals in general wherever possible.

Another strategy to minimize exposure to xenoestrogens is to use natural plant-based estrogens to tie up estrogen receptor sites. Phytoestrogens are chemicals in plants that also bond to estrogen receptor sites. However, phytoestrogens have a much weaker estrogenic effect than natural estrogens or xenoestrogens. The theory is that by consuming foods rich in phytoestrogens, receptor sites will be tied up, resulting in less estrogen stimulation.

Soy products and other legumes (beans and peas) are rich in phytoestrogens. We do not, however, recommend large quantities of soy, especially for men, because soy has a very strong estrogenic effect of its own. So, we recommend using a variety of legumes, if you can tolerate them. Other good sources include dark green vegetables and whole grains. Herbal sources include *Phytoestrogen Blends*, red clover, licorice and hops.

Because our exposure to chemicals is so high in modern society, it is also wise to support the liver's ability to detoxify estrogens. Indole-3 Carbinol, SAM-e, cruciferous vegetables, onions and garlic all support the detoxification pathways that rid the body of excess estrogens. *Hepatoprotective* and *Liver Tonic Formulas* may also be helpful.

The therapy *Avoid Xenoestrogens* helps deal with *Toxic Overload*, one of the root causes of disease.

Bone Broth

Bone broth is a nourishing food that supplies nutrients and minerals needed for the health of bones, teeth, joints and the gastrointestinal tract. It is used to help heal the GI tract in Leaky Gut Syndrome, Irritable Bowel Syndrome, Inflammatory Bowel Diseases and Small Intestinal Bacterial Overgrowth. It is also helpful for arthritis, joint problems and osteoporosis.

Here are the directions for making bone broth.

Ingredients

2 lbs beef or chicken bones (organic grass fed are best, but chicken necks or oxtails can be used also)

About three gallons of cold filtered water

1/2 cup Braggs Apple Cider Vinegar

1 tablespoon of good sea salt

You can optionally add vegetables, and it's okay if these vegetables are slightly wilted. This is a good way to use up vegetables that are still good but a little past their prime.

3 onions, coarsely chopped

3 carrots coarsely chopped

3 celery sticks coarsely chopped

You can also optionally add seasonings, such as:

Several sprigs of fresh thyme, tied together

1 tsp. dried green peppercorns, crushed

1 bunch parsley

Instructions

When using beef bones with meat still on them, it works best to roast the bones in the oven until the meat is slightly cooked. This is an optional, but not essential step.

Place the bones in a very large stockpot with the vinegar and cover with the water. Let stand for one hour, then add the vegetables to the stock pot. Bring the pot to a boil and allow to boil for about 20-30 minutes. A large amount of scum (looks like bubbles/oil slick) will come to the top. This needs to be skimmed off with a spoon and discarded.

After you have skimmed off the scum, reduce the heat and add the seasonings. A crockpot can also be used to simmer the stock if you are leaving the house for extended periods of time.

Simmer for at least 12 hours and up to 72 hours (about 24 is good). Add fresh parsley in the final 10 minutes.

Finally, remove bones with tongs and discard. Strain the rest of the stock into a large bowl. Place the pot in the sink and surround with cold water and/or ice to partially cool, then place in the refrigerator until cold. Fat will congeal at the top and can be skimmed off. Stock may thicken with the natural gelatin in it. This is normal. Stock can be kept in the refrigerator for 7-10 days or placed into containers and frozen for later use. (Be sure to allow room for expansion during freezing.)

Stock can be warmed and consumed as is or can be used as a base for soups.

The therapy *Bone Broth* helps deal with *Nutritional Deficiencies*, one of the root causes of disease.

Castor Oil Pack

Castor oil packs are used topically to break up congestion and help to soften hardened tissue. To make a castor oil pack you will need:

1/4 cup castor oil

8 drops essential oil such as lavender (optional)

A soft cloth

Combine the castor oil and the essential oils. Soak the cloth in the oil so the cloth is saturated, but not dripping. Fold the cloth and place it in a baking dish and put the dish in the oven at 350 degrees for about 20 minutes. It should be warm, but not hot. As an alternative, you can heat the oil and the cloth in a crock pot. This is slower, but produces a more steady heat.

Place folded cloth directly over painful area. Cover with a towel to keep it warm. You can also put a hot water bottle over the pack. Use the pack once a day for 30 to 60 minutes. Rinse off the oil after each use.

The therapy *Castor Oil Pack* helps deal with *Toxic Overload*, one of the root causes of disease.

Colon Cleanse

Every day our body manufactures waste in the process of metabolism. Every day we also ingest substances through food, water and air that are potentially harmful for our system. Fortunately, the body has the capacity to deal with this problem. The body rids itself of metabolic waste and chemical irritants through various eliminative systems.

Although medical science tends to discredit the idea of cleansing, natural healers have long stressed the importance of maintaining good elimination for better health. After all, it makes sense that the body will be healthier if waste and toxins are eliminated quickly. In fact, just about any system or machine needs some kind of regular cleaning to run properly.

Plumbers know that pipes can get clogged and drains need to be cleaned. Auto mechanics realize that oil and other fluids need to be regularly changed to keep engines running smoothly. Even electronic equipment needs to be cleaned periodically to keep dust from damaging circuits. It makes sense that this is also true for our bodies.

Most of us strive to keep the outside of the body clean, but few pay much attention to keeping clean on the inside. Most people who have done some internal cleansing, however, have noted numerous improvements in their general health.

Cleansing is about two things. One is minimizing your exposure to toxins in the first place and the other is using herbs, supplements, hydrotherapy, fasting or other natural means to improve the function of eliminative organs.

Since, cleansing is the process of getting rid of what is no longer useful, doing a cleanse simply involves supporting the body's natural detoxification systems to eliminate metabolic waste and environmental toxins more efficiently. Generally, this means using herbs that have been found historically or scientifically to improve liver and kidney function, bind toxins, increase lymphatic flow, open the sweat glands and encourage elimination from the bowels. It may also involve destroying harmful organisms (yeast, bacteria or parasites).

Here are the basic elements of a good cleanse.

Water

The most important tool for cleansing is water, because all eliminative processes require water. Most people do not drink enough water. Experts suggest we should have about 1/2 ounce of water per pound of body weight each day. On a cleanse, one might need a little more. Since the quality of water is also important, drink the purest water you can find.

Fiber

The second most important tool for cleansing is fiber. Dietary fiber binds toxins in the intestinal tract and bulks the stool to promote normal and healthy elimination. Most Americans do not get enough fiber in their diet, so a good *Fiber Blend Formula* should be part of any good cleanse.

Detoxifying Herbs

The third tool needed for a good cleanse is a blend of herbs that support the liver, kidneys, colon and lymphatics. The liver utilizes enzyme systems that neutralize toxins and prepare them to be flushed through the kidneys or colon (via the gallbladder). Water and fiber then carry these toxins away.

Many good herbal formulas for supporting this process are available. These formulas are listed in the book as *General Detoxifying Formulas. Blood Purifier Formulas* can also be used for this purpose.

For people with extremely sluggish elimination, a *Stimulant Laxative Formula* may also be helpful. However, herbal laxatives should not be used long term because people tend to become dependent on them. For long-term problems with sluggish elimination, consider using a *Gentle Laxative Formula*, which will help to tone and rebuild the intestinal system. Magnesium and vitamin C are also helpful for restoring normal bowel tone and function.

Depending on your specific needs, herbal and nutritional formulas that help destroy yeast, parasites or bacteria may also be used as part of a cleanse. So, also consider *Antiparasitic*, *Antibacterial* and *Antifungal Formulas. Heavy Metal Cleansing* and *Liver Tonic Formulas* can also be part of a cleanse if the situation calls for it. Consult a professional herbalist for advice.

Diet

Traditionally, a cleanse has involved fasting or at least partially fasting. In fact, fasting for 24 hours consuming only water one day per month is a good practice for general health. A modified form of fasting is called the juice fast. You can read more about fasting and juice fasting under Fasting in the Therapy Section.

Since most cleansing programs last two weeks or more, it is better to adopt a semi-fasting state during the cleanse. Simply avoid all refined and processed foods during the cleanse and eat lots of fresh fruits and vegetables. This aids the cleansing process by not burdening the body with more cooked, processed foods and chemical additives.

The nice thing about making this a time to clean up your diet is that cleaning out the body tends to reduce your craving for junk food, anyway. So, by the time you have finished the cleansing program it will be easier to maintain a healthy eating program. It can also help you identify foods that cause allergic reactions.

Other Suggestions

Cleansing can also be aided by various forms of hydrotherapy. For instance, enemas and colonics can be helpful as long as they aren't overdone. Generally speaking, enemas and colonics shouldn't be done more than once or twice per week and never for a period longer than a few months without taking a break.

Sweat baths, steam baths or saunas are also useful as they encourage detoxification through the skin. These may be done more frequently.

Foot soaks or foot spa baths are also helpful to the detoxification process. Again, once or twice a week for a limited period of time is more than enough.

Remember that cleansing takes the good out with the bad, so you should alternate cleansing with a program of rebuilding and good nutrition. When it comes to cleansing more is not better.

Sample Cleansing Programs

There are prepackaged cleansing programs, some of which can be found under General Detoxifiers, but it's also fairly easy to put together your own. Here are two basic cleansing programs to chose from:

Basic Cleanse

Here's a great basic two to four week cleansing program. For two weeks take the following.

- 2 capsules of a *General Detoxifying Formula* two or three times daily.
- 1-2 capsules or a *Digestive Enzyme Blend* or a digestive enzyme supplement with each meal
- Once per day at breakfast time take one or two heaping teaspoons of a *Fiber Blend Formula* or bulk psyllium hulls in a large glass of water or juice. Start with 1/2 teaspoon and gradually increase to a larger amount to help the body get used to taking the fiber.
- Drink 1/2 ounce of purified water per pound of body weight each day. If you do not drink enough water, the fiber will actually constipate you.

The above supplies the three main items needed in a cleanse. Optionally, you can add the following:

If the bowels move less than 2-3 times daily add:

- 2-4 capsules of a *Gentle Laxative Formula* or 1-2 capsules of a *Stimulant Laxative Formula* before bedtime. Another option is to take 500-1,000 mg of magnesium and 1,000-5,000 mg of vitamin C to encourage bowel movements.

If yeast or bacterial infections are a problem, add:

• *Antifungal Formula* as directed on the label
If parasites may be a problem, add:

• *Antiparasitic Formula* as directed on the label.

These are only basic suggestions; both the amounts and the products may be varied to account for individual circumstances.

This cleanse should be done for a maximum of two to four weeks. It is rarely necessary or wise to continue a cleanse longer than this. Over cleansing can be a problem as cleansing depletes the body of nutrients as well as eliminating toxins.

Daily Internal "Housekeeping"

Doing a complete cleansing program is like doing a major cleanup job in your home, washing walls and carpets while throwing away things you no longer need. However, we also do little housekeeping chores every day to keep our homes clean, such as washing dishes, vacuuming or putting away clothes.

Our body also needs to do its daily cleaning for us to stay in good health. We can help our body do its "housekeeping" by taking some supplements that keep the colon and eliminative organs working properly. This prevents the buildup of toxins in the first place. Drinking plenty of water and making sure we get enough fiber are the most important aspects of daily cleansing.

Ivy Bridge, an herbalist in Tustin, California has long recommended a once a day cleansing program called Ivy's Recipe. Her basic program is:

• 2 tbsp. aloe vera juice
• 2 tbsp. liquid chlorophyll
• 1 heaping tsp. *Fiber Blend Formula*

These ingredients are blended in a glass of apple juice and taken first thing in the morning. Ivy also recommended taking 2 capsules of cascara sagrada, but using *Stimulant Laxative Formulas* or herbs daily isn't a wise idea. If you are having problems with constipation try a *Gentle Laxative Formula* with the cleanse.

There are lots of modifications you can make to the once-a-day cleansing drink. Besides aloe vera and liquid chlorophyll, you can add antioxidant juices, colloidal minerals, and other liquids to your fiber drink. The following products can also add to the effectiveness of this once-a-day cleanse.

• 2 capsules *Digestive Enzyme Formula*.
• 400 to 800 mg of magnesium to help relax the bowel and promote natural elimination in spastic colons.
• 2 capsules of a *Liver Tonic* or *Blood Purifier Formula*.

Of course, you wouldn't want to add all of these products, only the ones needed for a particular situation. There are no hard and fast rules here. There are many options available, and there is no harm in experimenting with what works best for each individual. Talk to a naturopath or a professional herbalist if you need help deciding the best cleansing program for your needs.

The therapy *Colon Cleanse* helps deal with *Toxic Overload*, one of the root causes of disease.

Colon Hydrotherapy

The fastest way to cleanse the bowel is with an enema or colonic. Clearing the colon in this manner can be helpful in a wide range of conditions. The procedures are simple, safe and effective.

For older children and adults you will need an enema bag. Adults can also use stronger enema solutions.

You can use just plain water as an enema solution; however, I recommend that you use purified water, not tap water. An enema is more effective, though, when you use an herbal solution. One of the most effective enema solutions is garlic 'tea'. Garlic is nature's most powerful antibiotic, as powerful as penicillin without the side effects. It also helps induce perspiration, and elimination through the lungs, so a garlic enema actually helps open up three of the four eliminative channels.

You can make a garlic enema solution in any of the following ways.

1. Blend a small clove of fresh garlic with a pint of warm water in the blender and then strain to remove the pulp. (This may, however, leave a residual garlic smell/taste in some blenders, especially plastic ones.)

2. Make a garlic tea by steeping two or three capsules of garlic powder, or about a quarter teaspoonful, in a cup of boiling water. Strain through a fine cloth to remove fiber particles.

3. Put a couple of droppers full of garlic oil (the garlic oil has been diluted in an olive oil base) into a teacup full of warm water and add a few of drops of a natural liquid soap (like Dr. Bronner's Supermild Baby Soap). The soap helps emulsify the oil so it will dissolve in the water. Stir the solution thoroughly. A small amount of the oil may continue to float on the surface, but this is fine. There is no need to strain this solution.

If you can't stand the smell of garlic, here are some other options. Make a tea of any of the following (or use an extract and use about 1/2 to 1 teaspoon per quart of water: Catnip (one of the best), fennel, peppermint, chamomile, blue vervain, lobelia, Oregon grape, *Catnip and Fennel For-*

mulas, Cold and Flu Formulas, Goldenseal & Echinacea Formulas. Coffee has also been used as an enema solution and has a very cleansing effect on the colon and liver.

Always test the enema solution to make sure it is warm, not hot or cold. If you place a couple of drops on your wrist, it should feel neutral in temperature (like testing a baby bottle).

Fill the enema bag with purified, lukewarm water or an enema solution. Lay on your left side. Lubricate the end of the enema tip and the rectal area and gently insert the tip into the rectum. Allow the solution to flow into the colon. If there is any sense of pressure or pain, stop the flow immediately and gently massage the area where you feel the discomfort. If it does not go away after a minute or two, get up and expel. If it does go away, release a little more fluid into the colon.

Once the fluid flows freely into the colon while lying on your side, you can move to your back and continue the procedure. Finish the procedure by lying on your right side. Remember, any time you feel pain or discomfort, massage that area and then expel the liquid and start again. You may need to fill the bag and repeat the process three or four times before you will really begin to get the colon clean. In fact, the first few times you try this, you may not be able to cleanse the entire colon. You may encounter spasms or other obstructions that won't want to move. Don't be discouraged, it took me several months of doing an enema once per week before I was able to get fluid past the halfway point in my colon due to a muscle spasm in my transverse colon. I finally learned to use lobelia or lavender oil to relax that spasm and clean out the entire length of the colon.

An even more effective method of cleansing the colon is to get a colonic from a colon therapist. A colonic is much more effective than an enema for cleansing the colon. You can also obtain a colonic board that you can use in your own home.

Giving Enemas to Children

To give an enema to a baby or a young child you will need a bulb syringe, some petroleum jelly or similar lubricant and an enema solution. For children, a weaker solution of garlic or herbs like catnip, fennel, chamomile and blue vervain work well.

For an older child you can use an enema bag in place of the bulb syringe. Before giving any child an enema, however, we urge you to try the procedure on yourself.

Place a towel on the floor and lay the child on his or her back or left side on the towel. When doing this with a baby, place a diaper on top of the towel. Explain to the child that this procedure will be uncomfortable, but it will help him or her feel better. Be gentle, but firm. If you were taking the child to the doctor, the child might have to get a shot or have blood drawn which would hurt far more, but you'd probably make them hold still for that anyway. An enema is nowhere near as uncomfortable as a shot, and I've often told children that. I have always talked to my children in a loving, but firm manner when doing this procedure.

Lubricate the anal opening and the tip of the syringe. Fill the syringe with the enema solution by squeezing the syringe and then sucking up the solution. Turn the syringe upright and squeeze any remaining air out of it. Refill the rest of the way, so that the syringe is completely full. Gently insert the tip of the syringe into the anus. Then give a gentle squeeze. If you encounter strong resistance, or the child seems to be in pain, stop squeezing and withdraw the syringe. Make sure you don't "suck" with the syringe as you withdraw.

If nothing comes out, repeat the process again. It may take several tries before anything passes, but don't be concerned, just patient. Putting in a small amount of fluid every five minutes will not hurt the bowel. In fact, small children often get dehydrated when they are feverish from not drinking enough fluids, so the body could be absorbing all of the liquid that you have put into the bowel.

With an older child, tell them they can go "potty" if they feel that they need to. If they don't, then repeat the process. Then wait a minute or two and put a little more fluid in.

With a baby, on the other hand, put a diaper on the baby's bottom after putting one syringe-full into the rectum and then wrap the diaper in a towel. (Enemas can make the stool "runny" and you don't want it to leak onto you.) Then cuddle and hold the baby for a few minutes. Again, if nothing comes out after about ten to twenty minutes, repeat the procedure.

The stool should be soft. If only a small amount of hard stool is passed, you may still need to repeat the process again, until a soft stool passes. The trick is to get the bowel to move freely.

The therapy *Colon Hydrotherapy* helps deal with *Toxic Overload*, one of the root causes of disease.

Compress

A compress is simply a cloth pad (like a washcloth or clean hand towel) or piece of cotton (like a cotton ball) soaked in a hot herbal extract and applied to the painful area. It is used to accelerate healing of wounds or muscle injuries. A cold compress is sometimes used for headaches. Infusions, decoctions, and tinctures diluted with water may be used for a compress. To make compress:

1. Submerge cloth or cotton in the herbal liquid, or apply a tincture directly to a cotton ball or gauze pad.
2. Squeeze out the excess liquid, if any.
3. Hold the pad against the affected area.
4. When it cools or dries, repeat the process using hot mixture.

Examples of herbs used in compresses:

Chamomile (soothing and anti-inflammatory)

Elderflower (cooling and anti-inflammatory)

Yarrow (anti-inflammatory, shrinks swelling, stops bleeding)

Comfrey (speeds tissue healing, reduces swelling)

Plantain (draws poisons, speeds healing)

White Oak (astringent, reduces swelling, dries tissue)

Calendula (astringent, stops bleeding, dries tissue)

The therapy *Compress* helps deal with *Physical Trauma*, one of the root causes of disease.

Deep Breathing

Oxygen is the most important "nutrient" the body needs for healing, and yet, we seldom think about oxygen when we think about health. However, chronically ill people are almost always shallow breathers.

Healthy cells require a highly oxygenated environment. A low oxygen environment in the body favors infections and can ultimately lead to the development of cancer. Oxygen helps the body stay more alkaline and makes metabolism more efficient so we get more energy out of the food we eat. Deep breathing also pumps the lymphatic system which removes waste material from around the cells.

Ideally, a person should be able to take a deep breath from their diaphragm, which means their stomach will rise up as they breathe in and fall as they breathe out.

To practice deep breathing, start by laying on your back on the floor. Inhale slowly and deeply for the count of four. If you are breathing correctly, your belly should rise as you inhale. Hold your breath for the count of four and then exhale for the count of four. Your belly should fall as

you exhale. Then pause for a count of four before taking another breath.

If your belly does not rise as you inhale and fall as you exhale and you have to move your chest to breathe deeply you probably have a hiatal hernia. Do the exercises for correcting this so you can open up your diaphragm and breathe more freely.

After practicing inhaling and exhaling for the count of four, see if you can gradually increase the count on your inhalation and exhalation. You do not need to hold for longer than the count of four after the inhalation and exhalation. A trick to strengthening your diaphragm and deepening your capacity to breathe is to force as much air out of your lungs as possible when you exhale. This allows you to take an even deeper breath on the next inhalation.

If you practice deep breathing at least once per day for 15-20 minutes you will find that your breathing naturally becomes slower and deeper. You will feel emotionally calmer and more centered, too. You may also notice an increase in mental clarity and energy.

The therapy *Deep Breathing* helps deal with *Mental and Emotional Stress*, one of the root causes of disease.

Dietary Fiber

If people were eating fruits and vegetables every day, including edible skins and seeds, and if they were eating only whole grains, then they'd probably be getting enough fiber. However, very few people do this.

Fiber has numerous benefits. It absorbs bile from the gallbladder to help reduce cholesterol levels, slows the release of sugar into the blood to regulate hypoglycemia and diabetes, absorbs toxins in the intestinal tract to help detoxify the body, reduces inflammation in the gut and provides food for friendly bacteria. Fiber also reduces the risk of colon cancer and prevents diverticulitis and hemorrhoids. And, of course, it helps assure regular elimination.

Many people think that cleansing the colon means taking a stimulant laxative. These products just stimulate peristalsis, which is something that is rarely needed. Most people are constipated from lack of fiber, lack of water, and magnesium deficiency. Besides, fiber is what really cleanses the colon, because fiber is what binds the toxins so they can't be absorbed into the bloodstream. So, fiber is the one cleansing product that can be taken regularly by most Americans.

Taking just one heaping teaspoonful of a *Fiber Blend Formula*, first thing in the morning, along with a large glass of water, can make a dramatic difference. The only problem you might run into with fiber is if you don't drink enough water with it. Without water, fiber can actually bind you, so make certain you drink plenty of water when you take fiber. Stay hydrated. If you are taking fiber and stop having regular bowel movements, discontinue the fiber and drink plenty of water. You many need to take a *Stimulant Laxative* or a *Gentle Laxative Formula* to get the colon working properly again.

The natural way to get more fiber is to eat more fresh fruits and vegetables, beans and whole grains. Foods like apples, beans, prunes and figs are especially helpful.

The therapy *Dietary Fiber* helps deal with *Toxic Overload*, one of the root causes of disease.

Drawing Bath

A drawing bath is used to draw or pull toxins from the body, primarily through the oil glands on the skin. Sweat baths help eliminate water soluble toxins, while drawing baths help eliminate fat soluble toxins. Drawing baths are useful for skin eruptive diseases and heavy metal detoxification.

There are a couple of ways to make a drawing bath. For instance, decoctions of blood purifying herbs can be used in baths. Simmer a handful of the herb or herbs you want to use in a large pot with a couple of gallons of water in it for about 20-30 minutes. Strain and add to the bath.

You can also use commercially prepared liquid herbal extracts in a bath. You need a full two-ounce bottle in a bath, however, so while convenient, it can be rather expensive. Both blood purifying herbs and some mucilaginous herbs can be used. Oatmeal also makes a good drawing bath.

The best agent for a drawing bath, however, especially when detoxifying heavy metals, is clay. A fine clay like Redmond clay can be added to the bath water. Use about one cup for a standard bath. Soak for 20-30 minutes and then rinse off. The clay is fine enough that it won't clog drains if you flush a lot of water down the drain after the bath. Hydrated bentonite can also be used in drawing baths.

The therapy *Drawing Bath* helps deal with *Toxic Overload*, one of the root causes of disease.

Eliminate Allergy-Causing Foods

An underlying cause of many people's health problems is food allergies. Food allergies can cause migraine headaches, irritability, hyperactivity, inflammatory diseases of all kinds and can contribute to respiratory congestion.

The most common foods that cause allergic reactions are grains containing gluten (wheat, rye and barley) and dairy products. Corn, eggs, oranges and other citrus fruits, nuts, peanuts, sulfites, food additives, dyes, chocolate, strawberries, shellfish and soy products are others. Interestingly many of these foods have been highly "tampered with" through genetic modification, modern agricultural methods and/or excessive processing.

If you suspect that some of your health problems may be related to food allergies, you can start by trying a simple experiment. Stop eating foods that you suspect allergies to and see if your symptoms subside. The foods listed above are a good place to start.

Wait at least seven days, then reintroduce suspected foods one at a time to see if symptoms reappear. Wait 24 hours and watch for reactions. Look for these signs, as they indicate a probable reaction to a food: dark circles under the eyes; redness of the ears, face or eyes; a glassy look; an increased pulse rate or mood changes. If no changes or symptoms occur, try introducing another suspect food.

You can also fast for a few days, consuming only water or juice. If symptoms improve, then food allergies may be involved. Again, reintroduce the suspect foods one at a time and watch for reactions.

Still another method for isolating suspected food allergies is muscle response testing. Simply name each of the suspected allergy-causing foods and muscle test for it. A weak response indicates the body is not handling that food very well. In one case, muscle testing revealed that a person with a wheat allergy wasn't allergic to wheat at all. He was allergic to the pesticide residues on the grain. By switching to organically grown wheat, the problem disappeared.

If you don't know how to muscle test, another method is to take the pulse, eat a small amount of a food, and test the pulse again. Any food that raises the pulse more than six beats per minute after ingestion is probably an allergen.

Another thing to watch for in identifying food allergens is by paying attention to food cravings. Food allergy is generally linked with food addiction. It is much like any other addiction, cigarettes, alcohol or even refined sugar. Although the substance isn't good for the body, it adapts to its presence. When the substance is withdrawn and the body starts to "cleanse" itself of the irritant, the person feels "dis-ease". It is a type of healing crisis.

Many nutritionists say that the best way to combat food allergies is to adopt a "rotation diet." This means that a person's diet should be increased to include a wide variety of non-allergenic fruits and vegetables, seeds and nuts, and grains such brown rice, millet, amaranth, and barley. Eat one food one day, then you should wait three or four days to eat that particular food again. Increasing the types of foods eaten, as well as rotating them through the diet, will help to greatly reduce food allergy responses.

The therapy *Eliminate Allergy-Causing Foods* helps deal with *Toxic Overload*, one of the root causes of disease.

Eliminate Gluten

Gluten is a protein structure found in wheat and other grains. The inability to handle gluten causes Celiac disease, but is also involved in other inflammatory bowel disorders. Gluten intolerance can cause inflammation in the joints, skin, respiratory tract and brain without any obvious gut symptoms. Gluten may also trigger autoimmune reactions in Hashimoto's disease, rheumatoid arthritis and other problems.

Since there are no nutrients in gluten-containing foods that you can't get more easily and efficiently from foods that don't contain gluten there are no nutritional deficiencies one could develop by avoiding gluten. There are, however, many potential health benefits to avoiding or eliminating it.

Foods containing gluten include: wheat (includes bulgur, durum flour, farina, graham flour, semolina), barley (malt, malt flavoring and malt vinegar are usually made from barley), rye, triticale (a cross between wheat and rye), spelt and kamut.

Alternatives to gluten-bearing grains include all of the following non-gluten grains and grain alternatives: amaranth, buckwheat, coconut flour, corn (hominy and cornmeal), flax, millet, potato flour, quinoa, rice, sorghum, soy flour and teff.

Many foods contain wheat or other gluten grains, so you need to be vigilant in looking at ingredients. Look for foods that say "gluten-free" on the package. Ask about gluten in foods when eating out at restaurants.

The therapy *Eliminate Gluten* helps deal with *Toxic Overload*, one of the root causes of disease.

Emotional Healing Work

Research shows that positive thoughts and emotions enhance healing. The tools of affirmation and visualization are helpful for creating positive thoughts, but our emotional state is not based solely on our thoughts as many believe. While it is true that our thoughts influence our emotions, it is also true that our emotions influence our thoughts.

Emotional healing is about learning to work through our negative emotions. It is NOT about making our negative emotions go away, as many people try to do. This is because both our positive and our negative emotions play an important role in our lives. The goal is not to eliminate negative emotions, but to turn them into positive opportunities for growth and healing.

Negative emotions are like pain. We may not like pain, but if we didn't feel pain, we wouldn't know what was harmful to the body. Without pain to warn us we would injure ourselves and never know it. Without the discomfort associated with disease symptoms we would not know that we were sick and would not be motivated to seek healing. So, whether we like it or not, pain is a necessary part of our lives.

What pain does for the body, negative emotions do for the soul. Negative emotions tell us when something is wrong in our lives, which needs to be identified and healed. Feeling angry, sad or even depressed is a sign that a particular behavior or attitude is harmful to us. So, just like pain can teach us to avoid injuring our body or cause us to seek help, negative emotions can teach us how to stop harming our soul or cause us to seek help for unresolved emotional wounds.

Unfortunately, few people learn the lessons that pain and negative emotions are trying to teach. When it comes to pain, most people seek symptomatic treatment. Without identifying the cause of the pain (or their disease symptoms) they take drugs that merely address the symptoms. This provides temporary relief, but the real problems are never resolved and overall health deteriorates over time. This form of medicine is known as allopathy, which literally means "against the symptom."

As explained in the beginning of this book, one of the hardest tasks a natural healer faces is to help people understand that natural healing is not designed to provide symptomatic relief. Natural healing is about identifying the root causes of health problems and fixing them. The true natural healer doesn't treat diseases, per se, but rather looks at the habits and lifestyle of the person to determine what they are doing that is harming their body. The "cure" is to fix the cause and in the case of emotions these causes involve how we relate to other people and situations.

When the cause is addressed, the effect (the disease symptoms) disappears. When the cause of the emotion is identified and the person takes steps to change their attitudes and behaviors (NOT the attitudes and behaviors of others), healing can take place.

Just as allopathic medicine is targeted and suppressing symptoms, our culture practices "emotional allopathy," meaning people are taught to just try to make the negative feelings go away without understanding what is causing them. People do this in a variety of ways. For example, they may take drugs to suppress their depression or anxiety, but they may also seek to numb their emotional pain through alcohol, eating, sex or other addictions.

There are also more subtle ways people practice emotional allopathy on themselves or others. For instance, most of us have been taught to suppress one or more emotional responses by denying what we are feeling. We may also learn to project the responsibility for what we feel outward through blame. That is, we seek to restore our sense of well being through attacking others, playing the victim or otherwise trying to make others responsible for our happiness.

Our Hearts Hold the Key

All of this is unfortunate, because the feelings we experience in our heart are the key to discovering our ultimate happiness. Just as pain can help us realize something is wrong and cause us to seek to healing, our negative emotions can motivate us to make the changes in our life that will ultimately bring us joy, love, peace and happiness. We just have to be willing to listen to our heart and understand what these feelings are trying to tell us.

Unfortunately, most of us have been told over and over again that we can't trust our heart and our emotions. Instead of learning to listen to our negative feelings and understand them, we're encouraged to deny, ignore or suppress them, in which case we often react to them unconsciously. Rarely are we helped to understand and use them in constructive ways.

Running away from our emotions is like running away from the monster in a childhood nightmare. As long as we deny, suppress or otherwise try to "get rid of" a feeling, it will continue to chase us. As the title of a book by Carol Truman so eloquently states, *"Feelings Buried Alive, Never Die."*

Denying one's feelings isn't the only way one may try to deal with them. One may also try to blame what they feel on others. Now, it is true that we can have a negative emotional reaction to the behavior of others. For instance, I'm sure that all of us would be scared if someone was pointing a gun to our head and threatening our life, but these reactions to the behavior of others are temporary emotional reactions. Our overall mood and our typical emotional reactions (or personality) are based on what is inside of us, not what is happening in the world around us.

To demonstrate the truth of this idea, think about someone you dislike. It is quite likely that there are other people who love that person. It is also likely that others may dislike people you love. What is true for people is also true for life events. A situation that might evoke feelings of hurt or anger in you might not provoke the same reaction in someone else. You might be scared to death in a situation that another person might view as an interesting challenge.

As you contemplate this, you will see that your emotional reactions are not primarily caused by the world around you, they are primarily the result of what is inside of you. More specifically, your emotional reactions are caused by how you choose to respond to a given situation.

Emotional healing work involves learning to get in touch with our emotions and acknowledge rather than deny them. It involves learning to feel what our heart is telling us, rather than just blaming what we feel on everyone else and insisting that they change so we can feel good.

If you are lucky enough to find someone who can help you through the process of understanding your emotions, it is certainly worth seeking out there help. For example, you may wish to utilize a counselor or a minister to help you work through your unresolved emotional wounds. If you do not have someone you can work with, here are some self-help techniques extracted from Steven Horne's book *The Heart's Key to Health, Happiness and Success.*

Step One: Practice making your mind shut up so you can listen to your heart.

If you already practice some form of meditation, this step won't be hard for you. If you've never tried meditating, it takes some practice to learn how to quiet the mind. Most of the time our minds are constantly "chattering with words." These words express our worries, cares, desires, plans, schemes and an endless stream of social conditioning.

There are many techniques for reaching this meditative state of mind and you are free to use any technique that works for you. However, if you do not currently have a technique, here is a very simple one that I use.

First, find a quiet environment. Ideally, this is done in the wilds of nature, but most modern people don't have easy access to wilderness environments, so a private room or place of worship is fine.

Second, you need to get into a comfortable position and allow your body to relax. When first getting started it can be helpful to lie down and allow every part of your body to sink deeply into the floor or the earth. However, it is also easy to fall asleep when doing this, so you may find that it is easier to quiet the mind and stay awake while sitting up. The way I do this is to sit or lie down and allow my body to sink into the earth. I imagine gravity as the arms of "mother earth" and relax into the embrace of it.

Third, you will need a focal point for your mind. Some people gaze at a candle or repeat a phrase, verse, scriptural passage, mantra or one of the names of Deity over and over again. Dr. Herbert Bensen, M.D. and author of *The Relaxation Response*, suggested repeating the word "one" over and over again in your mind. However, breathing alone can be an effective focus point.

Simply start by breathing slowly and deeply making the inhalation, exhalation and the pauses in between them equal. Directions for doing this can be found under *Deep Breathing* in this *Therapy Section*. The breathing and counting become the point of focus for the mind that stills the monkey chatter in the brain.

Fourth, you will need to adopt a passive attitude. This means that whatever comes to your mind, you observe it passively without judging or analyzing it. You just notice it and then return to your single point of focus. It is especially important to not judge or analyze how well you're doing in the process. Just relax and "let go."

The goal is to reach the state where there are no words in your mind, where you are "thinking" without language. Yes, this is possible. This is the state of mind where you can observe your own thoughts, feelings and actions as if you were an objective, outside party.

Step Two: Tune into your feelings and bodily sensations.

Once you learn to quiet your mind, this exercise is the next step. Even if you haven't been able to completely quiet your mental chatter, as long as you have reached a relaxed state of body, you can try this. In fact, tuning into your body and your feelings can be used as a point of focus to reach this quiet state of mind.

Simply ask yourself, "What am I feeling?" or "How do I feel?" while you continue to breathe deeply. Stay focused on your body. Your head will often want to provide an immediate answer in words, but this is not the real answer to the question you are asking. What you want is not words, but sensations in your body. You want to actually feel something in your body.

Don't be surprised if you have a hard time feeling your bodily sensations and answering the question, "How do I feel?" We are so used to the idea that their feelings don't matter (and that nobody cares how we feel) that it can be

difficult for us to connect with our feelings. This shows how disconnected from our hearts we can be and is a sign of deeply buried emotions.

To help you tune into your feelings, it may help to get more specific. Think about a problem, worry or concern that you have and then ask, "How does this make me feel?" Breathe deeply and again, notice any sensations that arise in your body.

When you actually do get in touch with a bodily sensation, feeling or emotion, you should turn your attention to it. Allow yourself to just experience the sensation or emotion without trying to make it go away or change it.

It helps to breathe into the area of your body where you are feeling it. You do this by imagining your breath moving into that part of your body as you inhale. This works because it sends energy to that part of the body, enlivening it and intensifying the feeling. Your awareness will also follow your breath.

If the feeling is an actual emotion, then notice where you feel that emotion. Is it in your heart, your stomach or your gut? What does the feeling feel like? All feelings are experienced through bodily sensations. Is the feeling warm or cool, tense or relaxed, pleasant or painful? Whatever it is, turn your attention on it and just experience it.

What you feel may not be an emotion. It may be a physical sensation such as pain or tension. If this is the case, treat it the same way you would an emotion. Don't resist it or fight it, just allow it to be. Breathe deeply into the area where you feel the tension or pain. Then, as you exhale, imagine that pain or tension flowing back out of your body with your breath.

You may even try asking the pain or tension, "What do you want?" or "What are you trying to tell me?" If your brain tries to answer, ignore it, keep breathing and keep asking the part of your body that's in discomfort the question. You may need to do this for several minutes, but don't be surprised when your body actually answers you. Oh, and you will know that it was your body (not your head) that answered the question, because often the pain and tension will dissipate once it has delivered its message.

Step Three: Use questions and question-affirmations to deepen your understanding of your emotions and find healing.

The most powerful tool for emotional healing is something Steven calls the question-affirmation. To understand this tool, you first have to know what an affirmation is. An affirmation is a present tense statement that affirms what I want as if I actually had it. See *Affirmation and Visualization* for more information.

A question-affirmation is an affirmation that is used to explore your feelings about that affirmation. It turns the affirmation into a question by asking, "How would I feel if…". This allows you to explore and uncover negative belief systems surrounding the affirmation.

Here's an example of how this technique works. The story is a composite of several real case histories.

A woman went to a nutritionist for help with a weight problem. She wanted to be attractive so she could get married. She was put on a weight loss program that worked beautifully for a few weeks. Then, suddenly, the weight came back on and she wound up even heavier than before. This had happened every time she tried to lose weight.

The nutritionist was also familiar with emotional healing techniques. He did some investigation and probed into the woman's past to see when she had first started to gain weight. It was discovered that when she was five, an uncle had attempted to sexually molest her. Fortunately, he had been caught before he could actually perpetrate the deed.

However, it was a very emotionally upsetting time. In the midst of this pain and trauma, her mother had blurted out, "It's a shame she's not fat! Fat girls never get molested." Within the year, the girl had started to gain weight.

Since our subconscious mind is wired to avoid pain and suffering, the girl's mind laid hold on the mother's words. To protect her from being molested in the future, it caused her to gain weight. She couldn't lose weight because her subconscious mind was programmed with a belief that the weight was necessary to protect her from pain and suffering. Of course, it didn't protect her from pain and suffering, so the belief was an illusion or a lie.

The problem with regular affirmations is that in situations like these, they will actually backfire. If the woman starts to affirm, "I am thin and beautiful," the subconscious fear that says, "being thin and beautiful means you will get sexually molested," kicks in gear, which can sabotage her efforts to lose weight.

The question-affirmation would allow her to uncover the buried feelings surrounding the weight issue by asking, "What would it feel like if I were thin and beautiful?" By examining this question, the feelings of fear and pain will surface and the illusions, which underlie these buried emotions, are forced to reveal themselves. By bringing them to the light of awareness, they can be changed and healed.

When the subconscious mind sees that a particular belief is a lie, it instantly reprograms itself, because we are hard-wired to want happiness. As soon as we perceive that a changed course of action will result in positive emotions, the desire for these positive emotions kicks in gear and behavior patterns start to change naturally.

Examples of question-affirmations would include:

What would it feel like if it was all right for me to cry?

What would it feel like if it was okay for me to feel my fears?

What would it feel like if I was free to laugh?

The possible uses of this tool are endless, so be creative with it and remember that whatever comes up, just try to feel it and accept it. Don't try to make it go away.

Questions in general are useful for healing, even when they aren't linked to a positive affirmation. For example, one time Steven had an earache that lasted for over a month. Nothing he tried seemed to help, including going to a medical doctor. So, he went into a quiet, meditative state and asked himself the question, "What would I hear if I could hear clearly?" He only had to ask himself this question twice when he suddenly knew why his emotions were shutting down his hearing. As soon as he resolved to do something to change the situation, his ears started to heal.

For help in identifying emotional issues that may be linked with your health problems, consider getting the book, *You Can Heal Your Life* by Louise L. Hay. More information on emotional healing can also be found on at *modernherbalmedicine.com*.

The therapy *Emotional Healing Work* helps deal with *Mental and Emotional Stress*, one of the root causes of disease.

Epsom Salt Bath

Epsom salt is magnesium sulfate. Soaking in a warm to hot bath containing this salt of magnesium is a great way to reduce stress, ease muscle tension, eliminate toxins and relax. To take an Epsom salt bath simply add two cups of Epsom salt to the bath water. You can add 5-10 drops of one of your favorite essential oils. Good choices for relaxing include lavender and rose. Be sure to mix the essential oils with a small amount of a natural, unscented soap like Dr. Bronner's Supermind Baby soap, so they will disperse in the water. Soak in the bath for 15-20 minutes. Feel free to light candles and listen to relaxing music, too.

The therapy *Epsom Salt Bath* helps deal with *Physical Trauma*, one of the root causes of disease.

Exercise

Over the past few decades, Americans have become increasingly sedentary. Many of us work 40 hours a week (or more) at a desk job and then come home to watch TV, play video games or surf the web.

Statistics suggest that children and adults alike spend 20-40 hours a week at these sedentary activities. Participation in outdoor activities has diminished. Because of safety concerns, many parents don't let their children play outside and explore anymore. Even state and federal parks are seeing fewer visitors each year as people find all their entertainment inside their homes.

This trend is dangerous to our health. No matter how well we eat or what supplements we take, nutrition alone is not enough to ensure good health. Physical activity is essential to maintain optimum weight, regulate blood sugar, maintain emotional health, and reduce the risk of degenerative diseases, like heart disease.

So, to be healthy, we need to get out of our chairs and get involved in more physical activities. Yes, we're talking about exercise. We all know we should get regular exercise, but how many of us actually do it? Judging by the number of Americans who are out of shape, overweight and depressed, a large percentage of us are not getting the physical activity we need to stay healthy.

For many of us, the thought of exercise is hard to bear. There are many reasons to loath exercising. It might remind you of sweaty high school gym classes. You may feel too busy or too stressed to exercise. Some of us are just too embarrassed by how out of shape we are. You may believe that exercise is all "no pain, no gain" and has to be difficult and grueling. And some of us have injuries or illnesses that make exercise very difficult. Well, if you shudder at the thought of exercise for any of these (or other) reasons, then here is some good news—you don't have to do anything that difficult. You just have to get moving.

One of the best forms of exercise is simply walking. If you walk for just 30 minutes a day, you activate enzymes that help the body burn fat. You can also try swimming or playing any kind of a sport several times a week. If that's too difficult, you can just start lymphasizing.

Lymphasizing

What is lymphasizing? It's a term coined in the early 1980s by Lymphologist Dr. C. Samuel West to describe gently bouncing up and down on a mini-trampoline without having your feet leave the mat. This gentle up and down movement is similar to the motion we make when we bounce a crying baby up and down. This gentle movement does wonders for health because it doesn't take strenuous physical activity and provides most of the health benefits of exercise.

It's called lymphasizing because this type of movement stimulates lymphatic flow. This is important because unlike the circulatory system, the lymphatic system lacks a pump, so lymph flow is largely passive. Gently bouncing up and down on a mini-trampoline greatly increases lymphatic flow, hence "lymphasizing."

Of course, you don't really need a mini-trampoline to get the benefits of lymphasizing. Any kind of activity that gets you moving and breathing deeply is a form of lymphasizing, including just taking a walk. Yoga and Tai Chi can also be thought of as lymphasizing because they involve non-strenuous movement performed with deep breathing. Any activity that just gets you moving without stress and pain while breathing deeply can be considered lymphasizing. Doing this non-stressful activity for just 20-30 minutes a day will make a big difference in your health.

Why is Lymphasizing So Valuable to Our Health?

When cells are damaged due to trauma, toxins or nutritional deficiencies, a process called inflammation is started. We now know that inflammation is the "mother of all diseases," meaning that heart disease, cancer, diabetes, arthritis, asthma, dementia and a host of other chronic and degenerative diseases are all linked to chronic inflammation.

Part of the inflammatory process is the movement of fluid and protein out of the blood stream and into the tissue spaces. This is the cause of one of the four classic symptoms of inflammation—swelling. The other three are heat, redness and pain. Once you realize that the only way for the fluid and protein causing this swelling to be removed is through the lymphatic system, you understand why lymphasizing, i.e., physical movement and deep breathing, is essential to staying healthy. You cannot reduce inflammation and properly detoxify your cells without it.

When you remove the excess fluid from around your cells, they are able to get more oxygen and nutrients. Your cells' energy production increases, which gives you more energy. The more sedentary you are, the less energy you will have, which will contribute to fatigue and depression.

For someone who is chronically ill or "burned-out" from stress, rigorous exercise can actually be counterproductive because it increases the output of stress hormones and may further damage already weakened tissues. Lymphasizing, on the other hand, will rebuild health, even if you are seriously ill. The key is to start slowly and build up gradually, but be consistent about it.

If you can only walk or bounce on a mini-trampoline for five minutes the first day without feeling tired or stressed, then do it for five minutes. Then try it for six minutes the next day and seven minutes the day after that. This regular physical movement will gradually detoxify your cells and renew your health and energy. It will also elevate your mood and mental abilities. Have you ever noticed how your head "clears" when you take a walk?

Lymphasizing (gentle movement coupled with deep breathing) is something everyone can do, but if you're well enough to do so, a little resistance training is also beneficial. Lift some weights to strengthen your muscles or participate in a sport or dancing or gardening or anything that gets you using your muscles. This has been proven to help reverse type II diabetes, improve cardiovascular tone, reduce the risk of heart disease and aid in weight reduction by increasing metabolism (muscle burns more energy than fat).

With all these benefits, don't wait to get started. Get out of that chair or off that couch and start exercising today.

The therapy *Exercise* helps deal with *Mental and Emotional Stress*, one of the root causes of disease.

Fast or Juice Fast

Have you ever noticed that little children and animals tend to shun food when they are sick? There is a reason for this. In most acute illness, the body is congested, and when the body is congested it does little good to put more food into it. It just clogs the system more.

Think of it this way. Suppose the drain in your kitchen sink got plugged up and you were unable to wash dishes. You wouldn't continue to make more meals and dirty more dishes until you'd gotten the drain unplugged, right? Well, when you are sick, it's often a sign that one or more of the "drains" in your body are clogged. If you take time to unclog the drain before you resume eating, your food will digest better and the body will metabolize it more efficiently.

Okay, maybe you're not into the kitchen stuff, so here's another analogy for those of you who are more mechanically inclined. Think of what happens to a car when the air filter is dirty, the oil needs to be changed and the carburetor and spark plugs are getting fouled. The car no longer burns fuel efficiently, which reduces performance. It also increases the amount of "gunk" being generated by the engine, which causes the engine to get even more clogged up. If one takes the time to clean the carburetor, change the oil and replace the spark plugs and filters, the engine will burn cleaner and more efficiently.

Just like an automotive engine or our household plumbing, the body gets "clogged" periodically. When this happens, the body needs a nutritional "lube, oil and filter service" or an herbal "drain opener" to clean it out so that it can run efficiently again.

Of course, we're not suggesting that cleansing is the only thing we need to keep the body healthy. Obviously, the body also needs exercise, rest and good nutrition. But, the body isn't going to be able to utilize good nutrition properly if it's congested, and you won't feel like exercising when your metabolic "engine" isn't running efficiently. You probably won't sleep very well when the body's drains are plugged, either. So, in many cases, if you want to improve your health, a good place to start is by doing a cleanse.

The most basic of all cleanses is a fast. In fact, fasting is one of the oldest and most effective natural healing techniques. As mentioned earlier, it's also instinctive, since small children and animals don't eat when they don't feel well.

"Starving" Illness

Some of us have been taught to "eat to keep up your strength" when we're sick, but this is bad advice. Even though everyone has heard the sage wisdom of the famous Greek physician Hippocrates, "Feed a cold and starve a fever," practically nobody understands what it means. His advice becomes clearer if you render it as "if you feed a cold, you will have to starve a fever." In other words, it's not wise to feed a cold or a fever. Both need to be "starved" out with fasting because these illnesses are signs the body is congested with metabolic waste.

Many modern Western herbalists and naturopaths have discovered the incredible value of "starving" colds, flu, fevers and other acute ailments. So, next time you feel a cold or flu coming on, stop eating and do some cleansing! Putting food into the body when you're ill is like running more water into a sink with a plugged drain—it's just going to make the problem worse.

Of course, while water is not likely to help a plugged kitchen drain, water is exactly what the body needs when its "drains" are clogged. The old adage, "Go to bed, rest and drink plenty of fluids," is probably the best advice ever written as basic therapy for acute illness. Every eliminative channel of the body needs water to function properly. Simply resting and flushing the system with liquids will help you get over most colds, flu, and other minor ailments faster than an OTC (over-the-counter) medication.

A 24-hour fast once per month is a good basic health-building practice. Periodically, longer fasts can be utilized. For most people, a three-day fast is sufficient, but people have fasted for as long as 40 days. We don't recommend long fasts for health purposes.

Juice Fasting

People who are hypoglycemic, that is, they suffer from low blood sugar, have a hard time fasting. If you're one of these people, it's probably better to do a juice fast. It's also better to do a juice fast if you're going to fast for more than 24 hours. A juice fast involves abstaining from solid food, and drinking some kind of fresh fruit or vegetable juice whenever you feel hungry. Plenty of water should also be consumed while on a juice fast. The famous herbalist, Dr. John Christopher, described this type of juice fast cleansing in his booklet, *Dr. Christopher's Three-Day Cleansing Program*.

When juice fasting, it's important to have a supply of fresh, raw juice. This means one will either need to own a juicer, or have a source to buy fresh, unpasteurized juice. It is best to stick with one type of juice for the duration of the fast. Raw unfiltered apple juice is a good choice because it has a mild laxative action. However, if one has blood sugar issues it should be diluted half and half with water, or the person should opt to use vegetable juices, as they don't raise blood sugar levels as much.

One of the easiest (and most effective) juice fasts is to drink lemon water sweetened with real maple syrup. Grade B maple syrup has a higher mineral content than grade A maple syrup, which is more sugary. However, you can use either. You can make the lemon drink anyway you want, but a good recipe is the juice of four lemons in a half gallon of water with about an equal amount of maple syrup as lemon juice.

Lemon is great because it helps both the liver and the kidneys flush toxins. If you're interested in learning more about this cleanse, read *The Master Cleanser*, by Stanley Burroughs, which explains how to do this type of juice fasting.

The 24- hour fast or a two or three day juice fast once a month can have many health benefits. First, it eliminates allergy-causing foods from the diet, which results in the elimination of allergy-induced health symptoms. Juice fasting can help reduce chronic pain, relieve digestive upset, clear thought processes, create stronger resistance to disease and increase energy.

A fast should always be broken by eating a meal of fresh fruits or vegetables. Never "pig out" when breaking a fast! Eat light at first and gradually reintroduce heavier foods.

People with serious gut health issues should probably not juice fast or do long total fasts. Instead, they can do a "fast" using bone broth for 24-48 hours. See Gut Healing Diet for more information on this type of diet.

The therapy *Fast or Juice Fast* helps deal with *Toxic Overload*, one of the root causes of disease.

Fresh Fruits and Vegetables

If you've ever cut an apple and left it sitting on the counter, you've seen oxidation at work. Oxidation is what causes a cut apple to turn brown. It's also what causes a fire to burn, oils to go rancid, iron to rust and copper to develop a green patina. Most researchers now believe that oxidation is also what causes the body to deteriorate and develop degenerative diseases as we age. The free radicals that cause oxidative stress can be thought of as tiny "arsonists" waiting to start little inflammatory "fires" in the body.

Experts suggest that about 50-80% of all chronic and degenerative diseases, including heart disease, cancer, diabetes, arthritis, macular degeneration, Alzheimer's and dementia are caused by oxidative stress, are caused by free radical damage. Free radical damage also causes the cosmetic problems we associate with aging, dry skin, wrinkles, age spots and so forth.

Oxidation is not bad per se. The body uses oxidation to break down the food we eat and convert it to energy. The immune system also uses oxidation to destroy microbes and fight infection. Free radicals are also produced during the process the body uses to break down toxins for elimination.

Just like an automobile needs a cooling system (radiator) to keep the heat generated by the engine from destroying the engine parts, the body needs a cooling system to keep the oxidative processes it generates under control. Antioxidants can be thought of as the body's radiator cooling system.

Antioxidant nutrients are abundant in fresh plant foods. For example, fresh wheat contains an antioxidant called vitamin E, but this vitamin deteriorates within a few days after grinding the grain. Similar processes take place in all the foods we eat. So, because so little of the food we eat is fresh, most of us don't get enough antioxidant nutrients to keep our body's cooling system working properly. This allows oxidative stress and the resulting inflammation to "burn up" our health.

To compound this problem, we actually eat foods that increase oxidation and inflammation. Refined sugar, white flour, hydrogenated oils, trans fats and food additives put additional stress on our already overtaxed cooling system and further overheat the body's metabolic engine.

Fortunately, just like the car has a temperature gauge that warns you when the engine is getting too hot, the body also has warning indicators that tell you the metabolic engine is overheating. These warnings include: chronic, low grade aches and pains, fatigue (especially after exercise), constipation, headaches, difficulty concentrating ("brain fog"), excess weight, carbohydrate cravings, gum disease and loss of energy.

If these warning lights are going off in your body, don't ignore them. It's time to add some antioxidant "coolants" to protect your metabolic engine from continuing to "overheat" because of oxidative stress and chronic inflammation. The best way to do this is to eat 5-7 servings of fresh fruits and vegetables every day. And no, the ketchup and lettuce on that hamburger and those greasy french fries don't count! We're talking about eating generous portions (about 1/2 cup) of 5-7 different fresh fruits and vegetables every day.

The fact is, most people primarily eat processed (canned and frozen) produce—if they eat produce at all. Studies suggest that the average American consumes only 1-1/2 servings of vegetables and no servings of fruit in a typical day.

While eating processed produce is better than not eating produce at all, much of the antioxidant potential of these foods is lost in processing. And as for that word "fresh," how much of the produce at your local mega-mart is actually fresh? It typically takes 7-14 days to ship produce from the farm to the store, so many foods like tomatoes and peaches are picked green, which means they've never been allowed to develop their full nutritional value or flavor.

That's part of the reason most of us don't eat more fresh fruits and vegetables; the produce at mega-mart doesn't really taste that good. If you've ever eaten home-grown tomatoes or tree-ripened peaches, you'll know what we're talking about. That fresh, fully ripe flavor that makes these foods so delicious is actually a sign that the food is loaded with nutritional (including antioxidant) value.

For these reasons, it's probably a good idea to supplement with extra antioxidant nutrients in many situations. We should still eat those 5-7 servings of the best produce (fresh, frozen or even canned) we can find, because supplements are meant to supplement, not replace, a healthy diet. If you do want to supplement, you can try an *Antioxidant* or *Superfood Formula* that contains a variety of antioxidant berries and fruits.

The therapy *Fresh Fruits and Vegetables* helps deal with *Nutritional Deficiencies*, one of the root causes of disease.

Friendly Flora

Most of us associate bacteria with disease. We think of bacteria as something to be eliminated and destroyed. This has created an almost obsessive use of disinfectants in our culture. But, not all bacteria are bad. It is the action of bacteria, for example, that allows milk to be fermented to create cheese, yoghurt and kiefer. Bacteria also create other fermented foods such as sauerkraut and tofu. Another benefit of bacteria is that they breakdown minerals in the soil and make them available to the roots of plants.

Our "roots," i.e., the place where we absorb water and nutrients, is our intestinal tract, and bacteria play an important role in our "root" system, too. In fact, there are about three to four pounds of friendly microorganisms living in the intestinal tract, most of them bacteria. A proper balance of these microbes is essential to one's health, because we live in a symbiotic relationship with microorganisms. Many strains of bacteria are actually part of our body's natural ecosystem. They serve to help protect the body against unfriendly microbes.

There are many different species of beneficial bacteria inhabiting our intestines. Many belong to the genus *Lactobacillus*. These include *L. acidophilus*, one of the first strains sold as a supplement. Another genus containing species of friendly bacteria is *Bifidobacterium*, sometimes referred to as bifidophilus. A third major group belong to the *Streptococcus* genus. There are many others.

The good bacteria inhabiting the intestines are called *friendly flora* or *probiotics*. *Biotic* is from a Greek word that refers to life. So *pro*-biotic means favorable to life. This is in contrast to the word *anti*-biotic, which literally means against life.

Antibiotics weaken the immune system because they destroy the friendly flora. These friendly flora are actually part of the immune system. Friendly bacteria enhance the immune system in several ways. First of all, they form a sort of living "blanket" that coats the intestinal tract and inhibits other species of microorganisms from "gaining a foothold" on the intestinal mucosa. They compete with other microbes for food, which also holds down the growth of infectious organisms.

Friendly bacteria even produce chemicals that are deadly to harmful forms of bacteria, so they act as natural antibiotic agents against harmful bacteria. Another benefit of friendly bacteria is that they have a stimulating effect on the body's immune system. For instance, animal studies showed that *S. thermophilus* and *L. bulgaricus* increased proliferation of lymphocytes, stimulated B lymphocytes and activated macrophages.

A well-known benefit of friendly flora is their ability to keep yeast such as *Candida albicans* in check. When antibiotics, chemotherapy, chlorine or other chemicals or drugs destroy the friendly flora, yeasts multiple out of control. The yeast secrete a toxin that weakens the intestinal membranes and reduces the immune response. Probiotics are the antidote to this problem, helping to restore a healthy intestinal microflora.

Probiotics also help overall colon health. They reduce the risk of inflammatory bowel disorders such as colitis, Crohn's disease, and irritable bowel syndrome. They also reduce the risk of colon cancer. They should be used as part of a natural treatment plan for these diseases.

Healthy intestinal microflora improve the body's ability to digest fats and proteins. Probiotics synthesize certain vitamins the body needs, including B1, B2, B6, B12, folic acid and biotin. The synthesis of B12 by probiotics is particularly important for vegetarians who are not getting this vitamin in their diets.

The friendly flora also help detoxify certain poisons in the digestive tract. For instance, they help break down ammonia, cholesterol and excess hormones.

Finally, about 70% of the energy requirements of the intestinal mucosa come from fatty acids produced as a by-product of bacterial fermentation. This means that the intestinal microflora actually helps feed the intestinal lining demonstrating how vital this synergistic relationship is to health.

In fact, a healthy intestinal microflora is such an important part of total health, that some health researchers feel it should be considered as an independent body system. The intestinal microflora is a highly adaptable system, as it changes constantly, adapting itself to one's diet and environment. It is easy to see why a balanced intestinal microflora is such an important factor in a healthy body.

Probiotics can be obtained from yoghurt, keifer and other fermented dairy foods containing live bacterial cultures. They can also be found in naturally fermented pickles, kim chi and sauerkraut in the refrigerated section of the health food store. Fermented soy products like miso can also help. There are many good recipes for fermented foods in *Nourishing Traditions* by Sally Fallon.

When looking for a probiotic product, look for one that contains several strains of bacteria such as acidophilus, bifidophilus, etc. Make certain that the product is stored in the refrigerator, as the bacteria are living organisms and will die quickly when stored a room temperatures.

The therapy *Friendly Flora* helps deal with *Nutritional Deficiencies*, one of the root causes of disease.

Gall Bladder Flush

The gall bladder flush is a natural procedure that has been used to ease gall bladder attacks and potentially pass gall stones. It has been around for years and many people have had good success in using it. How it works isn't totally clear, but one explanation is that the large amount of olive oil ingested on the gall bladder flush sends the gall bladder into spasms which eject small stones and may also clear bile ducts.

The procedure is controversial and there is a slight risk, which is that a large stone may get stuck in the bile ducts resulting in the need for surgery. However, in nearly 30 years of experience I have only had one report of this happening. Besides, surgery is the standard treatment for this condition and surgery carries a much higher risk than this procedure, which makes me think that it is worth trying first. If it fails, then go for the surgery.

Here's the standard way to do a gall bladder flush. Start by fasting for 24 to 48 hours on fresh, raw apple juice or fresh squeezed grapefruit juice to clear the colon. Malic acid, an ingredient in the apple juice, is reported to soften the stones, but persons with hypoglycemia or yeast infections will do better on grapefruit juice. If using grapefruit juice, supplement with magnesium and malic acid for a similar effect.

Just before going to bed at the close of the fast, drink 1/2 cup of olive oil and 1/2 cup of lemon (or grapefruit) juice. Mix these together thoroughly like you would shake up a salad dressing. The lemon juice cuts the olive oil and makes it more palatable. It sounds and smells worse than it tastes. Next, lie on your right side for a half hour before going to sleep. In the morning, if you don't have a bowel movement, take an enema. This procedure may need to be repeated 2 days in a row.

Generally, you will pass some dark black or green objects that look like shriveled peas the day after drinking the olive oil and lemon juice. These objects are not gallstones. Gallstones that can be passed are much smaller than this, generally less than 2 millimeters in diameter. Chemical analysis of these objects shows they are composed of soap, and are created by the bile interacting with the oil.

The controversy of this procedure is whether the stones actually pass, or it just eases the pain and discomfort of the gall bladder attack and allows the problem to become asymptomatic again. You see, most people with gallstones don't know they have them, because they cause no symptoms. Whether stones are passing or not, this procedure typically eases gall bladder pain and allows the person to resume a normal life without surgery.

Therapies

I have seen a number of versions of this procedure, but they all rely on olive oil. This may be because olive oil acts as a solvent of cholesterol, the chief constituent of most gall stones. Some gall stones, however, are calcium based.

One variation that seems to work particularly well is to take a dose of Epsom salt about two or three hours prior to taking the olive oil and lemon juice. Follow the directions on the box of Epsom salts as per the dosage.

Certain herbs may also enhance the procedure. Herbs called cholagogues increase the flow of bile and help to dissolve stones slowly over a period of weeks and months. Herbs that have this property include dandelion root, artichoke, barberry bark, yellow dock root, fringetree bark, turmeric and celandine. A *Chologogue Formula* containing any of these can be taken before attempting the gallbladder flush to increase its effectiveness, or afterwards to continue improving gallbladder function.

In fact, taking these herbs regularly for a year or more may even help to dissolve larger stones. I would recommend a combination of artichoke, barberry, fringetree and turmeric, as these seem to especially good at helping the gallbladder to heal and potentially removing stones.

If gall stones are calcium-based, then hydrangea and magnesium will be helpful in dissolving them. Take these herbs during the fast and for several months after the gall bladder flush.

If the procedure does not bring relief, medical help should be sought.

The therapy *Gall Bladder Flush* helps deal with *Toxic Overload*, one of the root causes of disease.

Gut Healing Diet

In people with healthy GI tracts, food is completely digested, the nutrients absorbed, and the non-nutritive components eliminated. In people with impaired digestion and intestinal irritation, however, undigested food proteins are absorbed into the blood stream, causing an inflammatory immune response that can manifest as a host of other disorders including migraines, autoimmune diseases, allergies, Hashimoto's thyroiditis, GERD, Inflammatory Bowel Disease (IBD) and Irritable Bowel Syndrome (IBS).

Diet is absolutely essential to healing the gastrointestinal tract. There are three main diets one can follow, which will help the gut to heal. They are the Specific Carbohydrate diet, the Gut and Psychology Syndrome diet (GAPS) and the Paleo diet. Each of these diets is a little different, but all are well-known for their GI healing abilities. There are some commonalities between these diets, which should be a basic starting point for anyone with GI tract problems.

For starters, all simple sugars and refined carbohydrates should be eliminated from the diet. This includes refined sugars of all kinds, white flour and white rice. All gluten-bearing grains should also be eliminated, which include wheat, spelt, kamut, rye and barley. In fact, it is a good idea to eliminate all grains from the diet, at least in the beginning until the gut has healed.

Dairy may also be problematic because the bacteria love to feast on the sugar in dairy, lactose. Many people also have problems with a milk protein called A1 Beta-Casein. Modern dairy cows (Holstein) have this protein, which releases a peptide called BCM 7. This protein can cause neurological impairment, autoimmune reactions (including type 1 diabetes), inflammation of the blood vessels, reduced intestinal motility and excess mucus secretion. Goat milk products and some traditional breeds of cattle do not have A1 Beta-Casein. So, goat milk products and cultured dairy foods can be beneficial for some people, yet other people may have to eliminate all dairy foods.

Also eliminate all processed foods. Instead, eat a diet comprised exclusively of fresh, nutrient dense vegetables, fruits, and proteins (fish, eggs and meat). Cultured foods, especially cultured vegetables, are especially beneficial.

While on this diet, the following supplements can be used to help heal the gut:

Digestive Bitters Formula taken about 15-20 minutes before every meal with a large glass of water.

Digestive Enzyme supplements and/or Betaine Hydrochloric Acid supplements taken with meals.

Probiotic supplements and/or cultured foods with every meal.

2 tsp. daily of cod liver oil (for the omega-3 fatty acids EPA and DHA).

2 cups of bone broth per day or supplementation with 3000 mg of L-glutamine in powdered form twice daily.

Here are the basics of the three diets mentioned earlier and resources for learning more about them.

Specific Carbohydrate Diet (SCD)

The Specific Carbohydrate Diet works well for people who need a black and white list of foods they can and cannot eat. It has allowed (legal) foods and not allowed (illegal foods). The list can be found at: *breakingtheviciouscycle.info*

The diet allows meat, fats, non-starchy vegetables, ripe fruit, nuts and seeds, some beans and lactose-free dairy. It also allows glucose and honey. The inclusion of dairy foods and honey make this diet easier for some people to follow.

Foods that are eliminated (or reduced) include: processed foods, grains, starch, starchy vegetables, some beans, sugar, lactose, oligosaccharides, gums and thickeners. Starchy vegetables like potatoes, sweet potatoes, yams, parsnip and turnips are not allowed, while rutabaga, beets, celery root, carrots and squashes are allowed. Vegetables should be peeled, seeded and cooked as fiber can be irritating to damaged GI membranes.

There is a 75%-84% success rate for people following this diet rigidly. Improvement should be seen in a month if the diet is going to work. If it doesn't switch to another diet. It should be followed for one year past the point of having no symptoms. For more information on the Specific Carbohydrate Diet you can check out the websites: *www.breakingtheviciouscycle.info*, *www.SCDLifestyle.com* and *www.scdiet.org* or the following books:

Healing Foods by Sandra Ramacher,
Recipes for the SCD by Raman Prasad,
Grain-Free Gourmet by Bager & Lass
Eat Well Feel Well by Kendall Conrad.

GAPS (Gut and Psychology Syndrome) Diet

The GAPS diet differs from the SCD diet because it doesn't allow dairy products, honey, gelatin or store bought fruit juice. GAPS also allows vegetables in soups. The GAPS diet has stages in an introductory diet that should be followed before moving into the full GAPS diet. It depends on the severity of the condition of the GI tract how fast or slow a person can move through the stages.

The following is a simple overview of the allowed foods at each of the stages. At each stage one can use all the foods from previous stages.

Stage I

Stock or bone broth
Simmered meat
Simmered vegetables
1 teaspoon daily of a probiotic liquid or food (this should be gradually increased)
Herbal Tea sweetened with honey

Stage II

Raw egg yolks and then whole soft boiled eggs
Sautéed meat
Baked meat
Fermented fish
Ghee
If experiencing constipation drink carrot juice with cod liver oil

Stage III

Avocado
Nut butters
Squash
Fried or scrambled eggs
Fermented vegetables

Stage IV

Roasted meat
Grilled meat
Olive oil
Fresh vegetable juice
Nut flour bread

Stage V

Cooked apple puree
Fresh fruit juice (no citrus)
Raw vegetables

Stage VI

Raw peeled apple, gradually other fruits
More honey
Dried fruit

Typically you spend 1-2 days to a full week on each stage. People with severe gut problems might need up to four weeks on each stage. It is best not to skip the stages as this program helps to heal the gut, making it possible to digest and absorb other foods without problems. If you do go directly to the full GAPS diet, remember that about 85% of everything you eat should be meats, fish, eggs, fermented dairy and vegetables (some well-cooked, some fermented and some raw). Homemade meat stock, soups, stews and natural fats are not optional – they should be dietary staples. Fermented vegetables are also an important part of the GAPS diet, as fermenting eliminates the oligosaccharides that feed intestinal bacteria.

For more resources on GAPS you can go to the following websites: *gutandpsychologysyndrome.com* (Introductory Diet), *gaps.me*, *gapsguide.com* and *gapsdiet.com*.

You can also check out the following books: *GAPS* by Dr. Natasha Campbell-McBride and *Gaps Guide* by Baden Lashkov.

Paleo Diet

Unlike SCD and GAPS, Paleo isn't a set diet. Instead, it's a philosophy about eating, with several variations. The idea is to eat foods that were traditionally eaten by hunter-gatherer people for thousands of years before modern agriculture and processed foods. Strict Paleo is grain free, legume free and dairy free, but as people get healthier there are several variations of Paleo that allow and encourage certain dairy products.

A great resource for following the Paleo diet is *Practical Paleo* by Diane Sanfilippo. It explains both the why and the how of the Paleo diet and has 30-day meal plans focused on a variety of health issues. The recipes are detailed, tasty and easy to follow.

For more information on the Paleo diet you can check out the following websites and books:

> *marksdailyapple.com everydaypaleo.com, lifeasaplate. com* and *nomnompaleo.com*
> *Primal Body Primal Mind* by Nora Gedgaudas and *Primal Blueprint* by Mark Sisson.

Another good resource on eating traditional foods is *Nourishing Traditions* by Sally Fallon. Her recommendations are not as strict as other diets, and they include many delicious recipes with sensible guidelines. It also contains guidance about eating whole natural foods and includes a recipe section for making naturally fermented vegetables and beverages.

The therapy *Gut Healing Diet* helps deal with *Nutritional Deficiencies*, one of the root causes of disease.

Healthy Fats

Contrary to all the propaganda that suggests otherwise, we need fats in our diet to stay healthy. Fats play critical roles in our health. Brain and nerve tissue, for instance, requires the proper kind of fats, and low fat diets can lower the intelligence of children. The heart burns fat as its primary source of fuel. Fats are burned to keep the body warm in cold weather and are necessary for the production of many hormones.

Extremely low fat diets aren't good for us and can actually raise cholesterol, since about half of the cholesterol in our body is used to make bile to digest fats. However, we need to get the right kinds of fats in our diet. Unfortunately, most Americans are eating the wrong kind of fats, which include margarine, shortening, processed vegetable oils and animal fat from non-organically raised animals.

Americans tend to get too many Omega-6 fatty acids and not enough Omega-3 fatty acids in their diets. Omega-3 fatty acids protect us against heart disease. They also benefit the immune system because they help control the chronic inflammation that underlies the development of hardening of the arteries, arthritis, memory loss in aging and other degenerative disease. The best sources of Omega-3 are wild game, grass fed beef, eggs and poultry and deep ocean fish (not farm raised). Avocados and nuts, especially walnuts, also contain good fats.

Because most Americans get too many bad fats, and not enough good fats, most Americans can benefit from supplementing their diet with Omega-3 essential fatty acids. The best way to get Omega-3 fatty acids is through fish oil supplements. While flax seed and hemp seed oil contain Omega-3s, they are shorter chain fatty acids and must be converted to the longer chain DHA and EPA Omega-3s. Many people have problems with this conversion.

You also need some medium chain saturated fats in the diet. The best source for these is coconut oil and organic butter from grass-fed cows. You can make a great soft-spread butter by mixing softened butter with flax seed oil, getting the benefit of all your essential fats at the same time. Use half as much flax seed oil as butter.

The therapy *Healthy Fats* helps deal with *Nutritional Deficiencies*, one of the root causes of disease.

Heavy Metal Cleanse

Heavy metal detoxification is important for anyone who has worked around a lot of chemicals in their job (including painters beauticians, lab technicians, dry cleaners, carpet cleaners, farmers and factory workers in many industries). It's also a good thing for people suffering from any kind of chronic inflammatory disorder or problem that involves nerve damage.

Because the body is naturally exposed to small amounts of heavy metals, even in natural foods, it has defensive mechanisms to help it eliminate these toxic elements, as well as other harmful substances, from our body. By nutritionally supporting these mechanisms, while keeping the body's channels of elimination open, one can help the body remove excess heavy metals from the system.

One of the principal detoxifying agents in the body is a substance called glutathione. It is an antioxidant, produced in the liver from three amino acids: cysteine, glutamic acid and glycine. Glutathione helps cells eliminate drugs and heavy metals and protects the body from damage from smoking, radiation and alcohol.

N-acetyl-cysteine (NAC) contains the amino acid cysteine, which is a building block for glutathione, a powerful antioxidant that protects tissues including the liver, respiratory and immune systems, and the eyes. NAC helps increase glutathione levels, which protects healthy cells from damage by heavy metals and other toxic chemicals.

L-methionine is a sulfur bearing amino acid that acts as a powerful antioxidant. It is needed in extra amounts when toxins are present in the body because it protects glutathione. It can also be converted into cysteine to help produce more glutathione.

Another nutrient that helps the body detox from heavy metals is alpha lipoic acid, a powerful antioxidant. Because it is soluble in both water and fat, it has an especially wide range of protective actions. Even more, it enhances the function of other antioxidants like vitamin C, vitamin E, and glutathione. It also helps increase energy production in the cells.

An herb that is commonly used to help detoxify heavy metals is cilantro. This is based on research that showed eating cilantro increased the excretion of mercury (and possibly other toxic metals) from the body.

Heavy Metal Cleansing Formulas are used to help the body eliminate heavy metals. These formulas typically contain cilantro as a key ingredient. Other key herbs for heavy metal detoxification include lobelia and milk thistle.

Heavy metals (and many other environmental toxins) are not water-soluble. This means the body uses cholesterol to bind and transport them in the blood. So, make sure you are supplementing the diet with good fats when trying to remove heavy metals from the system. Consider taking cod liver oil, coconut oil, krill oil or some other good fatty acid supplement.

Enzyme systems, primarily located in the liver, convert the heavy metals into a water soluble form. Typically, they are too heavy to be flushed through the kidneys, so the liver eliminates them by binding them to cholesterol in the bile and flushing them out of the gall bladder into the small intestines. Fiber is needed to bind the cholesterol and heavy metals so they will be carried out of the body. While any kind of fiber helps, a particular form of mucilage known as sodium alginate is especially good at binding heavy metals. Sodium alginate is a mucilaginous fiber derived from kelp. Kelp is a purifier of the oceans because the alginate in it bonds to heavy metals and other toxins to neutralize them. Sodium alginate binds to heavy metals such as lead and mercury in the intestinal tract and carries them out of body with regular bowel movements. Apple pectin can also help bind heavy metals.

If you know or suspect you have heavy metal poisoning it's probably a good idea to work with an experienced doctor, naturopath or herbalist to custom design a program for your individual needs. However, as a starting point, here's a basic mercury and heavy metal detox program:

- 1 Tablespoon of coconut oil twice daily
- 1 capsule of a *Heavy Metal Cleansing Formula* twice daily
- 2-4 Algin three times daily or 1 Tablespoon of a *Fiber Blend Formula* in a glass of water or juice twice daily
  Drink 1/2 ounce of water per pound of body weight daily while on the cleanse.

Make certain the bowels are moving at least two to three times per day. If not, you may wish to take *Stimulant Laxative* or *Gentle Laxative Formula*.

If you develop a strong cleansing reaction (rash, diarrhea, nausea, dizziness, weakness, etc.) while on the cleanse, stop taking it for a couple of days. You can use a drawing bath to help the body detoxify more rapidly. In fact, doing a drawing bath once or twice a week while doing heavy metal cleansing will help you avoid any adverse reactions.

The therapy *Heavy Metal Cleanse* helps deal with *Toxic Overload*, one of the root causes of disease.

Hiatal Hernia Correction

Due to stress and repeated bouts of bloating and gas, or chronic nervous tension, the stomach may move up into the diaphragm creating a hiatal hernia. In a simple hiatal hernia, tension is holding the stomach up. In more severe cases, the stomach may adhere, requiring surgery. Because doctors use muscle relaxants when testing for a hiatal hernia, the simple kind often goes undetected. The instructions here are for the simple hiatal hernia where there are no adhesions.

A hiatal hernia stresses the stomach by inhibiting the vagus nerve and blood flow to the stomach. Protein digestion is impaired and the resulting lack of essential amino acids causes glandular malfunction, immune system deficiency, poor muscle tone, excessive weight loss or gain, cold limbs and general physical weakness.

Symptoms of a hiatal hernia include the inability to breath from the diaphragm, tension in the solar plexus, difficulty swallowing capsules, the sensation of a "lump" in throat and an over-stimulated thyroid gland (high metabolism). Chronic intestinal gas may occur as the ileocecal valve becomes permanently swollen and irritated and unable to close properly. Most people suffering from general poor health have this condition.

This problem can be overcome using a variety of self-help techniques.

Check your breathing. As a first step in treating the hiatal hernia, perform this simple test to assess your pattern of breathing. Put your hand on your abdomen as you breathe. If your abdomen moves in and out more than your chest, you are probably handling your stress well, or at least, you aren't letting stress control you.

If you are breathing from the top of your lungs, just sit back and relax to allow your breathing apparatus to revert to normal abdominal breathing. If it doesn't, then you need to relax the diaphragm. To do this, take lobelia essence or blue vervain in liquid form. Then, practice breathing from the abdomen again. You can also practice abdominal breathing while relaxing in a bath with lavender oil.

Find healthy ways to vent your repressed anger and frustration. This releases tension from the diaphragm and will help defuse much of the tension maintaining the hiatal hernia problem. For example, try taking a long, slow deep breath and feel the tension build up in your diaphragm (like you are starting to get angry). Make your hands into fists and raise them up in front of you as if you want to punch somebody. Exhale forcefully with an angry "huh!" sound while shaking your fists downward like you are hitting something. Do this several times, safely discharging your inner tension and frustrations.

Other methods of dealing with stress include changing your environment, finding new ways to resolve problems and communicating your thoughts and feelings honestly with others.

You can also find a chiropractor or a massage therapist who knows how to manually manipulate a hiatal hernia. It usually takes 4-6 treatments combined with self-help techniques to bring down a hiatal hernia.

As an alternative to having someone work on the problem for you, you can use the following technique.

Drink a pint of warm water first thing in the morning. Next, stand on your toes and drop suddenly to your heels several times. The force of this little jump and the weight of the water helps pull the stomach down in place while the warm temperature of the water relaxes the stomach area. Taking a dropperful of lobelia essence with the water will relax the stomach and make the treatment more effective.

If you're adventurous, jump off a chair or down a short flight of stairs to get the same effect. The idea behind this technique is to get your stomach to "drop" as if you were in an elevator that suddenly started going down.

If this doesn't solve the problem, place both hands under your breastbone in the center of your ribcage. Take a deep breath, press your fingers firmly into the solar plexus area (just under the breastbone). As you forcefully exhale, push your fingers downward and bend forward slightly. Be careful not to push your fingers up under the ribcage. Repeat this action several times. Do this before meals on an empty stomach.

You can find more information on dealing with a hiatal hernia, including a video demonstrating how to work on the problem in the article database at *modernherbalmnedicine.com*. The videos can also be found on YouTube.

The therapy *Hiatal Hernia Correction* helps deal with *Nutritional Deficiencies*, one of the root causes of disease.

Hydration

We don't often think of water as a nutrient, but it is the most important thing the body's needs besides oxygen. We can survive for weeks without food, but without water we would last a few days at best. A loss of just 15-20% of our body's water can be fatal. Only a lack of oxygen could kill us faster. Adequate intake of pure water is one of the simplest and cheapest health insurance policies you can buy. Without water, you don't have the ability to properly utilize either the food you eat or the supplements you take.

It has been estimated that 75% of all Americans are chronically dehydrated. So, of all underlying causes of ailments, dehydration is probably the most common and frequently overlooked. In about one-third of all Americans, the thirst mechanism is so weak that it is often mistaken for hunger. In one University of Washington study, a glass of water eliminated hunger in almost 100% of all the dieters studied.

Dehydration contributes to a wide variety of ailments, including indigestion, colitis, appendicitis, heart burn, rheumatoid arthritis, back and neck pain, headaches, stress, depression, high blood pressure, asthma, fatigue, memory loss and allergies. Many people have found that increasing their water intake reduces pain of all kinds, but especially headache, back and neck pain. Preliminary research indicates that 8-10 glasses of water a day could significantly ease back and joint pain for up to 80% of sufferers. Lack of water is the number one trigger of daytime fatigue.

Drinking water can also help to prevent disease. Water is necessary to flush waste products, particularly acid waste products, from the system. There is research to suggest that drinking five glasses of water daily could decrease the risk of colon cancer by 45%. Increased water intake could also slash the risk of breast cancer by 79% and reduce bladder cancer risk by 50%.

The brain is 80% water, so proper hydration is essential to its function. A mere 2% drop in body water can trigger fuzzy short-term memory, trouble with basic math, and difficulty focusing on the computer screen or on a printed page.

How much water do you need? A good rule of thumb is to divide your body weight in half and drink that many ounces of water per day. So, if you weigh 160 pounds, you need to drink about 80 ounces of water each day. There are 32 ounces in a quart, so this would equate to a little less than three quarts of water per day.

If you aren't drinking 1/2 ounce of water per pound of body weight per day and don't feel thirsty, you really need to drink more water anyway. When the human body is sufficiently dehydrated, its thirst mechanism shuts off.

This means that senior citizens are at greater risk for dehydration than younger people because their bodies are less effective at letting them know when they need water.

However, it isn't just the amount of water that is important. The kind of water we drink is critical, too. Increasingly, our water supplies are being polluted and poisoned with disastrous consequences to our health and well-being. So, drink the purest water you can find. Here are some options to consider:

Bottled Water

We can buy bottled water, but this is expensive and varies widely in quality. There are no government standards for bottled water. Some bottled water is simply tap water run through a carbon filter, others are waters bottled from various springs or natural sources. Unfortunately, the plastic containers bottled water comes in also leach chemicals into water, especially if they are left in a warm place. Still, some of the better brands of bottled water, especially if bottled in glass, can be good options for drinking water when traveling.

Carbon Filtration

Carbon filters are helpful in improving water quality and taste. In particular, they are very effective at removing chlorine and chlorine by-products. Carbon filters can be put on your shower heads or on the intake system for your whole house to remove these types of chemicals from the water you bath and wash in, as well as drink. Unfortunately, however, there are two major downsides to carbon filters.

First, they do not remove contaminants such as heavy metals, and secondly, they are prone to periodic dumping. That is, unless changed regularly, they can become saturated and dump previously removed contaminants back into your drinking water. Carbon filtration also works better the longer the water is able to be in contact with the carbon, so when water is passed too rapidly through a carbon filter, it is less effective.

However, at the very least you should use a carbon filter for your drinking water. As long as you change it regularly, it will greatly improve the quality of the water you drink.

Distillation

Distilling water is another great way to purify drinking water. With the exception of a few volatile chemicals which also evaporate in the distillation process, distilling water removes all contaminants. By running distilled water through a carbon filter after distillation, even these volatile substances can be removed. The major drawbacks to distillation are expense, cleanup and taste. Distillation is an expensive way of purifying water and requires considerable cleanup. The taste of distilled water is flat, but can be improved through aeration.

Reverse Osmosis

Reverse osmosis (RO) is the all-around best way to treat water for home use. Like distillation, RO removes all contaminants from water except for a few gases like chlorine, which are easily removed by carbon filtration. Reverse osmosis is a very inexpensive way to treat water, too, since it requires no other energy source except for the pressure in the tap. And, unlike distilled water, RO water has a fresh clean taste that makes you want to drink more. Many families have discovered that making RO water reduces their food budget for sodas, juices and other beverages because the water tastes so good. The only drawback of reverse osmosis is that it does not deal with bacteria, so RO units are suitable for use with treated tap water only.

RO water has a couple of drawbacks. It tends to be slightly acidic, so it is not very good at alkalizing the body. This drawback can be overcome by increasing magnesium and potassium intake. The other drawback is that it is not as healthy a water structure as ionized water. Still, it is a very good choice for cleaning up drinking water at home.

Ozone

Ozone is a more recent technology used to purify water. Ozone is a natural element created by ultraviolet light. Ozone oxidizes toxic substances. In fact, it destroys microorganisms in water 3,000 faster than chlorine and without chlorine's toxic effects. Ozone even helps to remove chlorine. E. coli, salmonella, giardia, cryptosporidium, parasites, bacteria, cysts, molds and a variety of others pollutants are all neutralized by ozone. In fact, washing produce in ozonated water will help to kill any of these organisms that might be present on your fruits and vegetables.

Ozone water can be very therapeutic, but it does not taste as good as the RO water. It also requires electricity, though it does not use even a fraction of the energy consumed in distillation.

Ozone is already being used in place of chemicals for hot tubs and swimming pools. Someday, this technology may replace the use of chemicals like chlorine in the treatment of municipal water supplies as well. So, where bacteria or microorganisms are a concern, such as with well water, ozonation would be the ideal choice.

Ionized Water

Research from Japan has shown that ionized water is by far the healthiest water to drink. Ionized water can be produced at varying degrees of alkalinity, which helps to counteract acid waste in the body. It also has antioxidant properties. Another advantage of properly ionized water is that it has the same structure as glacial runoff water, the healthiest water in the world. This is one of the factors that makes it superior for healing over reverse osmosis water. Carbon filtration is still needed in ionizing units to remove chemicals.

One of the biggest drawbacks of ionized water is the cost of the machines needed to produce it. The machines cost thousands of dollars and do require electricity. Machines that produce ionized water are also highly variable in quality. If you do decide to invest in one of these units, do your research and make sure you get a high quality unit.

The therapy *Hydration* helps deal with *Nutritional Deficiencies*, one of the root causes of disease.

Low Glycemic Diet

The single biggest problem with our modern diet is the huge amount of refined carbohydrates we consume. There are many problems with this obsession we have with refined sugars, white flour and processed grains. Here's why:

The pancreas, adrenals and liver work together to maintain a stable blood sugar level for healthy body and brain function. When you get up in the morning, your body has been fasting all night and your blood sugar is low. You "break your fast" by eating breakfast. And how you break-fast in the morning will set your metabolism for the day.

If you start off with coffee and donuts or other pastries, sugar sweetened breakfast cereal or other simple carbohydrates, you raise your blood sugar level quickly, but it comes at a cost. Your blood sugar goes too high and your pancreas has to secrete high levels of insulin to get this sugar out of your bloodstream. Insulin causes the body to store carbohydrates in the liver and fat cells (causing weight gain). Insulin also increases inflammation, which is the root cause of heart disease, cancer and numerous other degenerative ailments.

Normally, when blood sugar levels drop, another pancreatic hormone called glucagon steps in to mobilize sugar stores in the liver to keep the blood sugar level stable. However, high levels of insulin, depress the release of glucagon. So, once that sugar is low you crave your next high carbohydrate and/or caffeine fix. This low blood sugar is called hypoglycemia. 'Hypo' meaning low, 'gly' for sugar and 'cemia' referring to the bloodstream.

When blood sugar levels start to dip below normal, the body gives certain subtle clues that it needs help. These may include suddenly feeling cold or getting a cold nose, strong craving for sweets or caffeine, sudden fatigue or mental confusion, the inability to concentrate, a mild headache, or sense of pain around the eyes. If not dealt with soon, the symptoms may worsen into irritability, severe fatigue, dizziness or shakiness.

As the above symptoms suggest, hypoglycemia affects far more than our physical bodies. It also affects our mind and emotions. As the sugar in candy and chocolate rushes into the blood stream, it produces a sugar "high." Once the sugar drops the person experiences a corresponding "downer." As one again consumes sugary and starchy foods, the body goes on a blood sugar roller coaster ride, with your energy and mood going up and down with it.

Refined carbohydrates also rob your body of vitamins and minerals, since it requires these nutrients to process the carbohydrates into energy. This steadily reduces nutrient stores and depletes the health not only of bones and teeth, but the brain, heart, liver and other vital organs.

Probably half of most people's health problems would go away if they just stopped eating refined carbohydrates and processed fats. And, although this sounds hard, it's actually easier to make this change than most people think. It starts with that breakfast we referred to earlier.

Instead of starting the day with sugary, starchy foods and caffeine, start the day with some high quality fat and protein. Eggs, avocados, organic meats or unsweetened, whole milk yoghurt are all good choices. If you're in a hurry, take a spoonful of coconut oil and make a protein shake with a protein powder or a whole food meal replacement powder. These products are available in any health food store.

Protein and good fats cause your pancreas to secrete glucagon. Glucagon mobilizes sugar stored in your liver to enter the blood stream. This raises your blood sugar, but it also sets your metabolism to start burning fats instead of storing them. The result, your blood sugar stays more stable throughout the day and so does your energy and mood.

You can also reduce sugar cravings by taking two licorice root capsules at breakfast, two again at lunch, and two in the mid-afternoon. Energy Boosting Blends taken in the morning and again at lunch time can also help.

It also helps to eat low glycemic foods during the day. A low glycemic food is one that does not trigger high levels of insulin. Starchy foods like potatoes and whole grains have a higher glycemic index than non-starchy vegetables. Low glycemic vegetables include: green leafy vegetables, zucchini squash, green beans, cruciferous vegetables (broccoli, cabbage, cauliflower, etc.), tomatoes, onions, asparagus, cucumbers, peppers and turnips. You can lower the glycemic index of potatoes by mashing equal parts of cooked cauliflower with cooked potatoes.

It's also important to avoid eating an excess of sugary fruits. Fruit juices tend to have a high glycemic index. Fruits with lower glycemic indexes include apples, apricots, cherries, grapefruit, lemons, limes, peaches, pears and plums. If you are trying to lose weight or balance blood sugar in hypoglycemia or diabetes, it may be wise to avoid all fruits for a period of time until your body becomes more stable.

When foods are combined, it can lower the glycemic load. For example, adding fat, like butter or sour cream to a baked potato will lower the amount of insulin released. When looking at prepackaged foods, you can calculate the glycemic load of the food using the following formula. Take the total carbohydrates and subtract the amount of fiber and half of the fat. This gives you the glycemic load. You want to keep this under 10 grams.

So, for example. If you have a food that has 12 grams of carbohydrates, 2 grams of fiber and 2 grams of fat, the glycemic load would be 9. That's 12 minus 2 for the fiber and 1 for the fat.

It takes about two weeks to get over the cravings for sugar. However, once you've done so, you'll be pleased with how much your overall mood, energy and health will improve. Try it!

The therapy *Low Glycemic Diet* helps deal with *Nutritional Deficiencies*, one of the root causes of disease.

Mineralization

Since our bodies are literally composed of minerals (i.e., we are made of the "dust of the earth"), healthy bodies are connected to healthy soil. If any element is missing from the soil, then it will be missing from the foods we eat and as a result, we will not be properly nourished.

Unfortunately, our commercial methods of agriculture are not only depleting the soil of precious trace minerals, they are also destroying the ability of plants to be able to utilize those elements. Hence, our food is nutritionally deficient right from the start. To make matters worse, as our food gets refined, more of its nutritional content is removed.

Modern food is lacking in minerals because modern farming methods reduce mineral content in food. This is partly because chemical fertilizers focus on three nutrients: nitrogen, phosphorus and potassium, while neglecting other elements needed in the soil for healthy plants. Agricultural chemicals and a lack of organic matter in the soil also reduce mineral availability. This is because minerals are made available to plants through microorganisms in the soil.

Bacteria in the soil break down organic material from dead animals and plants to recycle it for use by other plants. Mycorrhiza fungi, which grow on the roots of plants, protect growing plants against these bacteria (fungus and bacteria are natural antagonists). Both these fungi and the bacteria in the soil help the plants assimilate the minerals they need. Chemical agriculture destroys these microbes.

This is why most people need something to supplement their mineral intake. When seeking to obtain minerals, the first source people should be encouraged to use is mineral-rich plants. This is because the minerals in plants are more bioavailable to the body. Consider using an herbal *Mineral Formula*.

Another way human beings get minerals is through water. Mineral springs have long been sought out for their healing benefits. Colloidal mineral supplements are generally a form of concentrated mineral water and can also be used to increase mineral intake. There are many of these products in the marketplace.

The therapy *Mineralization* helps deal with *Nutritional Deficiencies*, one of the root causes of disease.

Poultice

A poultice is a mixture of crushed fresh herbs or dried herbs moistened with water to make a paste. The crushed herbs or paste are applied topically. It is similar to a compress but plant parts are used rather than liquid extraction. To make a poultice with fresh herbs, simply crush, chop or mash the fresh plant parts and apply topically. To make a poultice with dried herbs, use a base of mucilaginous herbs like comfrey root, slippery elm or marshmallow and add other herbs to it. Add enough water to form a thick paste. Apply the paste directly to the skin. Poultices can be covered with a gauze bandage or other dressing. Change the poultice once or twice daily.

Herbs to consider for poultices include:
Slippery Elm (binding and drawing agent, cooling, soothing, nutritive)
Comfrey leaf (vulnerary, soothing, absorbs, mild astringent, not for deep wounds)
Comfrey root (binding and drawing agent, soothing, moistening)
Marshmallow (binding, soothing, cooling, moistening)
Flaxseed (lubricating, emollient, softening, nutritive, warming)
White oak bark (astringent, cooling, drying)
Psyllium seeds (binding, mildly drawing, absorbs moisture)

Plantain (drawing, anti-inflammatory, mildly astringent, antipoisonous, stimulates lymphatic drainage)

Lily of the Valley (very drawing, pulls slivers and pus, disinfecting)

Pine gum (very drawing, pulls slivers, disinfectant, warming, drying and astringent)

Lobelia (antipoisonous, stimulates lymphatic drainage, relaxing)

Calendula (astringent, cooling, drying, styptic, good for deep/infected wounds)

Yarrow (astringent, drying, stimulating, good for deep/infected wounds)

Goldenseal (astringent, vulnerary, antiseptic, good for ulceration)

Aloe Vera (good for moistening other herb powders in place of water to bind poultice, cooling, moisturizing, anti-inflammatory)

Clay (drying, drawing and binding)

Charcoal (draws toxins)

Instant potato flakes can be mixed with the juice of a fresh herb for an instant poultice (plantain juice or fresh plant tincture).

The therapy *Poultice* helps deal with *Physical Trauma*, one of the root causes of disease.

Stress Management

Worry. Tension. Stress. In modern society, it's difficult to avoid stress. From debts and unpaid bills to traffic jams and deadlines at work, everyday we're faced with situations that can cause us to "tense up" or start worrying. It has been estimated that 75-90% of all visits to primary care physicians are for stress-related health problems. So, learning how to manage the stress in our lives is a major key to maintaining good health.

To understand how to manage stress, we first need to understand what stress is. When the brain perceives stress, it sends a chemical message to the pituitary via the hypothalamus which triggers the release of the adrenocorticotropic hormone (ACTH). ACTH causes the adrenals to start producing hormones like epinephrine (adrenaline) and cortisol. Epinephrine is both a hormone and neurotransmitter. It tenses our muscles, increases our heart rate and blood pressure, dilates the bronchials and speeds up our breathing, shuts down digestion and other functions not essential to immediate survival, and otherwise prepares the body for action.

Cortisol reduces inflammation, enabling us to deal better with injury and pain. Although it's role in reducing inflammation is important, too much cortisol causes premature aging, depresses immune function and causes us to lose muscle and gain weight. These stress hormones also cause a rise in blood sugar levels and an increase in blood clotting factors.

With this understanding, it's easy to see how chronic, long term stress can become a factor in numerous health problems, including poor digestive function, constipation, tension headaches, neck and shoulder pain, low back pain, ulcers, high blood pressure, blood clotting, increased risk of infections, asthma, diabetes, excess weight and even cancer and autoimmune disorders. In fact, it is probable that a large percentage of all the illness we experience has a stress component.

If stress can cause so many health problems, it's obvious that we need to learn how to reduce stress in our lives. We may not be able to eliminate the stressful situations in our life, but we can reduce the stressful effects these problems cause in our body.

Here are seven keys to reducing the effects of stress on the body.

1. Breathe Deeply

One of the simplest things you can do to reduce your stress level, calm your anxiety and relieve the tension in your body is to just breathe. If you stop and notice what happens when you are feeling stressed, you will probably notice that you are either holding your breath or breathing very rapidly and shallowly. By concentrating on breathing slowly and deeply, you will activate the parasympathetic nervous system and help reduce your stress levels. You can also try breathing in while thinking, "I am," and out while thinking, "relaxed." See Deep Breathing therapy for more information.

2. Practice the Relaxation Response

You can take the breathing a step further by utilizing what Dr. Herbert Benson dubbed "The Relaxation Response." In 1975, Dr. Benson published his book of that title showing how a simple, non-religious meditation technique could help patients with insomnia, heart problems, high blood pressure and chronic pain. Dr. Benson demystified the subject, showing that all one needed to do was consciously relax the muscles, breathe slowly and deeply, and find a repetitive phrase to keep the brain occupied (such as repeating the word "one" in one's mind).

Taking just 20 minutes a day for this process will dramatically reduce one's stress level. Start by finding a comfortable place to sit or lie down. Consciously allow all the muscles of your body to relax. Start breathing slowly and deeply while counting your breath (in, one, two, three, four and out, one, two, three, four). Then pick a single focus for your mind, such as the word "one" or "peace" and

Therapies

simply repeat this word over and over again in your mind. This causes the "monkey chatter" in the brain to stop and quiets the mind.

3. Avoid Caffeine and Sugar

Have you ever noticed how attracted you are to junk food when you are under stress? Sugar and caffeine may give you a quick "pick up," but they'll let you down just as fast. Even worse, they tend to further stress the adrenal glands, which eventually will tire and give you that "burned-out" feeling. To reduce stress, avoid sugar-sweetened, high carbohydrate snacks in favor of snacks high in protein and good quality fats (like nuts). If you feel tired without caffeine, consider taking Adrenal Tonics to rebuild your adrenals and increase your energy.

4. Hydrate

This may seem strange, but drinking more water can actually make your nerves feel calmer and help you sleep more soundly. Dehydration increases anxiety levels, so drink plenty of purified water when you are under stress. See Hydration therapy for more information.

5. Exercise

What are those stress hormones for? They're gearing your body up to take physical action, and that's what makes modern stress such a big problem. The stress hormones gear our body to run, fight or physically work to combat the problem, but our sedentary lifestyle doesn't allow us to burn off these stress hormones in physical activity. Exercise gives us the opportunity to "work off" those stressful feelings. See Exercise therapy for more information.

6. Feed Your Nerves and Take Adaptogens

Nerves, like any other part of the body need nutrition. For starters, nerves need good quality fats like butter, coconut oil, nuts, olive oil, flax seed oil and Omega-3 essential fatty acids.

Vitamins are also important for nerve functions. Many people have found that B-complex vitamins help them cope with stress more easily. Vitamin C and pantothenic acid are also helpful because they support the adrenal glands. Silica, found in horsetail and dulse, key ingredients in many *Mineral Formulas*, helps the nerves become more resilient because it strengthens the myelin sheath.

There is a specific class of herbs that has been shown to greatly reduce the impact of stress on our health. These herbs are called adaptogens. Adaptogenic herbs modulate the signals that are sent from the hypothalamus and pituitary glands causing a reduction of adrenal output of adrenaline and cortisol, thus lowering overall stress levels. They help to break the damaging fight-or-flight chain reaction patterns in which the body gets stuck due to chronic stress. By reducing cortisol levels, these herbs also help boost the immune system.

Eleuthero root was the first to be identified as an adaptogen. Russian studies proved it helps increase stamina, endurance and energy, improve concentration and stimulate male hormone production. It also helps the immune system response.

Other single herbs that have been identified as possessing adaptogenic properties include gotu kola, American and Korean ginseng, suma and schizandra berries. Use *Adaptogen Formulas* to help reduce the output of stress hormones and calm your nerves.

7. Make Time for Rest and Relaxation

Telling someone to reduce stress is like telling them to avoid death and taxes. It just isn't going to happen. The good news is one doesn't have to try to avoid stress to reduce its effects. It turns out that a pleasurable experience causes the release of hormones and neurotransmitters that counteract the effects of stress. And, a pleasurable experience creates more positive benefits than a stressful experience causes harm. So, instead of reducing stress, we should be deliberately creating pleasure and enjoyment in our lives.

It's likely that a major part of the reason anxiety-related disorders are epidemic in our society is because we are just too busy. We are constantly on the go, and take very little time for pleasure and recreation. Making sure we plan time to do enjoyable things is very important to our emotional and physical health.

Many people feel they are too busy for this. Well, the truth is, that the busier you are, the more important it is for you to make time for rest and relaxation. If a woodcutter doesn't take time to sharpen his saw or his axe, he will find himself working harder and harder while becoming less and less productive. Rest and relaxation is "saw-sharpening" time, it makes you more productive with the rest of your day. If you are busy, you can't afford to not take time for rest and relaxation.

Watching TV doesn't count. Generally speaking, TV is designed to be stimulating, not relaxing. Instead, look for activities that feel pleasurable to the body, such as a warm bath, a soak in a hot tub, a massage, listening to relaxing music or taking a walk in the park. Find things that make you laugh and awaken a childlike delight in life. Slow down when you eat and really enjoy the flavor of the food. Remember that anything that brings a sensation of bodily pleasure counteracts the effects of stress and reduces anxiety.

Part of this is also making sure you are getting a good night's sleep. If you aren't, look up Insomnia in the Conditions Section and follow some of the suggestions for getting a good night's sleep.

Practicing these principles of stress management will not only help you stay healthy, it will also help you heal more quickly if you are sick.

The therapy *Stress Management* helps deal with *Mental and Emotional Stress*, one of the root causes of disease.

Sweat Bath

Many people in temperate climates the world over have used sweating both to prevent and treat disease. Scandinavians built saunas; Native Americans built sweat lodges. Samuel Thomson would wrap a person sitting in a chair in blankets and place a hot stone in a pail at his feet. By pouring water into the pail, the steam would come up under the blankets until the patient started to perspire.

During his college years Thomas Easley used a hot plate with a pan of water on it. By administering a sudorific formula with extra lobelia and steaming fellow students for about 20 minutes, they were able to knock out all kinds of acute illnesses.

With modern hot running water and bathtubs, inducing perspiration to clear toxins isn't that difficult. Start by drinking plenty of fluids.

Sudorific herbs are herbs that enhance perspiration. They move blood to the surface of the skin and help to open the sweat glands to promote elimination. You can also make a warm tea of any sudorific herb or use a *Sudo-*rific Formula with warm liquids. Some of the best herbs for this purpose include yarrow, capsicum, ginger, catnip and blue vervain.

After drinking the tea, draw a bath as hot as can be comfortably tolerated. Add to the water a couple of tablespoons of ginger powder, a handful of yarrow, rosemary or mint leaves or other aromatic herbs. Put the herbs in a cloth bag so the leaves don't get all over in the tub. Another, even easier, sweat bath water treatment is to put 5-10 drops of an essential oil such as lavender, tea tree, eucalyptus, or peppermint in the bath. Dissolve the oils in a little liquid soap before putting them into the bath water so they will mix with the water and not just float on the surface.

After getting out of the bath, don't dry off. Wrap up in a cotton sheet and go to bed. Pile on the blankets and allow the sweat to come freely. It's fine to fall asleep. When done, take a cool shower to cleanse the skin and close your pores. Don't allow chilling during the process.

With small children, don't put them into a really hot bath. Use a warm bath, and gently wash the child's body down with some natural soap (such as Dr. Bronners) and a wash cloth to make certain the pores are open. Adding just a small amount of lavender essential oil or tea tree essential oil to the bath, or using a natural soap will help to stimulate the circulation and draw the blood to the extremities.

Sweat baths can be helpful for all types of acute ailments, especially colds, fevers, flu, sinus congestion, rashes and earaches. Sweat baths are not recommended for people who are infirm, elderly or have heart conditions.

The therapy *Sweat Bath* helps deal with *Toxic Overload*, one of the root causes of disease.

Herbal Formulas Section

A Guide to Herbal Formulas in Capsules, Tinctures, Glycerites, Teas and Other Dosage Forms

This section lists over 1200 formulas, indicating the name of the company that makes it, the dosage form(s) the product comes in and the herbal and non-herbal ingredients. To help you find formulas that may be helpful for you, we've broken these products down into 102 categories. Each category is based on the idea of key herbs, which are herbs with specific therapeutic actions and effects on body systems. Formulas whose main ingredients fit the key herbs that define that product category were listed under that category, whether the name of the product matched the category or not.

Although many formulas could fit in several categories, we've listed the formula only in the one (or ocassionally two) categories that it's key herbs and/or name matched the best. There is an appendix where you can look up formulas by name and see which category or categories they are listed under. Many categories are subcategories of each other, so you can also look up formulas in related product categories for more options.

We've provided a brief description of how formulas in each category might be used and a list of the key herbs that define that category. To make it easier to review the formulas, we've highlighted these key herbs in the ingredient lists of the products.

We also did some standardizing of herb names and plant parts, so the label may use a slightly different name for a particular herbal ingredient (i.e. say blossoms instead of flowers). We've tried to include all commonly used names for that herb in parenthesis after the main trade name the plant is sold under. All herbs are listed in the order they appear on the product label. This does not mean that the first ingredient is the main herb in the formula and the last herb is in the least amount. Some companies choose to keep their formulas proprietary and don't list ingredients in order based on what percentage you will find them in the formula.

Also keep in mind that companies change product names, ingredients and dosage forms on a regular basis. We did our best to double check the accuracy of this information before going to press, but expect some discrepancies and always double-check the actual product labels before purchasing any product.

Adaptogen Formulas

See also *Adrenal Tonic Formulas*

Adaptogens are herbs that reduce the output of stress hormones from the adrenal glands. They work by affecting the hypothalamus/pituitary/adrenal (HPA) axis in the glandular system, reducing hormones from the hypothalamus and pituitary that stimulate the release of cortisol from the adrenal glands. In this manner, they mediate the stress response, which helps the body maintain normal function under mental, physical, emotional or even chemical stress.

Adaptogenic Formulas enhance immunity, increase stamina, reduce anxiety and improve mental and physical performance. Because both affect the adrenal glands, *Adaptogenic Formulas* and *Adrenal Tonics* are closely related and contain many of the same key herbs. However, *Adrenal Tonics* are generally more targeted at building up the health of the adrenal glands, while *Adaptogenic Formulas* are more targeted at reducing stress. They can often, however, be used interchangeably.

Key Herbs: Ashwaganda, Astragalus, Cordyceps, Eleuthero (Siberian ginseng), Ginseng (American), Ginseng (Asian, Korean), Holy Basil, Rhodiola, Schisandra (Schizandra) and Suma

Zand
Active Herbal (Capsule and Liquid)
Eleuthero root, **Astragalus**, **Ginseng (American)**, Ginkgo, Codonopsis root, He Shou Wu (Fo-Ti), Licorice

Herbalist & Alchemist
Adrenal Balance Compound™ (Alcohol Extract)
Eleuthero root, **Schisandra**, Devil's Club root bark, **Holy Basil**, Oat seed (milky), Sarsaparilla

Solaray
Adrenal Caps™ (Capsule)
Eleuthero root, Licorice, Gotu Kola aerial parts, Clove

Gaia Herbs
Adrenal Health (Liquid Phyto-Caps)
Ashwagandha, **Holy Basil**, **Rhodiola**, **Schisandra**, Oat seed

Gaia Herbs
Astragalus Supreme (Alcohol Extract)

Astragalus, **Schisandra**, Ligustrum berry

Irwin Naturals
Body-Type Vata (Softgel)

Pumpkin seed, Chebulic Myrobalan fruit, **Ashwagandha root**, Bacopa (Water Hyssop) whole plant, **Holy Basil leaf**, Long Pepper (Pippali), Ginger; Non-Herbal: Shilajit extract

Herbs Etc.
Deep Health® (Deep Chi Builder) (Alcohol Extract or Softgel)

Reishi (Ganoderma), Shiitake Mushroom, California Spikenard root, **Astragalus root**, Maitake Mushroom, **Ashwagandha root**, Eleuthero root, **Schisandra berry**, **Cordyceps**, Ginger root

Urban Moonshine
Energy Tonic (Alcohol Extract)

Rhodiola root, He Shou Wu (Fo-Ti), Eleuthero, **Ginseng (American)**, Hawthorn leaf and berry & flower, **Schisandra**, Licorice root, Cinnamon, Ginger

Solaray
Ginseng and Damiana (Capsule)

Ginseng (Korean, Asian), Eleuthero root, Damiana leaf

Gaia Herbs
Ginseng Schisandra Supreme (Alcohol Extract)

Ginseng (American), Scullcap (Skullcap), Kola (cola) nut, Damiana, Eleuthero root, Licorice, Prickly Ash (Zanthoxylum americanum), **Schisandra**, Oat seed

Gaia Herbs
Ginseng Supreme (Alcohol Extract)

Ginseng (American), Eleuthero root

Yogi Tea
Ginseng Vitality™ (Tea)

Cinnamon bark, Honeybush, Licorice, Ginger, Eleuthero root, **Ginseng (Korean, Asian)**, Alfalfa leaf, Dong Quai, Black Pepper, Hibiscus, **Astragalus**

Herbalist & Alchemist
Ginseng/Schisandra Compound™ (Alcohol Extract)

Eleuthero root, Oat seed (milky), **Schisandra**, Gotu Kola, **Rhodiola**, **Ginseng (American)**

Irwin Naturals
Ginza-Plus (Softgel)

Maca root, **Rhodiola root**, **Schisandra berry**, **Ginseng (Korean, Asian)**, **Cordyceps**, Black Pepper, Ginger, Turmeric; Non-Herbal: Fish oil, soy lecithin, annatto, St. John's bread

Solaray
Pituitary Caps™ (Capsule)

Eleuthero root, Gotu Kola aerial parts, Clove

New Chapter
Stress Advantage (Softgel)

Schisandra, **Ginseng (American)**, Eleuthero root, **Rhodiola**, Temulawak rhizome, Turmeric, **Astragalus**, Galangal rhizome, Ginger

Herb Pharm
Stress Manager™ (Alcohol Extract)

Eleuthero root, Reishi (Ganoderma), **Holy Basil leaf**, **Rhodiola root**, **Schisandra berry**

Herbs Etc.
Stress ReLeaf® (Alcohol Extract or Softgel)

Holy Basil, Passionflower, Valerian root, Oat seed (milky), **Ashwagandha root**, Black Cohosh root, Scullcap (Skullcap), Betony

Gaia Herbs
Stress Response (Liquid Phyto-Caps)

Rhodiola, **Holy Basil**, **Ashwagandha root**, **Holy Basil leaf**, Oat seed (milky), **Schisandra**

New Chapter
Stress Take Care™ (Softgel)

Schisandra, **Ginseng (American)**, Eleuthero root, **Rhodiola**, Temulawak rhizome & essential oil, Turmeric, **Astragalus**, Galangal rhizome, Ginger

Solaray
Tonic Blend™ SP-28™ (Capsule)

Sarsaparilla, Eleuthero root, **Astragalus**, He Shou Wu (Fo-Ti), Gotu Kola aerial parts, Saw Palmetto root, Licorice, Kelp, Alfalfa aerial parts, Ginger, Stillingia (Queen's Root)

Herbs Etc.
Ultimate Ginseng™ (Alcohol Extract or Softgel)

Ginseng (American) root, Ginseng (Red) root, **Ginseng (Korean, Asian) root**, Tienchi Ginseng root, Eleuthero root

Adrenal Tonic Formulas

See also *Adaptogen Formulas*

These formulas are targeted at strengthening the adrenal glands. Long-term stress, especially when coupled with a diet high in sugar and caffeine, can severely deplete the adrenal glands, resulting in adrenal fatigue. When the adrenals are fatigued, a person will feel tired, exhausted and burned-out, but have difficulty relaxing and sleeping at night. They may have lapses in short term memory, experience difficulty concentrating and be easily confused. They will also be emotionally sensitive and vulnerable and feel like they "just can't take it any more." People who experience post-traumatic stress syndrome, once known as "shell shock" or "battle fatigue," typically suffer from severe adrenal fatigue.

The adrenals produce cortisol, a hormone that controls excessive inflammation and keeps the immune system in check. When the adrenals are exhausted, they may not produce enough cortisol. This can make adrenal fatigue a factor in autoimmune diseases, asthma and other problems involving chronic inflammation. Corticosteroid drugs mimic this hormone and are often used to control symptoms in these types of conditions, but restoring adrenal health (and normal cortisol levels) is a more permanent solution.

Various adaptogens are the key ingredients in *Adrenal Tonic Formulas*, which share many of the same key herbs and *Adaptogenic Formulas*. *Adrenal Tonics* may also contain nutrients like vitamin C and pantothenic acid. In severe cases of adrenal fatigue, adrenal glandulars may be required. See *Adrenals (exhaustion, weakness or burnout)* in the *Conditions Section* for more information on adrenal fatigue.

Key Herbs: Borage, Eleuthero (Siberian ginseng), Ginseng (American), Ginseng (Asian, Korean), Gotu kola, Holy Basil, Licorice and Schisandra (Schizandra)

Vitanica
Adrenal Assist™ (Capsule)

Rhodiola, Astragalus, Ashwagandha root, **Holy Basil leaf**, **Ginseng (Korean, Asian)**, **Schisandra**, Eleuthero; Non-Herbal: Vitamin C, Vitamin B6, Vitamin B5, Magnesium, Zinc

Solaray
Adrenal Caps™ (Capsule)

Eleuthero root, **Licorice**, **Gotu Kola aerial parts**, Clove

RidgeCrest Herbals
Adrenal Fatigue Fighter (Capsule)

Eleuthero root, **Ginseng (Korean, Asian) root**, **Schisandra fruit**, Suma root, Astragalus root, **Ginseng (American) root**, Ashwagandha, **Holy Basil**; Non-Herbal: GABA, Taurine, vitamins B1, B2, B3, B5, B6 and B12, biotin, folic acid

Christopher's
Adrenal Formula (Capsule)

Mullein leaf, Lobelia, **Ginseng (Korean, Asian)**, **Gotu Kola**, Hawthorn berry, Capsicum (Cayenne) root, Ginger

Herb Pharm
Adrenal Support™ (Alcohol Extract)

Eleuthero root, **Licorice root**, Oat seed (milky), Sarsaparilla root, Prickly Ash bark

Herbs Etc.
Adrenotonic™ (Alcohol Extract)

Black Currant leaf, Astragalus root, Eleuthero root, **Licorice root**, **Ginseng (American) root**, **Schisandra berry**, Sarsaparilla root, He Shou Wu (Fo-Ti) root

Western Botanicals
Ginseng Plus Formula (Capsule and Alcohol Extract)

Ginseng (American), Astragalus, Milk Thistle seed, **Ginseng (Korean, Asian)**, **Ginseng (Korean, Asian)**, Eleuthero root, Echinacea (angustifolia) root, Mullein leaf & flower

Planetary Herbals
Schizandra Adrenal Complex™ (Tablet)

Schisandra, Chinese Yam rhizome, Poria Mushroom, Asian Water Plantain rhizome, Rehmannia, Dodder seed, Asian Water Plantain, Raspberry (Palm-Leaf) fruit, Lycium (Wolfberry/Gogi), Asiatic Dogwood berry; Non-Herbal: Calcium, Sodium

Western Botanicals
Super Adrenal Support (Alcohol Extract)

Maca, **Licorice**, Eleuthero root, Ashwagandha root

Herbs Etc.
Vibrant Energy™ (Alcohol Extract or Softgel)

Ginseng (Red) root, He Shou Wu (Fo-Ti) root, **Gotu Kola**, Eleuthero root, Damiana (diffusa) leaf, **Ginseng (American) root**, **Licorice root**, Prickly Ash bark, Peppermint, Ginger root, Capsicum (Cayenne) fruit

Allergy-Reducing Formulas

See also *Anti-Inflammatory* and *Decongestant Formulas*

These are blends that counteract allergic reactions. Allergic reactions occur when the body's immune system overreacts to minor irritants, causing the release of histamine, a pro-inflammatory chemical messenger. This histamine causes other immune cells to overreact, resulting in an inflammatory cascade. Because of the relationship between the digestive and respiratory membranes, an allergic reaction in the digestive tract can cause respiratory symptoms and an allergic reaction in the respiratory system can cause digestive upset.

Antihistamine drugs focus on neutralizing histamine after it has been released, but there are herbs and nutrients that can make the immune system less sensitive so that it doesn't overreact. Besides key herbal ingredients, there are several key nutrients that can be beneficial in combating allergies—vitamin C, quercitin and bromelain.

In addition to these key herbs and nutrients, *Allergy-Reducing Formulas* usually contain herbs that reduce inflammation and decongest respiratory passages, so they are related to *Decongestant* and *Anti-Inflammatory Formulas*. For more ideas on how to deal with allergies, see *Allergies (food)* and *Allergies (respiratory)* in the *Conditions Section*.

Key Herbs: Burdock, Eyebright, Nettle (Stinging) and Osha

Gaia Herbs
Aller-Leaf (Liquid Phyto-Caps)

Turmeric, **Nettle (Stinging) leaf**, **Eyebright**, Bayberry bark, Chinese Scullcap (Scute/Huang Qin), Goldenseal, Yarrow flower, Feverfew

Grandma's Herbs
Allergy Defense (Capsule)

Eyebright, Bilberry (Myrtilli fructus), Myrica bark, Raspberry (Red) leaf, Goldenseal, Rue, Labiatae, Fennel, Chamomile flower, Capsicum (Cayenne); Non-Herbal: Lutein

Western Botanicals
Allergy Formula (Capsule)

Astragalus, Marshmallow, **Nettle (Stinging) leaf**, Brigham (Mormon) Tea

Western Botanicals
Allergy Formula Syrup (Glycerine Extract)

Astragalus, Marshmallow, **Nettle (Stinging) leaf**, Peppermint leaf & essential oil; Non-Herbal: Pure Honey

Zand
Allergy Season Formula (Capsule)

Nettle (Stinging) leaf, Turmeric, Milk Thistle seed, Grape seed, Pueraria root, Coptis (Chinese Goldthread,Huang Lian) rhizome, Schisandra, Oat straw, Dandelion root, Ginger; Non-Herbal: Pantothenic Acid, Bromelain, Quercetin

Herbs Etc.
Allertonic® (Alcohol Extract)

Nettle (Stinging), Licorice root, **Eyebright**, Horehound, **Osha**, Horsetail, Mullein leaf, Elecampane root, Plantain leaf

Solaray
Histamine Blend™ SP-33 (Capsule)

Horehound aerial parts, Mullein leaf, Cherry (Wild) bark, Barberry root, Peppermint aerial parts; Non-Herbal: Montmorillonite Clay

Eclectic Institute
Nasal Support (Capsule)

Nettle (Stinging) leaf, **Eyebright flower & leaf**, Horseradish

Eclectic Institute
Nettles - Eyebright
(Alcohol Extract and Glycerine Extract)

Nettle (Stinging) leaf, **Eyebright flower and leaf**, Mullein leaf

Herbs for Kids
Nettles & Eyebright (Glycerine Extract)

Echinacea (purpurea) root, **Eyebright**, Peppermint, Oregon Grape, Sage, **Nettle (Stinging) leaf**, Chamomile flower, Milk Thistle seed

Herb Pharm
Pollen Defense™ (Alcohol Extract)

Eyebright flowering herb, Goldenseal rhizome and root, Horseradish root, **Nettle (Stinging) seed**, Yarrow flower

Herbalist & Alchemist
Respiratory Calmpound™ (Alcohol Extract)

Ginkgo, Khella seed, Reishi (Ganoderma), Licorice, Lobelia flower, Lobelia seed; Non-Herbal: Apple cider vinegar

Analgesic Formulas

See also *Anti-Inflammatory*, *Antispasmodic*, *Joint Healing* and *Topical Analgesic Formulas*

People who are used to modern fast-acting pain-relieving drugs may be disappointed when they first try herbal *Analgesic Formulas*. Herbs tend to be milder in their pain relieving effects than modern drugs, but they also have fewer side effects and a more cumulative action. In other words, they become more effective when taken over time. This is probably because they actually promote tissue healing, which permanently eases pain.

Pain is a symptom of inflammation and tissue damage. Simply "killing" the pain signal doesn't relieve the cause. One always needs to examine the cause of the pain and try to heal it, not just numb the pain. (See introductory material in this book)

Still, we all need something to ease pain from time to time, and *Analgesic Formulas* can be very effective for headaches, arthritic pains and muscle pain. They typically reduce inflammation, so they are closely related to *Anti-Inflammatory Formulas*. There is also a subclass of *Analgesic Formulas* that are aimed more specifically at migraines and headaches (see *Migraine/Headache Formulas*).

Many of the key herbs in *Analgesic Formulas* contain various forms of salicylic acid, the herbal precursor to aspirin (acetylsalicylic acid). Salicylic acid was first derived from meadowsweet in 1860 by a German chemist named Kolbe. It was subsequently synthesized in 1899 by the Bayer Company and became known as aspirin.

Salicylic acid inhibits the formation of cyclooxygenases (COX-1 and COX-2 inflammatory mediators) inside the cells. Because it lacks the acetyl group found in aspirin, these natural salycilates don't thin the blood.

Salicylic acid rarely occurs in plants in its free form. It usually occurs as a glycoside, ester or salt. Salicylic acid-containing herbs are used as analgesics, anti-inflammatories and febrifuges. Some have an anti-clotting effect, but it is much milder than that of aspirin. Because of this, herbs containing salicin don't cause the stomach bleeding problems that aspirin causes.

Herbs containing these compounds have a long history of use for relief of pain and inflammation. Remember that just because an herb contains salycilates doesn't mean it acts like other herbs that contain them. Each herb is a complex mixture of many compounds and has its own unique properties.

Major salycilate-bearing plants and key herbs for *Analgesic Formulas* include white willow bark, meadowsweet and black cohosh. Other key herbs found in these formulas have other types of analgesic, nervine or anti-inflammatory actions.

Also consider *Topical Analgesic Formulas*, which share many of the same key herbs. See *Pain (general remedies for)* in the *Conditions Section*.

Key Herbs: Black Cohosh, California Poppy, Corydalis, Feverfew, Indian Pipe, Jamaican Dogwood, Kava-kava, Lavender, Lobelia, Meadowsweet, Turmeric, Valerian, Wild Lettuce and Willow

Herbalist & Alchemist
Aspirea Compound™ (Alcohol Extract)

Meadowsweet flowering tops, St. John's Wort flower, **Willow bark**, **Corydalis rhizome**, **Indian Pipe**, **Jamaican Dogwood bark**

Eclectic Institute
Black Cohosh-Kava Kava (Alcohol Extract)

Black Cohosh, **Kava Kava**, **Jamaican Dogwood root**, Ginger

Gaia Herbs
Feverfew Jamaican Dogwood Supreme (Alcohol Extract)

Feverfew, **Jamaican Dogwood bark**, Cramp Bark, St. John's Wort flowering tops, Blue Vervain, **Valerian**, Ginger

Herbs Etc.
Herbaprofen® (Alcohol Extract)

Jamaican Dogwood bark, **Black Cohosh root**, Wood Betony (betonica), **Meadowsweet**, Passionflower, Devil's Claw root, Licorice root, Stevia leaf

Planetary Herbals
Inflama-Care™ (Tablet)

Turmeric, Boswellia, Ginger, **Turmeric**, Scullcap (Skullcap), Hops flower, **Corydalis tuber**, Holy Basil leaf, Rosemary, Japanese Knotweed (Hu Zhang) root, Pine bark, Grape seed, Green Tea leaf, Black Pepper fruit; Non-Herbal: Bromelain, Papain, Quercetin, Lecithin

Herb Pharm
Inflamma Response™ (Alcohol Extract)

Turmeric, Chamomile flower, **Meadowsweet leaf & flower**, Licorice, St. John's Wort flowers and buds

Christopher's
Nerve Comfort Formula (Glycerine Extract)

Wild (Prickly) Lettuce, **Valerian**

Western Botanicals
Pain Relief Formula (Capsule and Alcohol Extract)

Valerian, **Willow (White) bark**, **Jamaican Dogwood root**, **California Poppy**, **California Poppy flower**, Wild Yam, **Lobelia**, **Lobelia seed**, **Black Cohosh**, Devil's Claw, **Meadowsweet**, Chamomile flower, Clove, Capsicum (chinense)

Grandma's Herbs
Pain-Aid (Capsule)

Feverfew, **Valerian**, Chamomile, **Lavender**, **Willow (White) bark**, Wood Betony (betonica), Lemon Balm, Scullcap (Skullcap), **Bladder Pod**, Linden (Basswood, Tilia) flower, Ginkgo, Catnip, Peppermint, Passionflower, Blue Vervain, Peruvian bark

Solaray
Relief Blend™ SP-10™ (Capsule)

Willow (White) bark, Vervain aerial parts, **Feverfew leaf**, Rosemary, Scullcap (Skullcap) aerial parts, Kelp

Christopher's
Stop-Ache (Capsule)

Willow (White) bark, **Feverfew**, Clove, **Valerian**, **Wild (Prickly) Lettuce**, Hops flower, Wood Betony (betonica), **Lobelia**

Eclectic Institute
White Willow - Feverfew (Capsule)

Willow (White) bark, Ginger, **Black Cohosh**, **Black Cohosh**, **Feverfew flower & leaf**, **Kava Kava**

Nature's Answer
White Willow with Feverfew Std. (Capsule)

Willow (White) bark, Feverfew aerial parts

Planetary Herbals
Willow Aid™ (Tablet)

Willow bark, **Corydalis tuber**, Dong Quai, **Valerian**, Boswellia, Guggul; Non-Herbal: Calcium, Fiber

Herb Pharm
Willow Pain Response™ (Alcohol Extract)

Jamaican Dogwood bark, St. John's Wort flowers and buds, **Meadowsweet leaf and flower**, **Willow bark**

Antacid Formulas

See also *Catnip & Fennel, Digestive Bitter Tonic* and *Digestive Enzyme Formulas*

Antacids and acid blockers are very popular remedies for acid indigestion, heartburn and acid reflux. Unfortunately, most people who are suffering from acid indigestion do not have excess stomach acid. Instead, they suffer from a deficiency of stomach acid and enzymes. The acid burning they experience is due to poor digestion.

Acid deficient indigestion starts as a dull burning pain about 30-60 minutes after eating. It typically happens in people over 30. Digestion is poor and food sits heavily on the stomach.

In real over-acid conditions, pain starts shortly after eating and is sharp. Food digests rapidly and does not sit heavily on the stomach.

A person who suffers from gastro-esophogeal reflux disorder (GERD), also known as acid reflux or heartburn, usually has a hiatal hernia that is inhibiting the closing of the valve at the top of the stomach. When this is corrected, the acid stays where it belongs—in the stomach.

Neutralizing the stomach acid (or worse, blocking its production) is usually a bad idea because we need acid to digest protein and assimilate minerals like calcium. The hydrochloric acid in the stomach is also part of our immune system—it kills bacteria, yeast and parasites that may be in our food.

Herbal *Antacid Formulas* can normalize stomach acid production. When acid is high they calm the stomach, and when acid is low they stimulate digestion. This helps with the digestion process and relieves acid burning.

Catnip & Fennel Formulas can also be used as herbal *Antacid Formulas*. Where acid indigestion is due to low stomach acid consider *Digestive Bitter Tonic* or *Digestive Enzyme Formulas*. See *Acid Indigestion (Heartburn, Acid Reflux)* in the *Conditions Section* for more information on natural ways to regulate stomach acid.

Key Herbs: Catnip, Fennel, Gentian, Goldenseal, Meadowsweet and Turkey Rhubarb

Eclectic Institute
Neutralizing Cordial (Alcohol Extract and Glycerine Extract)

Turkey Rhubarb, Cinnamon (cassia) bark, **Goldenseal**, Peppermint essential oil; Non-Herbal: Potassium Bicarbonate

Herb Pharm
Neutralizing Cordial (Alcohol Extract)

Turkey Rhubarb, Cinnamon (aromaticum) bark, **Goldenseal rhizome and root**, Peppermint leaf and essential oil

Gaia Herbs
Reflux Relief (Tablet)

Aloe vera vera gel, Licorice, Chamomile flower, Marshmallow, Barley seed; Non-Herbal: Sugar Cane

Yogi Tea
Stomach Ease (Tea)

Licorice, Cardamom seed, **Fennel**, Coriander seed, Barley malt, Peppermint leaf, Ginger, Black Pepper

Herbs Etc.
Stomach Tonic™ (Alcohol Extract)

Chamomile flower, **Catnip flowering tops**, **Fennel seed**, Lavender (angustifolia) flower, Anise seed, Cardamom seed, **Gentian root**, Angelica root, Prickly Ash bark

Anti-Alcoholic Formulas

These formulas are used to help people stop drinking and to ease symptoms of alcoholic hangovers. The key herb here is kudzu, which has been shown to reduce alcoholic cravings and ease hangover symptoms like headaches, dizziness, upset stomach and vomiting.

See *Addictions (alcohol)* in the *Conditions Section* for more suggestions.

Key Herbs: Kudzu

Planetary Herbals
Kudzu Recovery™ (Tablet)

Kudzu root & flower, Hovenia fruit, Coptis (Chinese Goldthread,Huang Lian) root, Poria Mushroom, Zhu-Ling, Atractylodes (Bai-Zhu) rhizome, Codonopsis root, Cardamom fruit, Ginger

Nature's Sunshine Products
Kudzu/St.John's Wort (Capsule)

St. John's Wort aerial parts, Alfalfa aerial parts, **Kudzu root**

Anti-Diarrhea Formulas

See also *Fiber Blend* and *Intestinal Toning Formulas*

This formulas is to help arrest diarrhea. There are no key herbs for this category. *Fiber Blend Formula* and *Intestinal Toning Formulas* can also be helpful for diarrhea. See *Diarrhea* in the *Conditions Section* for more information.

Renew Life
DiarEASE™ (Bulk Powder)

Rice, Carob, Cinnamon, Ginger, Cardamom, Clove

Anti-Inflammatory Formulas

See also *Analgesic*, *Anti-Alcoholic* and *Antioxidant Formulas*

Inflammation is the body's natural response to irritation and tissue damage. Whenever your body gets cut, burned, bruised, bumped or bitten by an insect, an inflammatory response follows. Inflammation also occurs with sore throats, earaches, headaches and other common ailments. The term "itis" is Latin for inflammation, so many common disease names are simply naming parts of the body that are inflamed, such as bronchitis, appendicitis, tonsillitis, etc.

Inflammation is characterized by four symptoms—heat, swelling, redness and pain. Normally, the body repairs the damage and tissue returns to normal within a few days. However, inflammation can also become chronic and create long term damage in the body. Recent research suggests that heart disease, cancer, Alzheimer's, Parkinson's, dementia and other serious diseases are the result of chronic inflammation.

Inflammation is associated with both pain and oxidative damage in the body. For this reason, *Antioxidant Formulas* are usually anti-inflammatory and *Anti-Inflammatory Formulas* usually have some antioxidant effects. Also, *Analgesic Formulas* are typically anti-inflammatory and vice-versa. Hence, you will find common herbal ingredients in all three of these formula categories.

The various key herbs in these formulas have their own unique mode of action, so a blend will generally be more effective against inflammation than using them as singles. Consider using an *Anti-Inflammatory Formula* for conditions like arthritis pain, pain associated with autoimmune diseases, headaches, inflammatory bowel disorders, muscle pain or recovery from surgery or injury.

Key Herbs: Boswellia, Chamomile (English and Roman), Devil's Claw, Ginger, Meadowsweet, Turmeric, Willow and Yucca

Western Botanicals
Anti-Inflammation Formula (Capsule)
Turmeric, **Boswellia**, **Ginger**, **Devil's Claw**

NOW Foods
D-Flame™ (Capsule)
Holy Basil leaf, **Turmeric**, **Ginger**, Green Tea leaf, **Boswellia**, Chinese Scullcap (Scute/Huang Qin) root, Japanese Knotweed (Hu Zhang) root, Barberry root; Non-Herbal: Bromelain

Eclectic Institute
Devil's Claw - Yucca (Glycerine Extract)
Devil's Claw, **Yucca**, **Ginger**, Dandelion whole plant, Black Cohosh

Gaia Herbs
Ginger Supreme (Liquid Phyto-Caps)
Ginger, **Turmeric**

Gaia Herbs
Infla-Profen (Liquid Phyto-Caps)
Jamaican Dogwood bark, **Turmeric root**, Burdock root, **Devil's Claw root**, Feverfew flower and leaf, **Ginger rhizome**, Nettle (Stinging) seed, Nettle (Stinging) leaf

Planetary Herbals
Inflama-Care™ (Tablet)
Turmeric, **Boswellia**, **Ginger**, **Turmeric**, Scullcap (Skullcap), Hops flower, Corydalis tuber, Holy Basil leaf, Rosemary, Japanese Knotweed (Hu Zhang) root, Pine bark, Grape seed, Green Tea leaf, Black Pepper fruit; Non-Herbal: Bromelain, Papain, Quercetin, Lecithin

Nature's Answer
Inflama-Dyne (Capsule)
Rosemary, Holy Basil, **Ginger essential oil**, Green Tea leaf, **Turmeric**, Barberry root, **Devil's Claw**, Scullcap (Skullcap), Coptis (Chinese Goldthread,Huang Lian) root, Japanese Knotweed (Hu Zhang) root, Oregano leaf; Non-Herbal: Curcumin

Herb Pharm
Inflamma Response™ (Alcohol Extract)
Turmeric, **Chamomile flower**, **Meadowsweet leaf & flower**, Licorice, St. John's Wort flowers and buds

Gaia Herbs
Joint Health (Liquid Phyto-Caps)
Devil's Claw, Green Tea leaf, **Turmeric**, Brown Seaweed, Hawthorn berry, **Ginger**, Hops, Rosemary

Herbalist & Alchemist
Muscle/Joint Tonic™ (Alcohol Extract)
Sarsaparilla, **Turmeric**, **Devil's Claw**, Bupleurum, **Ginger**, Sichuan Teasel, **Willow bark**

Nature's Answer
Turmeric & Ginger (Liquid Capsule)
Turmeric, **Turmeric**, **Ginger**

Gaia Herbs
Turmeric Supreme (Liquid Phyto-Caps)
Turmeric, **Turmeric**, Black Pepper fruit

New Chapter
Zyflamend® Breast (Capsule)
Broccoli, Reishi (Ganoderma), Rosemary, **Turmeric**, Pomegranate, **Ginger**, Holy Basil leaf, Green Tea leaf, Japanese Knotweed (Hu Zhang) root & rhizome, Coptis (Chinese Goldthread,Huang Lian) root, Barberry root, Oregano leaf, Chinese Scullcap (Scute/Huang Qin)

New Chapter
Zyflamend® Nighttime (Softgel)
Holy Basil leaf, **Turmeric**, Chinese Scullcap (Scute/Huang Qin), Lemon Balm leaf, **Chamomile flower**, Hops flower, **Ginger**, Valerian

New Chapter
Zyflamend® Tiny Caps™ (Capsule)
Rosemary, **Turmeric**, **Ginger**, Holy Basil leaf, Green Tea leaf, Japanese Knotweed (Hu Zhang) root & rhizome, Coptis (Chinese Goldthread,Huang Lian) root, Barberry root, Oregano leaf, Chinese Scullcap (Scute/Huang Qin)

New Chapter
Zyflamend® Whole Body (Softgel)
Rosemary, **Turmeric**, **Ginger**, Holy Basil leaf, Green Tea leaf, Japanese Knotweed (Hu Zhang) root & rhizome, Coptis (Chinese Goldthread,Huang Lian) root, Barberry root, Oregano leaf, Chinese Scullcap (Scute/Huang Qin)

Anti-Itch Formulas

See also *Allergy-Reducing* and *Topical Vulnerary Formulas*

Itchy skin can be very uncomfortable, and constant scratching of mosquito bites, chicken pox sores, rashes and other itchy skin irritations can severely damage skin tissue. Fortunately, there are herbs that can be applied topically that can ease itchy feelings in the skin that form the basis for *Anti-Itch Formulas*. Where itching is due to allergic reactions, an *Allergy-Reducing Formula* might also be helpful when used both internally and externally.

Key Herbs: Chickweed, Plantain and Witch Hazel

Herbs Etc.
Bug Itch Releaf® (Spray)
Echinacea (angustifolia) root, Calendula (Marigold) flower, Propolis gum, **Plantain leaf**, Licorice root

Christopher's
Itch Ointment (Salve)
Chickweed, Olive oil; Non-Herbal: Beeswax

Herbs Etc.
Ivy Itch ReLeaf® (Spray)
Jewelweed, Grindelia (Gumweed) flower, **Plantain leaf**, Licorice root, Echinacea (angustifolia) root

Herbal Formulas

Antibacterial Formulas

See also *Echinacea Blend, Goldenseal & Echinacea* and *Immune Stimulating Formulas*

Antibiotics were a lifesaving discovery. Unfortunately, the overuse of these drugs, especially for viral infections like colds, has contributed to the development of antibiotic resistant strains of bacteria. Furthermore, broad spectrum antibiotics can destroy the friendly bacteria that live in our digestive tract. These bacteria help protect our body against infection and inhibit yeast overgrowth.

As the disadvantages of antibiotics become more widely known, many people are looking for more natural alternatives. Fortunately, there are many herbal remedies that can be very effective in treating bacterial infections. One of the advantages of these remedies is that, unlike antibiotics which only work on bacterial infections, most of these agents also fight against viral and fungal infections and won't contribute to the development of fungal infections.

Herbal antibacterial agents also don't have such destructive effects on the friendly flora of the intestinal tract. In many cases, these herbs also strengthen the immune system, thereby enhancing the body's natural resistance to infection and making you less susceptible to future infections.

Antibacterial Formulas are herbal blends where the primary agents are antibacterial in nature. This doesn't mean they will only work on bacterial infections; it simply means that their ingredients are a little more targeted to bacterial infections.

One of the secrets to using *Antibacterial Formulas* effectively is to use frequent doses. With many products you can take 1-2 capsules or 30-60 drops as often as ever two hours. This works much better than taking the formula only once or twice a day.

Of course, antibiotics are still a viable option for serious bacterial infections, but considering the problems of antibiotic resistant microbes and yeast infections, it seems wise to try an herbal remedy first. If it isn't powerful enough you can always get an antibiotic, but you'll probably be pleased with how often the herbal antibacterial agents work effectively by themselves.

If you are prone to frequent infections, you may also want to consider *Immune Stimulating Formulas*. See *Infections (bacterial)* in the *Conditions Section* of this book for additional information.

Key Herbs: Echinacea, Garlic, Goldenseal, Myrrh, Oregon Grape and Wild Indigo (Baptista)

Nature's Answer
Allertone (Glycerine Extract)

Echinacea (angustifolia) root, **Goldenseal**, Red Clover flowering tops, Bayberry bark, Mullein leaf

NOW Foods
AlliBiotic Non-Drowsy CF™ (Softgel)

Elder (Black) berry, Olive leaf, Oregano oil, **Garlic**, Larch (Larix), Rosemary oil

Planetary Herbals
Andrographis Respiratory Wellness™ (Tablet)

Andrographis aerial parts, **Echinacea (purpurea) root**, **Echinacea (pallida) root**, Olive leaf, Isatis (Woad) root, **Goldenseal**, Dandelion root, **Garlic**, Ginger, Licorice

Western Botanicals
Anti-Plague (Capsule and Liquid)

Garlic, Gravel Root root, Marshmallow, White Oak bark, Hydrangea, Elecampane root, Wormwood leaf, Uva Ursi, Cherry (Wild) bark, Black Walnut hulls, Lobelia, Lobelia seed, Scullcap (Skullcap), Mullein leaf, Aloe vera vera gel; Non-Herbal: Apple Cider Vinegar

Herbalist & Alchemist
Astragalus/Echinacea Compound™ (Alcohol Extract)

Echinacea (purpurea) root, Andrographis, Astragalus, Eleuthero root, **Oregon Grape**, **Myrrh**

Vitanica
CandidaStat™ (Capsule)

Garlic, **Oregon Grape**, Milk Thistle, Grapefruit seed; Non-Herbal: Lactobacillus acidophilus, Vitamin E, Calcium, Caprylic Acid

Herbs Etc.
Early Alert™ (Alcohol Extract or Softgel)

Andrographis, **Echinacea (angustifolia) root, herb and flower**, **Echinacea (pallida) root**, **Echinacea (purpurea) root, herb, flower and seed**, Olive leaf, Elder (canadensis) berry, Spilanthes

Herb Pharm
Echinacea Goldenseal (Alcohol Extract)

Echinacea (purpurea) root, **Goldenseal rhizome and root**, Osha root, Spilanthes flowering herb, Yerba Santa leaf, Horseradish root, Elder (Black) berry, Ginger root, Yarrow flower, **Baptisia (Wild Indigo) root**

Gaia Herbs
Echinacea Goldenseal Supreme, Alcohol-Free (Glycerine Extract)

Echinacea (purpurea) root, **Oregon Grape**, **Echinacea (angustifolia) root**, St. John's Wort flowering tops, Barberry root bark, **Goldenseal**, **Echinacea (purpurea) seed & aerial parts**

Gaia Herbs
Echinacea Goldenseal Supreme, Extra-Stength (Alcohol Extract)

Echinacea (purpurea) aerial parts, **Echinacea (angustifolia) root**, **Goldenseal**, **Oregon Grape**, Barberry root bark, St. John's Wort flower bud and tops, Propolis

Gaia Herbs
Echinacea Red Root Supreme (Alcohol Extract)

Echinacea (angustifolia) root, **Echinacea (purpurea) aerial parts, root & seed**, Indigo, Prickly Ash, Red Root, Stillingia (Queen's Root), Thuja

Eclectic Institute
Echinacea-Oregon Grape (Alcohol Extract)

Echinacea (purpurea) root and seed, **Oregon Grape**

Herbs for Kids
Echinacea/GoldenRoot™ Blackberry (Glycerine Extract)

Blackberry, **Echinacea (purpurea) root**, **Oregon Grape**

Herbs for Kids
Echinacea/GoldenRoot™ Orange (Glycerine Extract)

Echinacea (purpurea) root, **Oregon Grape**, Orange

Nature's Way
Garlicin® CF (Tablet)

Echinacea (purpurea) stem, leaf & flower, **Garlic**; Non-Herbal: Vitamin C, Calcium, Zinc

Herbalist & Alchemist
Healthy Kid's Compound™ (Glycerine Extract)

Echinacea (angustifolia) root, Elder (Black) berry, Lemon Balm; Non-Herbal: Orange extract

Herb Pharm
Herbal Detox™ (Alcohol Extract)

Red Clover leaf & flower, Licorice, Buckthorn bark, Burdock seed, **Oregon Grape**, Stillingia (Queen's Root) root, Poke Root (Phytolacca), **Baptisia (Wild Indigo) root**, Prickly Ash; Non-Herbal: Potassium Iodide, USP

Zand
HerbalMist (Spray)

Echinacea (angustifolia) root, Licorice, Sage, Hyssop, **Goldenseal**, Isatis (Woad) root & leaf, Marshmallow, Peppermint, Tea Tree essential oil, Thyme essential oil

Solaray
Immuboost Blend™ SP-21™ (Capsule)

Echinacea (purpurea) root, **Goldenseal**, **Myrrh**, **Garlic**, Licorice, Vervain aerial parts, Butternut bark, Kelp

Nature's Answer
Immune Support (Glycerine Extract)

Osha, **Baptisia (Wild Indigo) root**, **Echinacea (angustifolia) root**, **Echinacea (purpurea)**, Thuja, Maitake Mushroom

New Chapter
Immune Support Echinacea Ginger Tonic (Liquid)

Ginger, **Echinacea (purpurea) leaf**, **Echinacea (angustifolia) root**, Lemon essential oil, Ginger

Herb Pharm
ImmuneAttack™ (Alcohol Extract)

Echinacea (purpurea) root, Spilanthes, **Baptisia (Wild Indigo) root**, **Myrrh (abyssinica) tears**

Christopher's
Infection Formula (Capsule)

Plantain, Black Walnut, **Goldenseal**, Bugleweed, Marshmallow, Lobelia

Zand
Insure™ Immune Support (Capsule and Liquid)

Echinacea (angustifolia) root, **Echinacea (purpurea)**, **Goldenseal**, Red Clover, Sage, Burdock root, Peppermint leaf, Parsley leaf, Fennel, Ginger, Elecampane root, Bayberry bark, Chamomile flower, Valerian, Barberry bark, Blessed Thistle, Capsicum (Cayenne)

Zand
Insure™ Organic Immune Support Unflv (Liquid)

Echinacea (angustifolia) root, **Echinacea (purpurea)**, **Goldenseal**, Red Clover, Sage, Burdock root, Peppermint leaf, Parsley leaf, Fennel, Ginger, Elecampane root, Chamomile flower, Valerian, Bayberry bark, Blessed Thistle, Capsicum (Cayenne)

Zand
Kids Insure Herbal Formula Orange-Banana (Liquid)

Echinacea (angustifolia) root, **Goldenseal**, Red Clover, Sage, Burdock root, Peppermint leaf, Parsley leaf, Fennel, Ginger, Elecampane root, Chamomile flower, Valerian, Barberry bark, Blessed Thistle, Capsicum (Cayenne); Non-Herbal: Orange-Banana flavor

Zand
Kids Insure Herbal Formula Raspberry (Liquid)

Echinacea (angustifolia) root, **Goldenseal**, Red Clover, Sage, Burdock root, Peppermint leaf, Parsley leaf, Fennel, Ginger, Elecampane root, Chamomile flower, Valerian, Barberry bark, Blessed Thistle, Capsicum (Cayenne); Non-Herbal: Raspberry flavor

Herbs Etc.
Lymphatonic™ (Alcohol Extract, Glycerine Extract or Softgel)

Echinacea (angustifolia) root, Red Root root, Ocotillo stem bark, Burdock root, Licorice root, Dandelion root, Yellow Dock root, **Baptisia (Wild Indigo) root**, Blue Flag root, Stillingia (Queen's Root) root

Grandma's Herbs
Nature's Biotic (Capsule)

Garlic, **Goldenseal**, **Echinacea**, **Myrrh**, Plantain, Propolis

NOW Foods
Olive Leaf Extract with Echinacea (Capsule)

Olive leaf, **Echinacea (angustifolia) root**

Zand
Organic Herbalmist Throat Spray

Licorice, **Echinacea (angustifolia) root**, **Echinacea (purpurea)**, **Goldenseal**, Hyssop, Marshmallow, Peppermint, Tea Tree essential oil, Thyme

Gaia Herbs
Osha Supreme (Alcohol Extract)

Echinacea (angustifolia), **Echinacea (purpurea)**, Elecampane, **Goldenseal**, Grindelia (Gumweed), Irish Moss, Licorice, Mullein, Oregano, Osha

Herbs Etc.
Phytocillin® (Alcohol Extract or Softgel)

Usnea, Yerba mansa root, Propolis gum, **Echinacea (angustifolia) root**, Licorice root, **Oregon Grape root**, Hops strobile

NOW Foods
Propolis Plus Extract (Glycerine Extract)

Forsythia fruit, Licorice, Slippery Elm, **Goldenseal**, **Myrrh**, **Echinacea (purpurea) root**, Clove (aromaticum), Propolis

Gaia Herbs
Quick Defense (Liquid Phyto-Caps)

Echinacea (purpurea) root, **Echinacea (angustifolia) root**, Andrographis leaf, Elder (Black) berry, Ginger

Christopher's
Respiratory Relief Syrup

Onion, **Garlic**, Fennel, Nettle (Stinging) leaf, Mullein leaf, Chickweed

Christopher's
Super Garlic Immune Formula (Syrup)

Garlic, Wormwood, Lobelia, Marshmallow, White Oak bark, Black Walnut, Mullein leaf, Gravel Root root, Plantain, Aloe vera vera gel; Non-Herbal: Apple Cider Vinegar, Glycerine, Honey

Herbs for Kids
Super Kids Throat Spray™

Echinacea (purpurea) root, Rose hips, Licorice, Thyme leaf, Peppermint

Gaia Herbs
Urinary Support (Liquid Phyto-Caps)

Coptis (Chinese Goldthread,Huang Lian), **Echinacea (angustifolia) root**, **Echinacea (purpurea) aerial parts, root & seed**, Usnea, Uva Ursi

Gaia Herbs
Usnea Uva Ursi Supreme (Alcohol Extract)

Coptis (Chinese Goldthread,Huang Lian), **Echinacea (angustifolia) root**, **Echinacea (purpurea) aerial parts, root & seed**, Usnea, Uva Ursi

Christopher's
X-Ceptic (Alcohol Extract)

White Oak bark, **Goldenseal**, **Myrrh**, Comfrey root, **Garlic**, Capsicum (Cayenne)

Anticancer Formulas

See also *Blood Purifier, Essiac, Immune Stimulating* and *Mushroom Blend Formulas*

Herbs have been used successfully for thousands of years in the treatment of cancer. When used as part of a comprehensive program they can be very helpful in recovery. They can also be used as supporting agents to modern cancer treatments.

All the traditional herbal *Anticancer Formulas* in this book are also *Blood Purifier Formulas* and can be helpful for the same kinds of health problems. Likewise, many *Blood Purifier Formulas* can also be useful in anticancer programs. There is also a subcategory of herbal anticancer remedies—*Essiac Formulas*. Essiac is a popular anticancer blend that also acts as a blood purifier.

Unlike the modern medical approach to cancer, which is targeted at killing cancer cells, herbal therapy for cancer is aimed at altering the internal environment of the body to make it unfriendly to the growth of cancer.

Cancer cells thrive in a low oxygen, acidic environment in the body. Cancer can also be triggered by exposure to environmental toxins, which these types of herbs help to flush from the system.

Even in modern cancer therapy, as cancer cells are killed, the body must eliminate them or the system becomes overly toxic. So, these formulas are often helpful when used between rounds of radiation or chemotherapy to help rebuild the system.

The NIH reports that burdock may have anticancer properties, and herbalists have used it effectively for this purpose for decades. It is one of the most common herbs in traditional formulas for cancer and seems to work by deeply nourishing the body to promote better health while blocking the effect of cancer causing substances.

Herbal remedies that enhance the immune system, such as *Mushroom Blend Formula* and *Immune Stimulating Formulas*, can also be helpful. For more information on natural methods of treating cancer see *Cancer (natural therapies for)* in the *Conditions Section*. Because of the serious nature of cancer, competent help should be sought to design a treatment approach that is appropriate for the individual cancer patient.

Key Herbs: Burdock, Chaparral, Poke Root, Red Clover and Sheep Sorrel

Herbalist & Alchemist
Alterative Compound™ (Alcohol Extract)

Buckthorn bark, **Burdock root**, **Red Clover flower**, Licorice, Oregon Grape, Stillingia (Queen's Root), Poke Root (Phytolacca), Prickly Ash, Quassia wood; Non-Herbal: Potassium Iodide

Grandma's Herbs
Blood Cleanser Phase II (Capsule)

Red Clover, **Chaparral (Creosote)**, Licorice, Stillingia (Queen's Root), Prickly Ash, **Burdock root**, Poke Root (Phytolacca), Oregon Grape, Buckthorn

Grandma's Herbs
Blood Cleanser Phase III (Capsule)

Burdock, Cascara Sagrada, **Red Clover root**, Plantain, **Chaparral (Creosote)**, Raspberry (Red), Buckthorn, Marshmallow, Calendula (Marigold), Aloe vera, Licorice

Herb Pharm
Herbal Detox™ (Alcohol Extract)

Red Clover leaf & flower, Licorice, Buckthorn bark, **Burdock seed**, Oregon Grape, Stillingia (Queen's Root) root, Poke Root (Phytolacca), Baptisia (Wild Indigo) root, Prickly Ash; Non-Herbal: Potassium Iodide, USP

Gaia Herbs
Hoxsey Red Clover Supreme (Alcohol Extract)

Barberry, Buckthorn, **Burdock root**, Cascara Sagrada, Licorice, Nettle (Stinging) leaf, Poke Root (Phytolacca), Prickly Ash (Zanthoxylum americanum), **Red Clover**, Stillingia (Queen's Root); Non-Herbal: Sweet Orange essence

Western Botanicals
Immune-Virus Tea

Echinacea (angustifolia) root, **Chaparral (Creosote)**, **Chaparral (Creosote) flower**, Pau d'Arco, **Red Clover flower**, Lobelia, Lobelia seed

NOW Foods
Ojibwa Herbal Cleansing Tea

Red Clover flower, **Burdock root**, **Sheep Sorrel**, Licorice, Slippery Elm, Dandelion root, Barberry root bark, Turkey Rhubarb root

Gaia Herbs
Scudder's Alterative Compound (Alcohol Extract)

Alder, Corydalis, Figwort, Mayapple, Yellow Dock

Antidepressant Formulas

Although depression has many different causes (which need to be addressed for a permanent cure), one common denominator in most cases of depression is that energy production is reduced. *Antidepressant Formulas* tend to increase energy and lift one's mood. They also help to reduce anxiety and relax the nerves.

The most popular key herb in *Antidepressant Formulas* is St. John's wort because of the publicity it has received, but there are many other herbs that work in various ways to elevate mood and lift depression. A blend of several antidepressant herbs may be more helpful than a single herb like St. John's wort, because each of the key herbs in these blends are helpful for different root causes of depression. See *Depression* in the *Conditions Section* for more information and suggestions.

Key Herbs: Black Cohosh, Bupleurum, Damiana, Ginkgo, Kava-kava, Lemon Balm, Mimosa (Albizia, Silk Tree) and St. John's wort

Western Botanicals
Depression Formula (Capsule and Alcohol Extract)

St. John's Wort flowering tops, **Ginkgo**, Oat, Ginseng (American), Schisandra, Eleuthero root, Wood Betony (betonica), Ginger, Capsicum (chinense)

Herbs Etc.
Deprezac™ (Alcohol Extract)

St. John's Wort bud, **Lemon Balm**, Kola (cola) nut nut, Oat seed (milky), Peppermint, Valerian root, Eleuthero root, Rosemary leaf, **Damiana (diffusa) leaf**, Stevia leaf

Herbalist & Alchemist
Emotional Relief™ (Alcohol Extract)

St. John's Wort flower, **Lemon Balm**, **Mimosa (Albizia, Silk Tree) bark**, **Black Cohosh**, Holy Basil, Lavender (angustifolia) flower, Night Blooming Cereus (Cactus) stem

Herb Pharm
Good Mood (Alcohol Extract)

St. John's Wort flowering tops, Ashwagandha root, Scullcap (Skullcap), Prickly Ash

Herbalist & Alchemist
Grief Relief Compound™ (Alcohol Tincture)

Mimosa (Albizia, Silk Tree) bark, Rose petals, Hawthorn fruit, Hawthorn flower

Nature's Way
Mood Aid™ (Capsule)

St. John's Wort stem, leaf & flower, **Lemon Balm leaf**, Ginseng (Korean, Asian); Non-Herbal: L-5-Hydroxytryptophan

Eclectic Institute
Mood Balance (Capsule)

St. John's Wort flower & leaf, **Lemon Balm leaf**, Oat seed (milky)

Solaray
Mood Blend™ SP-39™ (Capsule)

St. John's Wort aerial parts, Velvet Bean, Griffonia bean, Gotu Kola aerial parts, Eleuthero root, Butternut bark, Violet seed, Ginger, Kelp

Traditional Medicinals
St. John's Good Mood® (Tea)

St. John's Wort, **Lemon Balm leaf**, Lavender flower, **St. John's Wort essential oil**, Oat straw, **Damiana**, Beebalm (Bergamot), Sage, Spearmint, Lemongrass leaf, Licorice

Eclectic Institute
St. John's Wort - Lemon Balm (Alcohol Extract and Glycerine Extract)

St. John's Wort flower & leaf, **Lemon Balm leaf**, Oat seed, **Kava Kava**

Yogi Tea
St. John's Wort Blues Away™ (Tea)

St. John's Wort leaf & flower, Fennel, Cinnamon bark, Spearmint, Cardamom seed, Ginger, Lavender flower, Fenugreek, Licorice, Clove, Black Pepper

Planetary Herbals
St. John's Wort Emotional Balance™ (Tablet)

St. John's Wort tops, Jujube seed, **Bupleurum**, Tree Peony, Atractylodes (Bai-Zhu) rhizome, Dong Quai, Poria Mushroom, **Lemon Balm leaf**, Cypress rhizome, Licorice, Ginger; Non-Herbal: sodium, calcium

Irwin Naturals
Sunny Mood (Softgel)

Rhodiola, **Lemon Balm**, Passionflower, **Damiana**, Saffron, Black Pepper, Ginger; Non-Herbal: Vitamin D3, Magnesium, Chromium Picolinate, Fish oil, L-Theanine, soy lecithin, riboflavin

Vitanica
Uplift™ (Capsule)

St. John's Wort, Rhodiola, **Ginkgo**, **Lemon Balm leaf**; Non-Herbal: Vitamin B6, Folate, Vitamin B-12

Vitanica
Woman's Passage™ (Capsule)

Hops, **St. John's Wort**, **Black Cohosh**

Antifungal Formulas

See also *Immune Stimulating Formulas*

Many people have problems with yeast infection, especially vaginal yeast infections, athlete's foot, jock itch and nail fungus. These infections may indicate that there is yeast overgrowth (such as *Candida albicans*) in the intestinal tract as well. The overuse of antibiotics and other medications that disrupt normal intestinal flora has been a major factor in causing these yeast infections.

When accompanied by appropriate dietary changes, *Antifungal Formulas* can be very helpful for all kinds of yeast and fungal infections. Since simple sugars feed yeast, best results will be obtained if all simple sugars, including natural ones like honey and fruit juice, are completely eliminated from the diet for at least a month or two. It is also wise to eliminate all simple starches such as white flour and polished rice while taking *Antifungal Formulas*.

Normally, the friendly lactobacteria in the colon protect us against yeast infections, but it is wise to include probiotic supplements such as acidophilus or bifidophilus while taking *Antifungal Formulas*. You can also eat yoghurt or other fermented foods with live bacterial cultures.

Liquid blends can be applied topically to control yeast infections, but should also be taken internally. Rebuilding the immune system with Immune Stimulating Formulas may also be helpful when treating yeast infections. Many symptoms blamed on yeast, however, are actually due to bacteria. For more information see *Small Intestinal Bacterial Overgrowth (SIBO)* and *Fungal Infections* in the *Conditions Section*.

Key Herbs: Garlic, Oregano, Pau d' Arco, Spilanthes, Tea Tree and Usnea

Herbalist & Alchemist
AF Compound™ (Alcohol Extract)

Black Walnut hulls, Yellow Root, **Spilanthes aerial parts**, Myrrh, **Usnea**, Cardamom seed

NOW Foods
Candida Clear™ (Capsule)

Pau d'Arco bark, Black Walnut hulls, **Oregano essential oil**, **Garlic**, Olive leaf, Cat's Claw root, Wormwood; Non-Herbal: Caprylic Acid, Magnesium, Biotin

Zand
Candida Quick Cleanse (Capsule)

Garlic, Goldenseal, **Oregano leaf**, Turmeric seed, Cinnamon bark, Cabbage, Clove, Oat seed, Coptis (Chinese Goldthread,Huang Lian) root, Dong Quai, Gentian, Ginger, Nettle (Stinging) leaf, Parsley leaf, Thyme leaf; Non-Herbal: Caprylic Acid

Vitanica
CandidaStat™ (Capsule)

Garlic, Oregon Grape, Milk Thistle, Grapefruit seed; Non-Herbal: Lactobacillus acidophilus, Vitamin E, Calcium, Caprylic Acid

Renew Life
CandiGONE™ (Capsule and Liquid)

Uva Ursi, **Garlic**, Grapefruit seed & rind, **Pau d'Arco**, **Pau d'Arco**, Barberry root, **Oregano leaf**, Orange peel, Oregon Grape, **Pau d'Arco**, **Pau d'Arco**, Cinnamon bark, Clove, Peppermint leaf, Neem leaf, Olive leaf; Non-Herbal: Magnesium Caprylate (Caprylic Acid), Calcium Undecylenate (Undecylenic Acid), Berberine Sulphate

Irwin Naturals
Candistroy® (Tablet)

Goldenseal, **Garlic**, **Pau d'Arco bark**, Oregon Grape root, Barberry root, Cassia bark, Clove, Licorice root, Orange peel, Peppermint leaf, Thyme leaf; Non-Herbal: Calcium Carbonate, Zinc Oxide

Herb Pharm
Fungus Fighter™ (Alcohol Extract)

Usnea, **Oregano leaf & flower**, **Spilanthes whole plant**, **Pau d'Arco (impetiginosa)**

Eclectic Institute
Pau d'Arco - Usnea (Alcohol and Glycerine Extract)

Pau d'Arco, **Usnea**, Black Walnut hulls, Yerba mansa, White Pond Lilly; Non-Herbal: glycerine version has cherry concentrate

Herbs Etc.
Phytocillin® (Alcohol Extract or Softgel)

Usnea, Yerba mansa root, Propolis gum, Echinacea (angustifolia) root, Licorice root, Oregon Grape root, Hops strobile

Vitanica
Yeast Arrest Suppositories™ (Capsule)

Cocoa (Cacao) butter, Neem oil, Oregon Grape, **Tea Tree essential oil**; Non-Herbal: Homeopathic Ingredients: Borax, Hydrastis Canadensis, Berberis Aquifolium, Kreosotum; Other Ingredients: Boric acid, Lactobacillus acidophilus,Triglycerides, Vitamin E.

Eclectic Institute
Yeast Balance (Capsule)

Pau d'Arco, **Spilanthes**, Goldenseal, Black Walnut

Solaray
Yeast Blend™ SP-7A™ (Capsule)

Goldenseal, Witch Hazel leaf, Plantain, Myrrh, **Pau d'Arco**, Slippery Elm, Blue Cohosh, Uva Ursi, Juniper berry

Herbs Etc.
Yeast ReLeaf® (Alcohol Extract or Softgel)

Pau d'Arco bark, Quassia wood wood, Licorice root, Echinacea (angustifolia) root, Myrrh gum resin, Yerba mansa root, Black Walnut hulls, Thuja leaf, Astragalus root, **Garlic bulb**

Antioxidant Formulas

See also *Anti-Inflammatory Formulas*

Experts suggest that about 50-80% of all chronic and degenerative diseases, including heart disease, cancer, diabetes, arthritis, macular degeneration, Alzheimer's and dementia are caused by oxidative stress, or free radical damage. Free radical damage also causes the cosmetic problems we associate with aging, dry skin, wrinkles, age spots and so forth.

Oxidation is not bad per se. The body uses oxidation to break down the food we eat and convert it to energy. The immune system also uses oxidation to destroy microbes and fight infection. Free radicals are produced in this process. They are also produced in the process of breaking down toxins for elimination.

Just like an automobile needs a cooling system (radiator) to keep the heat generated by the engine from destroying the engine parts, the body needs a cooling system to keep the oxidative processes it generates under control. Antioxidants can be thought of as the body's radiator or cooling system.

Fortunately, just as the car has a temperature gauge that warns you when the engine is getting too hot, the body has warning indicators that tell you the metabolic engine is overheating. These warnings include: chronic, low grade aches and pains, fatigue (especially after exercise), constipation, headaches, difficulty concentrating ("brain fog"), excess weight, carbohydrate cravings, gum disease and loss of energy.

If these warning lights are going off in your body, don't ignore them. It's time to add some antioxidant "coolants" to protect your metabolic engine from overheating due to oxidative stress and chronic inflammation. The best way to do this is to eat 5-7 servings of fresh fruits and vegetables every day, but *Antioxidant Formulas* can also help.

Key Herbs: Açaí, Bilberry (Blueberry, Huckleberry), Ginkgo, Lycium (Wolfberry, Gogi), Mangosteen, Rosemary and Tea (Green or Black)

Irwin Naturals
Açaí Power Berry Pure-Body Cleanse (Tablet)

Açaí, Blueberry, Cranberry, Lychee, **Mangosteen**, Pomegranate, Cascara Sagrada, Slippery Elm, Ginger; Non-Herbal: Calcium Carbonate

Celestial Seasonings
Antioxidant Green Tea

Green Tea, **White Tea**, Rose hips, **Eleuthero**, Alfalfa; Non-Herbal: Rebiana (sweetener from Stevia), Vitamin A palmitate, Ascorbic acid

New Chapter
E & Selenium Food Complex™ (Capsule)

Cinnamon bark, Fenugreek, Oregano leaf, Cumin, Coriander seed, **Rosemary**, Clove, Allspice, Peppermint leaf, Spinach, Blueberry, Turmeric, Ginger; Non-Herbal: Vitamin E, Selenium

Yogi Tea
Green Tea Energy™ (Tea)

Green Tea leaf, Anise, Ginseng (Korean, Asian), Lemongrass, Spearmint, **Eleuthero**, Kombucha

Yogi Tea
Green Tea Goji Berry (Tea)

Green Tea leaf, Green Matcha Tea leaf, **Lycium (Wolfberry/Gogi) berry**

Yogi Tea
Green Tea Kombucha (Tea)

Green Tea leaf, Lemongrass, Spearmint, Kombucha

Yogi Tea
Green Tea Kombucha Decaf (Tea)

Green Tea leaf, Lemongrass, Spearmint, Kombucha

Yogi Tea
Green Tea Pomegranate (Tea)

Dandelion root, **Green Tea leaf**, Hibiscus, Peppermint leaf, Burdock root

Yogi Tea
Green Tea Rejuvenation™ (Tea)

Green Tea leaf, Lemongrass, Spearmint, Cat's Claw root, Kombucha

Yogi Tea
Green Tea Super Antioxidant (Tea)

Lemongrass, **Green Tea leaf**, Licorice, Alfalfa leaf, Burdock root, Dandelion root, Grape seed, Emblic fruit, Irish Moss

New Chapter
LycoPom® (Capsule)

Tomato, Pomegranate, Sea Buckthorn seed, Rose hips, Turmeric, Saffron, **Rosemary**, Calendula (Marigold) flower

Celestial Seasonings
Moroccan Pomegranate Rooibos Tea

Rooibos (Redbush), Hibiscus, Pomegranate

Planetary Herbals
PlantiOxidants™ (Tablet)

Pomegranate seed, Pine (White) bark, Amla (Indian Gooseberry), **Green Tea leaf**, Japanese Knotweed (Hu Zhang) root, **Mangosteen**, **Lycium (Wolfberry/Gogi)**, Cherry (Sweet), Elder (canadensis) berry, Grape seed, **Rosemary**, Turmeric, Milk Thistle seed, **Açaí berry**, Raspberry (Red) leaf, **Bilberry**; Non-Herbal: Bioflavonoids, Red Wine extract

Celestial Seasonings
Pomegranate Green Tea

Green Tea, **White Tea**, Pomegranate; Non-Herbal: Ascorbic acid

New Chapter
Smoke Take Care™ (Capsule)

Turmeric, **Green Tea leaf**, Clove, Ginger, Parsley leaf & seed, Peppermint leaf, **Rosemary**

NOW Foods
Super Antioxidants (Capsule)

Green Tea leaf, Milk Thistle seed, Turmeric, Cranberry, **Rosemary leaf**, Grape seed, **Ginkgo**, Ginger, Hawthorn berry, **Bilberry fruit**; Non-Herbal: Quercetin, Bromelain

New Chapter
Supercritical Antioxidants (Softgel)

Turmeric, Turmeric oil, **Green Tea leaf**, Clove, Ginger, Parsley leaf & seed, Peppermint leaf, **Rosemary**

Celestial Seasonings
Sweet Açaí Mango Zinger Ice Herbal Tea

Hibiscus, Rose hips, Orange peel, Blackberry leaf, **Açai berry**; Non-Herbal: Rebiana (sweetener from Stevia)

Celestial Seasonings
Sweet Wild Berry Zinger Ice Herbal Tea

Hibiscus, Rose hips, Chicory, Orange peel, Blackberry leaf, Black Raspberry berry, Strawberry, Blueberry, Raspberry (Red), Cranberry, Cherry; Non-Herbal: Rebiana (sweetener from Stevia)

Solaray
Very Berry® Antioxidant Blend (Capsule)

Cranberry, Blueberry, Elder (canadensis) berry, Blackberry, Raspberry (Palm-Leaf) berry, **White Tea**, Apple, **Rosemary**

New Chapter
Zyflamend® Breast (Capsule)

Broccoli, Reishi (Ganoderma), **Rosemary**, Turmeric, Pomegranate, Ginger, Holy Basil leaf, **Green Tea leaf**, Japanese Knotweed (Hu Zhang) root & rhizome, Coptis (Chinese Goldthread,Huang Lian) root, Barberry root, Oregano leaf, Chinese Scullcap (Scute/Huang Qin)

Antiparasitic Formulas

See also *Digestive Bitter Tonic*, *Gentle Laxative* and *Stimulant Laxative Formulas*

These formulas contain herbs that have been used historically to destroy intestinal parasites, such as tapeworms, ring worms and pin worms. They may also help with single-celled parasites like giardia. *Antiparasitic Formulas* will also act as *Digestive Bitters Tonic Formulas* when taken in a liquid form. This means they will also stimulate digestive secretions.

These formulas often contain stimulant laxative herbs or are taken with *Stimulant Laxative Formulas* for enhanced effectiveness. *Antiparasitic Formulas*, especially those con-taining tansy, wormwood, male fern and quassia should be avoided during pregnancy and nursing.

See various types of parasites in the *Conditions Section* for more specific information.

Key Herbs: Black Walnut, Clove, Elecampane, Garlic, Male Fern, Pumpkin Seed, Quassia, Sweet Annie (Ching-Hao) and Wormwood

Western Botanicals
Anti-Parasite Formula (Alcohol Extract)

Black Walnut hulls, Lavender flower, Pumpkin seed, Wormseed seed, Cramp Bark, Grapefruit peel, Black Currant fruit & leaf, Olive leaf, **Quassia wood**, **Sweet Annie tops**, **Wormwood leaf**

Herbalist & Alchemist
AP Compound™ (Alcohol Extract)

Black Walnut hulls, **Elecampane root**, Long Pepper (Pippali), **Quassia wood**, **Sweet Annie**

Nature's Answer
Black Walnut & Wormwood (Glycerine Extract)

Black Walnut hulls, **Wormwood leaf & flowering tops**, **Sweet Annie leaf & flowering tops**

Nature's Answer
Black Walnut & Wormwood (Liquid Capsule)

Black Walnut hulls, Clove, **Wormwood aerial parts**, **Sweet Annie**

Nature's Answer
Black Walnut Complex (Capsule)

Black Walnut hulls, **Sweet Annie aerial parts**, **Quassia (amara) bark**, Red Clover tops, **Wormwood leaf**

Eclectic Institute
Black Walnut-Wormwood G (Glycerine Extract)

Black Walnut hulls, **Wormwood flower & leaf**, Thyme leaf, Cascara Sagrada, Cinnamon (cassia) bark, **Quassia wood**, Cinnamon essential oil

Eclectic Institute
Black Walnut-Wormwood O (Alcohol and Glycerine Extract)

Black Walnut hulls, **Wormwood flower & leaf**, Thyme leaf, Cascara Sagrada, Cinnamon (cassia) bark, **Quassia wood**, Cinnamon essential oil

NOW Foods
Fresh Green Black Walnut Wormwood Complex (Glycerine Extract)

Black Walnut hulls, **Wormwood**, **Clove bud**

Christopher's
Herbal Parasite Syrup

Wormwood leaf, Wormseed seed, Sage, Fennel, Malefern leaf, Papaya

Solaray
Intestinal Blend™ SP-24™ (Capsule)

Garlic, **Black Walnut hulls**, Butternut bark, Myrrh, Irish Moss

Eclectic Institute

Intestinal Support (Capsule)

Black Walnut, Wormwood flower & leaf, Clove

Herb Pharm

Intestinal Tract Defense™ (Alcohol Extract)

Black Walnut hulls, Wormwood, Quassia wood, Clove, Cardamom seed, Ginger

Gaia Herbs

Para-Shield (Liquid Phyto-Caps)

Pomegranate seed, Black Walnut hulls, Wormwood, Sweet Wormwood, Coptis (Chinese Goldthread,Huang Lian) root, Ginger, Gentian, Clove essential oil

Herbs Etc.

ParaFree™ (Alcohol Extract or Softgel)

Black Walnut hulls, Wormwood, Quassia wood wood, Clove flower bud, Malefern root

Renew Life

ParaGONE for Kids™ (Capsule and Liquid)

Black Walnut hulls & seed, Quassia (amara) wood, Wormwood leaf & stem, Pau d'Arco, Clove, Pumpkin seed, Garlic, Long Pepper (Pippali), Rosemary, Rosemary stem, Thyme leaf & stem, Marshmallow, Orange peel

Renew Life

ParaGONE™ (Capsule)

Black Walnut hulls, Quassia (amara) wood, Wormwood, Aloe vera, Garlic, Pau d'Arco, Clove, Grapefruit seed & rind, Pumpkin seed, Long Pepper (Pippali) seed, Rosemary, Rosemary stem, Thyme leaf & stem, Marshmallow, Orange peel; Non-Herbal: Caprylic Acid, Undecylenic Acid, Bismuth Citrate

Grandma's Herbs

Parasites & Worms (Capsule)

Tansy, Wormwood, Black Walnut, Garlic, Pomegranate, Hyssop, Pumpkin seed, Blue Vervain, Senna, Chaparral (Creosote), Bayberry bark

Irwin Naturals

Parastroy™ (Capsule)

Black Walnut kernel & hulls, Garlic, Cascara Sagrada, Fennel seed, Wormwood leaf, Clove, Epazote seed, Pumpkin seed, Slippery Elm, Capsicum (Cayenne), Onion, Sage leaf, Tansy, Thyme, Black Pepper; Non-Herbal: Betaine Hydrochloride, Bromelain

Gaia Herbs

Wormwood Black Walnut Supreme (Alcohol Extract)

Black Walnut, Clove, Coptis (Chinese Goldthread,Huang Lian), Gentian, Ginger, Pomegranate, Sweet Wormwood, Wormwood

Antispasmodic Formulas

See also *Bronchialdilator, Menstrual Cramp* and *Relaxing Nervine Formulas*

These formulas relax muscle cramps and spasms. They constitute the basic remedy for all conditions involving constriction—one of the six tissue terrains discussed in the introduction to this book.

Antispasmodic Formulas have broad uses. They can relieve Charlie horses, restless leg syndrome, tension headaches and back pain due to muscle tension. They are specifically helpful for conditions like torticollis, sciatica, back pain from muscle cramps, trigeminal neuralgia, Bell's palsy and facial tics and may also be helpful for tics associated with Tourette's syndrome.

Digestive problems where antispasmodic remedies may be helpful include adult colic, intestinal cramping, and easing pain associated with gall bladder attacks. When passing kidney stones they may also ease pain and make the passage easier. They can also be helpful for easing pain during labor and delivery.

For respiratory problems, *Antispasmodic Formulas* can be combined with *Cough Remedies* to ease whooping cough or other coughs with a spastic characteristic. They can also be helpful for asthma and COPD.

Liquid *Antispasmodic Formulas* can be applied topically to relax tense muscles, relieve cramps and ease pain. They can be warmed to body temperature and used as ear drops they can relieve earache pain. They can be massaged into the chest and back when children have a spastic cough or asthma attack. They can be rubbed into the pelvic area for menstrual cramps. Combined with *Topical Analgesic Formulas* they can be applied to the back to relax tense muscles, ease back pain and make chiropractic adjustments hold longer.

Two sub-categories of antispasmodic remedies are *Menstrual Cramp* and *Bronchialdilator Formulas*. These can also be considered *Antispasmodic Formulas*, but are listed separately because they are more targeted to the reproductive or respiratory system. With the many uses of a good antispasmodic remedy, it is a good idea to have at least one in your home medicine chest for use whenever cramping or spastic conditions occur.

For more information, see *Cramps (leg), Cramps (menstrual)* and *Cramps and Spasms (general)* in the *Conditions Section*.

Key Herbs: Black Cohosh, Black Haw, Blue Cohosh, Cramp Bark, Khella, Lobelia, Skunk Cabbage, Valerian and Wild Yam

Herbal Formulas

Christopher's
Antispasmodic Formula (Alcohol Extract)

Scullcap (Skullcap), **Lobelia**, Capsicum (Cayenne), **Valerian**, **Skunk Cabbage**, Myrrh, **Black Cohosh**

Eclectic Institute
Black Cohosh-Kava Kava (Alcohol Extract)

Black Cohosh, Kava Kava, Jamaican Dogwood root, Ginger

Herbs Etc.
Cramp ReLeaf® (Alcohol Extract or Softgel)

Black Haw stem bark, **Cramp Bark bark**, Bethroot root, Clove flower bud, Cinnamon (verum) bark, **Wild Yam root**, Cardamom seed, Orange peel

Christopher's
Ear & Nerve Formula (Alcohol Extract)

Black Cohosh, **Blue Cohosh**, Blue Vervain, Scullcap (Skullcap), **Lobelia**

Herbalist & Alchemist
J. Kloss Anti-Spasmodic Compound (Alcohol Extract)

Black Cohosh, Myrrh, Scullcap (Skullcap) flowering tops, **Skunk Cabbage**, **Lobelia flower**, **Lobelia seed**, Capsicum (Cayenne); Non-Herbal: Apple cider vinegar

Herb Pharm
Lobelia/Skunk Cabbage (Alcohol Extract)

Lobelia, **Skunk Cabbage**, Scullcap (Skullcap), **Black Cohosh**, Myrrh tears, Capsicum (Cayenne)

Western Botanicals
Nerve Calm Formula (Capsule and Alcohol Extract)

Black Cohosh, **Valerian**, **Blue Cohosh**, **Wild Yam**, Hops flower, Passionflower, Scullcap (Skullcap), **Lobelia**, **Lobelia seed**, Chamomile flower, Wood Betony (betonica)

Christopher's
Nerve Formula (Glycerine Extract)

Black Cohosh, **Blue Cohosh**, Blue Vervain, Scullcap (Skullcap), **Lobelia**

Eclectic Institute
Skullcap - Oats (Alcohol Extract and Glycerine Extract)

Scullcap (Skullcap) flowering tops, Oat seed, Licorice, **Lobelia leaf & seed**, Yerba Santa

Antiviral Formulas

See also *Antibacterial, Cold* and *Flu* and *Goldenseal & Echinacea Formulas*

One therapeutic area where modern medicine has few effective drugs is in fighting viral infections. The plant kingdom has far more effective antiviral remedies than modern medicine.

Many *Antiviral Formulas* can also be helpful for bacterial infections, and *Antibacterial* and *Goldenseal & Echinacea Formulas* can also be helpful for viral infections. When it comes to treating colds and flu, however, there are some other plant remedies that can really help besides those with antiviral activity. (Check out *Cold and Flu Formulas* for even more options). You can also look up specific viral problems in the *Conditions Section*.

Key Herbs: Astragalus, Echinacea, Elder, Isatis, Lemon Balm, Lomatium, Olive and St. John's wort

NOW Foods
AlliBiotic Non-Drowsy CF™ (Softgel)

Elder (Black) berry, **Olive leaf**, Oregano oil, Garlic, Larch (Larix), Rosemary oil

Traditional Medicinals
Cold Care P.M.® (Tea)

Linden (Basswood, Tilia) flower, Chamomile flower, Passionflower, Peppermint leaf, Yarrow flower, Eucalyptus leaf, Licorice

Eclectic Institute
Compound Biotic (Glycerine Extract)

Rose hips, Cherry (Wild) bark, Licorice, **Echinacea (purpurea) root & seed**, Peppermint leaf, Red Clover flower, **Astragalus**, Osha, **Lomatium**, **Elder (canadensis) flower**, Calendula (Marigold) flower, **Lemon Balm leaf**, Myrrh, Lemon essential oil, Lime essential oil; Non-Herbal: Ascorbic Acid

Eclectic Institute
Compound Herbal Biotic (Liquid)

Rose hips, Cherry (Wild) bark, Licorice, Red Clover flower, Peppermint leaf, **Elder (canadensis) flower**, Calendula (Marigold) flower, **Echinacea (purpurea) root & seed**, **Astragalus**, Osha, **Lomatium**, **Lemon Balm leaf**, Myrrh

Solaray
Echinacea and Elderberry (Capsule)

Echinacea (purpurea) root, **Elder (canadensis) berry**

Traditional Medicinals
Echinacea Elder Herbal Syrup

Echinacea, **Elder (canadensis) berry**

Traditional Medicinals
Echinacea Plus® Elderberry (Tea)

Echinacea (purpurea), **Elder (canadensis) flower**, **Echinacea root**, **Elder (canadensis) berry**, Ginger, Chamomile flower, Yarrow flower, Peppermint leaf

Planetary Herbals
Echinacea-Elderberry Syrup (Glycerine Extract)

Elder (canadensis) berry, **Echinacea (purpurea) root**, **Isatis (Woad) root**, Honeysuckle flower, Forsythia fruit, Platycodon, Boneset aerial parts, Licorice, Apricot seed; Non-Herbal: Honey

Herbs for Kids
Echinacea/Astragalus™ (Glycerine Extract)

Echinacea (purpurea) root, **Astragalus**, Peppermint leaf, Cleavers (Bedstraw), **Lemon Balm**, Burdock root

Eclectic Institute
Elderberry - Red Root (Spray)

Elder (canadensis) berry, Red Root, Echinacea (purpurea) root and seed, Slippery Elm, Capsicum (Cayenne); Non-Herbal: available in kids version without capsicum

NOW Foods
Elderberry, Zinc & Echinacea Syrup

Elder (Black) flower & berry, Echinacea (purpurea) root; Non-Herbal: Zinc Citrate

Gaia Herbs
GaiaKid's® Sniffle Support Herbal Drops

Elder (Black) berry, Elder (canadensis) flower, Eyebright, Plantain, Fenugreek, Thyme leaf, Anise seed

Herbalist & Alchemist
Healthy Kid's Compound™ (Glycerine Extract)

Echinacea (angustifolia) root, Elder (Black) berry, Lemon Balm; Non-Herbal: Orange extract

Eclectic Institute
Herbal Biotic (Liquid)

Osha, Rose hips, Cherry (Wild) bark, Licorice, Echinacea (purpurea) root & seed, Peppermint leaf, Red Clover flower, Astragalus, Lomatium, Calendula (Marigold) flower, Lemon Balm leaf, Myrrh, Lemon essential oil, Lime essential oil

Zand
HerbalMist (Spray)

Echinacea (angustifolia) root, Licorice, Sage, Hyssop, Goldenseal, Isatis (Woad) root & leaf, Marshmallow, Peppermint, Tea Tree essential oil, Thyme essential oil

Eclectic Institute
Immune Support (Capsule)

Elder (canadensis) berry, Larch (Larix), St. John's Wort flower & leaf, Lemon Balm leaf, Echinacea (purpurea) flower & leaf

Eclectic Institute
Lomatium - Osha (Alcohol Extract)

Osha, Lomatium, Licorice, Yarrow flower & leaf, Lemon Balm leaf

Eclectic Institute
Lomatium - Osha Spray

Osha, Lomatium, Echinacea (angustifolia) root, Echinacea (purpurea) root, flower, leaf & seed, Slippery Elm, Licorice, Lemon Balm leaf, Yarrow flower & leaf, Echinacea (pallida) root, Echinacea root; Non-Herbal: Kosher vegetable glycerin, Organic Grape Alcohol (28%)

Nature's Answer
Lomatium & St. John's Wort (Alcohol Extract)

Lomatium, St. John's Wort flowering tops, Shiitake Mushroom, Lemon Balm aerial parts, Licorice

Herbs Etc.
Loviral™ (Alcohol Extract or Softgel)

Lomatium root, Umckaloabo root, Osha root, Elder (canadensis) berry and flower, Andrographis, Boneset, Honeysuckle flower, Grindelia (Gumweed) flower, Elecampane root, Echinacea (angustifolia) root, Licorice root, Yarrow flowering tops, Lobelia

Vitanica
Lysine Extra™ (Capsule)

St. John's Wort, Lemon Balm, Astragalus, Oregon Grape, Myrrh; Non-Herbal: Vitamin C, Zinc, L-lysine HCL

NOW Foods
Olive Leaf Extract with Echinacea (Capsule)

Olive leaf, Echinacea (angustifolia) root

Zand
Organic Herbalmist Throat Spray

Licorice, Echinacea (angustifolia) root, Echinacea (purpurea), Goldenseal, Hyssop, Marshmallow, Peppermint, Tea Tree essential oil, Thyme

Nature's Way
Sambucus Immune Syrup

Echinacea (angustifolia) root, Echinacea (purpurea) flower, Propolis, Elder (Black) berry; Non-Herbal: Fructose, Natural Raspberry flavor, Vitamin C, Zinc

Herb Pharm
Soothing Throat Spray (Alcohol Extract)

Echinacea (purpurea) root, Propolis, Hyssop leaf & flower, Sage, St. John's Wort flowering tops

Herbs for Kids
Vi Protection Blend™ (Glycerine Extract)

Echinacea (purpurea) root, Hyssop root, Lemon Balm, Thyme leaf, Lemongrass, Ginger

Herb Pharm
Virattack™ (Alcohol Extract)

Lomatium, St. John's Wort flowers and buds, Echinacea (purpurea) root, Olive leaf, Lemon Balm leaf

Herbalist & Alchemist
VX Immune Support™ (Alcohol Extract)

Elder (canadensis) berry, Hyssop, Isatis (Woad) root, Japanese Honeysuckle flower, Lemon Balm, Lomatium, St. John's Wort flower

Planetary Herbals
Well Child™ (Glycerine Extract)

Honeysuckle flower, Lemon Balm leaf, Chamomile flower, Catnip aerial parts, Echinacea (purpurea) leaf, Cinnamon (cassia) twig, Licorice

Blood Purifier Formulas

See also *Anticancer, Cholagogue, General Detoxifying, Hepatoprotective, Liver Tonic* and *Lymphatic Drainage Formulas*

The concept of a blood purifier (also known as an alteratives) is unique to herbal medicine. Blood purifiers are herbs that have been used traditionally to cleanse the body without having a pronounced laxative or diuretic effect. The name "alterative" comes from their ability to alter the internal environment of the body, without producing strong diuretic or laxative actions.

Herbal Formulas

Blood Purifier Formulas ease stagnation, one of the six basic tissue imbalances discussed in the introduction to this book. This makes them useful for a wide variety of health problems.

Blood purifiers aid liver function, tend to increase the flow of bile and aid in the digestion and metabolism of fats. They have been traditionally used to clear up skin conditions, especially skin eruptive diseases like acne, rashes, hives, measles and chicken pox. They are also used to treat wounds containing pus. Many have also been used as anticancer remedies.

Herbal blood purifiers or alteratives are also key herbs in *Anticancer, Cholagogue, General Detoxifying, Hepatoprotective, Liver Tonic, Lymphatic Drainage* and *Skin Healing Formulas*. All of these categories of formulas have blood purifying effects and relieve stagnation, as well. They are just more targeted to specific organs and systems through the addition of other herbs.

Key Herbs: Burdock, Chaparral, Dandelion, Echinacea, Goldenseal, Oregon Grape, Pau d' Arco, Red Clover, Sarsaparilla and Yellow Dock

Herbalist & Alchemist
Alterative Compound™ (Alcohol Extract)

Buckthorn bark, **Burdock root**, **Red Clover flower**, Licorice, **Oregon Grape**, Stillingia (Queen's Root), Poke Root (Phytolacca), Prickly Ash, Quassia wood; Non-Herbal: Potassium Iodide

Yogi Tea
Berry DeTox (Tea)

Ginger, Fennel, Hibiscus, Orange peel, **Yellow Dock**, Turkey Rhubarb, Honeybush, Açai berry, Emblic fruit

Solaray
Blood Blend™ SP-11A™ (Capsule)

Capsicum (Cayenne), Kelp, **Dandelion root**, **Yellow Dock**, **Sarsaparilla**, **Burdock root**, **Echinacea (purpurea) root**, Licorice

Grandma's Herbs
Blood Cleanser Phase II (Capsule)

Red Clover, **Chaparral (Creosote)**, Licorice, Stillingia (Queen's Root), Prickly Ash, **Burdock root**, Poke Root (Phytolacca), **Oregon Grape**, Buckthorn

Grandma's Herbs
Blood Cleanser Phase IV (Capsule)

Burdock, **Pau d'Arco**, Cleavers (Bedstraw), Licorice, Slippery Elm, Black Walnut, Buckthorn, Calendula (Marigold), Canaigre, Aloe vera

Western Botanicals
Blood Cleansing Tea

Chaparral (Creosote) flowering herb, **Echinacea root**, Elder (canadensis) flower, **Red Clover flower**, Raspberry (Red) leaf, Yarrow flowering tops, **Yellow Dock**, Hyssop leaf, Plantain, **Sarsaparilla**, **Burdock root**, Chamomile flower, Corn Silk, **Pau d'Arco**, Sassafras leaf and root, Licorice, Valerian, Stevia

Western Botanicals
Blood Detox Formula (Capsule and Alcohol Extract)

Burdock root, **Oregon Grape**, Baptisia (Wild Indigo) root, **Yellow Dock**, **Chaparral (Creosote)**, **Chaparral (Creosote) flower**, **Red Clover flower**, Garlic, Lobelia, Lobelia seed, Capsicum (chinense)

Christopher's
Blood Stream Formula (Capsule)

Red Clover, Cat's Claw, Cat's Claw, **Pau d'Arco**, Licorice, Poke Root (Phytolacca), Peach bark, Oregano, Stillingia (Queen's Root), Cascara Sagrada, **Sarsaparilla**, Prickly Ash, **Burdock**, Buckthorn

Eclectic Institute
Blood Support (Capsule)

Burdock root, **Red Clover flower**, **Yellow Dock**, Nettle (Stinging) leaf, **Dandelion root**

Herbalist & Alchemist
Burdock/Red Root Compound™ (Alcohol Extract)

Burdock root, **Echinacea (purpurea) root**, Figwort, **Red Clover flower**, Red Root, Violet

Gaia Herbs
Cleanse & Detox Tea

Aloe vera, Artichoke, **Burdock**, Fennel, Licorice, Peppermint, Star Anise

Yogi Tea
DeTox (Tea)

Sarsaparilla, Cinnamon, Ginger, Licorice, **Burdock**, **Dandelion root**, Cardamom, Clove, Black Pepper, Juniper berry, Long Pepper (Pippali), Amur Cork Tree (Phellodendron) bark, Turkey Rhubarb, Scullcap (Skullcap), Coptis (Chinese Goldthread,Huang Lian) root, Forsythia fruit, Gardenia fruit, Japanese Honeysuckle flower, Wax Gourd seed

NOW Foods
Detox Support™ (Capsule)

Bladderwrack, Beet, **Red Clover flower & leaf**, **Dandelion root**, **Oregon Grape**, Milk Thistle fruit & seed; Non-Herbal: MSM, Sodium Alginate, Organic Chlorella, Alpha Lipoic Acid

NOW Foods
Echinacea & Goldenseal Plus (Glycerine Extract)

Echinacea (purpurea) root, **Goldenseal**, **Red Clover aerial parts & flower**, **Burdock root**, Peppermint leaf, Bayberry fruit, Capsicum (Cayenne)

Traditional Medicinals
EveryDay Detox® Lemon (Tea)

Burdock, Nettle (Stinging), Cleavers (Bedstraw), **Dandelion**, Lemon Myrtle

Vitanica
HepaFem™ (Capsule)

Burdock root, Milk Thistle seed, Celandine leaf, Fringetree, Beet

Herb Pharm
Herbal Detox™ (Alcohol Extract)

Red Clover leaf & flower, Licorice, Buckthorn bark, **Burdock seed**, **Oregon Grape**, Stillingia (Queen's Root) root, Poke Root (Phytolacca), Baptisia (Wild Indigo) root, Prickly Ash; Non-Herbal: Potassium Iodide, USP

Western Botanicals
Immune-Virus Tea

Echinacea (angustifolia) root, **Chaparral (Creosote)**, **Chaparral (Creosote) flower**, **Pau d'Arco**, **Red Clover flower**, Lobelia, Lobelia seed

Grandma's Herbs
Liver (Capsule)

Dandelion, Barberry, Milk Thistle, Plantain, **Burdock**, **Oregon Grape**, Yarrow, Cleavers (Bedstraw), Uva Ursi, Blue Flag, Beet

Western Botanicals
Liver Detox Tea

Dandelion root, Cardamom seed, Black Pepper seed, Cinnamon bark, **Burdock root**, Fennel, Clove, Juniper berry, Licorice, Orange peel, **Pau d'Arco**, Sassafras root, Ginger, Uva Ursi, Horsetail, **Dandelion leaf**, Parsley leaf

Nature's Answer
Liver Support (Capsule)

Oregon Grape, **Dandelion root**, **Goldenseal**, Milk Thistle fruit & seed, **Red Clover flowering tops**, Turkey Rhubarb, Gentian, Prickly Ash

Western Botanicals
Liver/Gallbladder Formula (Capsule and Alcohol Extract)

Milk Thistle seed, Barberry root, Turkey Rhubarb, **Burdock root**, **Dandelion root**, Juniper berry, **Pau d'Arco**, Garlic, Ginger, Parsley root, Uva Ursi, **Oregon Grape**, Black Walnut hulls, Fennel, Fringetree, Gentian, Wormwood leaf

Gaia Herbs
Milk Thistle Yellow Dock Supreme (Alcohol Extract)

Burdock root, Echinacea (angustifolia) root, **Echinacea (purpurea) root, seed & aerial parts**, Milk Thistle seed, **Oregon Grape**, Sarsaparilla, **Yellow Dock**

Celestial Seasonings
Natural Detox Wellness Tea

Milk Thistle seed, **Dandelion root**, **Echinacea (purpurea)**, **Red Clover**, Chicory, Licorice, **Sarsaparilla**, Green Rooibos, Carob

Vitanica
Opti-Recovery™ (Capsule)

Horse Chestnut, **Dandelion leaf**, **Echinacea (angustifolia) root**, **Echinacea (purpurea) root**, Cleavers (Bedstraw), Blue Flag; Non-Herbal: Vitamin C, Zinc, Bromelain

Renew Life
Organic Essential Detox (Capsule)

Burdock root, Slippery Elm, Sheep Sorrel, Watercress, Turkey Rhubarb, Blessed Thistle, **Red Clover**, Kelp, Astragalus, Milk Thistle seed, **Dandelion root**, Oat straw, Peppermint leaf, Hawthorn berry, Ginger, Mullein leaf

Planetary Herbals
Pau D'Arco Deep Cleansing™ (Tablet)

Burdock root, **Pau d'Arco**, **Pau d'Arco**, **Echinacea (pallida)**, **Red Clover tops**, Poria Mushroom, Astragalus, Licorice, Ginger, Ginseng (American), Reishi (Ganoderma); Non-Herbal: calcium, fiber, Potassium Iodide

Eclectic Institute
Red Clover - Burdock (Alcohol and Glycerine Extract)

Red Clover flower, **Burdock root & seed**, **Oregon Grape**, Stillingia (Queen's Root), Licorice, Cascara Sagrada, Prickly Ash; Non-Herbal: Potassium Iodide

Planetary Herbals
Red Clover Cleanser™ (Tablet)

Honeysuckle flower, **Echinacea (purpurea) root**, **Echinacea (pallida) root**, **Yellow Dock**, Siler, Coptis (Chinese Goldthread,Huang Lian) rhizome, **Sarsaparilla**, **Red Clover tops**, Chinese Scullcap (Scute/Huang Qin), Ginseng (American), Ginger, Licorice; Non-Herbal: Sodium, fiber

NOW Foods
Red Clover Plus Extract (Glycerine Extract)

Red Clover aerial parts & flower, **Dandelion root**, **Oregon Grape**, Licorice, Buchu leaf, **Burdock root**, Buckthorn bark

Gaia Herbs
Red Clover Supreme (Alcohol Extract)

Red Clover tops, **Burdock root**, **Yellow Dock**, Nettle (Stinging) leaf, Yarrow flower, Plantain, Licorice, Cleavers (Bedstraw), Prickly Ash (Zanthoxylum americanum)

Nature's Way
Red Clover with Prickly Ash Bark (Capsule)

Red Clover stem, leaf & flower, Prickly Ash (Zanthoxylum americanum), Buckthorn bark, **Sarsaparilla**, **Burdock root**, Licorice, Barberry root bark, **Echinacea (purpurea) stem, leaf & flower**, Cascara Sagrada, Sheep Sorrel stem, leaf & flower, Rosemary

Solaray
Skin Blend™ SP-4™ (Capsule)

Burdock root, Gotu Kola aerial parts, **Yellow Dock**, **Dandelion root**, Milk Thistle seed, Irish Moss, **Red Clover flower**, Capsicum (Cayenne), Kelp, **Sarsaparilla**

Nature's Way
Thisilyn® Cleanse (Mineral) (Capsule)

Cranberry, Asparagus root, Parsley leaf, **Burdock root**, **Red Clover flower**, Cleavers (Bedstraw), **Oregon Grape**, Milk Thistle seed, Artichoke leaf, Turmeric, **Dandelion root**, Psyllium hulls, Oat bran, Guar gum, Flax seed, Grapefruit pectin, Peppermint leaf, Ginger, Fennel, Marshmallow, Triphala, Amla (Indian Gooseberry), Haritaki, Bibhitaki (Behada); Non-Herbal: Magnesium Hydroxide, Fructooligosaccharides

Zand
Thistle Cleanse Formula (Capsule and Liquid)

Milk Thistle seed, **Dandelion root**, Chinese Salvia root, **Yellow Dock**, Barberry bark, Bayberry bark, **Burdock root**, Hyssop leaf, **Red Clover**, Bupleurum, Ginger, Licorice, Sage, Chrysanthemum flower, Honeysuckle flower

Irwin Naturals
Ultimate Cleanse™ (Tablet)

Alfalfa leaf, Fenugreek seed, **Dandelion root**, Fennel seed, Yarrow flower, Eleuthero, Green Tea, Hawthorn fruit, Horsetail, Licorice, Marshmallow root, Peppermint leaf, **Red Clover aerial parts**, Raspberry (Red) leaf, Safflower seed, Scullcap (Skullcap), **Burdock**, Chickweed, Mullein leaf, Papaya leaf, Black Cohosh root, Club Moss aerial parts, Ginger, Ginkgo, Irish Moss whole plant, Kelp,

Herbal Formulas

Plantain leaf, Slippery Elm, **Yellow Dock**, Milk Thistle seed, Capsicum (Cayenne), **Echinacea (angustifolia)**; Non-Herbal: Calcium Carbonate, Iodine (from Kelp)

Blood Sugar Reducing Formulas

In type 2 diabetes, the pancreas is producing high amounts of insulin, but the cells have become resistant to its influence. *Blood Sugar Reducing Formulas* are used to reduce cellular resistance to insulin. When combined with appropriate dietary and lifestyle changes, *Blood Sugar Reducing Formulas* can help to manage type 2 diabetes and even reverse it. These formulas may also reduce the need for medication in type 1 diabetes.

Caution: These formulas should not be relied upon as the sole treatment for diabetes. Diabetes is a serious medical condition and should be monitored by a physician. Natural therapy for diabetes requires major dietary and lifestyle changes. See *Diabetes* in the *Conditions Section* for more information.

Key Herbs: Bitter Melon, Cinnamon, Devil's Club, Fenugreek, Ginseng (American), Goldenseal, Gymnema, Jambul, Juniper Berry and Nopal (Prickly Pear)

Eclectic Institute
Blood Sugar Balance (Capsule)

Devil's Club root, **Bitter Melon**, Bean pod, **Nopal (Prickly Pear) leaf**, Huckleberry leaf

Nature's Way
Blood Sugar with Gymnema (Capsule)

Cinnamon bark, **Fenugreek**, **Nopal (Prickly Pear)**, **Bitter Melon**, **Gymnema leaf**, Bilberry leaf; Non-Herbal: Vitamin A, Chromium

Planetary Herbals
Cinnamon Glucose Balance™ (Tablet)

Fenugreek, **Cinnamon bark**, **Bitter Melon**, **Gymnema leaf**, Holy Basil leaf, Blueberry leaf, Milk Thistle seed, Hawthorn berry, Chinese Salvia root

Solaray
GlucoCut Blend™ Sp-5 (Capsule)

Uva Ursi, Dandelion root, **Fenugreek**, Gentian, Huckleberry leaf, Parsley aerial parts

Gaia Herbs
Glycemic Health (Liquid Phyto-Caps)

Cinnamon (burmannii) bark, Turmeric, **Fenugreek**, Blueberry leaf, **Bitter Melon**, **Jambul**, Indian Ginger

Eclectic Institute
Huckleberry - Devil's Club (Alcohol Extract)

Huckleberry leaf, **Devil's Club root bark**, Dandelion whole plant, Burdock root & seed

Herbalist & Alchemist
Pancreaid™ (Alcohol Extract)

Blueberry leaf, **Cinnamon (cassia) bark**, Dandelion root, **Devil's Club root bark**, Gentian, **Gymnema**

Christopher's
Pancreas Formula (Capsule, Extract and Bulk)

Goldenseal, Uva Ursi, Capsicum (Cayenne), Cedar (Juniper) berry, Licorice, Mullein

Western Botanicals
Pancreas Support Formula (Capsule and Alcohol Extract)

Cedar (Juniper) berry, Burdock root, **Devil's Club root**, Eleuthero root, **Ginseng (American)**, Bilberry leaf, Mullein leaf, **Gymnema leaf**

Grandma's Herbs
Pancreas-Aid (Capsule)

Cedar (Juniper) berry, Licorice, Cascara Sagrada, Heal All, **Goldenseal**, Capsicum (Cayenne), Bladder Pod

Herb Pharm
Sugar Metabolism™ (Alcohol Extract)

Devil's Club root bark, **Gymnema leaf**, Blueberry leaf, Cinnamon (aromaticum) bark, Dandelion root, leaf & flower

Brain and Memory Tonic Formulas

As people age, they often develop problems with their memory. Fortunately, a number of herbs can help slow or reverse age-related memory loss. *Brain and Memory Tonic Formulas* are aimed at protecting the brain, improving memory and cognitive function and slowing age-related memory loss.

Besides the key herbs in these formulas, some key non-herbal ingredients that are helpful include huperzine A (from Chinese club moss), phosphatidylserine and phosphatidylcholine (precursors to acetylcholine) and vinpocetine. See *Memory and Brain Function*, *Alzheimer's Disease* and *Dementia* in the *Conditions Section* for more information.

Key Herbs: Bacopa (Water Hyssop), Ginkgo, Gotu kola, Periwinkle (Lesser), Rosemary and Sage

Planetary Herbals
Bacopa-Ginkgo Brain Strength™ (Tablet)

Bacopa (Water Hyssop) whole plant, Ashwagandha root, Cardamom fruit, Chebulic Myrobalan fruit, Valerian, **Ginkgo**, **Gotu Kola leaf**, Guggul gum resin

Herb Pharm
Brain & Memory™ (Alcohol Extract)

Gotu Kola, **Ginkgo**, Scullcap (Skullcap), **Sage**, **Rosemary**

Western Botanicals
Brain Circulation Formula (Capsule and Alcohol Extract)

Ginkgo, Kola (cola) nut, Calamus (Sweet Flag), Ginger, **Gotu Kola**, **Rosemary**, Capsicum (chinense)

NOW Foods
Brain Elevate™ (Capsule)

Ginkgo, **Rosemary leaf**, Firmoss, **Gotu Kola leaf**; Non-Herbal: Leci-PS® Phosphatidyl Serine (from soy), L-Glutamine, Choline

Nature's Answer
Brainstorm™ (Glycerine Extract)

Gotu Kola aerial parts, **Periwinkle aerial parts**, **Ginkgo**, Hawthorn berry, **Rosemary**, Prickly Ash, Capsicum (Cayenne)

Herbalist & Alchemist
Clarity Compound™ (Alcohol Extract)

Bacopa (Water Hyssop), **Ginkgo**, **Gotu Kola**, Lemon Balm, Schisandra, **Rosemary**

Eclectic Institute
Ginkgo - Gotu Kola (Capsule)

Ginkgo, **Gotu Kola leaf**

Eclectic Institute
Ginkgo - Gotu Kola (Alcohol and Glycerine Extract)

Ginkgo, **Gotu Kola leaf**, Oat seed, Eleuthero root; Non-Herbal: glycerite version contains grapefruit flavoring

Planetary Herbals
Ginkgo Awareness™ (Tablet)

Valerian, **Bacopa (Water Hyssop) whole plant**, Dendrobium stem, Polygala, Eclipta aerial parts, Nutmeg seed, Chinese Amomum fruit, **Gotu Kola leaf**, **Ginkgo**

NOW Foods
Ginkgo Biloba Extract (Glycerine Extract)

Ginkgo leaf, **Gotu Kola leaf**, Eleuthero root

Yogi Tea
Ginkgo Clarity™ (Tea)

Ginkgo, Peppermint leaf, Licorice, Spearmint, Lemongrass leaf, Basil leaf, Ginger, Lemon peel, Cinnamon bark, Lemon Myrtle, Amla (Indian Gooseberry), Belleric Myrobalan fruit, Chebulic Myrobalan fruit, Cardamom seed

Yerba Prima
Ginkgo Extra Strength (Capsule)

Ginkgo, Black Pepper

Gaia Herbs
Ginkgo Gotu Kola Supreme (Alcohol Extract)

Eleuthero root, **Ginkgo**, **Gotu Kola**, Peppermint, **Rosemary**, Oat seed

Solaray
Ginseng (Siberian) and Gotu Kola (Capsule)

Ginseng (Korean, Asian), Eleuthero root, **Gotu Kola aerial parts**

Eclectic Institute
Green Memory™ (Bulk Powder)

Spinach, **Ginkgo**, Oat, Hawthorn, Turmeric, Nettle (Stinging), Ginger

Christopher's
Master Gland Formula (Capsule)

Carrot leaf, **Gotu Kola**, **Ginkgo**, Mullein, Oregon Grape, Lobelia

Grandma's Herbs
Memory (Capsule)

Ginkgo, **Gotu Kola**, **Rosemary**, Scullcap (Skullcap), Blue Vervain, Capsicum (Cayenne), Eleuthero, Lady's Slipper, Yerba Mate, **Sage**

Solaray
Memory Blend™ SP-30™ (Capsule)

Peppermint aerial parts, Eleuthero root, **Gotu Kola aerial parts**, Kelp, **Rosemary aerial parts**, Damiana leaf, Butternut bark

Christopher's
Memory Plus Formula (Capsule)

Blue Vervain, **Gotu Kola**, Brigham (Mormon) Tea, **Ginkgo**, Blessed Thistle, Capsicum (Cayenne), Ginger, Lobelia

Gaia Herbs
Mental Alertness (Liquid Phyto-Caps)

Eleuthero root, Oat seed (milky), He Shou Wu (Fo-Ti) root, **Ginkgo leaf**, **Gotu Kola leaf**, Peppermint, **Rosemary leaf**; Non-Herbal: Vinpocetine (from Voacanga seed)

Vitanica
MindBlend™ (Capsule)

Ginkgo, Rhodiola, Blueberry, Ginseng (Korean, Asian), **Gotu Kola**; Non-Herbal: Vitamin C, Vitamin E, Folate, Vitamin B12, Huperzine A, Phosphatidylserine, Phosphatidylcholine, Phosphatidylinositol, Vinpocetine

Christopher's
MindTrac (Capsule)

Valerian, Scullcap (Skullcap), **Ginkgo**, Oregon Grape, St. John's Wort, Mullein, **Gotu Kola**, Sarsaparilla, Dandelion, Lobelia

New Chapter
NeuroZyme® (Softgel)

Ginkgo, **Gotu Kola leaf**, Ashwagandha root, Cat's Claw root, Lemon Balm leaf, **Bacopa (Water Hyssop) leaf**, **Rosemary**, Ginger, Chamomile flower, Turmeric, Peony (White, Chinese), Holy Basil leaf, **Sage**, Clove, Club Moss aerial parts

Irwin Naturals
Organic Brain Support (Tablet)

Ginkgo leaf, Blueberry, Ginseng (Korean, Asian), Ginseng (Korean, Asian), Grape seed, Ginger, Papaya

Herbs Etc.
Remember Now™ (Alcohol Extract)

Ginkgo leaf, **Periwinkle**, **Gotu Kola**, Peppermint, Oat seed (milky), St. John's Wort, Eleuthero root, **Rosemary leaf**, Prickly Ash bark

Traditional Medicinals
Think O2® (Tea)

Ginkgo, **Gotu Kola leaf**, **Sage**, Lemon Balm leaf, **Rosemary**, **Ginkgo**, Peppermint leaf, Eleuthero root, Lemon Myrtle leaf

Herbal Formulas

Brain Calming Formulas

Sometimes the brain is hyperstimulated or overactive and fires too much. This happens in epilepsy and attention deficit hyperactive disorder (ADHD). *Brain Calming Formulas* are used to help calm down the brain, improving concentration and mental focus.

In ADHD, the nervous system appears to work backwards because many of the nervine herbs that calm the average person are agitating to children and adults with ADHD. Instead of feeling more relaxed after taking the key herbs in *Relaxing Nervine Formulas*, the person suffering from ADHD feels more hyper and nervous. See *Attention Deficit Disorder* and *Epilepsy* in the *Conditions Section* for more information.

Key Herbs: Chamomile (English and Roman), Ginkgo, Hawthorn, Jujube, Lemon Balm and Oat

Western Botanicals
Attention Calm Formula (Capsule and Liquid)

Ginkgo, Passionflower flower, Oregon Grape, Black Cohosh, Valerian, Blue Cohosh, Wild Yam, St. John's Wort flowering tops, Grape seed, Hops flower, Scullcap (Skullcap), Lobelia, Lobelia seed, **Chamomile flower**, Wood Betony (betonica)

Western Botanicals
Attention Calm Syrup (Glycerine Extract)

Ginkgo, Passionflower flower, Oregon Grape, Black Cohosh, Valerian, Blue Cohosh, Wild Yam, St. John's Wort flowering tops, Grape seed, Hops flower, Scullcap (Skullcap), Lobelia, Lobelia seed, **Chamomile flower**, Wood Betony (betonica); Non-Herbal: Pure Honey

Gaia Herbs
Attention Daily Herbal Drops (Alcohol Extract)

Scullcap (Skullcap), **Chamomile**, Gotu Kola, Irish Moss, **Lemon Balm**, Passionflower, **Oat**

Western Botanicals
Attention Focus Formula (Alcohol Extract or Syrup)

Ginkgo, Passionflower, Passionflower flower, St. John's Wort flowering tops, Grape seed, Oregon Grape

Planetary Herbals
Calm Child™ (Tablet)

Jujube seed, **Hawthorn berry**, **Chamomile flower**, Catnip aerial parts, Long Pepper (Pippali) fruit, Licorice, **Chamomile flower**, Amla (Indian Gooseberry), Gotu Kola leaf, Anise fruit, Clove, Cinnamon (cassia) bark; Non-Herbal: Magnesium

Planetary Herbals
Calm Child™ Herbal Syrup (Glycerine Extract)

Chamomile flower, Jujube seed, **Hawthorn berry**, Catnip aerial parts, **Lemon Balm aerial parts**, Long Pepper (Pippali) fruit, Licorice, Amla (Indian Gooseberry), Gotu Kola aerial parts, Anise essential oil, Cinnamon (cassia) bark, Clove; Non-Herbal: Calcium, Magnesium

Herbalist & Alchemist
Focus Formula™ (Alcohol Extract)

Hawthorn berry, **Hawthorn flower**, **Lemon Balm flowering tops**, **Oat seed (milky)**, Bacopa (Water Hyssop), **Ginkgo**, Scullcap (Skullcap) flowering tops

Grandma's Herbs
Kid-e-Trac (Liquid)

Valerian, Scullcap (Skullcap), **Ginkgo**, Oregon Grape, St. John's Wort, Dandelion root, Wood Betony (betonica), Alfalfa, Barley, Wheat grass; Non-Herbal: Jurassic Green

Herbalist & Alchemist
Kid's Calmpound Glycerite™ (Glycerine Extract)

Catnip flowering tops, **Chamomile flower**, **Oat seed (milky)**, Scullcap (Skullcap) flowering tops

Herbs Etc.
Kidalin® (Alcohol Extract)

Catnip flowering tops, Damiana (diffusa) leaf, Kola (cola) nut nut, Lavender (angustifolia) flower, **Chamomile flower**, Periwinkle, **Lemon Balm**, Licorice root, **Oat seed (milky)**

Planetary Herbals
Positive Teens & Kids™ (Tablet)

Bacopa (Water Hyssop) leaf, St. John's Wort aerial parts, Passionflower leaf & flower, Jujube seed, **Lemon Balm aerial parts**, **Chamomile flower**, **Hawthorn berry**, Jujube fruit

Bronchialdilator Formulas

See also *Anti-Inflammatory, Antispasmodic, Cough Remedy* and *Decongestant Formulas*

When air passages are constricted due to asthma or chronic obstructive pulmonary disorder (COPD) air flow into the lungs is restricted. The inability to breathe can create fear and anxiety, which further inhibits breathing. *Bronchialdilator Formulas* are a subtype of *Antispasmodic Formulas*, specifically targeted at relaxing the bronchial passages to make breathing easier. They may also contain herbs that relieve bronchial inflammation and loosen deeply congested mucus.

Antispasmodic Formulas may also be used as bronchial dilators. Where inflammation is present, they may be combined with *Anti-inflammatory Formulas*. Where the lungs are congested, they may be combined with *Decongestant Formulas*. For whooping or spastic coughs, they may be combined with *Herbal Cough Remedy Formulas*. See *Asthma* and *Chronic Obstructive Pulmonary Disorder (COPD)* for more information.

Key Herbs: Grindelia (Gumweed), Khella, Licorice, Lobelia and Skunk Cabbage

Christopher's
Antispasmodic Formula (Alcohol Extract)

Scullcap (Skullcap), **Lobelia**, Capsicum (Cayenne), Valerian, **Skunk Cabbage**, Myrrh, Black Cohosh

Herb Pharm
Calm Breath™ (Alcohol Extract)
Khella seed, **Skunk Cabbage**, **Grindelia (Gumweed) leaf**, Turmeric, Thyme flower

Christopher's
Glandular System Formula (Capsule)
Mullein, **Lobelia**

Herb Pharm
Lobelia/Skunk Cabbage (Alcohol Extract)
Lobelia, **Skunk Cabbage**, Scullcap (Skullcap), Black Cohosh, Myrrh tears, Capsicum (Cayenne)

Herbalist & Alchemist
Lung Relief Antispasmodic Compound™ (Alcohol Tincture)
Mullein leaf, Cherry (Wild) bark, **Licorice**, Wild (Prickly) Lettuce, **Khella seed**, **Lobelia flower**, **Lobelia seed**; Non-Herbal: Apple cider vinegar

Eclectic Institute
Lung Support (Capsule)
Grindelia (Gumweed) flower and leaf, Green Tea leaf, **Lobelia leaf**, Turmeric; Non-Herbal: Arabinogalactan

Gaia Herbs
Nicotine Relief (Liquid Phyto-Caps)
Lobelia, **Lobelia seed**, Oat seed (milky), St. John's Wort flowering tops, Passionflower vine, **Licorice**

Herbalist & Alchemist
Respiratory Calmpound™ (Alcohol Extract)
Ginkgo, **Khella seed**, Reishi (Ganoderma), **Licorice**, **Lobelia flower**, **Lobelia seed**; Non-Herbal: Apple cider vinegar

Eclectic Institute
Skullcap - Oats (Alcohol Extract and Glycerine Extract)
Scullcap (Skullcap) flowering tops, Oat seed, **Licorice**, **Lobelia leaf & seed**, Yerba Santa

Cardiac Tonic Formulas

See also *Antioxidant, Cardiovascular Stimulant* and *Hypotensive Formulas*

The formulas are used to help reduce the risk of heart disease or aid in recovery from heart disease. These blends contain herbs that tonify and support the function of the heart, as well as remedies that aid the overall cardiovascular system.

Although two key herbs in these formulas, lily of the valley and night blooming cereus, can be toxic in large doses, they are safe when used in small amounts as part of a complete cardiac formula. If you do experience any unusual reactions to a formula containing these herbs, discontinue use and consult a professional herbalist for advice.

Cardiac Tonic Formulas will often contain many of the key herbs found in *Cardiovascular Stimulant Formulas* such as capsicum and garlic. They may also contain key herbs from *Hypotensive Formulas,* such as mistletoe and motherwort.

See *Cardiovascular Disease (Heart Disease), Arteriosclerosis (Atherosclerosis)* and *Hypertension* for more information.

Key Herbs: Arjuna, Hawthorn, Lily of the Valley and Night Blooming Cereus (Cactus)

Planetary Herbals
Arjuna CardioComfort™ (Tablet)
Hawthorn leaf & flower, Tienchi Ginseng, Guggul, Chinese Salvia root, **Arjuna bark**

A. Vogel
Cardiaforce Tonic (Alcohol Extract)
Lemon Balm essential oil, **Hawthorn berry**

Eclectic Institute
Circulatory Support (Capsule)
Hawthorn flower, leaf & berry, Ginkgo, Capsicum (Cayenne)

Nature's Way
Garlicin HC (Capsule)
Garlic, **Hawthorn**, Capsicum (Cayenne); Non-Herbal: Vitamin E, Calcium, Rutin

Eclectic Institute
Hawthorn - Cactus (Alcohol Extract and Glycerine Extract)
Hawthorn berry, leaf & flower, **Night Blooming Cereus (Cactus) stem and flower**, Ginkgo, Passionflower leaf

Western Botanicals
Hawthorn Berry Syrup (Glycerine Extract)
Hawthorn berry, leaf & flower, Motherwort, Ginkgo, Passionflower, Pau d'Arco, **Night Blooming Cereus (Cactus)**; Non-Herbal: Pure maple syrup, pure vegetable glycerine, brandy

Planetary Herbals
Hawthorn Heart™ (Tablet)
Tienchi Ginseng, **Hawthorn leaf & flower**, Chinese Salvia root, Polygala, Dong Quai, Codonopsis root, Dong Quai, Juniper berry, Longan fruit

Nature's Answer
Hawthorn Plus Extractacap (Liquid Capsule)
Hawthorn leaf, flower & berry, Linden (Basswood, Tilia) flower, Capsicum (Cayenne)

Herbalist & Alchemist
Healthy Heart Compound™ (Alcohol Tincture)
Hawthorn fruit, **Hawthorn flower**, **Night Blooming Cereus (Cactus) stem**, Chinese Salvia root, Prickly Ash (Zanthoxylum americanum) bark, Tienchi Ginseng

Solaray

Heart Blend™ SP-8™ (Capsule)

Hawthorn berry, Motherwort aerial parts, Rosemary, Capsicum (Cayenne), Kelp, Wood Betony (betonica) aerial parts, Shepherd's Purse aerial parts

Solaray

Heart Caps™ (Capsule)

Hawthorn berry, Clove, Motherwort leaf, Rosemary, Kelp, Capsicum (Cayenne)

Western Botanicals

Heart Formula (Capsule and Alcohol Extract)

Hawthorn berry, Ginger, Ginkgo, **Hawthorn leaf & flower**, Motherwort, Red Clover flower, Garlic, **Night Blooming Cereus (Cactus)**, Capsicum (chinense)

Herb Pharm

Heart Health (Alcohol Extract)

Hawthorn berry, **Night Blooming Cereus (Cactus) stem**, Motherwort leaf, Ginger rhizome

Grandma's Herbs

Heart Plus (Capsule)

Hawthorn berry, Motherwort, **Lily of the Valley**, Bugleweed, Bladder Pod, Canaigre

Traditional Medicinals

Heart Tea

Hawthorn leaf, flower & berry

Renew Life

Love Your Heart (Capsule)

Oat, **Hawthorn berry**; Non-Herbal: L-carnitine, Niacin, Magnesium, Coenzyme Q-10, Policosanol

Cardiovascular Stimulant Formulas

See also *Cardiac Tonic Formulas*

These formulas help to improve blood flow to the tissues of the body. In particular, they aid peripheral circulation, which can help decrease blood pressure, lower cholesterol, take stress off the heart and improve cardiovascular health in general. Since diabetes adversely affects circulation, they may also be useful for reducing some of the complications of diabetes. They may also help with wound healing in the extremities in the elderly or those with poor circulation.

Since a good blood supply is essential to the health of all body tissues, they can also have a general healing effect in people with symptoms of poor circulation, such as cold hands and feet, numbness and tingling sensations in the extremities and pale complexion. In fact, since most of the key ingredients in *Cardiovascular Stimulant Formulas* are pungent herbs, they are generally effective for tissue depression, discussed in the introduction.

Key Herbs: Capsicum (Cayenne), Garlic, Ginger, Ginkgo and Prickly Ash

Solaray

Artery Blend™ SP-9™ (Capsule)º

Garlic, Valerian, Black Cohosh, **Capsicum (Cayenne)**, Kelp, Blessed Thistle, Parsley

Christopher's

Blood Circulation Formula (Capsule's or Extract)

Capsicum (Cayenne), **Ginger**, Goldenseal, Parsley root, **Garlic**

Nature's Way

CapsiCool® (Capsule)

Capsicum (Cayenne), **Ginger**, Glucomannan root

Vitanica

CardioBlend™ (Capsule)

Garlic, Hawthorn berry, Grape seed, **Ginger**, **Ginkgo**; Non-Herbal: Vitamin C, Vitamin E, Riboflavin, Vitamin B6, Folic Acid, Vitamin B12, Magnesium, Co-enzyme Q-10

Nature's Way

Cayenne & Garlic (Capsule)

Capsicum (Cayenne), **Garlic**

Solaray

Cayenne & Ginger (Capsule)

Capsicum (Cayenne), **Ginger**, Marshmallow

Solaray

Cayenne With Garlic (Capsule)

Capsicum (Cayenne), **Garlic**

Solaray

Circulation Blend™ SP-11B™ (Capsule)

Capsicum (Cayenne), Butcher's Broom root, Kelp, Gentian, **Ginger**, Valerian aerial parts

Solaray

Cool Cayenne® (Capsule)

Capsicum (Cayenne), **Ginger**, Guar gum

Solaray

Cool Cayenne® with Butcher's Broom (Capsule)

Capsicum (Cayenne), Butcher's Broom root, **Ginger**, Guar gum

Nature's Way

Garlic & Parsley (Capsule)

Garlic, Parsley leaf

Solaray

Garlic and Parsley (Capsule)

Garlic, Parsley aerial parts

Nature's Answer

Garlic Super Complex (Capsule)

Garlic, Hawthorn leaf, Parsley leaf, **Capsicum (Cayenne)**; Non-Herbal: Vitamin E

Solaray

GarliCare™ with Cool Cayenne™ (Capsule)

Garlic, **Capsicum (Cayenne)**

Planetary Herbals
Ginger Warming Compound™ (Tablet)

Cinnamon (cassia) bark, **Ginger**, **Capsicum (Cayenne)**, Pine (White) bark, Clove, Bayberry bark, Marshmallow, Licorice; Non-Herbal: Calcium

A. Vogel
Heart & Circulatory Health Capsules

Garlic oil, Hawthorn flower, Passionflower; Non-Herbal: Vitamin E, glucose, beeswax, lecithin, lactose, silica, gelatin, glycerol, sorbitol, iron oxide

Western Botanicals
Herbal Super Tonic (Capsule and Liquid)

Horseradish, **Garlic**, Onion, **Ginger**, **Capsicum (Cayenne)**, Capsicum (chinense)

Celestial Seasonings
Honey Vanilla White Tea Chai Tea

White Tea, Black Tea, Chicory, Cinnamon bark, **Ginger**, Clove, Cardamom, Black Pepper, Nutmeg; Non-Herbal: Honey

Celestial Seasonings
India Spice Chai Tea

Black Tea, Cinnamon bark, **Ginger**, Clove, Cardamom, Nutmeg, Black Pepper, Star Anise, Chicory, Vanilla

Herb Pharm
Warming Circulation Tonic™ (Alcohol Extract)

Ginkgo, Eleuthero root, Rosemary flowering tops, **Ginger**, **Prickly Ash**, **Capsicum (Cayenne)**

Carminative Formulas

See also *Catnip & Fennel* and *Digestive Enzyme Formulas*

These formulas are used to help with gas and bloating in the intestinal tract. Carminatives are typically aromatic and pungent herbs that stimulate the secretion of digestive juices, enhance blood flow to digestive organs, improve downward motility of the GI tract and help to hold down bacterial growth in the intestines. So, *Carminative Formulas* aren't just for intestinal gas, they can also enhance the digestive process and the general health of the intestinal tract.

A key carminative blend is catnip and fennel, which is used to treat colic in infants, but can also be helpful for gas and bloating in adults. This blend is so famous that it is treated separately. (See *Catnip & Fennel Formulas.*)

Carminatives are also key ingredients in *Digestive Bitter Tonic Formulas*, which combine bitter herbs that stimulate digestion with carminatives. They are also treated separately. See *Colic, Gas and Boating* in the *Conditions Section* for more information.

Carminatives generally work best in liquid form and are usually more effective when taken as warm teas or as extracts with warm liquids. Many herbal tea blends are carminative, so this list contains a lot of herbal teas. Since these formulas are primarily aromatic in nature, they are general remedies for tissue depression, discussed in the introduction.

Key Herbs: Black Pepper, Cardamom, Catnip, Chamomile (English and Roman), Cilantro/Coriander, Fennel, Ginger and Peppermint

Eclectic Institute
Babies Tum-Ease (Glycerine Extract)

Dill essential oil, **Fennel essential oil**, **Ginger oil**; Non-Herbal: Sodium Bicarbonate

Celestial Seasonings
Bengal Spice® (Tea)

Cinnamon, Cinnamon, Chicory, Carob, Vanilla, **Ginger**, **Cardamom**, Black Pepper, Clove, Nutmeg

Herb Pharm
Breath Tonic Peppermint (Spray)

Peppermint essential oil, Cinnamon bark, **Ginger**, Clove (aromaticum)

Herb Pharm
Breath Tonic Spearmint (Spray)

Spearmint, **Ginger**, Cinnamon, **Fennel**, Clove (aromaticum)

Nature's Answer
Bubble-B-Gone (Liquid)

Chamomile flower, **Fennel**, **Catnip aerial parts**, Lemon Balm aerial parts

Herbalist & Alchemist
Carminitive Compound™ (Alcohol Extract)

Fennel, **Peppermint**, Wild Yam, **Chamomile flower**, **Ginger**

Yogi Tea
Chai Black (Tea)

Black Tea, **Cardamom seed**, Cinnamon bark, **Ginger**, Clove, Cinnamon essential oil, Black Pepper, **Ginger essential oil**, **Cardamom essential oil**

Yogi Tea
Chai Green (Tea)

Green Tea leaf, **Ginger**, **Cardamom seed**, Cinnamon bark, Clove, Cinnamon essential oil, **Ginger essential oil**, Black Pepper, **Cardamom essential oil**

Yogi Tea
Chai Rooibos (Tea)

Rooibos (Redbush), **Cardamom seed**, Cinnamon bark, **Ginger**, Clove

Eclectic Institute
Chamomile - Catnip kid (Glycerine Extract)

Chamomile flower & leaf, **Catnip flowering tops**, Lemon Balm leaf, Hyssop flower & leaf, **Peppermint leaf & essential oil**, Elder (canadensis) berry

Eclectic Institute
Chamomile - Catnip O (Alcohol and Glycerine Extract)

Chamomile flower & leaf, **Catnip flowering tops**, Elder (canadensis) flower, Lemon Balm, Hyssop flower & leaf, **Peppermint leaf**

Herb Pharm
Children's Herbal (Glycerite)

Chamomile flower, Lemon Balm leaf & flower, **Catnip leaf & flower**, **Fennel seed**

Celestial Seasonings
Cinnamon Apple Spice (Tea)

Cinnamon, Hibiscus, **Chamomile**, Chicory, Orange peel, Carob, Soybean; Non-Herbal: Apple flavor

Yogi Tea
Classic India Spice® (Tea)

Ginger, Chicory root, Carob, **Cardamom seed**, Cinnamon bark & essential oil, Clove, Black Pepper, **Ginger essential oil**

Celestial Seasonings
Decaf India Spice Chai Tea

Cinnamon bark, **Ginger**, Clove, **Cardamom**, Nutmeg, Black Pepper, Black Tea, Chicory, Vanilla

Western Botanicals
Digestion Aid Formula (Capsule and Alcohol Extract)

Ginger, Licorice, Dandelion root, **Fennel**, Gentian, **Chamomile flower**, **Peppermint leaf & essential oil**

Solaray
Digestion Blend™ SP-27™ (Capsule)

Papaya leaf, **Peppermint aerial parts**, **Fennel**, **Ginger**, Gentian, Capsicum (Cayenne), Irish Moss

Traditional Medicinals
Eater's Digest® (Tea)

Peppermint leaf, **Fennel fruit**, **Ginger**, Rose hips, Papaya leaf, Alfalfa leaf, Cinnamon bark

Traditional Medicinals
Eater's Digest® Peppermint (Tea)

Peppermint leaf, **Fennel fruit**, **Ginger**, Rose hips, Papaya leaf, Alfalfa leaf, Cinnamon bark

Yogi Tea
Egyptian Licorice Mint (Tea)

Peppermint leaf, Licorice, Cinnamon bark, **Cardamom seed**, **Ginger**, Clove, Black Pepper, Cinnamon essential oil, **Cardamom essential oil**, **Ginger essential oil**

Yogi Tea
Egyptian Licorice® (Tea)

Licorice, Cinnamon bark, Orange peel, **Ginger**, **Cardamom seed**, Tangerine, Black Pepper, Clove, Cinnamon essential oil

New Chapter
Energizer Green Tea Ginger Tonic™ (Liquid)

Ginger, **Ginger**, Green Tea leaf, Lemon essential oil; Non-Herbal: Honey

Gaia Herbs
GaiaKids® Tummy Tonic Herbal Drops

Lemon Balm, **Chamomile flower**, Spearmint, **Fennel**, **Catnip**, **Ginger**

Nature's Sunshine Products
Gall Bladder Formula (Capsule)

Oregon Grape, **Ginger**, Cramp Bark, **Fennel**, **Peppermint leaf**, Wild Yam, **Catnip**

Gaia Herbs
Gas & Bloating (Capsule)

Caraway, **Chamomile**, Cumin, **Fennel**, Lemon Balm leaf, Marjoram essential oil, **Peppermint essential oil**, Star Anise

Gaia Herbs
Gas & Bloating Tea

Caraway, **Chamomile**, **Fennel**, essential oil, **Licorice**, Peppermint leaf

Traditional Medicinals
Gas Relief™ (Tea)

Caraway fruit, **Coriander fruit**, **Chamomile flower**, Lemon Balm leaf, **Peppermint leaf**

Christopher's
Gas-Eze (Capsule)

Capsicum (Cayenne), Slippery Elm, Caraway seed, **Ginger**, **Catnip**; Non-Herbal: Papain

Nature's Way
Gastritix™ (Capsule)

Fennel, Wild Yam, **Ginger**, Slippery Elm, **Chamomile flower**, Marshmallow

Herb Pharm
Gastro Calm™ (Alcohol Extract)

Cinnamon (aromaticum) bark, Lavender (angustifolia) flower, **Ginger**, Clove, Nutmeg seed, **Peppermint**

Yogi Tea
Ginger (Tea)

Ginger, Lemongrass, Licorice, **Peppermint leaf**, Black Pepper

Traditional Medicinals
Ginger Aid® (Tea)

Ginger, Blackberry leaf, Stevia, Lemon Myrtle leaf

Traditional Medicinals
Golden Ginger® (Tea)

Ginger, **Chamomile flower**

Yogi Tea
Green Tea Lemon Ginger (Tea)

Green Tea leaf, **Ginger**, Lemongrass, **Ginger essential oil**, Lemon peel, Licorice, **Peppermint leaf**, Black Pepper; Non-Herbal: Citric Acid

Traditional Medicinals
Green Tea with Ginger (Tea)

Green Tea leaf, **Ginger**, Blackberry leaf

Yogi Tea
Himalayan Apple Spice (Tea)

Black Tea, Cinnamon bark, **Ginger**, Rooibos (Redbush), Nutmeg, Clove, Black Pepper

Celestial Seasonings
Honey Vanilla White Tea Chai Tea

White Tea, Black Tea, Chicory, Cinnamon bark, **Ginger**, Clove, **Cardamom**, Black Pepper, Nutmeg; Non-Herbal: Honey

Celestial Seasonings
India Spice Chai Tea

Black Tea, Cinnamon bark, **Ginger**, Clove, **Cardamom**, Nutmeg, Black Pepper, Star Anise, Chicory, Vanilla

Celestial Seasonings
Jammin' Lemon Ginger Herbal Tea

Ginger, Lemongrass, Lemon Verbena, Lemon, Rose hips, Chicory

Traditional Medicinals
"Just for Kids" Tummy Comfort® (Tea)

Lemon Balm leaf, **Chamomile flower**, **Peppermint leaf**

Herbalist & Alchemist
Kid's Tummy Relief™ (Glycerine Extract)

Catnip, **Chamomile flower**, **Ginger**, Lemon Balm, Dandelion root, **Peppermint essential oil**

Yogi Tea
Lemon Ginger (Tea)

Ginger, Lemongrass, Lemon peel, Licorice, **Peppermint leaf**, Black Pepper

Yogi Tea
Mayan Cocoa Spice™ (Tea)

Cocoa (Cacao) shells, Cinnamon bark, Chicory root, **Cardamom seed**, Cocoa (Cacao), **Ginger**, Clove, Black Pepper, Cinnamon essential oil, **Cardamom essential oil**, **Ginger essential oil**

Celestial Seasonings
Mint Magic® (Tea)

Spearmint, **Peppermint**, Chicory, Cinnamon, Orange peel

Herbs for Kids
Minty Ginger™ (Glycerine Extract)

Peppermint leaf, **Fennel**, **Chamomile flower**, Papaya leaf, **Ginger**, Orange peel

Vitanica
Nausea Ease™ (Capsule)

Ginger, **Ginger**, **Peppermint leaf**, Lemon Balm; Non-Herbal: Vitamin C, Vitamin K1, Vitamin B6

Yogi Tea
Peach DeTox (Tea)

Cinnamon bark, **Ginger**, **Cardamom seed**, Licorice, Clove, Orange peel, Bilberry leaf, Parsley leaf, He Shou Wu (Fo-Ti), Corn Silk, Dandelion root, Black Pepper, Cinnamon essential oil, **Cardamom essential oil**, Long Pepper (Pippali) berry, **Ginger essential oil**

NOW Foods
Queeze Ease™ Tea

Ginger, **Peppermint leaf**, Spearmint leaf, Licorice, **Fennel seed**

Herbs Etc.
Stomach Tonic™ (Alcohol Extract)

Chamomile flower, **Catnip flowering tops**, **Fennel seed**, Lavender (angustifolia) flower, Anise seed, **Cardamom seed**, Gentian root, Angelica root, Prickly Ash bark

Celestial Seasonings
Sugar Plum Spice (Tea)

Hibiscus, Barley, Chicory, Rose hips, **Chamomile**, **Ginger**, Carob, **Cardamom**

Planetary Herbals
Three Spices Sinus Complex™ (Tablet)

Ginger, Long Pepper (Pippali) fruit, Black Pepper seed; Non-Herbal: sodium, fiber, Dehydrated Honey

Western Botanicals
Tummy Tea

Peppermint leaf, **Ginger**, **Fennel**, Cinnamon bark, **Chamomile flower**, Orange peel, Licorice, Hibiscus

Catnip & Fennel Formulas

See also *Antacid* and *Carminative Formulas*

The blend of catnip and fennel is a time-tested remedy for colic in infants and indigestion in adults. It settles the stomach, expels gas from the colon and relaxes digestive spasms. It is a safe remedy for infants, but can also be helpful for adults who have acid indigestion and problems with gas and bloating. This blend is a sub-category of *Carminative Formulas*. See *Colic (children)* in the *Conditions Section*.

Key Herbs: Catnip and Fennel

Grandma's Herbs
Kid-e-Col (Liquid)

Catnip, **Fennel**

Christopher's
Kid-e-Col (Glycerine Extract)

Catnip, **Fennel**

Christopher's
Stomach Comfort (Alcohol Extract)

Catnip, **Fennel**

Cholagogue Formulas

See also *Cholesterol Balancing* and *Fiber Blend Formulas*

These formulas stimulate the flow of bile. They have similar properties to *Blood Purifier Formulas*, but they contain herbs that have a stronger impact on the gall bladder. These formulas help to reduce cholesterol when taken with *Fiber Blend Formulas* and many of the key ingredients in these formulas will also be found in *Cholesterol Balancing Formulas*.

Cholagogue Formulas can help a person digest fats better. They can help with clay-colored stools, greasy stools, indigestion after eating fats and gall bladder attacks. Taken over a long period of time with plenty of water and fiber, they may even help to clear the gallbladder of small stones. They can be used in conjunction with the gall bladder flush described in the *Therapies Section* of this book.

Key Herbs: Artichoke, Barberry, Blue Flag, Celandine, Culver's root, Dandelion and Fringe Tree

Gaia Herbs
Cleanse & Detox Tea

Aloe vera, **Artichoke**, Burdock, Fennel, Licorice, Peppermint, Star Anise

Vitanica
HepaFem™ (Capsule)

Burdock root, Milk Thistle seed, **Celandine leaf**, **Fringetree**, Beet

Christopher's
Liver & Gall Bladder Formula
(Capsule and Glycerine Extract)

Barberry root, Oregon Grape, Wild Yam, Cramp Bark, Fennel, Ginger, Catnip, Peppermint

Solaray
Liver Blend™ SP-13™ (Capsule)

Dandelion root, Milk Thistle seed, Burdock root, **Artichoke flower**, Kelp, Peppermint aerial parts

A. Vogel
Liver Gallbladder Drops
(Capsule and Alcohol Extract)

Milk Thistle seed, **Artichoke**, **Dandelion root**, **Dandelion**, Boldo leaf, Peppermint leaf

Herbs Etc.
Liver Tonic™
(Alcohol Extract, Glycerine Extract or Softgel)

Milk Thistle seed, Toadflax, Oregon Grape root, Echinacea (angustifolia) root, Licorice root, **Celandine**, **Fringetree root bark**, **Culvers root**, **Blue Flag root**

Western Botanicals
Liver/Gallbladder Formula/Tea Combo (Liquid)

Milk Thistle seed, Fennel, **Fringetree**, Oregon Grape, Black Walnut hulls, **Dandelion root**, Garlic, Gentian, Ginger, Wormwood leaf

RidgeCrest Herbals
LiverClean (Capsule)

Barberry root bark, Blessed Thistle, Boldo leaf, **Dandelion root**, Radish (Black) root, Wild Yam root, Fennel seed, Clove

Irwin Naturals
Milk Thistle Liver Cleanse® (Tablet)

Alfalfa leaf, Beet, Licorice, Capsicum (Cayenne), Black Pepper, Beet leaf, **Artichoke leaf**, **Dandelion root**, Milk Thistle seed, Turmeric, **Barberry**, Boldo leaf, **Celandine**, **Fringetree root**, Stone Breaker (Quebra Pedra) aerial parts, Kutki (Picorhiza kurroa) root, Schisandra; Non-Herbal: Soy Lecithin

Cholesterol Balancing Formulas

See also *Cardiovascular Stimulant, Cholagogue, Fiber Blend* and *General Detoxifying Formulas*

These are herbal blends used to help lower total cholesterol and/or raise HDL and lower LDL cholesterol. Since the main way the body gets rid of excess cholesterol is to use it to form bile, herbal formulas for lowering cholesterol often rely on key herbs that increase bile production. (See *Cholagogue Formulas*.) Once the cholesterol in bile enters the digestive tract, it is absorbed by fiber in the diet, so fiber products may also be included in these formulas.

Some of the formulas also contain red yeast rice, which inhibits cholesterol production in the liver. Statin drugs were developed from compounds in red yeast rice. This traditional Chinese remedy is a viable alternative to statin drugs, but we recommend that persons taking stain drugs or red yeast rice, should supplement Co-Q10 in their diet, as these products deplete Co-Q10—an essential antioxidant for the cardiovascular system.

Cardiovascular Stimulant Formulas and *Cholagogue Formulas* taken with *Fiber Blend Formulas* can also be used to naturally lower cholesterol. See *Cholesterol* in the *Conditions Section* for more information.

Key Herbs: Artichoke, Coleus, Garlic and Guggul

Vitanica
CholestBlend™ (Capsule)

Artichoke, **Guggul**, **Garlic**; Non-Herbal: Vitamin C, Pantethine, Policosanol,

Grandma's Herbs
Cholesterol (Capsule)

Garlic, Turmeric, Bayberry, Capsicum (Cayenne), Hawthorn berry, Fenugreek, Milk Thistle, Black Cohosh, Sassafras, Apple pectin, Alfalfa, Plantain, Bladderwrack, Speedwell, Turkey Rhubarb, Canaigre; Non-Herbal: Niacinamide, Lecithin, Otrus Pectin

Herb Pharm
Cholesterol Health (Alcohol Extract)

Artichoke leaf & flower, Hawthorn berry, leaf & flower, Turmeric, Fennel

Gaia Herbs
Cholesterol Maintenance (Liquid Phyto-Caps)

Arjuna bark, **Artichoke leaf**, **Coleus root**, Wild Yam root, Dandelion root; Non-Herbal: Policosanol, Pantethine

NOW Foods
Cholesterol Support (Capsule)

Garlic, Guar gum, **Guggul**; Non-Herbal: Chromium, Vitamin E (d-alpha Tocopherol), Alpha Tocotrienols, Beta Tocotrienols, Gamma Tocotrienols, Delta Tocotrienols, Policosanol (from Sugar Cane)

Planetary Herbals
CholestGar™ (Tablet)

Garlic, **Guggul**, Chinese Salvia root, Dong Quai, Gambier stem, He Shou Wu (Fo-Ti), Chebulic Myrobalan fruit, Capsicum (Cayenne), Amla (Indian Gooseberry), Belleric Myrobalan fruit, Ginger, Black Pepper fruit, Long Pepper (Pippali) fruit, Dill seed, Asafetida; Non-Herbal: Calcium

Planetary Herbals
Guggul Cholesterol Compound™ (Tablet)

Guggul, Chebulic Myrobalan fruit, Amla (Indian Gooseberry), Ginger, Black Pepper fruit, Long Pepper (Pippali) fruit, Dill seed, Asafetida; Non-Herbal: Calcium

Cold and Flu Formulas

See also *Antiviral, Cough Remedy, Decongestant, Ear Drop, Expectorant* and *Sinus Decongestant Formulas*

These are herbal blends formulated to help fight colds, flu and other acute viral infections. The formulas are generally "shotgun" approaches to the problem, formulated to address multiple aspects of colds and flu. For instance, they may contain antiviral remedies, expectorants and decongestants, immune stimulants and herbs to reduce fever and pain. Some formulas also contain cold-fighting nutrients like vitamin C and zinc in addition to their herbal ingredients.

There are so many blends, and they are so different, that you may need to experiment a little and find the formula(s) that work best for you. Besides these general remedies for colds and flu, you can find herbal formulas to deal with more specific cold and flu symptoms, by checking out related formula categories. Also look up *Colds* and *Flu* in the *Conditions Section*.

Key Herbs: Astragalus, Boneset, Capsicum (Cayenne), Echinacea, Elder, Garlic, Ginger, Lemon Balm, Rose and Yarrow

Christopher's
Chest Comfort (Capsule)

Bayberry bark, Clove, **Ginger**, **Capsicum (Cayenne)**, Pine (White) bark

Herb Pharm
Children's Herbal (Glycerite)

Chamomile flower, **Lemon Balm leaf & flower**, Catnip leaf & flower, Fennel seed

Herb Pharm
Children's Winter Health™ (Glycerite)

Echinacea (purpurea) root, **Elder (Black) berry**, Meadowsweet flower, Hyssop flower, **Ginger**, Horseradish, Thyme leaf, Cinnamon (verum) bark

Traditional Medicinals
Cold Care P.M.® (Tea)

Linden (Basswood, Tilia) flower, Chamomile flower, Passionflower, Peppermint leaf, **Yarrow flower**, Eucalyptus leaf, Licorice

Yogi Tea
Cold Season (Tea)

Ginger, Licorice, Eucalyptus leaf, Orange peel, Valerian, Peppermint leaf, Lemongrass, Basil leaf, Cardamom seed, Oregano leaf, Clove, Parsley leaf, **Yarrow flower**, Black Pepper, Cinnamon bark

Christopher's
Cold Season Immune Formula (Capsule)

Garlic, **Rose hips**, Watercress, Parsley

Solaray
Echinacea Root with Vitamin C & Zinc (Capsule)

Echinacea (angustifolia) root, **Echinacea (purpurea) root**, **Rose hips**; Non-Herbal: Vitamin C, Zinc, Citrus Bioflavonoid Complex, Hesperidin Complex, Rutin

Planetary Herbals
Echinacea-Elderberry Syrup (Glycerine Extract)

Elder (canadensis) berry, **Echinacea (purpurea) root**, Isatis (Woad) root, Honeysuckle flower, Forsythia fruit, Platycodon, **Boneset aerial parts**, Licorice, Apricot seed; Non-Herbal: Honey

NOW Foods
Elderberry, Zinc & Echinacea Syrup

Elder (Black) flower & berry, **Echinacea (purpurea) root**; Non-Herbal: Zinc Citrate

Western Botanicals
Flu and Virus Formula (Capsule)

Goldenseal, **Ginger**, Licorice, Capsicum (chinense)

Planetary Herbals
Ginger Warming Compound™ (Tablet)

Cinnamon (cassia) bark, **Ginger**, **Capsicum (Cayenne)**, Pine (White) bark, Clove, Bayberry bark, Marshmallow, Licorice; Non-Herbal: Calcium

Traditional Medicinals
Gypsy Cold Care® (Tea)

Elder (canadensis) flower, **Yarrow flower**, Peppermint leaf, Hyssop, **Rose hips**, Cinnamon bark, **Ginger**, Safflower petals, Clove, Licorice

Traditional Medicinals
"Just for Kids" Cold Care (Tea)

Elder (canadensis) flower, Linden (Basswood, Tilia) flower, Chamomile flower, Peppermint leaf

Christopher's
Kid-e-Well (Glycerine Extract)

Yarrow, **Elder (canadensis) flower**, Peppermint, **Echinacea (angustifolia) root**

Western Botanicals
Nature's C Complex (Capsule)

Acerola, **Rose hips**, Aloe vera, Lemon peel, Orange peel, Horseradish, Camu Camu berry

Olbas
Olbas Herbal Tea

Peppermint essential oil, Chamomile, Fennel, Thyme, Iceland Moss, Licorice, Lungwort, Star Anise, Calendula (Marigold), **Yarrow root**, **Elder (canadensis) flower**, Lime flower, Blackberry leaf, Sage, Plantain, Cyani (Cornflower) flower, Cowslip, Eucalyptus leaf, Mullein flower, Eucalyptus essential oil; Non-Herbal: Menthol, Grape Sugar, Sugar, Fruit Pectin

Herbs Etc.
Peak Defense™ (Alcohol Extract or Softgel)

Goldenseal root, **Echinacea (angustifolia) root**, Licorice root, Yerba mansa root, **Yarrow flowering tops**, **Elder (canadensis) berry and flower**, **Boneset**, Bayberry root bark, Dandelion root, Grindelia (Gumweed) flower, **Ginger root**, Red Root root, Osha root

Herbs for Kids
Temp Assure™ (Glycerine Extract)

Echinacea (purpurea) root, Peppermint leaf, **Yarrow flower**, Catnip

NOW Foods
TLC™ Tea

Elder (Black) berry, Licorice, Slippery Elm, Eucalyptus leaf, **Echinacea (purpurea)**, Holy Basil leaf, **Ginger**

Planetary Herbals
Well Child™ (Glycerine Extract)

Honeysuckle flower, **Lemon Balm leaf**, Chamomile flower, Catnip aerial parts, **Echinacea (purpurea) leaf**, Cinnamon (cassia) twig, Licorice

Planetary Herbals
Yin Chiao Classic™ (Tablet)

Forsythia fruit, Japanese Honeysuckle flower, Platycodon, Chinese Mint aerial parts, Lophatherum stem & leaf, Licorice, Schizonepeta aerial parts, Soybean, Burdock fruit, Phragmites rhizome

Cough Remedy Formulas

See also *Allergy-Reducing, Antispasmodic, Bronchialdilator, Decongestant, Drying Cough/Lung, Expectorant* and *Moistening Lung/Cough Formulas*

This category is a catch-all for formulas used to ease coughs. The problem is that not all coughs are the same. There are dry coughs, damp coughs, spastic coughs and irritated coughs, all of which respond best to different types of herbal remedies. So, to select a good cough remedy, it is helpful to first understand what is happening when you have a cough. See *Cough* in the *Conditions Section* for more information.

Cough Remedy Formulas generally combine expectorant and decongestant actions to loosen mucus and help the body expel it. They do not act as antitussives or cough suppressants the way that over-the-counter cough medicines do. The main goal is to make the cough productive so that the body can expel what is irritating it. If you need to calm down excessive coughing, look for formulas that contain coltsfoot or lobelia.

If the cough is dry and unproductive, select Cough Remedies with key ingredients that have a moistening energetic like elecampane, fritillary, licorice and marshmallow. See *Moistening Lung/Cough* and *Decongestant Formulas*.

If there is a lot of mucus and drainage, then select cough remedies that contain key ingredients that have a drying energetic like Osha, Thyme, Pine, Cherry (Wild) and Yerba Santa. See *Drying Cough/Lung* and *Expectorant Formulas*.

For coughs with a spastic or "whooping" quality use *Bronchialdilator* or *Antispasmodic Formulas*. Where coughs are due to allergies, consider *Allergy-Reducing Formulas*.

Key Herbs: Bayberry, Cherry (Wild), Coltsfoot, Elecampane, Eucalyptus, Fritillary, Horehound, Licorice, Lobelia, Marshmallow, Pine (White), Thyme and Yerba Santa

Nature's Answer
Broncitone™ (Glycerine Extract)

Elecampane root, Hyssop aerial parts, Goldenseal, **Bayberry bark**, Capsicum (Cayenne), **Coltsfoot leaf**

Herbs for Kids
Cherry Bark Blend™ (Glycerine Extract)

Thyme leaf, **Cherry (Wild) bark**, Mullein leaf, Peppermint leaf, Orange peel, Hops, **Horehound**, Pleurisy root, Oregon Grape, **Eucalyptus essential oil**

Gaia Herbs
GaiaKids® Cough Syrup with Honey & Lemon

Plantain leaf, Grindelia (Gumweed) flowering tops, Helichrysum flowering tops, Lemon essential oil, Orange essential oil, Myrtle essential oil

Eclectic Institute
Herb Cough Elixir (Liquid)

Licorice, Elecampane root, Red Clover flower, **Cherry (Wild) bark**, **Horehound flower & leaf**, **Black Cherry**, Grindelia (Gumweed) flower & leaf, **Lobelia leaf & seed**, Fennel, Lomatium, **Pine (White) bark**, Orange essential oil, Poplar bud

Traditional Medicinals
Herba Tussin® (Tea)

Eucalyptus leaf, **Licorice**, Slippery Elm, **Cherry (Wild) bark**, **Elecampane rhizome**, **Marshmallow**, Lemongrass leaf, Spearmint, Lemon peel, Lemon Myrtle leaf

Traditional Medicinals
Herba Tussin® Herbal Syrup

Spearmint, **Eucalyptus leaf**, **Licorice**, Slippery Elm, **Cherry (Wild) bark**, Lemongrass leaf, **Elecampane rhizome**, Lemon peel, Stevia, Lemon Myrtle leaf, **Marshmallow**; Non-Herbal: Honey

Christopher's
Herbal Cough Syrup

Cherry (Wild) bark, **Licorice**, **Marshmallow**, **Horehound**, Mullein leaf, Ginger, Anise seed, Lemon peel

Olbas
Olbas Cough Syrup

Chestnut oil, **Thyme**, **Licorice**, Plantain, Peppermint essential oil, **Eucalyptus essential oil**, Wintergreen essential oil, Juniper essential oil, Clove essential oil, Cajeput essential oil; Non-Herbal: Honey

Olbas
Olbas Pastilles (Lozenge)

Eucalyptus essential oil, Juniper essential oil, Wintergreen essential oil, Clove essential oil; Non-Herbal: Menthol, Chlorophyll

Grandma's Herbs
Respiratory Relief (Capsule)

Mullein, **Bayberry**, **Horehound**, **Bladder Pod**, Heal All, **Elecampane**, **Yerba Santa**, Plantain, Nettle (Stinging), **Coltsfoot**, Capsicum (Cayenne), Lungwort

Traditional Medicinals
Throat Coat® Lemon Echinacea (Tea)

Echinacea (purpurea) root, **Licorice**, **Licorice**, **Marshmallow leaf**, Lemon Myrtle leaf, **Marshmallow**, Fennel fruit, Orange peel, Cinnamon bark

Decongestant Formulas

See also *Cough Remedy* and *Sinus Decongestant Formulas*

These are herbal blends whose principle ingredients help to thin mucus and break up congestion. Many decongestant herbs are also expectorant and most expectorants are also somewhat decongestant. However to make it easier to find formulas that fit a person's needs, we've separated these two properties based on which herbs are best for each purpose.

Remedies that are more specifically targeted at decongesting the sinuses can be found under *Sinus Decongestant Formulas*, which is a subcategory of *Decongestant Formulas*. *Herbal Cough Remedy Formulas* have both decongestant and expectorant action, so you can also consider formulas under that category. For more information see *Congestion* and *Cough* in the *Conditions Section*.

Key Herbs: Eucalyptus, Garlic, Grindelia (Gumweed), Licorice, Plantain, Thyme and Yerba Santa

Yogi Tea
Breathe Deep (Tea)

Licorice, **Eucalyptus leaf**, Basil leaf, Ginger, Cinnamon bark, **Thyme leaf**, Elecampane root, Peppermint leaf, Cardamom seed, Mullein leaf

Traditional Medicinals
Breathe Easy® (Tea)

Licorice, **Eucalyptus leaf**, Fennel fruit, Peppermint leaf, Calendula (Marigold) flower, Pleurisy root, Ginger; Non-Herbal: Bi Yan Pian

Gaia Herbs
Bronchial Wellness Herbal Syrup

Plantain leaf, Helichrysum flowering tops, **Eucalyptus essential oil**, Star Anise seed, Lemon fruit

Gaia Herbs
Bronchial Wellness Tea

Peppermint leaf and essential oil, **Licorice root**, **Grindelia (Gumweed) aerial parts**, **Plantain leaf**, Star Anise fruit, **Thyme**, Helichrysum essential oil, **Eucalyptus essential oil**

Nature's Answer
Broncitone™ (Glycerine Extract)

Elecampane root, Hyssop aerial parts, Goldenseal, Bayberry bark, Capsicum (Cayenne), Coltsfoot leaf

Herbs for Kids
Cherry Bark Blend™ (Glycerine Extract)

Thyme leaf, Cherry (Wild) bark, Mullein leaf, Peppermint leaf, Orange peel, Hops, Horehound, Pleurisy root, Oregon Grape, **Eucalyptus essential oil**

Grandma's Herbs
Chest Rub (Salve)

Eucalyptus essential oil, Rosemary essential oil, Pine essential oil, Peppermint essential oil, Tea Tree essential oil; Non-Herbal: Camphor or Menthol

RidgeCrest Herbals
ClearLungs Chest Rub (Lotion)

Asparagus (Chinese) root, **Licorice (Chinese) root**, Chinese Scullcap (Scute/Huang Qin) root, Dong Quai root, Gardenia fruit, Luo han guo (Monk Fruit) fruit, Bitter Melon fruit, Ophiopogon root, Platycodon root, Poria Mushroom, Schisandra fruit, Tangerine peel, Mulberry (White) root bark, Fritillary bulb; Non-Herbal: Antimonium Tartaricum, Carbo Vegetbilis, Narum Sulphuricum, phosphorus

RidgeCrest Herbals
ClearLungs Classic (Capsule)

Dong Quai root, Ophiopogon root, Poria Mushroom, Asparagus (Chinese) root, Chinese Scullcap (Scute/Huang Qin) root, Gardenia fruit, Luo han guo (Monk Fruit) fruit, Platycodon root, Tangerine peel, Mulberry (White) root, Fritillary bulb, Schisandra fruit, **Licorice (Chinese) root**

Eclectic Institute
Compound Herbal Elixir (Liquid)

Licorice, Elecampane root, Red Clover flower, Cherry (Wild) bark, Horehound flower & leaf, **Grindelia (Gumweed) flower & leaf**, Lobelia leaf & seed, Fennel, Lomatium, Pine (White) bark, Poplar bud

Zand
Decongest Herbal Formula (Capsule)

Turmeric, Nettle (Stinging) leaf, Pueraria root, Coix, Ligustrum rhizome, Peony (White, Chinese), **Licorice**, Turkey Rhubarb; Non-Herbal: Vitamin B12, Vitamin B5, Zinc, Citrus Bioflavonoids Complex

Herb Pharm
Echinacea Goldenseal (Alcohol Extract)

Echinacea (purpurea) root, Goldenseal rhizome and root, Osha root, Spilanthes flowering herb, **Yerba Santa leaf**, Horseradish root,

Elder (Black) berry, Ginger root, Yarrow flower, Baptisia (Wild Indigo) root

Herbs for Kids
Eldertussin™ Elderberry Syrup
Echinacea (purpurea) root, Chamomile, Horehound, Cherry (Wild) bark, Raspberry (Red)

Gaia Herbs
GaiaKids® Cough Syrup with Honey & Lemon
Plantain leaf, **Grindelia (Gumweed) flowering tops**, Helichrysum flowering tops, Lemon essential oil, Orange essential oil, Myrtle essential oil

Nature's Way
HAS® Original Blend (Capsule)
Brigham (Mormon) Tea leaf & stem, Marshmallow, Burdock root, Capsicum (Cayenne), Goldenseal, Elecampane root, Parsley leaf, Rosemary, Cleavers (Bedstraw) stem, leaf & & flower

Traditional Medicinals
Herba Tussin® (Tea)
Eucalyptus leaf, **Licorice**, Slippery Elm, Cherry (Wild) bark, Elecampane rhizome, Marshmallow, Lemongrass leaf, Spearmint, Lemon peel, Lemon Myrtle leaf

Traditional Medicinals
Herba Tussin® Herbal Syrup
Spearmint, **Eucalyptus leaf**, **Licorice**, Slippery Elm, Cherry (Wild) bark, Lemongrass leaf, Elecampane rhizome, Lemon peel, Stevia, Lemon Myrtle leaf, Marshmallow; Non-Herbal: Honey

Herb Pharm
Herbal Respiratory Relief (Alcohol Extract)
Cherry (Wild) bark, Umckaloabo root, Skunk Cabbage rhizome and root, **Licorice root**, **Thyme leaf & flower**

Western Botanicals
Herbal Snuff Powder (Bulk Powder)
Bayberry, Goldenseal, Horseradish, **Garlic**, Capsicum (chinense)

Planetary Herbals
Loquat Respiratory Syrup for Kids (Glycerine Extract)
Loquat leaf, Fritillary bulb, Black Cherry bark, Slippery Elm, Platycodon, Trichosanthes seed, Polygala, Poria Mushroom, Schisandra, **Licorice**

Herbalist & Alchemist
Lung Relief Cold/Damp Compound™ (Alcohol Extract)
Thyme, Ginger, Orange peel, **Yerba Santa**, Osha

Eclectic Institute
Lung Support (Capsule)
Grindelia (Gumweed) flower and leaf, Green Tea leaf, Lobelia leaf, Turmeric; Non-Herbal: Arabinogalactan

Western Botanicals
Lungs Plus Formula (Alcohol Extract)
Lobelia, Lobelia, Coffee bean, Peppermint leaf, Brigham (Mormon) Tea, Bitter Orange, Peppermint essential oil

Planetary Herbals
Mullein Lung Complex™ (Tablet)
Platycodon, Ophiopogon, Long Pepper (Pippali) fruit, Elecampane root, Mullein leaf, Black Cherry bark, **Licorice**, Ginger, Cinnamon (cassia) twig; Non-Herbal: Sodium, Fiber

Olbas
Olbas Inhaler (Vapor)
Peppermint essential oil, Cajeput essential oil, **Eucalyptus essential oil**; Non-Herbal: Menthol

Olbas
Olbas Lozenges
Eucalyptus essential oil; Non-Herbal: Menthol, Black Currant Flavor, Vitamin C

Planetary Herbals
Old Indian Syrup for Kids™ (Glycerine Extract)
Yerba Santa, Elecampane flower & root, **Grindelia (Gumweed) flower bud**, Platycodon, Horehound leaf, Hyssop aerial parts, **Thyme leaf**, Mullein leaf, Nettle (Stinging) leaf, Pine (White) bark, Angelica root, Loquat leaf, Fritillary bulb, Marshmallow, Irish Moss, **Licorice**, Black Cherry bark

Gaia Herbs
Osha Supreme (Alcohol Extract)
Echinacea (angustifolia), Echinacea (purpurea), Elecampane, Goldenseal, **Grindelia (Gumweed)**, Irish Moss, **Licorice**, Mullein, Oregano, Osha

Gaia Herbs
Respiratory Defense (Liquid Phyto-Caps)
Osha root, Oregano leaf, **Grindelia (Gumweed) flower and leaf**, Echinacea (purpurea) root, flowering tops & seed, Echinacea (angustifolia) root, Irish Moss fronds, Lobelia herb and seed, Mullein leaf, Oregon Grape root, Hyssop flower, St. John's Wort flower bud and tops, Barberry root, Goldenseal rhizome

Irwin Naturals
Respiratory Support & Defense™ (Tablet)
Fenugreek seed, Marshmallow root, Mullein leaf, Scullcap (Skullcap) leaf, Watercress aerial parts, **Garlic**, Onion, Pleurisy root, Turnip, **Thyme leaf**, **Licorice root**, Alfalfa aerial parts, Capsicum (Cayenne), Black Pepper; Non-Herbal: N-Acetyl-L-Cysteine (NAC), PABA

Christopher's
Sen Sei Menthol Rub (Salve)
Olive oil, **Eucalyptus essential oil**, Cajeput essential oil, Camphor; Non-Herbal: Menthol

Herbs Etc.
Singer's Saving Grace® (Spray)
Yerba mansa root, Collinsonia (Stoneroot) root, **Licorice root**, Jack-in-the-Pulpit root, Propolis gum, Echinacea (angustifolia) root, Ginger root, Osha root

New Chapter
Sinus & Respiratory (Softgel)
Garlic, Oregano essential oil, Echinacea (purpurea) leaf & flower, Echinacea (angustifolia) root, Elder (canadensis) berry, Goldenseal, Andrographis leaf, Green Tea leaf, Astragalus, Lemon Balm, Lemon Balm leaf, Myrrh, Wintergreen, Ginger, **Eucalyptus essential oil**, Peppermint leaf, Meadowsweet, Purple Willow

Traditional Medicinals

Throat Coat® Lemon Echinacea (Tea)

Echinacea (purpurea) root, **Licorice, Licorice**, Marshmallow leaf, Lemon Myrtle leaf, Marshmallow, Fennel fruit, Orange peel, Cinnamon bark

Gaia Herbs

Throat Shield Tea

Fennel, **Grindelia (Gumweed), Licorice**, Marshmallow, Peppermint essential oil, Sage essential oil, Sage

Planetary Herbals

Yin Chiao-Echinacea Complex™ (Tablet)

Notopterygium root, Yin Chiao Classic™, Echinacea (pallida) root, Echinacea (purpurea) root, Horehound aerial parts, Boneset aerial parts, Elecampane root, Isatis (Woad) root & leaf; Non-Herbal: Calcium

Digestive Bitter Tonic Formulas

See also *Antacid, Blood Purifier, Carminative, Digestive Enzyme* and *Digestive Tonic Formulas*

When we taste something bitter, our digestive "juices" are stimulated. Bitter herbs increase the production of hydrochloric acid in the stomach and bile from the liver, which aids the digestion of heavy fats and proteins.

The Western tradition of eating a salad with slightly bitter greens at the beginning of a meal comes from the ability of bitter greens to aid in the digestive process. The traditional vinegar dressing used with these greens also aids digestion. Unfortunately, a salad consisting of iceberg lettuce and creamy dressing won't trigger beneficial digestive secretions.

Bitter Digestive Tonic Formulas do the same thing a traditional salad does. By taking them 15-20 minutes prior to the main meal, they trigger the flow of digestive "juices." They can also be taken after a meal to settle the stomach and relieve indigestion and dull acid burning.

People with poor digestion often benefit from taking a *Digestive Bitter Tonic Formula*. These blends are also helpful for easing belching, as bitters tend to promote the downward flow of energy in the body. These formulas also have a mild laxative effect and act as blood purifiers (See *Blood Purifier Formulas*).

Bitters can help your body absorb more nutrients from the food you eat by signaling the stomach to secrete gastrin—the hormone that controls how much acid your stomach produces. These formulas also contain aromatic herbs that also stimulate digestive secretions and promote better peristalsis or motility in the digestive tract.

Aromatics and bitters that stimulate digestion are often combined with digestive enzymes and papaya to form *Digestive Enzyme Formulas*. While not herbal formulas in the strict sense, the combination of digestive enhancing herbs combined with digestive enzymes like proteases, amylases and lipases in these *Digestive Enzyme Formulas* is also extremely helpful for poor digestion. Also consider digestive enzyme supplements.

Key Herbs: Angelica, Cardamom, Chamomile (English and Roman), Dandelion, Fennel, Gentian, Ginger, Goldenseal and Orange Peel

Herbalist & Alchemist

Bitters Compound™ (Alcohol Extract)

Artichoke leaf, **Dandelion root**, Gentian, **Angelica root**, **Orange peel**, Peppermint

Vitanica

Bitters Extra™ (Capsule)

Artichoke leaf, **Dandelion root**, Yellow Dock, **Gentian, Ginger**, Burdock root, **Fennel, Chamomile flower**, Turmeric, **Cardamom seed**; Non-Herbal: Protease, Amylase, Lipase, Cellulase, Lactase, Phytase, Invertase, Bromelain

Solaray

Digestion Blend™ SP-27™ (Capsule)

Papaya leaf, Peppermint aerial parts, **Fennel, Ginger, Gentian**, Capsicum (Cayenne), Irish Moss

A. Vogel

Digestive Aid (Alcohol Tincture)

Yarrow, **Dandelion**, Lemon Balm, **Gentian**, Blessed Thistle, **Angelica root**, Centaury

Herb Pharm

Digestive Bitters (Alcohol Extract)

Angelica root, Hyssop leaf & flower, Juniper berry, **Cardamom seed, Ginger, Gentian rhizome and root**, Anise seed, Cinnamon bark, Myrrh, Peppermint essential oil

Planetary Herbals

Digestive Grape Bitters™ (Alcohol Extract)

Gentian, Angelica root, Astragalus, Atractylodes (Bai-Zhu) rhizome, Dill fruit, **Goldenseal**, Juniper berry, Oregon Grape, Yerba Santa, **Cardamom seed**, Yarrow flowering tops, Coriander seed, Galangal rhizome, **Ginger**, Anise essential oil, **Orange essential oil**, Grape

Eclectic Institute

Digestive Support (Capsule)

Gentian, Angelica root, Ginger, Artichoke leaf

Eclectic Institute

Gentian-Angelica Bitters (Alcohol Extract and Glycerine Extract)

Fennel, Elecampane root, Licorice, **Gentian, Angelica root, Goldenseal**

Solaray

GI Blend™ SP-20™ (Capsule)

Goldenseal, Licorice, Papaya leaf, **Gentian**, Myrrh, Irish Moss, Fenugreek, **Ginger**, Aloe vera

Gaia Herbs
Herbal Digest Tea
Caraway, **Gentian**, **Ginger**, Lemon Verbena, Licorice, Peppermint leaf, Star Anise, Yarrow leaf

Nature's Way
NatureWorks® Swedish Bitters™ (Liquid)
Manna Grass stem, **Angelica root**, Zedoary root, Aloe vera leaf, Turkey Rhubarb, Senna, Myrrh stem, Carline Thistle root, Camphor, Black Snakeroot root, Valerian, Cinnamon bark, **Cardamom fruit**, Saffron

Eclectic Institute
Neutralizing Cordial
(Alcohol Extract and Glycerine Extract)
Turkey Rhubarb, Cinnamon (cassia) bark, **Goldenseal**, Peppermint essential oil; Non-Herbal: Potassium Bicarbonate

Herb Pharm
Neutralizing Cordial (Alcohol Extract)
Turkey Rhubarb, Cinnamon (aromaticum) bark, **Goldenseal rhizome and root**, Peppermint leaf and essential oil

Urban Moonshine
Original Bitters (Alcohol Extract)
Dandelion leaf and root, **Angelica root**, Burdock, Yellow Dock, **Gentian root**, **Orange peel**, **Fennel seed**, **Ginger**; Non-Herbal: Organic essential oils, gum arabic

NatureWorks
Swedish Bitters (Capsule)
Aloe vera, Manna Grass, Senna, Turkey Rhubarb, Zedoary root, Theriac Venezian root, **Angelica root**, Carline Thistle root, Myrrh, Camphor, Saffron

Gaia Herbs
Sweetish Bitters Elixir (Alcohol Extract)
Turmeric, Milk Thistle seed, Wild Yam, **Fennel**, Kelp, **Dandelion root**, **Gentian**, **Cardamom seed**, **Ginger**, Amla (Indian Gooseberry), Anise seed, Bitter Orange essential oil

Digestive Enzyme Formulas

See also *Carminative* and *Digestive Bitter Tonic Formulas*

Digestive Enzyme Formulas are herbal blends for digestion that also contain enzymes like proteases, amylases and lipases. Protease enzymes help break down protein, amylase enzymes break down starches and lipase enzymes break down fats. The only key herb found in these formulas is papaya, which contains a natural protein-digesting enzyme called papain. These formulas may also contain bromelain, a protein-digesting enzyme from pineapple.

Digestive Enzyme Formulas are excellent for people who have problems with food sitting heavily on their stomach after meals or who suffer from frequent indigestion. Elderly people often suffer from weakening digestive function and can benefit from taking enzymes, but younger people whose diets consist mainly of cooked and processed foods can also benefit from them.

For more information and suggestions see *Digestion (Poor)* in the *Conditions Section*. Also consider supplementing with betaine hydrochloric acid (HCl) and/or digestive enzymes as described in the *Nutrients Section*.

Key Herbs: Papaya

Vitanica
Bitters Extra™ (Capsule)
Artichoke leaf, Dandelion root, Yellow Dock, Gentian, Ginger, Burdock root, Fennel, Chamomile flower, Turmeric, Cardamom seed; Non-Herbal: Protease, Amylase, Lipase, Cellulase, Lactase, Phytase, Invertase, Bromelain

Vitanica
Colon Motility Blend™ (Capsule)
Gentian, Triphala, Dandelion root; Non-Herbal: Magnesium, Protease, Amylase, Lipase, Cellulase, Invertase, Lactase, Bromelain

Christopher's
Gas-Eze (Capsule)
Capsicum (Cayenne), Slippery Elm, Caraway seed, Ginger, Catnip; Non-Herbal: Papain

Renew Life
Indigestion STOP (Capsule)
Gentian, Ginger, Meadowsweet, Peppermint leaf; Non-Herbal: Digestive Enzymes

Zand
Quick Digest (Capsule)
Papaya, Parsley leaf, Stevia; Non-Herbal: Papain, Amylase, Cellulase, Bromelain, Lipase, dextrose, calcium carbonate, vegetable stearic acid, vegetable magnesium stearate, citrus flavor, croscarmellose sodium

Zand
Quick Digest™ Citrus (Tablet)
Papaya, Parsley leaf, Stevia; Non-Herbal: Papain, Amylase, Cellulase, Bromelain, Lipase

Digestive Tonic Formulas

See also *Digestive Enzyme Formulas*

As we age, one of the problems we can develop is increasing difficulty in digesting food and assimilating and utilizing nutrients. This can lead to wasting, a gradual loss of muscle tone and density. Wasting can also occur in certain diseases like cancer and AIDS. Some people have chronically poor digestion, meaning they have a difficult time digesting proteins and may be excessively skinny no matter how much they eat.

There are a number of herbs that tonify digestion and improve the body's ability to absorb nutrients. These herbs enhance what is called in Chinese medicine the "spleen chi." Spleen chi enables us to transform the food we eat into flesh, particularly muscle. Herbs that tonify digestion and aid this process, and thus become key herbs in these formulas, which also typically contain key ingredients found in *Digestive Bitter Tonic Formulas*.

Digestive Tonic Formulas are different than digestive bitters because digestive tonics build up or nourish digestive organs, while digestive bitters simply stimulate digestive secretions. *Digestive Tonic Formulas* work well with *Digestive Enzyme Formulas*. See *Hiatal Hernia* and *Wasting* in the *Conditions Section* for additional information on dealing with poor digestion.

Key Herbs: Astragalus, Atractylodes, Ginger, Ginseng (American) and Licorice

Planetary Herbals
Candida Digest™ (Tablet)

Atractylodes (Bai-Zhu) rhizome, Asafetida, Caraway seed, Cumin, **Ginger**, Long Pepper (Pippali) fruit, Black Pepper fruit, Slippery Elm, Dandelion root; Non-Herbal: Sodium, Fiber, Calcium, Rock Salt

Planetary Herbals
Digestive Comfort™ (Tablet)

Poria Mushroom, Magnolia (acuminata) bark, Kudzu root, Chinese Giant Hyssop leaf, Job's Tears, **Atractylodes (Bai-Zhu) rhizome**, Angelica root, Wheat, Rice, Chrysanthemum flower, Gastrodia tuber, Chinese Mint leaf & stem; Non-Herbal: Calcium

Planetary Herbals
Ginseng Elixir™ (Tablet)

Astragalus, **Licorice**, Bupleurum, Chinese Cimicifuga rhizome, **Atractylodes (Bai-Zhu) rhizome**, Jujube fruit, Dong Quai, Dong Quai, **Ginger**; Non-Herbal: Molasses, Sodium, Fiber, Calcium

Planetary Herbals
Ginseng Revitalizer™ (Tablet)

Dong Quai, **Atractylodes (Bai-Zhu) rhizome**, Codonopsis root, Ginseng (Korean, Asian), He Shou Wu (Fo-Ti), **Licorice**, **Astragalus**, Eleuthero root, Poria Mushroom, Ginseng (Korean, Asian); Non-Herbal: Calcium, Sodium, Sugar

Planetary Herbals
Hinga Shtak (Tablet)

Atractylodes (Bai-Zhu) rhizome, Asafetida, Caraway seed, Cumin, **Ginger**, Long Pepper (Pippali) fruit, Black Pepper fruit, Slippery Elm, Dandelion root

New Chapter
Stamina Ginseng Ginger Tonic (Liquid)

Ginger, **Ginger**, **Ginseng (American)**, Lemon essential oil; Non-Herbal: Honey

Diuretic Formulas

See also *Kidney Tonic*, *Lithotriptic* and *Urinary Infection Fighting Formulas*

These formulas are used to stimulate kidney function to remove excess fluid from the body. Herbal *Diuretic Formulas* can be used in any situation where diuretic drugs might be used. They can be helpful in relieving edema,

lowering blood pressure, and may even be helpful as part of a treatment program for congestive heart failure.

There are several subclasses of diuretic formulas to consider. Those containing juniper as a principle ingredient are more suited to stimulating sluggish kidney function, but are not as useful when the kidneys are inflamed. When there is burning or painful urination, consider *Kidney Tonic Formulas*, or choosing a *Diuretic Formula* where cornsilk and marshmallow are primary ingredients.

For infection, consider *Urinary Infection Fighting Formulas*. You can also combine *Goldenseal & Echinacea* or *Antibacterial Formulas* with *Diuretic Formulas* for treating urinary tract infections.

When the kidneys are weak, *Kidney Tonic Formulas* are a good choice. These formulas contain herbs that are more soothing and supportive of the kidneys, rather than being stimulating.

Finally, for help in passing (or preventing the formation of) kidney stones, look to *Lithotriptic Formulas*. These formulas contain herbs that help dissolve calcification of tissues and flush calcium stones from the kidneys or gallbladder.

Key Herbs: Buchu, Dandelion, Juniper Berry, Pipsissewa and Uva Ursi

Christopher's
Bladder Formula (Capsule)

Parsley root, **Juniper berry**, Marshmallow, White Pond Lilly, Gravel Root root, **Uva Ursi**, Lobelia, Ginger, Black Cohosh

Irwin Naturals
Bloat-Away (Softgel)

Dandelion leaf, **Juniper berry**, **Uva Ursi leaf**, **Buchu leaf**, Cranberry, Hibiscus flower, Chamomile flower, Corn Silk, Grape seed, Parsley, Raspberry (Red) leaf, Black Pepper, Ginger; Non-Herbal: Potassium Citrate, Fish Oil

Solaray
GlucoCut Blend™ Sp-5 (Capsule)

Uva Ursi, **Dandelion root**, Fenugreek, Gentian, Huckleberry leaf, Parsley aerial parts

NOW Foods
Go With The Flow™ Tea

Spearmint leaf, Red Clover flower, Cinnamon (burmannii) bark, Lemon Myrtle leaf, **Dandelion leaf & root**, Chickweed, Milk Thistle seed, Stevia leaf

Gaia Herbs
Herbal Diuretic (Liquid Phyto-Caps)

Dandelion leaf, **Juniper berry**, Fenugreek, Parsley leaf & root, Cilantro leaf, Fennel, Bladderwrack

Nature's Herbs (TwinLab)
Juniper Berry Combination (Capsule)

Juniper berry, Marshmallow root, Goldenseal root, Papaya fruit, **Uva Ursi leaf**, Parsley aerial parts, Ginger root, Black Pepper fruit,

Rosemary oil; Non-Herbal: Gelatin, medium chain triglycerides, vitamin E

Grandma's Herbs
Kidney (Capsule)

Parsley, **Uva Ursi**, Marshmallow, **Juniper berry**, **Buchu**, Cleavers (Bedstraw), Corn Silk, **Dandelion**, Yarrow, Meadowsweet, Hydrangea

Solaray
Kidney Blend™ SP-6™ (Capsule)

Corn Silk, Parsley aerial parts, **Uva Ursi**, Cleavers (Bedstraw) aerial parts, Capsicum (Cayenne), **Juniper berry**, Kelp, **Buchu leaf**, Meadowsweet flower

Christopher's
Kidney Formula (Capsule and Glycerine Extract)

Juniper berry, Parsley, **Uva Ursi**, Marshmallow, Lobelia, Ginger, Goldenseal

Nature's Way
Kidney-Bladder (Capsule)

Juniper berry, Parsley leaf, Ginger, **Uva Ursi**, Marshmallow, Cramp Bark, Goldenseal

Western Botanicals
Kidney/Bladder Formula (Capsule and Alcohol Extract)

Juniper berry, Burdock root, Goldenrod flower, **Pipsissewa**, Gravel Root root, Hydrangea, **Uva Ursi**, **Dandelion leaf**, Horsetail, Marshmallow, Corn Silk

Western Botanicals
Kidney/Bladder Formula/Tea Combo (Liquid)

Juniper berry, Burdock root, Goldenrod flower, **Pipsissewa**, Gravel Root root, Hydrangea, **Uva Ursi**, **Dandelion leaf**, Horsetail, Marshmallow, Corn Silk

Western Botanicals
Kidney/Bladder Tea

Juniper berry, Gravel Root root, Orange peel, Hydrangea, Marshmallow, Parsley root, Peppermint leaf, **Uva Ursi**, Horsetail, Corn Silk, Parsley leaf, **Dandelion leaf**, Goldenrod flower

Christopher's
Male Urinary Tract Formula (Capsule)

Capsicum (Cayenne), Ginger, Goldenseal, Gravel Root root, **Juniper berry**, Marshmallow, Parsley root, **Uva Ursi**, Ginseng (American)

Traditional Medicinals
PMS Tea®

Dandelion root, Chicory root, Parsley leaf, Nettle (Stinging) leaf, **Uva Ursi**, Corn Silk, Carob, Barley, Oat straw, Cramp Bark

Irwin Naturals
Urinary Support & Flush™ (Capsule)

Cranberry, Aloe vera leaf, **Dandelion leaf**, **Juniper berry**, Marshmallow root, Corn Silk, Horsetail aerial parts, Rose hips

Eclectic Institute
Urinary Tract Support (Capsule)

Uva Ursi, Marshmallow, Goldenseal, Couchgrass (Quackgrass) root, Kava Kava, Corn Silk

Nature's Way
Urinary with Cranberry (Capsule)

Cranberry, **Dandelion leaf**, Marshmallow, Cleavers (Bedstraw) stem, leaf, fruit & flower, Corn Silk, Goldenseal

Planetary Herbals
Uva Ursi Diurite™ (Tablet)

Poria Mushroom, **Dandelion root**, Uva Ursi, Ginger, Marshmallow, Parsley root, **Uva Ursi**; Non-Herbal: Calcium

NOW Foods
Water Out™ (Capsule)

Uva Ursi, **Dandelion leaf**, Goldenrod, **Juniper berry**, **Buchu leaf**, Bladderwrack; Non-Herbal: Vitamin B6, Potassium

RidgeCrest Herbals
WaterX™ (Capsule)

Birch (White) leaf, Burdock root, **Dandelion root**, **Buchu leaf**, Couchgrass (Quackgrass) rhizome, **Juniper berry**; Non-Herbal: Betula Pendula Cortex, Lappa Major, Plantago Major, Taraxacum Officinale

Drawing Salve Formulas

See also *Anticancer* and *Topical Vulnerary Formulas*

As the name implies, a drawing salve is a remedy used to pull morbid material out of the body. *Drawing Salve Formulas* can be helpful for drawing slivers and for pulling pus and infection out of wounds.

Drawing Salve Formulas may have a mild escharotic quality. Escharotics are agents applied topically to destroy morbid tissue. They are typically used to destroy warts, moles and skin cancers. True escharotics should be used with caution and are best used under the direction of an experienced herbalist. The *Drawing Salve Formulas* listed in this section are safe for lay use.

If a *Drawing Salve Formula* does cause irritation, discontinue use and consult with a professional herbalist. It is often helpful to apply a *Topical Vulnerary Formula* to encourage healing after the drawing agent has completed its work.

One ingredient not found in these formulas that also has strong drawing ability is lily of the valley leaves. The crushed leaves of fresh lily of the valley can be applied to draw out slivers and pus. A useful thing to know if you have lily of the valley growing in your garden.

Key Herbs: Burdock, Chaparral, Lily of the Valley, Pine (White), Plantain, Poke Root and Red Clover

Christopher's
Black Drawing Ointment (Salve)

Chaparral (Creosote) leaf, Comfrey root, **Red Clover**, **Pine gum resin**, Mullein leaf, **Plantain**, Chickweed, Olive oil, Poke Root (Phytolacca); Non-Herbal: Mutton Tallow, Beeswax
Olive oil, **Chaparral (Creosote)**, White Oak bark, Chickweed, Comfrey, Lobelia, Marshmallow, **Red Clover**, Goldenseal, **Pine gum resin**, Tea Tree essential oil, Eucalyptus

Gaia Herbs
Plantain Goldenseal Salve (Salve/Ointment)

Black Walnut, **Burdock root**, **Chaparral (Creosote) leaf**, Eucalyptus essential oil, Goldenseal, **Plantain**, Thuja, Turmeric

Drying Cough/Lung Formulas

See also *Cough Remedy* and *Expectorant Formulas*

These are cough remedies whose key herbs make them more suitable for coughs where there is an excess production of mucus. They are also useful for respiratory problems aggravated by cold, damp weather. The key herbs in these formulas tend to help the body expel excess mucus or dampness from the lungs.

See *Cough (dry)* in the *Conditions Section* for more information.

Key Herbs: Cherry (Wild), Osha, Pine (White), Thyme and Yerba Santa

Gaia Herbs
GaiaKids® Cough Syrup for Wet Coughs

Anise, Cinnamon bark, Cramp Bark, Elecampane, Hyssop, Licorice, **Thyme**, **Cherry (Wild)**

Herbalist & Alchemist
Lung Relief Cold/Damp Compound™ (Alcohol Extract)

Thyme, Ginger, Orange peel, **Yerba Santa**, **Osha**

Herbalist & Alchemist
Lung Relief Hot/Damp Compound™ (Alcohol Tincture)

Ground Ivy, Japanese Honeysuckle flower, Chinese Scullcap (Scute/Huang Qin), Pleurisy root, White Sage

Western Botanicals
Lungs Plus Formula (Alcohol Extract)

Lobelia, Lobelia, Coffee bean, Peppermint leaf, Brigham (Mormon) Tea, Bitter Orange, Peppermint essential oil

Planetary Herbals
Old Indian Wild Cherry Bark Syrup™

Yerba Santa, **Osha**, Elecampane root & flower, Grindelia (Gumweed) flower bud, Echinacea (purpurea) root, **Black Cherry bark**, Horehound leaf, Hyssop leaf, Platycodon, Marshmallow, Apricot seed, Mullein leaf, Licorice, Nettle (Stinging) leaf, **Pine (White) bark**, Angelica root, Loquat leaf, Fritillary bulb

Herbs Etc.
Osha Root Cough Syrup

Osha root, **Pine (White) bark**, **Cherry (Wild) bark**, Spikenard root, Poplar, Bloodroot root

Ear Drop Formulas

See also *Lymphatic Drainage Formulas*

Mullein and garlic infused in olive oil is a traditional herbal remedy for earaches. Some companies add other ingredients to this basic mix, such as tea tree oil for infection or St. John's wort for its antiviral and anti-inflammatory actions.

These products are typically warmed to body temperate and then dropped in the ear (Do not drop them in the ear if they are too cold or hot). It can also be helpful to massage these oils into the side of the neck below the affected ear. This promotes lymphatic drainage and can lead to a faster recovery.

Lymphatic Drainage Formulas may also help with earaches. See *Ear Infection* or *Earache* in the *Conditions Section* for more information on natural therapy for earaches.

Key Herbs: Garlic and Mullein

Herbalist & Alchemist
Compound Mullein Oil

Mullein flower, St. John's Wort flower, **Garlic bulb**, Tea Tree essential oil, White Sage; Non-Herbal: Vitamin E

Eclectic Institute
Ear Drops (Oil)

Mullein flower, St. John's Wort flower & leaf, **Garlic oil**, Olive oil

Gaia Herbs
Ear Oil with Mullein & St. John's Wort

Olive oil, **Garlic**, **Mullein**, St. John's Wort flowering tops

Gaia Herbs
GaiaKids® Ear Drops (Oil)

Olive oil, **Garlic**, Goldenseal, Lobelia, **Mullein**, St. John's Wort bud

Christopher's
Glandular System Massage Oil (Essential Oil)

Mullein leaf, Lobelia, Olive oil

Western Botanicals
Herbal Ear Drops (Oil)

Garlic, **Mullein leaf & flower**, Lobelia herb and seed, Olive oil

Herb Pharm
Mullein/Garlic (Oil)

Calendula (Marigold) flower, St. John's Wort flower, **Mullein flower**, **Garlic**, Olive oil

Herbs Etc.
Mullein/Garlic Ear Drops (Oil)

Garlic bulb, **Mullein flower**, Olive oil; Non-Herbal: vitamin E

Herbal Formulas

Christopher's
Oil of Garlic (Oil)
Garlic, Olive oil, Tea Tree essential oil

Herbs for Kids
Willow/Garlic Ear Oil™ (Oil)
Olive oil, **Garlic**, Calendula (Marigold) flower, Willow bark, Usnea; Non-Herbal: Vitamin E

Echinacea Blend Formulas

See also *Immune Stimulating Formulas*

A number of herbal companies produce products that are blends of several species and plant parts of echinacea. These *Echinacea Blend Formulas* are useful for boosting the immune system. They can be taken when colds and flu are "going around" to reduce one's chance of getting sick. They can also be taken to boost the immune system when fighting off an infection. Echinacea has both antiviral and antibacterial properties, so it can be used on either type of infection, but it is more effective against bacterial infections than it is against viral infections.

Echinacea Blend Formulas are a subcategory of *Immune Stimulating Formulas*, which typically use echinacea as a key herb.

Key Herbs: Echinacea

Nature's Answer
E-KID-nacea (Glycerine Extract)
Echinacea (angustifolia) root, Echinacea (purpurea)

Eclectic Institute
E.P.B. (Glycerine Extract)
Echinacea (angustifolia) root, Echinacea (purpurea) root, leaf, flower & seed, Echinacea (pallida) root, Echinacea root, Blackberry; Non-Herbal: Ascorbic Acid. Comes in blackberry, lemon, orange, raspberry and tangerine flavors.

Yerba Prima
Echinace® (Capsule)
Echinacea (purpurea) herb and root, Echinacea (angustifolia) root, Black Pepper

NOW Foods
Echinacea 50/50 Ang./Purp. (Glycerine Extract)
Echinacea (angustifolia), Echinacea (purpurea)

Nature's Way
Echinacea Complex (Capsule)
Echinacea (purpurea) root, Echinacea (angustifolia) root

Traditional Medicinals
Echinacea Plus® (Tea)
Echinacea (purpurea), Echinacea (purpurea) root, Echinacea (angustifolia), Lemongrass leaf, Spearmint

Eclectic Institute
Echinacea Premium Blend (Glycerine Extract)
Echinacea (angustifolia) root, Echinacea (purpurea) root, leaf, flower & seed, Echinacea (pallida) root, Echinacea (tennesseensis) root

Solaray
Echinacea Purpurea, Angustifolia (Capsule)
Echinacea (angustifolia) root, Echinacea (purpurea) root

Gaia Herbs
Echinacea Supreme (Liquid Phyto-Caps)
Echinacea (purpurea) aerial parts & root, Echinacea (angustifolia) root, Echinacea (purpurea) seed

Gaia Herbs
Echinacea Supreme (Alcohol and Glycerine Extract)
Echinacea (angustifolia) root, Echinacea (purpurea) aerial parts, root & seed

Gaia Herbs
Echinacea Supreme, Extra-Strength (Alcohol Extract)
Echinacea (purpurea) root, aerial parts & seed, Echinacea (angustifolia) root

Herbs Etc.
Echinacea Triple Source™ (Alcohol Extract)
Echinacea (angustifolia) root, herb and flower, Echinacea (purpurea) root, herb, flower and seed, Echinacea (pallida) root

Yogi Tea
Green Tea Triple Echinacea (Tea)
Green Tea leaf, Lemongrass, Spearmint, **Echinacea (angustifolia) root, Echinacea (purpurea) root, Echinacea (pallida) root**

Herbalist & Alchemist
Ultimate Echinacea™ (Alcohol Extract)
Echinacea (angustifolia) root, Echinacea (pallida) root, Echinacea (purpurea) root & flower

Energy-Boosting Formulas

See also *Adaptogen, Adrenal Tonic, Exercise* and *Hypothyroid Formulas*

These formulas are useful for overcoming fatigue, enhancing energy, endurance and stamina, and aiding mental clarity. They rely on a variety of adaptogenic, immune-enhancing, nourishing and stimulating herbs. The key herbs used in these blends include caffeine-bearing plants like green tea or guarana. They may also include adaptogens and general tonics.

Low energy can be the result of adrenal exhaustion, low thyroid, depression, liver congestion, poor digestion and assimilation of nutrients, low grade infections or blood sugar issues. If you have consistent low energy, you need to seek help in identifying and correcting the underlying cause of your problem. Some other categories of remedies to consider for lack of energy include: *Adaptogenic, Adrenal Tonic, Exercise* and *Hypothyroid Formulas*. Also see *Fatigue* in the *Conditions Section*.

Key Herbs: Bee Pollen, Cordyceps, Eleuthero (Siberian ginseng), Ginseng (American), Ginseng (Asian, Korean), Gotu kola, Guarana, He Shou Wu (Ho Shou Wu, Fo-Ti), Kelp, Licorice, Rehmannia and Tea (Green or Black)

Christopher's
Bee Power Energy Formula (Capsule)

Eleuthero, **Bee Pollen**, **Licorice**, **Gotu Kola**, Brigham (Mormon) Tea, Yerba Mate, Ginger

Celestial Seasonings
Berry Enerji Green Tea Energy Shot

Green Tea, **Ginseng (American)**, Stevia; Non-Herbal: Evaporated Cane juice, Niacin, B-Vitamin blend, Inositol

Celestial Seasonings
Berry Kombucha Energy Shot (Tea)

Kombucha, **Guarana**, **Ginseng (Korean, Asian)**, Stevia; Non-Herbal: Evaporated Cane juice, Niacin, B-Vitamin blend, Inositol

Yogi Tea
Chai Black (Tea)

Black Tea, Cardamom seed, Cinnamon bark, Ginger, Clove, Cinnamon essential oil, Black Pepper, Ginger essential oil, Cardamom essential oil

Celestial Seasonings
Citrus ENERJI Green Tea Energy Shot

Green Tea, **Ginseng (American)**, Stevia; Non-Herbal: Evaporated Cane juice, Niacin, B-Vitamin blend, Inositol

Celestial Seasonings
Citrus Kombucha Energy Shot (Tea)

Kombucha, **Guarana**, **Ginseng (Korean, Asian)**, Stevia; Non-Herbal: Evaporated Cane juice, Niacin, B-Vitamin blend, Inositol

Planetary Herbals
Cordyceps Power CS-4™ (Tablet)

Cordyceps (militaris), Astragalus, Codonopsis root, Adenophora root, Eucommia (ulmoides) bark, Eleuthero root, Atractylodes (Bai-Zhu) rhizome, Ginger; Non-Herbal: Sodium

New Chapter
Energizer Green Tea Ginger Tonic™ (Liquid)

Ginger, Ginger, **Green Tea leaf**, Lemon essential oil; Non-Herbal: Honey

Gaia Herbs
Energy Vitality (Liquid Phyto-Caps)

Green Tea leaf, Eleuthero root, Schisandra, **Ginseng (Korean, Asian)**, Kola (cola) nut, Ginkgo, **Licorice**, Nettle (Stinging) seed, Prickly Ash

Celestial Seasonings
Fast Lane Caffeinated Black Tea

Black Tea, Cinnamon bark, Eleuthero, **Licorice**, Kola (cola) nut, Nutmeg

NOW Foods
Full Tilt™ Tea

Green Tea, Cinnamon (burmannii) bark, Ginger, Ashwagandha root, Eleuthero root, Yerba Mate leaf, Stevia

Traditional Medicinals
Ginger Yerba Maté (Tea)

Yerba Mate, Yerba Mate, Ginger, Lemon peel

NOW Foods
Ginseng & Royal Jelly (Capsule)

Ginseng (Korean, Asian), Royal Jelly, **Licorice**

Planetary Herbals
Ginseng Classic™ (Tablet)

Atractylodes (Bai-Zhu) root, Poria Mushroom, **Licorice**, **Ginseng (Korean, Asian)**

Yogi Tea
Ginseng Vitality™ (Tea)

Cinnamon bark, Honeybush, **Licorice**, Ginger, Eleuthero root, **Ginseng (Korean, Asian)**, Alfalfa leaf, Dong Quai, Black Pepper, Hibiscus, Astragalus

Yogi Tea
Green Tea Energy™ (Tea)

Green Tea leaf, Anise, **Ginseng (Korean, Asian)**, Lemongrass, Spearmint, Eleuthero, Kombucha

Christopher's
Herbal Thyroid Formula (Capsule)

Guarana, Eleuthero, **He Shou Wu (Fo-Ti)**, **Gotu Kola**, Mullein, **Kelp**

Celestial Seasonings
Honey Lemon Ginseng Green Tea

Green Tea, **White Tea**, Eleuthero root, **Licorice**, Lemon Verbena, Chicory, Ginger, Orange flower, **Ginseng (Korean, Asian)**; Non-Herbal: Honey

Solaray
OctaPower™ (Capsule)

Bee Pollen, Eleuthero root, Ginger; Non-Herbal: Octacosanol

Irwin Naturals
Oolong & Matcha Tea (Softgel)

Green Tea, Green Matcha Tea, Oolong Tea, **White Tea**, **Ginseng (Korean, Asian)**, Astragalus, **Kelp**, Schisandra, Peony (White, Chinese) root, Black Pepper, Ginger; Non-Herbal: Fish Oil

Celestial Seasonings
Pomegranate Xtreme ENERJI Green Tea Energy Shot (Liquid)

Green Tea, **Ginseng (American)**, Stevia; Non-Herbal: Evaporated Cane juice, Niacin, B-Vitamin blend, Inositol

Herbal Formulas

Celestial Seasonings

Pomegranate Xtreme Kombucha Energy Shot (Liquid)

Kombucha, **Guarana**, **Ginseng (Korean, Asian)**; Non-Herbal: Organic Evaporated Cane Juice, Citric Acid, Natural Pomegranate Flavor, Niacin (as Niacinamide), Rebiana (Sweetener from Stevia), Vitamins B6 [Pyridoxine Hydrochloride], B5 [Calcium Pantothenate] and B12 [Cyanocobalamine]), Inositol

Yogi Tea

Raspberry Passion Perfect Energy™ (Tea)

Black Tea, Hibiscus, Sage, **Green Tea**, **Gotu Kola**, Shank Pushpi leaf, Ashwagandha, Shatavari; Non-Herbal: L-Theanine Suntheanine®

Yogi Tea

Refreshing Mint Vital Energy™ (Tea)

Peppermint leaf, **Black Tea**, Spearmint, Cinnamon bark, Cardamom seed, Ginger, Black Pepper, **Guarana**, Kola (cola) nut, Clove

Planetary Herbals

Rehmannia Endurance™ (Tablet)

Rehmannia, Poria Mushroom, Tree Peony, Chinese Yam rhizome, Asian Water Plantain rhizome, **He Shou Wu (Fo-Ti)**, Chrysanthemum flower, Ligustrum fruit, Saw Palmetto, Lycium (Wolfberry/Gogi), Asiatic Dogwood berry; Non-Herbal: Calcium

Planetary Herbals

Rehmannia Vitalizer™ (Tablet)

Desert Broomrape aerial parts, **Rehmannia**, Psoralea fruit, Tree Peony, Chinese Yam rhizome, Dong Quai, Poria Mushroom, Schisandra, Asian Water Plantain rhizome, Saw Palmetto, Cinnamon (cassia) bark, Morinda (Noni) root, Dodder seed, **Ginseng (Korean, Asian)**, Epimedium (Horny Goat Weed) aerial parts, Asiatic Dogwood fruit, Lycium (Wolfberry/Gogi); Non-Herbal: Calcium

New Chapter

Stamina Ginseng Ginger Tonic (Liquid)

Ginger, Ginger, **Ginseng (American)**, Lemon essential oil; Non-Herbal: Honey

New Chapter

Supercritical Diet & Energy (Tablet)

Green Tea leaf, **White Tea**, Ginger, Maca, Capsicum (Cayenne), Rhodiola, Cinnamon (verum) bark, Fenugreek, Turmeric, Peppermint leaf, Clove, Rosemary, Sea Buckthorn, Sea Buckthorn seed, Calendula (Marigold) flower; Non-Herbal: Probiotic chromium

Yogi Tea

Sweet Tangerine Positive Energy™ (Tea)

Black Tea, **Green Tea leaf**, Lemongrass, Lemon Myrtle, Ashwagandha, Basil leaf, Shank Pushpi leaf, **Ginseng (Korean, Asian)**, Eleuthero root; Non-Herbal: Essential Oils, Citric Acid

Yogi Tea

Vanilla Spice Perfect Energy® (Tea)

Green Tea leaf, Cinnamon bark, **Black Tea**, Rooibos (Redbush), Honeybush, Ginger, **Licorice**, Vanilla bean, **Gotu Kola**, Ashwagandha, Shatavari, Shank Pushpi leaf; Non-Herbal: L-Theanine Suntheanine®

Herbs Etc.

Vibrant Energy™ (Alcohol Extract or Softgel)

Ginseng (Red) root, **He Shou Wu (Fo-Ti) root**, Gotu Kola, Eleuthero root, Damiana (diffusa) leaf, **Ginseng (American) root**, **Licorice root**, Prickly Ash bark, Peppermint, Ginger root, Capsicum (Cayenne) fruit

Essiac Formulas

See also *Anticancer* and *Blood Purifier Formulas*

The Essiac formula was introduced by a nurse named René Caisse (Essiac is Caisee spelled backwards). She claims it came from a Native American of the Ojibwa tribe. It's key ingredients are burdock and sheep sorrel, but it also contains slippery elm and turkey rhubarb. Like most anticancer formulas, *Essiac Formulas* are a subcategory of *Blood Purifier Formulas*.

For more information on natural methods of treating cancer see *Cancer (natural therapies for)* in the *Conditions Section*. Because of the serious nature of cancer, competent help should be sought to design a treatment approach that is appropriate for the individual cancer patient.

Key Herbs: Burdock and Sheep Sorrel

Eclectic Institute

Cleansing Support (Capsule)

Sheep Sorrel flower & leaf, **Burdock root**, Slippery Elm

Western Botanicals

Essiac Formula (Capsule, Alcohol Extract or Tea)

Burdock root, **Sheep Sorrel**, Slippery Elm, Turkey Rhubarb

Herbs Etc.

Essiac Tonic (Alcohol Extract, Glycerine Extract or Softgel)

Burdock root, **Sheep Sorrel**, Slippery Elm bark, Turkey Rhubarb root

NOW Foods

Ojibwa Tea Concentrate (Liquid)

Burdock root, **Sheep Sorrel leaf**, Slippery Elm, Turkey Rhubarb root

Exercise Formulas

See also *Adaptogen* and *Energy-Boosting Formulas*

As the category name suggests, these herbal formulas are used to aid athletes or people who are exercising. The herbal ingredients and exact uses of *Exercise Formulas* vary considerably.

Adaptogenic and *Energy-Boosting Formulas* are other categories to consider in enhancing exercise programs.

Key Herbs: Cordyceps, Eleuthero (Siberian ginseng) and Sarsaparilla

Herb Pharm
Athlete's Power (Alcohol Extract)

Sarsaparilla, Saw Palmetto, Eleuthero root, Gotu Kola

Planetary Herbals
Cordyceps Power CS-4™ (Tablet)

Cordyceps (militaris), Astragalus, Codonopsis root, Adenophora root, Eucommia (ulmoides) bark, Eleuthero root, Atractylodes (Bai-Zhu) rhizome, Ginger; Non-Herbal: Sodium

Herbalist & Alchemist
Fitness Formula™ (Alcohol Extract)

Eleuthero root, Schisandra, Hawthorn berry, Hawthorn flower, Reishi (Ganoderma), **Sarsaparilla**, Ashwagandha root, **Cordyceps**

Yogi Tea
Green Tea Muscle Recovery™ (Tea)

Green Tea leaf, Lemongrass, Blackberry leaf, Rose petals, Scullcap (Skullcap), Lemon Myrtle, Turmeric, Yucca, Ginseng (Korean, Asian), Ginseng (American), Eleuthero, Cat's Claw bark, Devil's Claw

Expectorant Formulas

See also *Cough Remedy Formulas*

The lungs and sinuses have tiny, hair-like projections called cilia that sweep mucus to the throat to be swallowed and eliminated. Expectorants aid this process by helping to eliminate mucus from the lungs and sinuses. The key herbs found in these blends are very good at loosening mucus that is not moving so the body get expel it.

Key Herbs: Cherry (Wild), Grindelia (Gumweed), Horehound, Lobelia, Osha, Pine (White) and Yerba Santa

Solaray
Bronchial Blend™ SP-22™ (Capsule)

Bayberry root bark, **Horehound aerial parts**, Ginger, Slippery Elm, Clove, Capsicum (Cayenne)

A. Vogel
Bronchosan (Syrup)

Thyme, Licorice, Anise essential oil, Eucalyptus essential oil

Eclectic Institute
Compound Elixir (Glycerine Extract)

Licorice, Elecampane root, Red Clover flower, **Cherry (Wild) bark**, **Horehound leaf & flower**, **Black Cherry**, **Grindelia (Gumweed) flower & leaf**, **Lobelia leaf & seed**, Fennel, Lomatium, **Pine (White) bark**, Poplar bud, Orange essential oil

Eclectic Institute
Compound Herbal Elixir (Liquid)

Licorice, Elecampane root, Red Clover flower, **Cherry (Wild) bark**, **Horehound flower & leaf**, **Grindelia (Gumweed) flower & leaf**, **Lobelia leaf & seed**, Fennel, Lomatium, **Pine (White) bark**, Poplar bud

Eclectic Institute
Herb Cough Elixir (Liquid)

Licorice, Elecampane root, Red Clover flower, **Cherry (Wild) bark**, **Horehound flower & leaf**, **Black Cherry**, **Grindelia (Gumweed) flower & leaf**, **Lobelia leaf & seed**, Fennel, Lomatium, **Pine (White) bark**, Orange essential oil, Poplar bud

Christopher's
Herbal Cough Syrup

Cherry (Wild) bark, Licorice, Marshmallow, **Horehound**, Mullein leaf, Ginger, Anise seed, Lemon peel

Western Botanicals
Herbal Super Tonic (Capsule and Liquid)

Horseradish, Garlic, Onion, Ginger, Capsicum (Cayenne), Capsicum (chinense)

Solaray
Histamine Blend™ SP-33 (Capsule)

Horehound aerial parts, Mullein leaf, **Cherry (Wild) bark**, Barberry root, Peppermint aerial parts; Non-Herbal: Montmorillonite Clay

Yogi Tea
Honey Lemon Throat Comfort® (Tea)

Honeybush, Lemongrass, Lemon Myrtle, Licorice, Peppermint leaf, **Cherry (Wild) bark**, Echinacea (angustifolia) root, Echinacea (purpurea) root, Echinacea (pallida) root, Black Pepper, Slippery Elm

Herbs for Kids
Horehound Blend™ (Glycerine Extract)

Mullein leaf, Astragalus, **Horehound**, Sage, Orange peel, Oregon Grape, Ginger, Eucalyptus essential oil

Traditional Medicinals
"Just for Kids" Throat Coat® (Tea)

Marshmallow, Sage, Calendula (Marigold) flower, Licorice, Cinnamon bark, **Cherry (Wild) bark**

Planetary Herbals
Loquat Respiratory Syrup

Loquat leaf, Fritillary bulb, **Black Cherry bark**, Slippery Elm, Platycodon, Trichosanthes seed, Polygala, Poria Mushroom, Schisandra, Licorice (Chinese), Peppermint essential oil; Non-Herbal: Honey, Blackstrap Molasses

Solaray
Lung Caps™ (Capsule)

Pleurisy root, **Cherry (Wild) bark**, Slippery Elm, Clove

Herbalist & Alchemist
Lung Relief Antispasmodic Compound™ (Alcohol Tincture)

Mullein leaf, **Cherry (Wild) bark**, Licorice, Wild (Prickly) Lettuce, Khella seed, **Lobelia flower**, **Lobelia seed**; Non-Herbal: Apple cider vinegar

Herbal Formulas

Herbs Etc.

Lung Tonic™
(Alcohol Extract, Glycerine Extract or Softgel)

Mullein leaf, **Horehound**, Elecampane root, **Grindelia (Gumweed) flower**, Echinacea (angustifolia) root, Pleurisy root, Passionflower, **Osha root**, **Lobelia**, **Yerba Santa leaf**

Planetary Herbals

Old Indian Syrup for Kids™ (Glycerine Extract)

Yerba Santa, Elecampane flower & root, **Grindelia (Gumweed) flower bud**, Platycodon, **Horehound leaf**, Hyssop aerial parts, Thyme leaf, Mullein leaf, Nettle (Stinging) leaf, **Pine (White) bark**, Angelica root, Loquat leaf, Fritillary bulb, Marshmallow, Irish Moss, Licorice, **Black Cherry bark**

Planetary Herbals

Old Indian Wild Cherry Bark Syrup™

Yerba Santa, **Osha**, Elecampane root & flower, **Grindelia (Gumweed) flower bud**, Echinacea (purpurea) root, **Black Cherry bark**, **Horehound leaf**, Hyssop leaf, Platycodon, Marshmallow, Apricot seed, Mullein leaf, Licorice, Nettle (Stinging) leaf, **Pine (White) bark**, Angelica root, Loquat leaf, Fritillary bulb

Herbs Etc.

Osha Root Cough Syrup

Osha root, **Pine (White) bark**, **Cherry (Wild) bark**, Spikenard root, Poplar, Bloodroot root

Herbs Etc.

Respiratonic® (Alcohol Extract or Softgel)

Echinacea (angustifolia) root, **Osha root**, Licorice root, Yerba mansa root, **Yerba Santa leaf**, Pleurisy root, **Grindelia (Gumweed) flower**, Ginger root

Christopher's

Respiratory Relief Syrup

Onion, Garlic, Fennel, Nettle (Stinging) leaf, Mullein leaf, Chickweed

Traditional Medicinals

Throat Coat® Herbal Syrup

Licorice, **Cherry (Wild) bark**, Fennel fruit, Cinnamon bark, Orange peel, Slippery Elm, Marshmallow, Licorice, Peppermint leaf; Non-Herbal: Honey

Yogi Tea

Throat Comfort® (Tea)

Licorice, Fennel, **Cherry (Wild) bark**, Cinnamon bark, Orange peel, Slippery Elm, Cardamom seed, Ginger, Mullein leaf, Clove, Black Pepper

Eye Wash Formulas

See also *Vision Supporting Formulas*

The famous Utah herbalist, Dr. John Christopher, created the original herbal *Eye Wash Formula*. It is made into a tea and used as an eye wash. It can also be dropped into the eyes or used as a compress. Be sure to strain the tea thoroughly so that no herb particles remain and make fresh tea every couple of days.

The formula is useful for sore, red and irritated eyes. It is also good for treating conjunctivitis and other eye infections. Dr. Christopher maintained that it would improve eyesight and dissolve cataracts when used daily. Few people have the determination to use this formula for the several months this is supposed to take.

Internally, the *Eye Wash Formula* is an herbal eye, ear, nose and throat soother. It can relieve itchy watery eyes, itchy, runny nose and redness and irritation of the upper respiratory system. It has some anti-allergy properties.

Vision Supporting Formulas are taken internally to help nourish the eyes. The nutrient, zeaxanthin, is very helpful for this purpose. See *Eye Infections* and *Eye Problems (general)* in the *Conditions Section*.

Key Herbs: Bayberry, Chamomile (English and Roman), Eyebright and Goldenseal

Nature's Sunshine Products

E-W (Capsule)

Bayberry root bark, **Goldenseal**, Raspberry (Red) leaf, **Eyebright aerial parts**

Christopher's

Herbal Eyebright (Capsule and Alcohol Extract)

Bayberry bark, **Eyebright**, **Goldenseal**, Raspberry (Red) leaf, Capsicum (Cayenne)

Western Botanicals

Herbal Eyewash Formula with Cayenne Pepper (Liquid)

Goldenseal, Bilberry, **Bayberry bark**, Raspberry (Red) leaf, **Eyebright**, Bilberry leaf, Capsicum (chinense)

Western Botanicals

Herbal Eyewash Formula without Cayenne Pepper (Liquid)

Goldenseal, Bilberry, **Bayberry bark**, Raspberry (Red) leaf, **Eyebright**, Bilberry leaf

Female Aphrodisiac Formulas

See also *Female Hormonal Balancing* and *Hypothyroid Formulas*

These formulas are a subcategory of *Female Hormonal Balancing Formulas*. They are more targeted at helping to balance female hormones to improve sexual desire and response. So, many *Female Hormonal Balancing Formulas* will have a similar effect.

Generally speaking, herbs aren't going to directly stimulate sexual desire. They can, however, improve hormonal balance and increase energy, making a woman more easily aroused and responsive.

Low sex drive in women can be due to low thyroid. See *Hypothyroid Formulas*. Also see *Sex Drive (low)* in the *Conditions Section* for more suggestions.

Key Herbs: Damiana, Eleuthero (Siberian ginseng), Ginseng (Asian, Korean), Maca, Muira Puama, Oat and Shatavari

Grandma's Herbs
Female Libido Enhancer (Capsule)

Oat straw, Nettle (Stinging), **Muira Puama**, Wild Yam, Epimedium (Horny Goat Weed), **Maca**, Corn Silk, Eleuthero, **Damiana (diffusa)**, Saw Palmetto, Tribulus, Cocoa (Cacao), Black Cohosh, Royal Jelly; Non-Herbal: L-Hstadine, L-Arginine, L-Tyrosine

Herb Pharm
Female Libido Tonic™ (Alcohol Extract)

Muira Puama stem, **Shatavari root**, **Ginseng (Korean, Asian) root**, Ginger rhizome, Cinnamon (aromaticum) bark

Christopher's
Herbal Libido Formula (Capsule)

Muira Puama, **Maca**, Yohimbe, Bee Pollen, Royal Jelly, Ginger, Eleuthero, Ginkgo, Nettle (Stinging), Guarana root; Non-Herbal: Be Pollen

Herbs Etc.
Passion Potion™ (Alcohol Extract)

Oat seed (milky), **Damiana (diffusa) leaf**, Passionflower, Hawthorn flower, leaf & berry, Ginseng (American) root, Licorice root, Nettle (Stinging), Parsley root, Stevia leaf

Gaia Herbs
Women's Libido (Liquid Phyto-Caps)

Tribulus fruit, **Oat seed (milky)**, Epimedium (Horny Goat Weed), **Damiana (diffusa) leaf**, **Maca root**, Blue Vervain, Sarsaparilla root

Female Hormonal Balancing Formulas

See also *Female Aphrodisiac, Menopause Balancing, Phytoestrogen* and *PMS Relieving Formulas*

This is a category of broad-acting formulas that are used to help balance a woman's hormones throughout her menstrual cycle. Like *Female Aphrodisiac Formulas*, they may help to improve sexual desire and responsiveness. They may be helpful in relieving or reducing symptoms of PMS like *PMS Relieving Formulas*. They may also be helpful in reducing problems associated with menopause like *Menopause Balancing Formulas*.

Because the ingredients in this class of formulas can very widely, it is important to understand some of the key herbs and what they do in order to select an appropriate remedy. You may have to experiment a little to find the blend that works right for you. Key herbs include black cohosh (an antispasmodic that also eases cramping and helps with hot flashes), chaste tree (which balanced estrogen and progesterone levels via the pituitary), dong quai and peony (which nourish the blood and support women's general health), red raspberry (which tones the uterus) and blessed thistle and milk thistle (which aid the liver in breaking down excess hormones).

See *PMS, Dysmenorrhea, Menorrhagia (Heavy Menstrual Bleeding), Menstrual Cramps* and *Menopause* in the *Conditions Section* for more suggestions on balancing specific female reproductive hormones.

Key Herbs: Black Cohosh, Blessed Thistle, Chastetree (Vitex), Dong Quai, False Unicorn (Helonias), Licorice, Milk Thistle, Peony, Red Raspberry and Rehmannia

Planetary Herbals
Avena Sativa Oat Complex™ for Women (Tablet)

Oat tops, **Dong Quai**, **Peony (White, Chinese)**, Chuan Xiong rhizome, **Chaste Tree (Vitex)**, Jujube fruit, Cinnamon (cassia) bark

Grandma's Herbs
Body Balance (Capsule)

Wild Yam, **Chaste Tree (Vitex)**, **Black Cohosh**, **Raspberry (Red)**, Sarsaparilla, St. John's Wort, Fenugreek, **Licorice**, Eleuthero, Valerian, Passionflower, **False Unicorn (Helonias, Chamaelirium)**, Heal All, **Dong Quai**, Nettle (Stinging), Suma, Motherwort, Bladder Pod, Horsetail, Capsicum (Cayenne)

NOW Foods
Chaste Berry-Vitex Extract (Capsule)

Chaste Tree (Vitex), **Dong Quai**

Eclectic Institute
Dong Quai - Wild Yam (Glycerine Extract)

Dong Quai, Wild Yam, Blue Cohosh, **Chaste Tree (Vitex)**

Gaia Herbs
Dong Quai Supreme (Alcohol Extract)

Dong Quai root, Saw Palmetto berry, **Black Cohosh root**, **False Unicorn (Helonias, Chamaelirium) root**, Squaw Vine (Partridge Berry) berry, **Licorice root**, Ginger root

Solaray
Dong Quai with Damiana (Capsule)

Dong Quai, Damiana leaf

New Chapter
Estrotone® (Softgel)

Evening Primrose oil, Schisandra, Ginger, **Black Cohosh**, **Black Cohosh**, **Chaste Tree (Vitex)**, Rosemary

Christopher's
False Unicorn & Lobelia (Capsule)

False Unicorn (Helonias, Chamaelirium), Lobelia

Vitanica
Fem Rebalance™ (Capsule)

Licorice, **Chaste Tree (Vitex)**, Rhodiola, Borage oil, **False Unicorn (Helonias, Chamaelirium) root**, Vervain root, Sarsaparilla, Wild Yam, **Black Cohosh**

Herbal Formulas

Grandma's Herbs
Fem-Aid (Capsule)

False Unicorn (Helonias, Chamaelirium), Wild Yam, Lady's Mantle, Squaw Vine (Partridge Berry), **Blessed Thistle**, **Raspberry (Red)**, St. John's Wort, **Dong Quai**, Chamomile, Blue Cohosh, Eleuthero, Cramp Bark, Sarsaparilla, Capsicum (Cayenne)

Gaia Herbs
Fem-Restore (Alcohol Extract)

Fraxinus bark, Red Root, **False Unicorn (Helonias, Chamaelirium) root**, Cinnamon bark, Mayapple root, Goldenseal root, Ginger rhizome, Lobelia herb and seed

Western Botanicals
Female Balance Formula (Capsule and Alcohol Extract)

Dong Quai, **Black Cohosh**, Wild Yam, **Chaste Tree (Vitex)**, Angelica root, Cramp Bark, Ginger, **Licorice**, Lobelia, Lobelia seed, Motherwort, Damiana leaf, Scullcap (Skullcap), Hops flower, Horsetail

NOW Foods
Female Balance™ (Capsule)

Borage oil, Wild Yam root, **Dong Quai root**, **Chaste Tree (Vitex) fruit**; Non-Herbal: Vitamin B-6, Folic Acid

Solaray
Female Caps™ (Capsule)

Dong Quai, Clove, **Black Cohosh**, **Licorice**, **Raspberry (Red) leaf**, Passionflower aerial parts, Chamomile flowering tops, Fenugreek

Nature's Answer
Female Complex™ (Capsule)

Dong Quai, **Raspberry (Red) leaf**, **Black Cohosh**, **Chaste Tree (Vitex)**

Solaray
Female Hormone Blend™ SP-7C™ (Capsule)

Black Cohosh, **Dong Quai**, Passionflower flower, **Raspberry (Red) leaf**, Fenugreek, **Licorice**, Cramp Bark, Chamomile flowering tops, Saw Palmetto, Wild Yam, Butternut bark, Kelp

Christopher's
Female Reproductive Formula (Capsule and Glycerine Extract)

Goldenseal, **Blessed Thistle**, Capsicum (Cayenne), Cramp Bark, **False Unicorn (Helonias, Chamaelirium) root**, Ginger, **Raspberry (Red) leaf**, Squaw Vine (Partridge Berry), Uva Ursi

Traditional Medicinals
Female Toner® (Tea)

Raspberry (Red) leaf, **Licorice**, Strawberry leaf, Nettle (Stinging) leaf, Angelica root, **Blessed Thistle**, Spearmint, Rose hips, Lemon Verbena, Lemongrass leaf, Ginger, Chamomile flower

Christopher's
Female Tonic Formula (Capsule)

Squaw Vine (Partridge Berry), **Raspberry (Red) leaf**, Nettle (Stinging) leaf, Dandelion leaf, Wild Yam, Cramp Bark, Chickweed, Dulse, **Chaste Tree (Vitex)**, Motherwort, Ginger

Solaray
Fertility Blend™ SP-1™ (Capsule)

Damiana leaf, Eleuthero root, Saw Palmetto, Buckthorn bark, Kelp, Sarsaparilla

Vitanica
HRT Companion™ (Capsule)

Garlic, Flax seed, Green Tea, **Milk Thistle**, Soybean; Non-Herbal: Vitamin C, Vitamin E, Vitamin B6, Folate, Vitamin B12, DIM (Diindolymethane), Phosphatidylserine,

Eclectic Institute
Motherwort - Black Cohosh G (Glycerine Extract)

Motherwort flowering tops, **Black Cohosh**, Alfalfa flower and leaf, Hops strobile, **Licorice**, Anise seed & essential oil

Eclectic Institute
Motherwort - Black Cohosh O (Alcohol Extract)

Motherwort flowering tops, **Black Cohosh**, Alfalfa flower and leaf, Hops strobile, Anise seed & essential oil

Solaray
Multi Gland Caps™ for Women (Capsule)

Ginger, Clove, **Dong Quai**, He Shou Wu (Fo-Ti), Dandelion root, Saw Palmetto

Vitanica
Pregnancy Prep™ (Capsule)

Tribulus, Rhodiola, **Chaste Tree (Vitex)**, **Raspberry (Red) leaf**, Alfalfa, **Dong Quai**, Motherwort, **False Unicorn (Helonias, Chamaelirium)**; Non-Herbal: Amylase, Protease, Lipase, Cellulose, Lactase

Herbalist & Alchemist
Uterine Tonic™ (Alcohol Extract)

Chaste Tree (Vitex), **Dong Quai**, **Peony (White, Chinese)**, Cinnamon (cassia) bark, Cypress root, Saw Palmetto, Shepherd's Purse

Gaia Herbs
Vitex Elixir (Alcohol and Glycerine Extract)

Bladderwrack, Blue Vervain, **Chaste Tree (Vitex)**, Cramp Bark, Dandelion leaf & root, Dulse, Kelp, Mugwort, Squaw Vine (Partridge Berry), Prickly Ash (Zanthoxylum americanum), **Raspberry (Red)**, Rose hips, Usnea; Non-Herbal: Sweet Grape syrup

Yogi Tea
Woman's Moon Cycle® (Tea)

Fennel, Ginger, Cinnamon bark, Chamomile flower, **Raspberry (Red) leaf**, Anise seed, **Dong Quai**, **Chaste Tree (Vitex)**, Juniper berry, Parsley leaf

Gaia Herbs
Women's Balance (Liquid Phyto-Caps)

Alfalfa leaf, Red Clover flower, **Chaste Tree (Vitex)**, Oat seed (milky), St. John's Wort flowering tops, Dandelion root & leaf, Blue Vervain, Sage

Herbalist & Alchemist
Women's Calmpound™ (Alcohol Extract)

Chaste Tree (Vitex), Motherwort flowering tops, Scullcap (Skullcap) flowering tops, Blue Vervain flowering tops, Pulsatilla root

Herbal Formulas

Planetary Herbals
Women's Dong Quai Tonifier™ (Tablet)

Dong Quai, **Peony (White, Chinese)**, Atractylodes (Bai-Zhu) rhizome, Codonopsis root, **Rehmannia**, Poria Mushroom, Chuan Xiong rhizome, **Licorice**; Non-Herbal: Molassas, Calcium

Planetary Herbals
Women's Dong Quai Treasure™ (Tablet)

Dong Quai, **Peony (White, Chinese)**, Cramp Bark, **False Unicorn (Helonias, Chamaelirium) root**, **Rehmannia**, **Dong Quai**, Atractylodes (Bai-Zhu) rhizome, **Chaste Tree (Vitex)**, Chuan Xiong rhizome, Tree Peony, Blue Cohosh, Ginger, Shatavari, Poria Mushroom; Non-Herbal: Calcium

Herbalist & Alchemist
Women's Formula™ (Alcohol Extract)

Motherwort flowering tops, **Raspberry (Red) leaf**, **Chaste Tree (Vitex)**, **Dong Quai**, Ginger, **Rehmannia**

Yerba Prima
Women's Renew® (Capsule)

Yellow Dock, Dandelion leaf & root, Red Clover flowering tops, **Chaste Tree (Vitex)**, Ginger, **Blessed Thistle**, **Dong Quai**, **Milk Thistle seed**, Plantain, Corn Silk; Non-Herbal: zinc, niacinamide, pantothenic acid, Vitamin B-6, folic acid, biotin, Vitamin B-12

Fiber Blend Formulas

See also *General Detoxifying Formulas*

Fiber has many important health benefits, and people on typical American diets generally don't get enough of it. Fiber absorbs water to help bulk, soften and lubricate the stool. When taken with enough water it has a cleansing effect on the colon and acts as a mild laxative. It is a safe remedy for constipation in pregnant women, nursing mothers and the elderly.

Fiber helps reduce cholesterol by absorbing cholesterol released in the bile and inhibiting its reabsorption. This means it also helps to prevent gallstones.

Fiber slows the release of sugars into the body so it can help control blood sugar problems. It also provides a feeling of fullness, making it useful in weight loss.

Fiber binds toxins in the intestinal tract and soothes intestinal irritation. This makes it useful for diarrhea as well as constipation.

Softer fibers like slippery elm and flax can be very helpful for healing inflammatory bowel disorders. Fiber also reduces the risk of diverticulitis and colon cancer and can promote the health of friendly bacteria in the gut, which enhances your immune system. *Fiber Blend Formulas* are essential to colon cleansing programs, which generally combine fiber with *General Detoxifying Formulas*.

Key Herbs: Flax Seed, Psyllium and Slippery Elm

Renew Life
Bowel Cleanse (Capsule)

Oat bran, **Flax seed**, Acacia fiber, Ginger, Fennel, Papaya leaf, Capsicum (Cayenne), Coriander seed, Cumin, Gentian, Black Pepper seed, Peppermint leaf, Spearmint, Marshmallow, **Slippery Elm**, Okra

Solaray
Cholesterol Blend™ SP-31™ (Capsule)

Apple pectin, Hawthorn berry, **Psyllium seed**, Devil's Claw, Juniper berry, Ginger

Zand
Cleansing Fiber (Capsule)

Psyllium seed & hulls, Rice bran, Apple pectin, Licorice, **Slippery Elm**, Pau d'Arco, Peppermint leaf

Yerba Prima
Colon Care Caps (Capsule)

Psyllium seed & hulls, Soybean, Acacia, Oat bran, Apple pectin; Non-Herbal: calcium carbonate, Fos probiotic growth complex, magnesium

Yerba Prima
Colon Care Formula (Bulk Powder)

Psyllium seed, Soybean, Oat bran, Acacia, Apple pectin; Non-Herbal: calcium carbonate, FOS probiotic growth complex, magnesium

Western Botanicals
Colon Detox Formula (Capsule and Bulk Powder)

Psyllium seed & hulls, **Flax seed**, Apple pectin, **Slippery Elm**, Marshmallow, Fennel, Willow charcoal; Non-Herbal: Bentonite Clay

Yerba Prima
Daily Fiber® Caps (Capsule)

Psyllium hulls, Acacia gum, Soybean fiber, Oat bran, Apple pectin

Yerba Prima
Daily Fiber® Formula (Bulk Powder)

Psyllium seed, Soybean, Oat bran, Acacia, Apple pectin

Solaray
Detox Blend™ SP-25™ (Capsule)

Apple pectin, **Psyllium seed**, Irish Moss, Alfalfa leaf, Kelp, Myrrh; Non-Herbal: Algin

Yerba Prima
Fiber Plus® Powder (Bulk Powder)

Psyllium seed, Soybean, Oat bran, Acacia, Apple pectin, Ginger, Red Clover flowering tops, Dandelion root & leaf, Senna

Renew Life
Fiber Smart (Capsule and Bulk Powder)

Flax seed, Guar gum seed, Fennel, Marshmallow, **Slippery Elm**, Triphala; Non-Herbal: Glutamine, Fructooligosaccharide (FOS), L.acidophilus, B.bifidum, B.infantis

Renew Life
Fiber-Tastic™ (Bulk Powder)

Prune, Raspberry (Red), Strawberry, Cranberry, Pomegranate, Apple, Soybean, Saw Palmetto, Grape seed, Bilberry, Barley, Green

Tea leaf, Wheat grass, Barley stem & leaf, Broccoli sprouts, Carrot, Spinach, Chlorella, Spirulina

Renew Life
Organic Triple Fiber (Capsule and Bulk Powder)

Flax seed, Oat bran, Acacia

Christopher's
Quick Colon Powder #2 (Bulk Powder)

Apple pectin, **Flax seed**, **Psyllium**, **Slippery Elm**, Marshmallow, Fennel leaf, Plantain

Gaia Herbs
Rejuve Gentle Daily Fiber (Bulk Powder)

Psyllium hulls, Triphala, Chia seed, Marshmallow, Licorice, Ginger, Cinnamon bark

Yerba Prima
Soluble Fiber Caps (Capsule)

Psyllium hulls, Acacia gum, Oat bran, Apple fiber & pectin

Yerba Prima
Soluble Fiber Formula (Bulk Powder)

Psyllium hulls, Acacia gum, Oat bran, Apple fiber & pectin

Nature's Way
Thisilyn® Daily Cleanse (Capsule)

Psyllium hulls, Oat bran, **Flax seed**, Grapefruit pectin, Milk Thistle seed, Artichoke leaf, Turmeric, Dandelion root, Guar gum; Non-Herbal: Fructooligosaccharides (FOS)

Planetary Herbals
Tri-Cleanse™ Complete Internal Cleanser (Bulk Powder)

Psyllium hulls, Triphala, **Flax seed**, Anise fruit, Guar gum, Wild Yam, Stevia, Ginger; Non-Herbal: Natural Licorice flavor

Irwin Naturals
Ultimate Fiber Cleanse™ (Bulk Powder)

Psyllium hulls, Marshmallow root, **Slippery Elm**; Non-Herbal: Lactobacillus acidophilus, Fructooligosaccharides (FOS)

General Detoxifying Formulas

See also *Blood Purifier* and *Stimulant Laxative Formulas*

The formulas classified as general detoxifiers are essentially blood purifier blends that also contain stimulant laxatives. These blends may also contain diuretics, fiber and lymphatic draining herbs. In short, these formulas are used as part of a general cleansing program for the whole body.

Key Herbs: Barberry, Buckthorn, Burdock, Cascara Sagrada, Dandelion, Pau d' Arco, Senna Leaves, Turkey Rhubarb and Yellow Dock

Irwin Naturals
15-Day Weight Loss Cleanse & Flush (Tablet)

Psyllium seed, Uva Ursi leaf, **Cascara Sagrada**, Fennel seed, Marshmallow root, Capsicum (Cayenne), Black Pepper, Juniper berry, Plum, Beet root, Grapefruit, Oat bran, Chickweed aerial parts, Chlorella, **Dandelion root**, Echinacea (angustifolia), Ginger,

Chamomile flower, Fenugreek seed; Non-Herbal: Calcium Carbonate, Fructooligosaccharides (FOS)

Grandma's Herbs
Blood Cleanser Phase I (Capsule)

Echinacea, Red Clover, Plantain, Chaparral (Creosote), Sage, Blue Flag, **Pau d'Arco**, **Dandelion**, **Burdock**, Sheep Sorrel, **Cascara Sagrada**, Black Walnut, Clove, Violet, **Yellow Dock**, Aloe vera, Celandine, Calendula (Marigold), Poke Root (Phytolacca), **Buckthorn**, Oregon Grape, Sassafras, Sarsaparilla

Grandma's Herbs
Blood Cleanser Phase II (Capsule)

Red Clover, Chaparral (Creosote), Licorice, Stillingia (Queen's Root), Prickly Ash, **Burdock root**, Poke Root (Phytolacca), Oregon Grape, **Buckthorn**

Grandma's Herbs
Blood Cleanser Phase III (Capsule)

Burdock, **Cascara Sagrada**, Red Clover root, Plantain, Chaparral (Creosote), Raspberry (Red), **Buckthorn**, Marshmallow, Calendula (Marigold), Aloe vera, Licorice

Grandma's Herbs
Blood Cleanser Phase IV (Capsule)

Burdock, **Pau d'Arco**, Cleavers (Bedstraw), Licorice, Slippery Elm, Black Walnut, **Buckthorn**, Calendula (Marigold), Canaigre, Aloe vera

Solaray
Cellular Blend™ SP-29™ (Capsule)

Red Clover flower, Licorice, **Pau d'Arco**, Bayberry root, Stillingia (Queen's Root), Sarsaparilla, Prickly Ash, **Cascara Sagrada**, **Burdock bark**, Kelp

Renew Life
CleanseSMART™ (Capsule)

Artichoke leaf, Ashwagandha root, Beet, Bupleurum, **Burdock root**, Celandine leaf, Corn Silk, **Dandelion root**, Hawthorn berry, Larch (Larix) gum, Milk Thistle seed, Mullein leaf, Red Clover leaf & stem, Turmeric, Aloe vera vera gel, **Turkey Rhubarb**, Slippery Elm, Marshmallow, Fennel, Ginger, Triphala, Chlorella

Renew Life
Daily Multi-Detox (Capsule)

Spirulina, Garlic, Green Tea leaf, Milk Thistle seed, Oat straw, Parsley leaf, Artichoke leaf, **Dandelion leaf**, Fenugreek, Marshmallow, Mullein leaf, Nettle (Stinging) leaf, Oregano leaf, Triphala, Turmeric, Red Clover, Slippery Elm, Ginger, Fennel, Papaya leaf, Capsicum (Cayenne), Coriander seed, Cumin, Gentian, Black Pepper seed, Peppermint leaf, Spearmint

Grandma's Herbs
Defense System (Capsule)

Agaricus, Echinacea (angustifolia), Black (seed), Astragalus, Sheep Sorrel, Red Clover tops, Plantain, **Pau d'Arco**, **Cascara Sagrada**, **Turkey Rhubarb**, Chaparral (Creosote), Wormwood, Blue Flag, White Oak bark, **Dandelion**, **Burdock root**

Renew Life
First Cleanse™ (Capsule)

Spearmint leaf, Parsley leaf, Artichoke leaf, Blessed Thistle, **Burdock root**, **Dandelion leaf & root**, Echinacea (angustifolia), Fenugreek, Garlic, Hawthorn berry, Horsetail, Kelp, Milk Thistle seed, Mullein leaf, Nettle (Stinging) leaf, Oat straw, Oregano leaf, Red Clover, Turmeric, Wormwood, Yarrow, **Yellow Dock**, Ginger, Fennel, Papaya leaf, Capsicum (Cayenne), Coriander seed, Cumin, Gentian, Black Pepper, Peppermint leaf, Spearmint, Flax seed, **Buckthorn bark**, **Turkey Rhubarb**, Marshmallow, Triphala, Slippery Elm, Ginger, Fennel, Capsicum (Cayenne), Cumin, Gentian, Black Pepper

Renew Life
Flush & Be Fit (Capsule)

Milk Thistle, Chlorella, **Burdock root**, **Dandelion**, Red Root bark, Horsetail, Red Clover, Turmeric, Indigo, Cranberry, Hibiscus, Yerba Mate, Ginseng (Korean, Asian), Ashwagandha, Green Tea, Rhodiola, Gotu Kola, Capsicum (Cayenne), Bitter Orange, Banaba, Horsetail, Aloe (cape) leaf, **Turkey Rhubarb**, **Buckthorn**, Marshmallow, Ginger, Fennel; Non-Herbal: Quercetin, Protease, Amylase, Lipase, S. boulardii, L. rhamnosus, L. reuteri

Yerba Prima
Kalenite® Cleansing Herbs (Tablet)

Acacia, Plantain, Blessed Thistle, Clove, Corn Silk, **Yellow Dock**, Red Clover flowering tops, **Buckthorn bark**

Yerba Prima
Men's Rebuild Internal Cleansing System (Capsule)

Psyllium hulls, Aloe vera, Ginger, Triphala, **Dandelion root and leaf**, **Yellow Dock**, Elecampane, **Senna**, Schisandra, Ginseng (Korean, Asian), Milk Thistle, Clove, Sarsaparilla, Cat's Claw, Black Walnut, Soybean fiber, Oat bran, Acacia gum, Blessed Thistle, Apple fiber, Plantain, Goldenseal, Saw Palmetto, Red Clover, Corn Silk; Non-Herbal: Bentonite, FOS, zinc

Irwin Naturals
Multi-Fiber Cleanse (Tablet)

Cascara Sagrada, Fennel seed, Psyllium hulls, Ginger, Acacia gum, Alfalfa, Apple pectin, Apple, Barley grass, Beet root, Karaya gum, Lemon peel, Oat bran, Peppermint, Raspberry (Red) leaf, Slippery Elm, Guar gum; Non-Herbal: Calcium Carbonate, Glucomannan, Lactobacillus acidophilus

Renew Life
Organic Total Body Cleanse™ (Capsule)

Burdock root, **Dandelion root**, Garlic, Milk Thistle seed, **Dandelion leaf**, Blessed Thistle leaf, Echinacea (angustifolia), Fennel, Kelp, Mullein leaf, Nettle (Stinging) leaf, Oat straw, Oregano leaf, Parsley leaf, Turmeric, **Yellow Dock**, Oat bran, Flax seed, **Turkey Rhubarb**, Fennel, Marshmallow, Slippery Elm, Acacia gum

Renew Life
Power Cleanse™ (Capsule)

Garlic, **Dandelion root**, Artichoke root & leaf, Turmeric, Milk Thistle seed, Aloe vera, **Turkey Rhubarb**, Slippery Elm, Marshmallow, Fennel, Ginger, Triphala; Non-Herbal: Vitamin A, Vitamin C, Vitamin E, Riboflavin, Niacin, Vitamin B6, Folic acid, Vitamin B12, Zinc, Selenium, Choline, L-Methionine, L-Taurine, NAC (N-Acetyl-Cysteine), Copper, Manganese, Magnesium

Irwin Naturals
Super Cleanse (Tablet)

Cascara Sagrada, Fennel seed, Licorice, Ginger, Irish Moss, Slippery Elm, **Barberry**, Capsicum (Cayenne), Chlorella, Marsh-

mallow root, Raspberry (Red) leaf, Triphala; Non-Herbal: Calcium Carbonate, Lactobacillus acidophilus (dairy-free)

Gaia Herbs
Supreme Cleanse (Capsule)

Alder, Radish (Black), **Burdock root**, Celandine, Chia, Corydalis, **Dandelion leaf & root**, Fenugreek, Figwort, Gentian, Ginger, Ginger, Licorice, Marshmallow, Mayapple, Milk Thistle, Psyllium, Red Root, Rooibos (Redbush), Triphala, Turmeric, **Yellow Dock**

Renew Life
Total Body Cleanse (Capsule)

Burdock root, **Dandelion root**, Garlic, Milk Thistle leaf, **Dandelion leaf**, Blessed Thistle leaf, Echinacea (angustifolia), Fenugreek, Kelp, Mullein leaf, Nettle (Stinging) leaf, Oat straw, Oregano leaf, Parsley leaf, Turmeric, **Yellow Dock**

Renew Life
Total Body Rapid Cleanse™ (Capsule and Bulk Powder)

Milk Thistle seed, **Burdock root**, **Dandelion leaf & root**, Fenugreek, Garlic, Mullein leaf, Oat straw, Oregano leaf, Nettle (Stinging) leaf, Turmeric, Aloe vera leaf, Bamboo leaf, **Turkey Rhubarb**, Marshmallow, Acacia, Slippery Elm, Triphala; Non-Herbal: Chlorophyll, Betaine Hydrochloride, L-Glycine, L-Glutamine, L-Methionine, N-Acetyl-Cysteine

Yerba Prima
Women's Renew® Internal Cleansing System (Capsule)

Psyllium hulls, Aloe vera, Ginger, Triphala, **Dandelion root and leaf**, **Yellow Dock**, Elecampane, **Senna**, Schisandra, Chaste Tree (Vitex), Milk Thistle seed, Clove, Dong Quai, Cat's Claw, Black Walnut, Soybean fiber, Oat bran, Acacia gum, Blessed Thistle, Apple fiber, Goldenseal, Red Clover, Plantain, Corn Silk; Non-Herbal: Bentonite, FOS, zinc, niacinamide, pantothenic acid, vitamin B-6, folic acid, biotin, vitamin B-12

Gentle Laxative Formulas

See also *Intestinal Toning* and *Stimulant Laxative Formulas*

Most laxative formulas rely on stimulant laxatives that contain anthraquinones, such as aloe, senna and cascara sagrada. These *Stimulant Laxative Formulas* are useful for occasional constipation or for a periodic bowel cleanse, but they are not the best choices for long term use as they tend to have a depleting effect on the bowel when used over long periods of time. They also stain the bowel tissue.

Gentle laxative formulas work primarily by toning and strengthening the bowel, rather than by directly stimulating peristalsis. The chief component of these products is triphala, a blend of three fruits used in Ayurvedic medicine as a gentle laxative, bowel tonic and blood purifier.

These three fruits are haritaki, bibhitaki and amalaki or Indian gooseberry. In various formulas these three fruits may also be referred to as belleric myrobalan fruit, chebulic myrobalan fruit and Indian gooseberry fruit, or as harada fruit, amla fruit and behada fruit.

Besides triphala these formulas may contain prunes. A non-herbal ingredient that contributes to the effectiveness of gentle laxative formulas is magnesium hydroxide.

Gentle Laxative Formulas can have some of the same properties as *Intestinal Toning Formulas*.

Key Herbs: Licorice, Triphala and Yellow Dock

Renew Life
Buddy Bear Gentle Lax™ (Tablet)

Prune, Fig, Turkey Rhubarb, Carob, Cocoa (Cacao), Lo han guo; Non-Herbal: Cane Juice Extract, Magnesium Hydroxide

Vitanica
Colon Motility Blend™ (Capsule)

Gentian, **Triphala**, Dandelion root; Non-Herbal: Magnesium, Protease, Amylase, Lipase, Cellulase, Invertase, Lactase, Bromelain

Irwin Naturals
Daily Gentle Cleanse (Softgel)

Triphala, Milk Thistle seed, Artichoke leaf, Dandelion leaf, Marshmallow root, Ginger, Black Pepper; Non-Herbal: Fish Oil

Yerba Prima
Herbal Guard® (Capsule)

Triphala, Elecampane root, Ginger, Schisandra, Clove, Dandelion leaf & root, Cat's Claw root, Black Walnut hulls, Goldenseal

Grandma's Herbs
Kid-e-Reg (Liquid)

Slippery Elm, **Licorice**, Fennel, Anise seed, Fig

Christopher's
Kid-e-Reg (Glycerine Extract)

Slippery Elm, **Licorice**, Anise, Fennel, Fig

Renew Life
KidLAX™ (Capsule)

Flax seed, Prune, Fig, Turkey Rhubarb, Peach leaf; Non-Herbal: Lactobacillus acidophilus, Bifidobacterium bifidum, Bifidobacterium infantis

Planetary Herbals
Legendary Intestinal Cleanser and Tonifier (Capsule and Tablet)

Chebulic Myrobalan fruit, Amla (Indian Gooseberry), **Belleric Myrobalan fruit**

Irwin Naturals
Soothing Coconut & Aloe Natural Laxative (Tablet)

Triphala, Aloe vera leaf, Coconut, Fennel seed, Ginger, Marshmallow root, Peppermint leaf, Coffee fruit; Non-Herbal: Fructooligosaccharides, Inulin, L-Glutamine, Bromelain, Papain

Planetary Herbals
Triphala (Capsule, Tablet and Powder)

Chebulic Myrobalan fruit, Amla (Indian Gooseberry), **Belleric Myrobalan fruit**

Gaia Herbs
Triphala Fruit (Capsule)

Amla (Indian Gooseberry), **Haritaki**, **Bibhitaki (Behada)**

Goldenseal & Echinacea Formulas

See also *Antibacterial, Antiviral* and *Cold* and *Flu Formulas*

The blend of goldenseal and echinacea is one of the most popular pairs in modern herbalism. Numerous companies offer this blend or variations of it. It is frequently used for colds, but many of the formulas listed under *Cold and Flu Formulas* are actually more effective for the early stages of a cold. *Goldenseal & Echinacea Formulas* are only useful for the later stages of colds where the mucus becomes thick and discolored.

The combination of goldenseal and echinacea is also a good remedy for bacterial infections in the sinuses, throat, bronchial passages, lungs and urinary passages. It can be helpful for chronic sinusitis, bronchitis, ear infections, sore throats, cystitis and urethritis. Check out *Antibacterial Formulas* for additional options, as most antibacterial formulas will contain both of these herbs plus additional antibacterial remedies.

The combination of these two herbs may be helpful for viral infections, but many of the blends listed under *Antiviral Formulas* may be much better for viral infections.

Key Herbs: Echinacea and Goldenseal

Eclectic Institute
Ech-Goldenseal (Glycerine Extract)

Echinacea (angustifolia) root, **Goldenseal**; Non-Herbal: Kosher vegetable glycerin, Ascorbic acid. This product is offered in orange and strawberry flavors.

Eclectic Institute
Ech-Goldenseal Spray

Echinacea (angustifolia) root, **Goldenseal**, Isatis (Woad) root, Cherry (Wild) bark, Slippery Elm, Orange essential oil

Nature's Answer
Echinacea & Goldenseal (Glycerine Extract)

Echinacea (angustifolia) root, **Echinacea (purpurea)**, **Goldenseal**

NOW Foods
Echinacea & Goldenseal Glycerite (Glycerine Extract)

Echinacea (purpurea) root, **Goldenseal**, St. John's Wort root, Boneset

NOW Foods
Echinacea & Goldenseal Plus (Glycerine Extract)

Echinacea (purpurea) root, **Goldenseal**, Red Clover aerial parts & flower, Burdock root, Peppermint leaf, Bayberry fruit, Capsicum (Cayenne)

Nature's Answer
Echinacea & Goldenseal Root (Capsule)

Echinacea (purpurea), **Echinacea (angustifolia) root**, **Goldenseal**

Gaia Herbs
Echinacea Goldenseal (Liquid Phyto-Caps)

Echinacea (purpurea) root, aerial parts, seed, Echinacea (angustifolia) root, Barberry root, **Goldenseal root**, Oregon Grape root, St. John's Wort flower bud and tops

Gaia Herbs
Echinacea Goldenseal Supreme (Alcohol Extract)

Echinacea (purpurea) root, Echinacea (angustifolia) root, Oregon Grape, St. John's Wort flowering tops, Barberry root bark, **Goldenseal, Echinacea (purpurea) seed & aerial parts**, Propolis

Solaray
Echinacea Root with Goldenseal Root (Capsule)

Echinacea (purpurea) root, Echinacea (angustifolia) root, Goldenseal

Eclectic Institute
Echinacea-Goldenseal (Alcohol and Glycerine Extract)

Echinacea (angustifolia) root, Goldenseal

Eclectic Institute
Echinacea-Goldenseal (Capsule)

Goldenseal, Echinacea (purpurea) root and tops

Eclectic Institute
Echinacea-Goldenseal (Capsule)

Echinacea (angustifolia) root, Echinacea (purpurea) flower, leaf and root, Echinacea (pallida) root, Echinacea (tennesseensis) root, Goldenseal

Planetary Herbals
Echinacea-Goldenseal Liquid Extract (Alcohol Extract)

Echinacea (purpurea) root, Goldenseal, Echinacea (purpurea) seed

Eclectic Institute
Echinacea-Goldenseal O (Alcohol Extract)

Echinacea (angustifolia) root, Goldenseal, Echinacea (purpurea) root, Echinacea (purpurea)

Planetary Herbals
Echinacea-Goldenseal with Olive Leaf (Tablet)

Echinacea (pallida) root, Goldenseal, Olive leaf, Garlic, Andrographis aerial parts, Isatis (Woad) root, Dandelion root, Licorice, Ginger

Nature's Way
Echinacea–Goldenseal (Glycerine Extract)

Goldenseal, Echinacea (purpurea) stem, leaf & flower, Echinacea (angustifolia) root, Burdock root, Gentian, Wood Betony (betonica) stem, leaf & flower, Capsicum (Cayenne)

Western Botanicals
Echinacea/Goldenseal (Capsule and Alcohol Extract)

Echinacea (angustifolia) root, Goldenseal

Herbalist & Alchemist
Echinacea/Goldenseal Compound (Alcohol Extract and Glycerine Extract)

Echinacea (purpurea) root, Goldenseal

Gaia Herbs
GaiaKids® Echinacea Goldenseal (Glycerine Extract)

Goldenseal root, Echinacea root, aerial parts, seed

Solaray
Thymus Plus Caps™ (Capsule)

Echinacea root, Goldenseal, Clove

Heavy Metal Cleansing Formulas

See also *Fiber Blend*, *Hepatoprotective* and *Liver Tonic Formulas*

Heavy metals like mercury, lead, arsenic and cadmium are common in modern society. These toxic metals can weaken the immune system and cause neurological damage. Heavy metals like mercury deplete glutathione, an intracellular antioxidant.

Cilantro is a key herb in formulas used to help the body detoxify heavy metals. Also look for these non-herbal ingredients as key aids for heavy metal detoxification: N-acytl-cysteine and alpha lipoic acid. Taking *Liver Tonic* or *Hepatoprotective Formulas* with *Fiber Blend Formulas* can also help detoxify the body of heavy metals.

See *Heavy Metal Poisoning*, *Lead Poisoning* and *Mercury Poisoning* in the *Conditions Section*.

Key Herbs: Cilantro/Coriander, Lobelia and Milk Thistle

Christopher's
Heavy Mineral Bugleweed Formula (Capsule)

Bugleweed, Yellow Dock, **Lobelia root**

New Chapter
Liver Take Care™ (Capsule)

Milk Thistle seed, Wasabi, Schisandra, Turmeric, **Cilantro leaf**, Artichoke leaf, Chokeberry fruit

Renew Life
MERC-Free Cleanse™ (Capsule)

Milk Thistle seed, Turmeric, **Cilantro leaf**, Parsley leaf, Chlorella; Non-Herbal: Vitamin C, Vitamin B-6, Zinc, Selenium, Copper, Molybdenum, N-Acetyl-Cysteine, Glycine, L-Glutamine,L-Methionine, L-Taurine, Alpha Lipoic Acid, Methylsulfonylmethane (MSM), L-Glutathione, Sodium, Potassium, Citrus Pectin, Sodium Alginate, Sodium Bicarbonate, Potassium Citrate, Potassium Bicarbonate

Herbal Formulas

Hepatoprotective Formulas

See also *Liver Tonic Formulas*

Modern medical research has shown that both milk thistle and schisandra have a powerful ability to protect the liver against environmental toxins. *Hepatoprotective Formulas* are *Liver Tonic Formulas* that contain one or both of these herbs as key ingredients.

Anyone who works around chemicals on a regular basis, such as beauticians, painters, auto mechanics, dry cleaners and carpet cleaners should consider taking a *Hepatoprotective Formula* on a regular basis to protect their liver against the toxins they are regularly exposed to. They should also consider using *Liver Tonic Formulas* regularly.

Key Herbs: Dandelion, Lycium (Wolfberry, Gogi), Milk Thistle and Schisandra (Schizandra)

Zand
Cleanse Today (Capsule)

Milk Thistle seed, Rosemary, Ginger, **Dandelion root**, Sage, Oat bran, Flax seed, Broccoli, Kale, Nettle (Stinging) leaf, Cabbage, Maitake Mushroom; Non-Herbal: Plant-based Enzymes (Amylase (2400DU), Cellulase (100CU), Invertase (140 SUMNER), Lactase (100 ALU), Lipase (40 FIP), and Malt Diastase (50 DP) 30 mg, Vegetable Cellulose Fiber, Alpha Lipoic Acid, L-Glutathione, Rice flour

Irwin Naturals
Daily Gentle Cleanse (Softgel)

Triphala, **Milk Thistle seed**, Artichoke leaf, **Dandelion leaf**, Marshmallow root, Ginger, Black Pepper; Non-Herbal: Fish Oil

Traditional Medicinals
EveryDay Detox® (Tea)

Chicory root, **Dandelion root**, **Schisandra**, **Schisandra**, **Lycium (Wolfberry/Gogi)**, Licorice, Ginger, Star Anise fruit, Green Tea twig

Yerba Prima
Liv-Cleanse Formula (Tablet)

Milk Thistle seed, **Dandelion root & leaf**, Yellow Dock

Solaray
Liver Caps™ (Capsule)

Milk Thistle seed, Burdock root, **Dandelion root**

A. Vogel
Liver Gallbladder Tablets

Milk Thistle seed, Artichoke, **Dandelion root**, Boldo leaf, Peppermint

Gaia Herbs
Liver Health (Liquid Phyto-Caps)

Turmeric root, **Schisandra berry**, Chinese Scullcap (Scute/Huang Qin) root, Licorice root; Non-Herbal: MSM

New Chapter
Liver Take Care™ (Capsule)

Milk Thistle seed, Wasabi, **Schisandra**, Turmeric, Cilantro leaf, Artichoke leaf, Chokeberry fruit

Western Botanicals
Liver/Gallbladder Formula/Tea Combo (Liquid)

Milk Thistle seed, Fennel, Fringetree, Oregon Grape, Black Walnut hulls, **Dandelion root**, Garlic, Gentian, Ginger, Wormwood leaf

Yerba Prima
Milk Thistle Extra Strength (Capsule)

Milk Thistle seed, Black Pepper seed

Irwin Naturals
Milk Thistle Liver Cleanse® (Tablet)

Alfalfa leaf, Beet, Licorice, Capsicum (Cayenne), Black Pepper, Beet leaf, Artichoke leaf, **Dandelion root**, **Milk Thistle seed**, Turmeric, Barberry, Boldo leaf, Celandine, Fringetree root, Stone Breaker (Quebra Pedra) aerial parts, Kutki (Picorhiza kurroa) root, **Schisandra**; Non-Herbal: Soy Lecithin

Eclectic Institute
Milk Thistle-Dandelion (Alcohol Extract and Glycerine Extract)

Milk Thistle seed, **Dandelion whole plant**, Red Root, Oregon Grape; Non-Herbal: Tangerine flavor in glycerine version

Herbalist & Alchemist
Thistles Compound™ (Alcohol Extract)

Blessed Thistle, **Dandelion root**, **Milk Thistle seed**, Turmeric, Watercress, Oregon Grape

Hyperthyroid Formulas

Sometimes the thyroid gland can become overactive. This condition is known as Grave's disease and can result in excessive nervous energy, rapid heartbeat, anxiety, insomnia and weight loss. The thyroid can also be overactive in Hashimoto's Disease, which is an autoimmune condition of the thyroid.

Hyperthyroid Formulas contain herbs that calm down thyroid activity. Both bugleweed and lemon balm contain compounds which attach to receptor sites for thyroid and inhibit signals from the pituitary that stimulate the thyroid. Motherwort is added to these formulas both to calm the thyroid and to slow rapid heart beat.

Hyperthyroid is a serious condition and should be treated under appropriate medical supervision. However, these herbal formulas may be helpful in management of symptoms. (See *Grave's Disease* and *Hashimoto's Disease* in the *Conditions Section* for more information.)

Key Herbs: Bugleweed, He Shou Wu (Ho Shou Wu, Fo-Ti) and Lemon Balm

Herb Pharm
Thyroid Calming™ (Alcohol Extract)

Bugleweed, Motherwort flowering tops, Night Blooming Cereus (Cactus) stem, **Lemon Balm leaf**

Herbalist & Alchemist
Thyroid Calmpound™ (Alcohol Extract)

Bugleweed, **Lemon Balm flowering tops**, Motherwort flowering tops

Hypoglycemic Formulas

Hypoglycemia is a condition characterized by extremely low blood sugar levels. It is a common side effect in diabetics, although it may also occur with metabolic syndrome or as a reaction to fasting. Normally, when a person's blood sugar levels begin to drop, your pancreas secretes glucagon to release sugar stores in the liver and normalize blood sugar levels. The adrenal glands can also release cortisol to convert proteins to sugars to restore normal blood sugar levels. Signs and symptoms of low blood sugar include vision problems, fatigue, malaise, increased heart rate, convulsions, cold sweats, headache, hunger, sugar cravings, irritability, confusion and trembling.

Hypoglycemic Formulas are used to aid the function of both the liver and the pancreas, thereby helping to keep blood sugar levels in the body stable. They can be used to reduce moodiness, stabilize energy levels, control hunger and sugar cravings and keep blood sugar levels more stable when fasting.

Key Herbs: Licorice

RidgeCrest Herbals
Blood Sugar Balance (Capsule)

Rice, Anemarrhena (Zhi-Mu) root, Eleuthero root, **Licorice (Chinese) root**; Non-Herbal: Calcium (from sulfate)

Yogi Tea
Healthy Fasting™ (Tea)

Fennel, **Licorice**, Barley malt, Cinnamon bark, Red Clover, Alfalfa leaf, Hawthorn berry, Garcinia (Brindleberry), Cardamom seed, Ginger, Clove, Burdock root, Dandelion root, Yellow Dock, Black Pepper; Non-Herbal: Essential oils

Nature's Sunshine Products
HY-A (Capsule)

Licorice, Safflower, Dandelion root, Horseradish

Hypotensive Formulas

See also *Adaptogen, Cardiac Tonic, Cardiovascular Stimulant* and *Relaxing Nervine Formulas*

These are remedies that help to reduce high blood pressure. These blends have many of the same properties as *Cardiac Tonic* and *Cardiovascular Stimulant Formulas* and contain many of the same herbs. There are a few key herbs that make these formulas more targeted towards normalizing blood pressure. High blood pressure has a variety of causes, so herbal formulas addressing it use a variety of herbs with different actions to help reduce it.

Arteries contain muscles that expand and contract to regulate blood flow. Tension in the arteries will constrict them, forcing the heart to raise pressure in order to move blood through the circulatory system. These formulas help to relax these blood vessels and reduce blood pressure. They may also help to reduce stress and tension.

Besides the key herbs listed below, nervines and adaptogens are also common ingredients in these blends. To work on the underlying causes of high blood pressure, also consider *Adaptogenic, Cardiac Tonic, Cardiovascular Stimulant* and *Relaxing Nervine Formulas*. See *Blood Pressure (high)* in the *Conditions Section* for more information.

Key Herbs: Garlic, Hawthorn, Linden, Mistletoe, Motherwort and Olive

Grandma's Herbs
Blood Pressure (Capsule)

Capsicum (Cayenne), **Garlic**, Black Cohosh, **Mistletoe**, Sassafras, Ginkgo, Valerian, Wild Yam, Nettle (Stinging), Horsetail, Bladderwrack, Hyssop, Ginseng (American), Bladder Pod, Dong Quai, Bayberry

RidgeCrest Herbals
Blood Pressure Formula (Capsule)

Gastrodia rhizome, Gambier vine, St. Paul's Wort (Xi Xian Cao) whole plant, Gardenia fruit, Scullcap (Skullcap) root, **Motherwort grass**, Achyranthes root, Eucommia (ulmoides) bark, **Mistletoe stem**, Japanese Knotweed (Hu Zhang) whole plant, Hoelen (Fu Ling, Tuckahoe, China Root), Alisma (Water Plantain) stem, Arnica; Non-Herbal: Abalone shell, Glonoinum (Nitroglycerine), Baryta carbonica

NOW Foods
Blood Pressure Health (Capsule)

Grape seed, **Hawthorn leaf & flower**

Herb Pharm
Blood Pressure Support (Alcohol Extract)

Hawthorn leaf, **Olive leaf**, **Linden (Basswood, Tilia) flower**, Bean pod, **Mistletoe**

New Chapter
Blood Pressure Take Care™ (Capsule)

Grape seed, **Hawthorn flower & leaf**, **Motherwort aerial parts**, Grape; Non-Herbal: L. bulgaricus, S. thermophilus, B. infantis

Western Botanicals
Cardio + (Alcohol Extract)

Gynostemma (Jiao Gu Lan), Chrysanthemum, **Olive leaf**, Maitake Mushroom, **Mistletoe**, Ginkgo, Passionflower

Herbalist & Alchemist
Cardio Calmpound™ (Alcohol Extract)

Hawthorn berry, Hawthorn leaf, Hawthorn flower, Linden (Basswood, Tilia) flower, Motherwort flowering tops, Olive leaf, Mistletoe

Nature's Answer
CardioNutriv (Glycerine Extract)

Hawthorn berry, **Linden (Basswood, Tilia) flower**, Capsicum (Cayenne)

Herbs Etc.
HB Pressure™ Tonic (Alcohol Extract or Softgel)

Linden (Basswood, Tilia) flower, **Mistletoe leaf and twig**, Dandelion leaf, Passionflower, **Hawthorn flower, leaf & berry**, Eleuthero root, Yarrow flowering tops, Scullcap (Skullcap), Prickly Ash bark

Western Botanicals
Vascular Support (Alcohol Extract)

Motherwort, Passionflower, Valerian, Dandelion root, **Hawthorn berry, leaf & flower**, Barberry root bark, Ginger, Nettle (Stinging) leaf, White Oak bark, Ginkgo, Lavender flower, Capsicum (chinense), Custard Apple (Ylang-Ylang) essential oil

Hypothyroid Formulas

Hypothyroid (low thyroid) is very common, especially in women. Herbal formulas that aid hypothyroid typically contain various seaweeds or sea vegetables, such as kelp, Irish moss or bladderwrack, as key ingredients. These plants serve as sources of iodine, an essential trace element needed to produce thyroid hormones. Even though iodine is needed in very small amounts, it is a hard element to obtain from the diet unless you eat a lot of foods from the sea. The iodine shortage is compounded by the fact that other halogens such as chlorine, bromine and flourides drive iodine from the body. So does the heavy metal, mercury.

Besides supplying natural iodine, many hypothyroid formulas contain herbs that help normalize thyroid function when taken regularly over long periods of time. See *Hypothyroid* and *Hasthimoto's Disease (thyroiditis)* in the *Conditions Section* for more information.

Key Herbs: Ashwaganda, Bladderwrack, Dulse, Irish moss and Kelp

Christopher's
Herbal Thyroid Formula (Capsule)

Guarana, Eleuthero, He Shou Wu (Fo-Ti), Gotu Kola, Mullein, **Kelp**

Vitanica
ThyroFem™ (Capsule)

Kelp, **Ashwagandha root**, Rhodiola; Non-Herbal: Vitamin C, Vitamin E, Vitamin B12, Zinc, L Tyrosine, Copper, Selenium

Grandma's Herbs
Thyroid (Capsule)

Kelp, **Bladderwrack**, Eleuthero, Bugleweed, Cleavers (Bedstraw), Iceland Moss, Gentian, Black Walnut, Burdock root, Watercress, Yellow Dock, Bladder Pod, Sage

Solaray
Thyroid Blend™ SP-26 (Capsule)

Capsicum (Cayenne), **Kelp**, **Irish Moss**, Eleuthero root, Gentian, Fenugreek

Nature's Answer
Thyroid Complete (Liquid Capsule)

Ashwagandha root, Coleus root, Velvet Bean, Schisandra, **Kelp**, **Bladderwrack**

Western Botanicals
Thyroid Formula (Capsule and Alcohol Extract)

Irish Moss, Black Cohosh, **Dulse**, Bayberry bark, **Bladderwrack**, Nettle (Stinging) leaf, Mullein leaf & flower

Herb Pharm
Thyroid Lifter™ (Alcohol Extract)

Bladderwrack, Eleuthero root, Nettle (Stinging) seed, Black Pepper seed, Prickly Ash

Planetary Herbals
Thyroid Lift™ (Tablet)

Guggul, **Ashwagandha root**, Holy Basil leaf, Astragalus, He Shou Wu (Fo-Ti), Coleus root; Non-Herbal: Vitamin A, Vitamin C, Vitamin D3, Vitamin E, Riboflavin, Niacin, Vitamin B6, Folate, Vitamin B12, Calcium, Pantothenic Acid, Iodine, Zinc, Selenium, Copper, Manganese, Acetyl-L-Tyrosine, Antler velvet

Christopher's
Thyroid Maintenance Formula (Capsule)

Kelp, Watercress, Mullein leaf, Parsley, Nettle (Stinging) leaf, **Irish Moss**, Iceland Moss, Sheep Sorrel

Gaia Herbs
Thyroid Support (Liquid Phyto-Caps)

Coleus root, **Ashwagandha root**, Schisandra, **Kelp (Mermaid's Bladder)**, **Bladderwrack**; Non-Herbal: L-Tyrosine

RidgeCrest Herbals
Thyroid Thrive (Capsule)

Suma root, Myrrh gum, Guggul, **Ashwagandha root**, **Bladderwrack**, Burdock root, Coleus root, Blue Flag root, **Kelp**; Non-Herbal: Vitamin C, vitamin B6, folic acid, selenium, copper, manganese, tyrosine

Immune Balancing Formulas

See also *Adaptogen*, *Anti-Inflammatory* and *Mushroom Blend Formulas*

In autoimmune conditions you don't want to stimulate the immune response as this can aggravate symptoms. Instead, you want to try to modulate or balance the immune system. This can be somewhat tricky, as some herbs may aggravate autoimmune conditions in some people and not in others. Generally speaking, the formulas listed in this section should be helpful in modulating immune function in autoimmune disorders. If a formula does appear to aggravate symptoms, simply stop using it for a few days. If symptoms improve, it is possible the remedy didn't work for you. To test this, try taking it again for a couple of days.

If it aggravates symptoms the second time, don't use it. If symptoms don't improve when you discontinue the formula, then the aggravation was caused by something else, so the formula is probably safe to take. Consult a professional herbalist if you have concerns.

In people who don't have autoimmune conditions, these formulas should help to boost immune responses in a similar manner to *Immune Boosting Formulas*. These formulas should also be helpful in improving immune responses in the elderly or people who get sick easily.

Key herbs in these formulas are adaptogens (astragalus, eleuthero and schizandra) and medicinal mushrooms (cordyceps, maitake and ganoderma). Adaptogens are good immune balancers, because they modulate immune reactions by modulating stress responses in the adrenal glands. This means that persons suffering from autoimmune disorders may also want to consider using *Adaptogenic Formulas*. Since medicinal mushrooms also have immune-modulating qualities, you can also consider *Mushroom Blend Formulas* for more options.

Since chronic inflammation is a problem in autoimmune conditions you may also want to consider *Anti-Inflammatory Formulas*. See *Autoimmune Disorders* in the *Conditions Section*. You can also look up specific autoimmune disorders in the *Conditions Section*.

Key Herbs: Ashwaganda, Astragalus, Bupleurum, Cordyceps, Eleuthero (Siberian ginseng), Maitake, Reishi (Ganoderma) and Schisandra (Schizandra)

Zand
Astragalus Formula (Capsule)
Astragalus, Codonopsis root, **Reishi (Ganoderma)**, Licorice, Ligustrum fruit & rhizome, Peony (White, Chinese), **Schisandra**

NOW Foods
Astragalus Plus Extract (Glycerine Extract)
Astragalus root, Codonopsis root, Atractylodes (Bai-Zhu) rhizome, **Schisandra fruit**, **Reishi (Ganoderma)**, Licorice root, Ligustrum fruit, Rehmannia root

Gaia Herbs
Astragalus Supreme (Alcohol Extract)
Astragalus, **Schisandra**, Ligustrum berry

Gaia Herbs
Astragalus Supreme (Liquid Phyto-Caps)
Astragalus, Ligustrum, **Schisandra**

Gaia Herbs
Deep Liver Support (Liquid Phyto-Caps)
Astragalus, Chinese Scullcap (Scute/Huang Qin), **Bupleurum**, **Reishi (Ganoderma)**, Maitake Mushroom, Licorice

Christopher's
Immucalm (Capsule)
Marshmallow, **Astragalus**

Herbalist & Alchemist
Immune Adapt Caps™ (Capsule)
Astragalus, Eleuthero root, **Reishi (Ganoderma)**, Licorice, Ligustrum berry, **Maitake Mushroom**, **Schisandra**

Herbalist & Alchemist
Immune Adapt™ (Alcohol Extract)
Codonopsis root, Eleuthero root, **Reishi (Ganoderma)**, **Schisandra berry**, **Astragalus**, Atractylodes root, Licorice, Ligustrum berry

Herbalist & Alchemist
Immune Balance Compound™ (Alcohol Tincture)
Reishi (Ganoderma), Turmeric, **Ashwagandha**, Chinese Scullcap (Scute/Huang Qin), Licorice, Rehmannia

NOW Foods
Immune Renew™ (Capsule)
Turkey Tail Mushroom, Sun Mushroom, **Maitake Mushroom**, **Cordyceps**, Mesima Mushroom, Lion's Mane Mushroom, **Reishi (Ganoderma)**, Shiitake Mushroom, **Astragalus**

Urban Moonshine
Immune Tonic (Alcohol Extract)
Astragalus root, **Reishi (Ganoderma)**, Codonopsis root, **Maitake Mushroom**, Eleuthero root, Licorice root, **Schisandra berry**, Ginger root

Nature's Answer
Immunotonic (Glycerine Extract)
Astragalus, **Reishi (Ganoderma)**, Ligustrum berry, Codonopsis root, Ginseng (Korean, Asian), Prickly Ash

Solaray
ImmuTain™ SP-40 (Capsule)
Astragalus, Eleuthero root, Shiitake Mushroom, **Reishi (Ganoderma)**, St. John's Wort; Non-Herbal: Iron Phosphate 3X, Potassium Phosphate 3X

Grandma's Herbs
Kid-e-Soothe (Liquid)
Astragalus, Marshmallow

Planetary Herbals
Reishi Mushroom Supreme™ (Tablet)
Reishi (Ganoderma), Shiitake Mushroom, **Schisandra**, **Astragalus**, Atractylodes (Bai-Zhu) rhizome, Zhu-Ling, Eleuthero root, Ligustrum fruit, Poria Mushroom, **Reishi (Ganoderma)**, Polygala, Ginger, Cypress root; Non-Herbal: Calcium

Immune Stimulating Formulas
See also *Adaptogen, Echinacea Blend* and *Mushroom Blend Formulas*

You can think of *Immune Stimulating Formulas* as non-specific, natural vaccines, because they boost your immune system's ability to resist infection. However, this analogy isn't completely accurate. A vaccine challenges your immune system to mount a response against whatever microbe or microbes it contains. If your immune system is strong enough, it will build up antibodies against the disease. If it isn't strong enough, it can "backfire" and make you sick.

Immune Stimulating Formulas create a non-specific immune reaction. Many of the key herbs in these blends contain complex polysaccharides (sugar chains) that trick the body into thinking infectious organisms are present. As a result, the body increases production of white blood cells. So, a better analogy might be to say that Immune Stimulating Formulas put your immune system on "red alert."

These formulas can be taken if you know you are going to be around sick people and want to avoid catching something. They can also be used to boost immune responses in people who get sick easily. Another use for these formulas is as an aid to helping the body fight off serious immune-related disorders like chronic viral infections or cancer.

The only case where this strategy might backfire is in autoimmune diseases, where stimulating the immune system can make symptoms worse. For this reason, be cautious with using formulas in this category with autoimmune disorders.

Key Herbs: Astragalus, Cordyceps, Echinacea, Goldenseal, Maitake, Reishi (Ganoderma) and Shiitake

Planetary Herbals
Andrographis Respiratory Wellness™ (Tablet)

Andrographis aerial parts, **Echinacea (purpurea) root**, **Echinacea (pallida) root**, Olive leaf, Isatis (Woad) root, **Goldenseal**, Dandelion root, Garlic, Ginger, Licorice

Zand
Astragalus Formula (Capsule)

Astragalus, Codonopsis root, **Reishi (Ganoderma)**, Licorice, Ligustrum fruit & rhizome, Peony (White, Chinese), Schisandra

Planetary Herbals
Astragalus Jade Screen™ (Tablet and Glycerite)

Astragalus, Atractylodes (Bai-Zhu) rhizome, Siler; Non-Herbal: Calcium, Fiber

NOW Foods
Astragalus Plus Extract (Glycerine Extract)

Astragalus root, Codonopsis root, Atractylodes (Bai-Zhu) rhizome, Schisandra fruit, **Reishi (Ganoderma)**, Licorice root, Ligustrum fruit, Rehmannia root

Herbalist & Alchemist
Astragalus/Echinacea Compound™ (Alcohol Extract)

Echinacea (purpurea) root, Andrographis, **Astragalus**, Eleuthero root, Oregon Grape, Myrrh

Eclectic Institute
Atomic Echinacea (Bulk Powder)

Larch (Larix), **Echinacea (purpurea) leaf & flower**

New Chapter
C Food Complex™ (Tablet)

Astragalus, **Shiitake Mushroom**, **Cordyceps (militaris)**, **Reishi (Ganoderma)**, **Maitake Mushroom**, Cinnamon bark, Fenugreek, Oregano leaf, Cumin, Coriander seed, Rosemary, Clove, Allspice, Peppermint leaf, Spinach, Blueberry, Ginger, Turmeric; Non-Herbal: Vitamin C

Planetary Herbals
Complete Cat's Claw Complex™ (Tablet)

Cat's Claw bark, Andrographis aerial parts, Isatis (Woad) root, Oldenlandia leaf, **Astragalus**, **Reishi (Ganoderma)**, **Echinacea (pallida) root**, Jujube fruit, Cardamom fruit

Herbs Etc.
Deep Health® (Deep Chi Builder) (Alcohol Extract or Softgel)

Reishi (Ganoderma), **Shiitake Mushroom**, California Spikenard root, **Astragalus root**, **Maitake Mushroom**, Ashwagandha root, Eleuthero root, Schisandra berry, **Cordyceps**, Ginger root

Grandma's Herbs
Defense System (Capsule)

Agaricus, **Echinacea (angustifolia)**, Black (seed), **Astragalus**, Sheep Sorrel, Red Clover tops, Plantain, Pau d'Arco, Cascara Sagrada, Turkey Rhubarb, Chaparral (Creosote), Wormwood, Blue Flag, White Oak bark, Dandelion, Burdock root

Herbs Etc.
Early Alert™ (Alcohol Extract or Softgel)

Andrographis, **Echinacea (angustifolia) root, herb and flower**, **Echinacea (pallida) root**, **Echinacea (purpurea) root, herb, flower and seed**, Olive leaf, Elder (canadensis) berry, Spilanthes

Eclectic Institute
Ech-Astragalus (Glycerine Extract)

Echinacea (purpurea) root & seed, **Astragalus**, Orange essential oil; Non-Herbal: Ascorbic acid

Planetary Herbals
Echinacea Defense Force™ (Tablet)

Schisandra, Ligustrum fruit, **Astragalus**, **Echinacea (purpurea) root**, **Echinacea (pallida) root**, Pau d'Arco (heptophylla), **Reishi (Ganoderma)**, Eleuthero root, Oregon Grape, Ginger, Garlic, Suma root; Non-Herbal: Calcium

Gaia Herbs
Echinacea Goldenseal Supreme (Alcohol Extract)

Echinacea (purpurea) root, **Echinacea (angustifolia) root**, Oregon Grape, St. John's Wort flowering tops, Barberry root bark, **Goldenseal**, **Echinacea (purpurea) seed & aerial parts**, Propolis

Yogi Tea
Echinacea Immune Support (Tea)

Peppermint leaf, Lemongrass, **Echinacea root**, **Echinacea (angustifolia) root**, **Echinacea (purpurea) root**, **Echinacea (pallida) root**, Cinnamon bark, Licorice, Spearmint, Fennel, Cardamom seed, Rose hips, Ginger, Burdock root, Clove, Mullein leaf, Black Pepper, **Astragalus**, Cinnamon essential oil, Cardamom essential oil, Ginger essential oil

Eclectic Institute
Echinacea-Astragalus (Alcohol Extract)

Echinacea (purpurea) root & seed, **Astragalus**

Eclectic Institute
Echinacea-Oregon Grape (Alcohol Extract)

Echinacea (purpurea) root and seed, Oregon Grape

Nature's Way
Echinacea, Astragalus & Reishi (Capsule)

Echinacea (purpurea) stem, leaf & flower, **Astragalus**, **Reishi (Ganoderma)**

NOW Foods
Feelin' Groovy™ Tea

Hibiscus flower, Lemon Myrtle leaf, Peppermint leaf, **Echinacea (purpurea)**, **Astragalus**, Ginger, Ashwagandha root, Stevia

Gaia Herbs
GaiaKids® Kids Defense Herbal Drops (Alcohol Extract)

Echinacea (purpurea) root, seed & aerial parts, Marshmallow, **Echinacea (angustifolia) root**, Elder (canadensis) flower, Bayberry root bark, Irish Moss, Ginger, Clove, Capsicum (Cayenne), Allspice, Cinnamon essential oil, Peppermint essential oil
Ginger, **Echinacea root**; Non-Herbal: Honey, Vitamin C
Astragalus, **Cordyceps**, Cat's Claw bark, Peony (White, Chinese), He Shou Wu (Fo-Ti), Licorice, Lycium (Wolfberry/Gogi), Chinese Salvia, Dong Quai, **Echinacea (purpurea)**, Ligustrum, Ginseng (Korean, Asian), Atractylodes (Bai-Zhu), Long Pepper (Pippali), Pantocrine, Lo han gou, Millet; Non-Herbal: Fructo-Oligosaccharides, MSM,

Nature's Answer
Immune Support (Glycerine Extract)

Osha, Baptisia (Wild Indigo) root, **Echinacea (angustifolia) root**, **Echinacea (purpurea)**, Thuja, **Maitake Mushroom**

Irwin Naturals
Immune Boost (Tablet)

Acerola fruit, **Echinacea (purpurea) root**, **Maitake Mushroom**, **Shiitake Mushroom**, **Reishi (Ganoderma)**, Ginger, Papaya; Non-Herbal: Vitamin C (from Acerola)

Western Botanicals
Immune Boost Formula (Capsule and Alcohol Extract)

Echinacea (angustifolia) root, **Echinacea (purpurea) root**, Eleuthero root, Garlic, Cat's Claw bark, Pau d'Arco, Usnea, Capsicum (Cayenne), Capsicum (chinense)

Western Botanicals
Immune Boost Syrup (Liquid)

Echinacea (angustifolia) root, **Echinacea (purpurea) root**, Pau d'Arco, Eleuthero root, Usnea, Cat's Claw bark, Cinnamon bark; Non-Herbal: Pure maple syrup

Herb Pharm
Immune Defense (Alcohol Extract)

Echinacea (purpurea) root, **Astragalus**, **Reishi (Ganoderma)**, Schisandra, Prickly Ash

Grandma's Herbs
Immune Enhancer (Capsule)

Echinacea, **Astragalus**, Eleuthero, Pau d'Arco, Suma, **Goldenseal**, Kelp, Bladder Pod, Plantain, **Reishi (Ganoderma)**, Capsicum (Cayenne)

Vitanica
Immune Symmetry™ (Capsule)

Licorice, Garlic, Eleuthero root, Oregon Grape, **Echinacea (angustifolia)**, **Echinacea (purpurea)**, Green Tea, **Astragalus**, Myrrh; Non-Herbal: Vitamin A , Vitamin A, Vitamin C, Vitamin E, Vitamin B6, Vitamin B12, Folic Acid, Zinc, Selenium, Citrus Bioflavinoids,

Christopher's
Immune System Formula (Capsule)

Astragalus, Eleuthero root, **Echinacea (purpurea)**, **Echinacea (purpurea) root**, **Reishi (Ganoderma)**

Urban Moonshine
Immune Zoom (Alcohol Extract)

Echinacea root, bud & flower, Elder (canadensis) berry & flower, Ginger root, Capsicum (Cayenne), Cinnamon; Non-Herbal: honey

Irwin Naturals
Immuno-Shield™ All Season Wellness (Softgel)

Echinacea (purpurea) root, Olive leaf, **Astragalus**, Andrographis, Cat's Claw bark, Oregano leaf, Black Pepper, Ginger, Turmeric; Non-Herbal: Vitamin C (Ascorbic Acid), Vitamin E (d-Alpha Tocopherol), Zinc, Selenium, Citrus Bioflavonoids, Beta glucans, Bifidobacterium bifidum, soy lecithin

Herbs Etc.
ImmunoBoost™ (Alcohol Extract)

Echinacea (angustifolia) root, herb and flower, **Echinacea (purpurea) root and seed**, **Astragalus root**, Osha root, **Echinacea (angustifolia) seed**, Calendula (Marigold) flower

Planetary Herbals
Kids' Immune Protect™ (Glycerine)

Astragalus, Atractylodes (Bai-Zhu) rhizome, Siler

Herbs for Kids
Super Kids Throat Spray™

Echinacea (purpurea) root, Rose hips, Licorice, Thyme leaf, Peppermint

Nature's Way
SystemWell® Ultimate Immunity (Capsule)

Garlic, **Cordyceps**, Capsicum (Cayenne), **Echinacea (purpurea) stem, leaf & flower**, **Astragalus**, Olive leaf, Myrrh, **Maitake Mushroom**, **Shiitake Mushroom**, Yamabushitake Mushroom, Oregon Grape, **Goldenseal**, Fenugreek, Horehound, Thyme leaf, Elecampane root, Eleuthero root, Guggul, Rosemary, Plantain, Gotu Kola stem & leaf, Aloe vera leaf; Non-Herbal: Dietary Fiber, Vitamin A, Vitamin C, Vitamin D, Zinc, Selenium, Inositol, Arabinogalactan, Fructooligosaccharides, Lactobacillus cultures, Bifidobacterium cultures

Planetary Herbals
Well Child™ Immune Chewable (Wafer)

Acerola f, **Echinacea (purpurea) root**, Kudzu root, Cassia twig, Elder (canadensis) berry, Marshmallow, **Astragalus**, **Maitake Mushroom**

Gaia Herbs
Whole Body Defense (Liquid Phyto-Caps)

Astragalus, **Echinacea (purpurea) aerial parts**, Larch (Larix) gum, **Maitake Mushroom**

Herbal Formulas

Planetary Herbals
Yin Chiao-Echinacea Complex™ (Tablet)

Notopterygium root, Yin Chiao Classic™, **Echinacea (pallida) root**, **Echinacea (purpurea) root**, Horehound aerial parts, Boneset aerial parts, Elecampane root, Isatis (Woad) root & leaf; Non-Herbal: Calcium

Intestinal Toning Formulas

See also *Anti-Inflammatory, Fiber Blend* and *Gentle Laxative Formulas*

Infections, parasites, toxins, antibiotics, NSAIDs and other factors can create inflammation in the gastro-intestinal tract that can cause the membranes of the intestinal tract to lose tone. This can make them excessively porous, allowing toxins and partially digested molecules to enter the blood and lymph that would normally be filtered out. This condition, known as leaky gut syndrome, is the root cause of many chronic health problems.

In this instance, the colon doesn't need to be cleansed so much as it needs to be soothed and toned. That's where Intestinal Toners are helpful. In addition to the key herbs for this category, the amino acid l-glutamine is known to help rebuild intestinal tone and can be very helpful.

Gentle Laxative and *Fiber Blend Formulas* work well with *Intestinal Toning Formulas* to help heal the gut lining. *Anti-Inflammatory Formulas* may also be helpful.

Key Herbs: Chamomile (English and Roman), Marshmallow and Slippery Elm

Western Botanicals
Colon Comfort Formula (Capsule)

Marshmallow, Wild Yam, Aloe vera resin, Ginger, **Slippery Elm**, Lobelia, Lobelia seed, Plantain, Capsicum (chinense)

Solaray
Comfree Pepsin with Algin (Capsule)

Marshmallow, Plantain, Aloe vera vera gel; Non-Herbal: Algin, Pepsin

Irwin Naturals
Internal Cleanse & Detox (Tablet)

Aloe vera leaf, Dandelion root, **Slippery Elm**, Cranberry, Ginger, Papaya

Renew Life
Intestinal Bowel Soother™ (Capsule)

Slippery Elm, **Chamomile flower**, Fenugreek, Fennel, Scullcap (Skullcap), Cranberry, Peppermint leaf, Atractylodes (Bai-Zhu) root, Yin Chen Hao, Codonopsis root, Job's Tears, Schisandra, Agastache, Licorice (Chinese), Chinese Thoroughwax (Chai Hu), Ginger, Korean Ash (Qin Pi), Magnolia bark, Amur Cork Tree (Phellodendron) bark, Poria Mushroom root, Psyllium seed, Coptis (Chinese Goldthread,Huang Lian), Peony (White, Chinese), Costus Root (Mu Xiang), Siler, Tangerine peel, Angelica root; Non-Herbal: MSM (methylsulfonylmethane)

Renew Life
Intestinal Bowel Support™ (Capsule)

Cranesbill (Wild Geranium) root, Ginger, Calendula (Marigold) flower, **Marshmallow**, Yin Chen Hao, Yin Chen Hao, Agastache, Chinese Thoroughwax (Chai Hu), Korean Ash (Qin Pi) bark, Amur Cork Tree (Phellodendron) bark, Coptis (Chinese Goldthread,Huang Lian), Costus Root (Mu Xiang), **Slippery Elm**, **Chamomile flower**, Fenugreek, Fennel, Scullcap (Skullcap), Cranberry, Peppermint leaf, Atractylodes (Bai-Zhu) root, Codonopsis root, Job's Tears, Schisandra, Licorice (Chinese), Ginger, Magnolia bark, Poria Mushroom, Psyllium seed, Peony (White, Chinese), Siler, Tangerine peel, Angelica root; Non-Herbal: L-Glutamine, N Acetyl D-Glucosamine, Gamma Oryzanol, MSM (methylsulfonylmethane)

Herbalist & Alchemist
Intestinal Calmpound™ (Alcohol Extract)

Catnip flowering tops, **Chamomile flower**, Sarsaparilla, Turmeric, Wild Yam, Yarrow flower

Renew Life
IntestiNew™ (Capsule and Bulk Powder)

Cranesbill (Wild Geranium) root, Ginger, Calendula (Marigold) flower, **Marshmallow**; Non-Herbal: L-Glutamine, N-Acetyl D-Glucosamine, Gamma Oryzanol

Traditional Medicinals
Throat Coat® (Tea)

Licorice, **Slippery Elm**, Licorice, **Marshmallow**, Cherry (Wild) bark, Fennel fruit, Cinnamon bark, Orange peel

Iron Formulas

Herbs can actually be more effective at restoring blood levels of iron than iron supplements, because iron is a difficult mineral to assimilate and utilize. Plants rich in iron appear to have co-factors that make the iron easier to absorb. They also contain co-factors that help build hemoglobin in the blood.

Herbal *Iron Formulas* are tonics for anemia and for building the blood after blood loss. The key herbs for this category are rich in iron and build up iron levels in the blood. Non-herbal ingredients like Vitamin C and Vitamin B12 can also aid assimilation and utilization of iron. See *Anemia* in the *Conditions Section.*

Key Herbs: Alfalfa, Beet Root, Nettle (Stinging) and Yellow Dock

Christopher's
Herbal Iron Formula (Capsule)

White Oak bark, Mullein root, **Yellow Dock**, Mullein leaf, Black Walnut leaf, Slippery Elm, Plantain root, Lobelia, Marshmallow

NatureWorks
Herbal Iron Yeast Free (Syrup)

Beet, Black Currant, Rose hips, Carrot, Spinach, Rosemary, Lemon Balm leaf, Gentian, Yarrow leaf, **Nettle (Stinging) leaf**, Sage; Non-Herbal: Vitamin C, Thiamin, Riboflavin, Vitamin B6, Iron

Herbalist & Alchemist
Iron Extract™ (Alcohol Extract)

Beet, Chickweed, Parsley, **Nettle (Stinging) leaf**, **Yellow Dock**, Ashwagandha root, Watercress; Non-Herbal: Blackstrap Molasses

Vitanica
Iron Extra™ (Capsule)

Yellow Dock, Dandelion root, **Alfalfa leaf**, **Nettle (Stinging) flowering tops**; Non-Herbal: Vitamin C, Folate, Vitamin B12, Iron

Joint Healing Formulas

See also *Analgesic, Anti-Inflammatory, Mineral* and *Tissue Healing Formulas*

These are herbal formulas used to help reduce pain and promote healing in arthritic joints. They are typically blends with analgesic, anti-inflammatory, tissue healing and remineralizing properties. They are related to *Analgesic Formulas, Mineral Formulas, Tissue Healing* and *Anti-inflammatory Formulas*, all of which can also be used to ease pain and promote joint healing.

The ingredients in these blends vary widely. See *Arthritis* in the *Conditions Section* for more information on natural remedies for healing the joints.

Key Herbs: Alfalfa, Boswellia, Burdock, Cats Claw (Una de Gato, Gambier), Devil's Claw, Hydrangea, Sarsaparilla, Turmeric, Willow and Yucca

Eclectic Institute
Devil's Claw - Yucca (Glycerine Extract)

Devil's Claw, **Yucca**, Ginger, Dandelion whole plant, Black Cohosh

Planetary Herbals
Flex-Ability™ (Alcohol Extract)

Gambier twig, Quince, Angelica root, Achyranthes root, Dong Quai, Chuan Xiong rhizome, Tienchi Ginseng, Sichuan Teasel, Siler, Lycium (Wolfberry/Gogi), Notopterygium root

Planetary Herbals
Flex-Ability™ (Tablet)

Angelica root, Achyranthes root, Chuan Xiong rhizome, Tienchi Ginseng, Quince, **Uncaria twig**, Lycium (Wolfberry/Gogi), Siler, Notopterygium root, Dong Quai; Non-Herbal: Sodium

Herb Pharm
Flexible Joint™ (Alcohol Extract)

Devil's Claw, **Sarsaparilla (Jamacian)**, Nettle (Stinging) mature seed, **Burdock seed**, Angelica root, Prickly Ash

Planetary Herbals
Glucosamine-MSM Herbal™ (Tablet)

Rehmannia, Wild Yam, Teasel root, Eucommia (ulmoides) bark, **Boswellia**, Drynaria rhizome, Myrrh; Non-Herbal: Calcium Citrate, Molybdenum, MSM, Glucosamine Sulfate

Gaia Herbs
Infla-Profen (Liquid Phyto-Caps)

Jamaican Dogwood bark, **Turmeric root**, **Burdock root**, **Devil's Claw root**, Feverfew flower and leaf, Ginger rhizome, Nettle (Stinging) seed, Nettle (Stinging) leaf

Solaray
Joint Blend™ SP-2™ (Capsule)

Devil's Claw, **Yucca stalk**, **Alfalfa aerial parts**, Wild Yam, **Sarsaparilla**, Kelp, **Willow (White) bark**, Capsicum (Cayenne), Horsetail, Chickweed aerial parts

Yogi Tea
Joint Comfort™ (Tea)

Lemongrass, Peppermint leaf, Green Tea leaf, **Alfalfa seed**, **Turmeric**, Celery seed, Spearmint, **Yucca**, **Cat's Claw bark**, **Devil's Claw**

Christopher's
Joint Formula (Capsule)

Brigham (Mormon) Tea, **Hydrangea**, **Yucca**, Chaparral (Creosote) leaf, Lobelia root, **Burdock seed**, **Sarsaparilla**, Wild (Prickly) Lettuce, Valerian, Wormwood root, Capsicum (Cayenne), Black Cohosh, Black Walnut bark

Gaia Herbs
Joint Health (Liquid Phyto-Caps)

Devil's Claw, Green Tea leaf, **Turmeric**, Brown Seaweed, Hawthorn berry, Ginger, Hops, Rosemary

Western Botanicals
Joint Relief Formula (Liquid)

Celery seed, Black Cohosh, Licorice, **Devil's Claw**, **Willow (White) bark**, **Cat's Claw bark**, **Alfalfa leaf**, Meadowsweet; Non-Herbal: Apple cider vinegar, pure honey

Planetary Herbals
Lower Back Support™ (Tablet)

Loranthus aerial parts, Achyranthes root, Eucommia (ulmoides) bark, Angelica root, Rehmannia, Chinese Yam root, Poria Mushroom, Asian Water Plantain rhizome, Psoralea fruit, Tree Peony, Asiatic Dogwood fruit; Non-Herbal: Calcium

Planetary Herbals
Neck and Shoulders Support™ (Tablet)

Kudzu root, Cinnamon (cassia) twig, Notopterygium root, Chuan Xiong rhizome, **Turmeric**, Dong Quai, Tree Peony, Astragalus, Evergreen Wisteria stem, Chinese Clematis root; Non-Herbal: Calcium

Kidney Tonic Formulas

See also *Diuretic, Hypotensive* and *Joint Healing Formulas*

This is a subclass of *Diuretic Formulas* that help nourish and support kidney function rather than just stimulating urine flow. These remedies also tend to be more soothing to urinary passages and are appropriate when there is kidney and bladder inflammation, burning urination or acute pain with the passage of urine.

Herbal Formulas

In Chinese medicine, the kidneys are said to "build the bones" because part of their role is to maintain the proper balance of fluids and minerals. The kidneys flush acid waste from the body. When this acid waste isn't properly eliminated, the body will borrow calcium, magnesium and potassium from bones, muscles and other tissues in order to neutralize the acid and maintain proper pH. This can lead to structural problems such as chronic back and neck pain, weakness of the legs and ankles, arthritis and osteoporosis.

Kidney Tonic Formulas help the kidneys flush acid waste and often supply mineral electrolytes that replenish mineral reserves. So, they both support the kidneys and strengthen weakened tissues to support the structural system. They can even be used in combination with *Joint Healing Formulas* for arthritic conditions.

Another important role of the kidneys is in helping to regulate blood pressure. *Kidney Tonic Formulas* may work well in combination with *Hypotensive Formulas* in lowering blood pressure.

Key Herbs: Cleavers (Bedstraw), Cornsilk, Goldenrod, Horsetail, Nettle (Stinging), Parsley and Pipsissewa

Herb Pharm
Calm Waters™ (Alcohol Extract)
Corn Silk, St. John's Wort leaf, Plantain, **Goldenrod**

Solaray
Continence® with Flowtrol (Capsule)
Butterbur root, Cranberry, Morinda (Noni) root, Psoralea fruit, Raspberry (Palm-Leaf) fruit, Alpinia

Nature's Sunshine Products
KB-C (Capsule)
Eucommia (almoides) bark, Broomrape stem, Achyranthes root, Teasel root, Drynaria rhizome, Hoelen (Fu Ling, Tuckahoe, China Root), Morinda (Noni) root, Rehmannia, Astragalus, Dogwood fruit, Dioscorea rhizome, Epimedium (Horny Goat Weed)

Christopher's
Kid-e-Dry (Glycerine Extract)
White Pond Lilly, Slippery Elm, Hydrangea, **Corn Silk**, **Parsley**, Lobelia, Catnip

A. Vogel
Kidney Bladder Complex (Alcohol Tincture)
Goldenrod aerial parts, Birch (White) leaf, Restharrow aerial parts, **Horsetail**

Solaray
Kidney Caps™ (Capsule)
Saw Palmetto, Dandelion root, Meadowsweet flower, Clove

Herbalist & Alchemist
Kidney Support Compound™ (Alcohol Extract)
Nettle (Stinging) seed, Astragalus, Rehmannia, **Nettle (Stinging) leaf**, Cordyceps (militaris)

Herbs Etc.
Kidney Tonic™ (Alcohol Extract or Softgel)
Dandelion leaf, Saw Palmetto berry, **Parsley root**, Couchgrass (Quackgrass) root, Boldo leaf, Buchu leaf, Juniper berry, Uva Ursi leaf, **Pipsissewa**, Cubeb berry

RidgeCrest Herbals
KidneyAid (Capsule)
Plantain leaf, **Goldenrod flower**, Fenugreek seed, **Horsetail**, Hydrangea root; Non-Herbal: Kidney substance

Herb Pharm
Urinary System Support (Alcohol Extract)
Goldenrod flowering tops, **Corn Silk**, **Horsetail**, Uva Ursi, Juniper berry

Lithotriptic Formulas

These blends are used to dissolve calcification. They can be helpful for kidney stones, calcium-based gall stones, bone spurs and calcification or hardening of any tissue. Although not an ingredient in any of these formulas, lemon water has lithotriptic action. See *Kidney Stones* in the *Conditions Section* for more information.

Key Herbs: Gravel root, Hydrangea and Stone Breaker

Western Botanicals
Kidney/Bladder Formula/Tea Combo (Liquid)
Juniper berry, Burdock root, Goldenrod flower, Pipsissewa, **Gravel Root root**, **Hydrangea**, Uva Ursi, Dandelion leaf, Horsetail, Marshmallow, Corn Silk

Western Botanicals
Kidney/Bladder Tea
Juniper berry, **Gravel Root root**, Orange peel, **Hydrangea**, Marshmallow, Parsley root, Peppermint leaf, Uva Ursi, Horsetail, Corn Silk, Parsley leaf, Dandelion leaf, Goldenrod flower

Herb Pharm
Stone Breaker (Alcohol Extract)
Stone Breaker (Quebra Pedra), **Hydrangea**, Celery seed, Burdock seed

Western Botanicals
Stone Dissolve Tea
Rose hips, **Hydrangea**, **Gravel Root root**, Marshmallow

Planetary Herbals
Stone Free™ (Tablet)
Turmeric, Dandelion root, **Gravel Root root**, Ginger, Lemon Balm leaf, Marshmallow, Parsley root, Licorice; Non-Herbal: sodium, fiber, sugar, calcium

Liver Tonic Formulas

See also *Hepatoprotective Formulas*

The liver is the biochemical mastermind of the body. It filters all the blood from the digestive tract, acting as a secondary line of immune defense to the mucus membranes of the gut. It stores nutrients and processes them for use by the tissues. It also plays a primary role in metabolizing toxins for elimination. The liver breaks down drugs, chemical additives in our food, microbial endotoxins, excess hormones, neurotransmitters and chemical solvents. It helps the body get rid of heavy metals as well.

Liver Tonic Formulas contain ingredients that aid general liver function. Many of these ingredients are the same key ingredients found in *Blood Purifier* and *Hepatoprotective Formulas*. These formulas may also include non-herbal ingredients that support the liver such N-acetyl-cysteine, alpha lipoic acid and amino acids, vitamins and minerals needed for healthy liver function.

Key Herbs: Beet Root, Blessed Thistle, Bupleurum, Dandelion, Milk Thistle and Oregon Grape

Zand
Allergy Season Formula (Capsule)

Nettle (Stinging) leaf, Turmeric, **Milk Thistle seed**, Grape seed, Pueraria root, Coptis (Chinese Goldthread,Huang Lian) rhizome, Schisandra, Oat straw, **Dandelion root**, Ginger; Non-Herbal: Pantothenic Acid, Bromelain, Quercetin

Planetary Herbals
Bupleurum Liver Cleanse™ (Tablet)

Cypress rhizome, Dong Quai, Fennel fruit, **Dandelion root**, **Milk Thistle seed**, Peony (White, Chinese), Wild Yam, **Bupleurum**, Lycium (Wolfberry/Gogi), Ginger, Chinese Scullcap (Scute/Huang Qin); Non-Herbal: Calcium

Herb Pharm
Cholesterol Health (Alcohol Extract)

Artichoke leaf & flower, Hawthorn berry, leaf & flower, Turmeric, Fennel

Zand
Cleanse Today (Capsule)

Milk Thistle seed, Rosemary, Ginger, **Dandelion root**, Sage, Oat bran, Flax seed, Broccoli, Kale, Nettle (Stinging) leaf, Cabbage, Maitake Mushroom; Non-Herbal: Plant-based Enzymes (Amylase (2400DU), Cellulase (100CU), Invertase (140 SUMNER), Lactase (100 ALU), Lipase (40 FIP), and Malt Diastase (50 DP) 30 mg, Vegetable Cellulose Fiber, Alpha Lipoic Acid, L-Glutathione, Rice flour

Renew Life
Critical Liver Support™ (Capsule)

Milk Thistle seed, Artichoke leaf, Green Tea leaf; Non-Herbal: Vitamin C, Selenium, N-Acetyl-Cysteine, L-Taurine, L-Isoleucine, Glycine, L-Methionine, L-Leucine, L-Valine, Alpha Lipoic Acid, Quercetin, Phosphatidylcholine, L-Glutathione

Gaia Herbs
Liver Cleanse (Liquid Phyto-Caps)

Milk Thistle seed, Turmeric, **Dandelion leaf & root**, Burdock root, Rooibos (Redbush), Radish (Black), Gentian, Fenugreek, Celandine seed, Red Root, Ginger

Planetary Herbals
Liver Defense™ (Tablet)

Astragalus, **Milk Thistle**, **Bupleurum**, Licorice, Jujube fruit, Schisandra, Chinese Scullcap (Scute/Huang Qin), Ginger; Non-Herbal: Sodium, Fiber

Renew Life
Liver Detox (Capsule)

Milk Thistle seed, Soybean, **Dandelion root**, Artichoke leaf, Green Tea leaf, Turmeric, Belleric Myrobalan fruit, Boerhavia Diffusa root, Eclipta root, Eclipta, Guduchi, Andrographis, Kutki (Picorhiza kurroa); Non-Herbal: Selenium, L-Methionine, L-Taurine, NAC (N-Acetyl-Cysteine), Alpha Lipoic Acid

NOW Foods
Liver Detoxifier & Regenerator™ (Capsule)

Milk Thistle seed, Artichoke leaf, **Beet**, Bladderwrack, Raspberry (Red) leaf, Grape seed, **Dandelion root**, Chinese Scullcap (Scute/Huang Qin), Schisandra, Barberry root bark, Turmeric; Non-Herbal: Pancreatin, L-Glutathione (Free-Form), N-Acetyl Cysteine, L-Carnitine, L-Methionine

Herb Pharm
Liver Health (Alcohol Extract)

Dandelion root, **Oregon Grape**, **Milk Thistle seed**, Artichoke leaf, Schisandra seed, Fennel

Eclectic Institute
Liver Support (Capsule)

Milk Thistle seed, **Dandelion whole plant**, Artichoke leaf, **Beet**, Goldenseal, Turmeric

Nature's Answer
Liver Support (Capsule and Glycerine Extract)

Oregon Grape, **Dandelion root**, Goldenseal, **Milk Thistle fruit & seed**, Red Clover flowering tops, Turkey Rhubarb, Gentian, Prickly Ash

Nature's Answer
Liver Tone (Glycerine Extract)

Sarsaparilla, **Milk Thistle seed**, **Dandelion root**, **Bupleurum**, Reishi (Ganoderma), Ginger, Turmeric

Christopher's
Liver Transition Formula (Capsule)

Ginseng (Korean, Asian), Rosemary, Ginkgo, **Oregon Grape**, **Milk Thistle**, Wild Yam, Scullcap (Skullcap)
Milk Thistle seed, Ginger, Artichoke leaf, Carrot, Spinach, Parsley, **Bupleurum**, Schisandra

Planetary Herbals
Shiitake Mushroom Supreme™ (Tablet)

Shiitake Mushroom, Reishi (Ganoderma), Lycium (Wolfberry/Gogi), Schisandra, Dong Quai, Chinese Salvia root, Turmeric, Ligustrum fruit, Rehmannia, Cypress root, **Milk Thistle seed**, Shiitake Mushroom, Reishi (Ganoderma)

Nature's Way
Super Thisilyn® (Capsule)

Milk Thistle seed, Artichoke leaf, Turmeric, **Dandelion root**, Broccoli, Spinach, Cabbage; Non-Herbal: N-Acetyl Cysteine, Alpha Lipoic Acid, L-Methionine

Lung and Respiratory Tonic Formulas

When the lungs get weak, a person may become susceptible to frequent respiratory infections. They may also suffer from wheezing and shortness of breath. *Lung and Respiratory Tonics* are formulas aimed at strengthening lung function. These remedies generally help hydrate the lungs and improve oxygenation in the body.

These blends can be beneficial for smokers, elderly people, people exposed to cold, dry air, and anyone who is extremely susceptible to respiratory infections like pneumonia. The key herbs in these formulas tend to hydrate and soften lung tissue.

Key Herbs: Astragalus, Codonopsis, Licorice, Mullein, Platycodon (Balloon Flower) and Schisandra (Schizandra)

RidgeCrest Herbals
ClearLungs Classic (Capsule)

Dong Quai root, Ophiopogon root, Poria Mushroom, Asparagus (Chinese) root, Chinese Scullcap (Scute/Huang Qin) root, Gardenia fruit, Luo han guo (Monk Fruit) fruit, Platycodon root, Tangerine peel, Mulberry (White) root, Fritillary bulb, **Schisandra fruit**, **Licorice (Chinese) root**

RidgeCrest Herbals
ClearLungs Extra Strength (Capsule)

Asparagus (Chinese) root, **Licorice (Chinese) root**, Chinese Scullcap (Scute/Huang Qin) root, Dong Quai root, Gardenia fruit, Luo han guo (Monk Fruit) fruit, Bitter Melon fruit, Ophiopogon root, Platycodon root, Poria Mushroom, **Schisandra fruit**, Tangerine peel, Mulberry (White) root bark, Fritillary bulb; Non-Herbal: Antimonium Tartaricum, Carbo Vegetabilis, Natrum Sulphuricum, phosphorus

RidgeCrest Herbals
ClearLungs Liquid

Dong Quai root, Poria Mushroom, Ophiopogon root, Luo han guo (Monk Fruit) fruit, Asparagus (Chinese) root, Tangerine peel, Fritillary bulb, Gardenia fruit, Mulberry (White) root bark, Platycodon root, Chinese Scullcap (Scute/Huang Qin) root, **Schisandra fruit**, **Licorice (Chinese) root**; Non-Herbal: vegetable glycerin, natural orange flavor

Traditional Medicinals
Lemon Echinacea Throat Coat® (Tea)

Echinacea (purpurea) root, **Licorice**, **Licorice**, Lemon Myrtle leaf, Marshmallow leaf, Marshmallow, Fennel fruit, Orange peel, Cinnamon bark

Christopher's
Lung & Bronchial Formula (Capsule and Glycerine Extract)

Marshmallow leaf, **Mullein**, Chickweed root, Lobelia root, Pleurisy root

Herbalist & Alchemist
Lung Relief Cold/Dry Compound™ (Alcohol Tincture)

Astragalus, Prince Seng root, Asparagus (Chinese) root, **Licorice**, Spikenard

Nature's Sunshine Products
Lung Support (Capsule)

Astragalus, Aster root, Gentian (Large Leaf), Platycodon, Anemarrhena (Zhi-Mu) rhizome, Bupleurum, Lycium (Wolfberry/Gogi), Ophiopogon, Ginseng (Korean, Asian), Angelica (Chinese) root, Atractylodes (Bai-Zhu) rhizome, **Schisandra**, Typhonium, **Licorice**

Herbs Etc.
Lung Tonic™ (Alcohol Extract, Glycerine Extract or Softgel)

Mullein leaf, Horehound, Elecampane root, Grindelia (Gumweed) flower, Echinacea (angustifolia) root, Pleurisy root, Passionflower, Osha root, Lobelia, Yerba Santa leaf

Planetary Herbals
Mullein Lung Complex™ (Tablet)

Platycodon, Ophiopogon, Long Pepper (Pippali) fruit, Elecampane root, **Mullein leaf**, Black Cherry bark, **Licorice**, Ginger, Cinnamon (cassia) twig; Non-Herbal: Sodium, Fiber

Solaray
Respiration Blend™ SP-3™ (Capsule)

Pleurisy root, Slippery Elm, Cherry (Wild) bark, Plantain leaf, Chickweed aerial parts, Horehound aerial parts, **Licorice**, **Mullein leaf**, Kelp, Ginger, Saw Palmetto

Herbs Etc.
Smoke Free® (Spray and Softgel)

Lobelia, Oat seed (milky), Osha root, **Licorice root**, Passionflower, Pleurisy root, Grindelia (Gumweed) flower, **Mullein leaf**, Ginger root

Lymphatic Drainage Formulas

See also *Blood Purifier Formulas*

The lymphatic system drains excess fluid and plasma proteins away from the tissue spaces and returns them to the circulatory system. The lymph passes through lymph nodes where white blood cells remove cellular debris and infectious organisms. Sometimes the lymphatic system becomes stagnant, resulting in poor lymph drainage. This can cause swollen lymph nodes and fluid retention in the tissues.

Poor lymphatic drainage is often seen with sore throats, earaches, respiratory congestion and dull pelvic pains and abdominal swelling with periods. Persons suffering from mumps, tonsillitis, lymphoma, cysts and certain tumors and skin conditions may benefit from *Lymphatic Drainage Formulas*.

Many of the key herbs in lymphatic drainage formulas are also considered blood purifiers or alteratives, such as burdock and red clover. However, these formulas contain herbs that are more specific for enhancing lymphatic flow and shrinking swollen lymph glands. Still, *Lymphatic Drainage Formulas* can have many of the same general health benefits as *Blood Purifier Formulas*.

Key Herbs: Burdock, Cleavers (Bedstraw), Echinacea, Lobelia, Mullein, Ocotillo, Red Clover, Red Root, Stillingia, Violet and Wintergreen

Herbalist & Alchemist
Burdock/Red Root Compound™ (Alcohol Extract)
Burdock root, Echinacea (purpurea) root, Figwort, **Red Clover flower, Red Root, Violet**

Gaia Herbs
Echinacea Red Root Supreme (Alcohol Extract)
Echinacea (angustifolia) root, Echinacea (purpurea) aerial parts, root & seed, Indigo, Prickly Ash, **Red Root, Stillingia (Queen's Root)**, Thuja

Christopher's
Glandular System Formula (Capsule)
Mullein, Lobelia

Christopher's
Glandular System Massage Oil (Essential Oil)
Mullein leaf, Lobelia, Olive oil

Herbs Etc.
Lymphatonic™ (Alcohol Extract, Glycerine Extract or Softgel)
Echinacea (angustifolia) root, Red Root root, Ocotillo stem bark, Burdock root, Licorice root, Dandelion root, Yellow Dock root, Baptisia (Wild Indigo) root, Blue Flag root, **Stillingia (Queen's Root) root**

Male Aphrodisiac Formulas

See also *Male Glandular Tonic Formulas*

This is a subcategory of *Male Glandular Tonic Formulas*. Both groups of formulas tend to enhance testosterone levels and male fertility, but *Male Aphrodisiac Formulas* are more specifically targeted toward problems relating to lack of desire and erectile dysfunction (impotency). See *Erectile Dysfunction* in the *Conditions Section* for more suggestions.

Key Herbs: Damiana, Ginseng (Asian, Korean), Horny Goat Weed (Epimedium), Maca, Muira Puama and Yohimbe

Solaray
Ginseng and Damiana (Capsule)
Ginseng (Korean, Asian), Eleuthero root, **Damiana leaf**

Christopher's
Herbal Libido Formula (Capsule)
Muira Puama, Maca, Yohimbe, Bee Pollen, Royal Jelly, Ginger, Eleuthero, Ginkgo, Nettle (Stinging), Guarana root; Non-Herbal: Be Pollen

Nature's Answer
Male Complex (Capsule)
Yohimbe, Muira Puama root, Tribulus fruit, Suma root, Nettle (Stinging) root, Oat Wild, Saw Palmetto, Prickly Ash, Yerba Mate, Red Clover flowering tops, Capsicum (Cayenne); Non-Herbal: Zinc, Boron

Eclectic Institute
Male Formula (Alcohol Extract)
Muira Puama root & stem, Catuaba Bark bark, Eleuthero root, Ginseng (American)

Gaia Herbs
Male Libido (Liquid Phyto-Caps)
Epimedium (Horny Goat Weed), Tribulus fruit, **Yohimbe**, Sarsaparilla root, Oat seed (milky), **Maca root**, He Shou Wu (Fo-Ti), Saw Palmetto

Grandma's Herbs
Male Libido Enhancer (Capsule)
Ginseng (Korean, Asian), Yohimbe, Maca, Muira Puama, Clavohuasca, Corn Silk, Tribulus, Saw Palmetto, Nettle (Stinging), **Epimedium (Horny Goat Weed), Damiana**, Velvet Bean; Non-Herbal: L-Arginine, Lycopine

Solaray
Male Stamina Blend Sp-15B (Capsule)
Yohimbe, Tribulus fruit, **Epimedium (Horny Goat Weed) root, Muira Puama root, Maca**, Fennel, Irish Moss, Sarsaparilla

NOW Foods
Men's Virility Power (Capsule)
Epimedium (Horny Goat Weed), Muira Puama, Maca root, Tribulus fruit, **Ginseng (Korean, Asian), Damiana (aphrodisiaca) leaf**, Ginkgo leaf, Capsicum (Cayenne) fruit

Western Botanicals
Sensual Enhancement Formula (Capsule and Alcohol Extract)
Saw Palmetto, Ginseng (American), Eleuthero root, **Maca, Muira Puama root**, Ashwagandha root, Ginkgo, Oat tops, Pygeum, Sarsaparilla, **Damiana leaf, Ginseng (Korean, Asian)**, Mullein leaf & flower, Pumpkin seed, Scullcap (Skullcap), Buchu leaf, Capsicum (chinense)

Irwin Naturals
Steel-Libido (Softgel)
Maca root, Ashwagandha root, **Epimedium (Horny Goat Weed) aerial parts**, Tribulus whole plant, **Yohimbe bark**, Ginger, Long Pepper (Pippali), Black Pepper; Non-Herbal: Fish Oil, L-Arginine, DMG (Dimethylglycine), L-Tyrosine, CDP-Choline, NADH (Nicotinamide Adenine Dinucleotide)

Irwin Naturals
Steel-Libido Red (Softgel)
Pumpkin seed, Velvet Bean seed, Ginkgo, **Ginseng (Korean, Asian)**, Capsicum (Cayenne), Black Pepper, Ginger; Non-Herbal:

Herbal Formulas

L-Citrulline, Medium-Chain Triglycerides, L-Theanine, Theobromine, Co-Q10, Superoxide Dismutase

NOW Foods
TestoJack 200™ (Capsule)

Tongkat Ali root, **Maca root**, **Epimedium (Horny Goat Weed) aerial parts & leaf**, Tribulus fruit, Ginseng (American), **Ginseng (Korean, Asian)**, **Muira Puama root and stem**

Solaray
Yohimbe and Saw Palmetto (Capsule)

Saw Palmetto, **Yohimbe**

Irwin Naturals
Yohimbe-Plus (Softgel)

Yohimbe bark, Ashwagandha root, **Damiana leaf**, Eleuthero root, **Epimedium (Horny Goat Weed) aerial parts**, **Muira Puama root**, Tribulus whole plant, Ginkgo, Black Pepper, Ginger; Non-Herbal: Fish Oil

Male Glandular Tonic Formulas

See also *Male Aphrodisiac* and *Prostate Formulas*

These are formulas used to balance glandular function in males and enhance testosterone production. Low levels of testosterone in men contribute to fatigue, excess body fat, loss of muscle tone, depression, anxiety, lack of self confidence and erectile dysfunction. *Male Glandular Tonics* can boost sexual performance and desire (like *Male Aphrodisiac Formulas*) and may be helpful for prostate problems (like *Prostate Formulas*). They may also enhance male fertility. See *Testosterone (low)* in the *Conditions Section* for more information and suggestions.

Key Herbs: Ginseng (Asian, Korean), Horny Goat Weed (Epimedium), Muira Puama, Sarsaparilla, Saw Palmetto, Tribulus and Yohimbe

Planetary Herbals
Avena Sativa Oat Complex™ for Men (Tablet)

Oat tops, **Saw Palmetto**, Damiana (aphrodisiaca) aerial parts, Nettle (Stinging) root, **Ginseng (Korean, Asian)**, Rose (laevigata) hips, Cinnamon (cassia) bark, Ginkgo; Non-Herbal: Calcium, Sodium

Planetary Herbals
Damiana Male Potential™ (Tablet)

Saw Palmetto, **Sarsaparilla**, Damiana (aphrodisiaca) aerial parts, Schisandra, Ophiopogon, **Ginseng (Korean, Asian)**, Cinnamon (cassia) bark, **Horny Goat Weed aerial parts**, Noni (Morinda) root, Ginkgo

Solaray
Fertility Blend™ SP-1™ (Capsule)

Damiana leaf, Eleuthero root, **Saw Palmetto**, Buckthorn bark, Kelp, **Sarsaparilla**

Herbalist & Alchemist
Gentle-Man™ (Alcohol Extract)

Oat seed (milky), Ashwagandha root, Mimosa (Albizia, Silk Tree) bark, **Saw Palmetto**, Black Cohosh, Pulsatilla root; Non-Herbal: Orange extract

Solaray
Male Caps™ (Capsule)

Clove, Eleuthero root, Damiana leaf, **Saw Palmetto**, Parsley leaf

Gaia Herbs
Male Libido (Liquid Phyto-Caps)

Epimedium (Horny Goat Weed), **Tribulus fruit**, Yohimbe, **Sarsaparilla root**, Oat seed (milky), Maca root, He Shou Wu (Fo-Ti), **Saw Palmetto**

Herb Pharm
Male Sexual Vitality™ (Alcohol Extract)

Ginseng (Korean, Asian), **Sarsaparilla**, Maca, Cardamom pod & seed

Christopher's
Male Tonic Formula (Capsule)

Eleuthero root, **Sarsaparilla**, Raspberry (Red) leaf, **Saw Palmetto**, Ginkgo, Pumpkin seed, Damiana leaf, Bee Pollen, Hops flower, Dandelion leaf, Hawthorn berry, Capsicum (Cayenne)

Herbalist & Alchemist
Men's Formula™ (Alcohol Extract)

Ashwagandha root, Cynomorium (Suo Yang), Maca, Ginseng (Red), **Epimedium (Horny Goat Weed)**, **Muira Puama root**

Yerba Prima
Men's Rebuild® (Capsule)

Yellow Dock, Dandelion leaf & root, **Ginseng (Korean, Asian)**, Red Clover flowering tops, Blessed Thistle, Ginger, **Sarsaparilla**, Milk Thistle seed, Plantain, **Saw Palmetto**, Corn Silk; Non-Herbal: zinc

Solaray
Multi Gland Caps™ for Men (Capsule)

Ginger, Clove, Eleuthero root, **Sarsaparilla**, Dandelion root, **Saw Palmetto**

Menopause Balancing Formulas

See also *Female Hormonal Balancing Formulas*

This is a subcategory of *Female Hormone Balancing Formulas* targeted at balancing women's hormones during menopause. Key herbs are very similar in both groups of formulas. (See *Female Hormone Balancers*). You can also look up *Menopause* in the *Conditions Section* for more suggestions on dealing with menopause.

Key Herbs: Black Cohosh, Chastetree (Vitex), Dong Quai, Ginseng (American) and Licorice

Nature's Way
Change-O-Life® (Capsule)

Black Cohosh, Sarsaparilla, Eleuthero root, **Licorice**, Blessed Thistle stem, leaf & flower, **Dong Quai**, Pomegranate seed

Zand
Changes for Women AM/PM Formula (Capsule)

Grape seed, **Black Cohosh**, Green Tea, Wild Yam, Peony (White, Chinese), Motherwort, Passionflower flower; Non-Herbal: Day Formula: Folic Acid, Vitamin B12, Pantothenic Acid, N-Acetyl L-Cysteine, Gama Amino Butyric Acid (GABA), Alpha lipoic acid. Night Formula: Magnesium, Gama Amino Butyric Acid (GABA), 5-HTP

Irwin Naturals
EstroPause™ Menopause Support (Softgel)

St. John's Wort flower, **Black Cohosh**, Red Clover aerial parts, Ginseng (Korean, Asian), Black Pepper; Non-Herbal: Calcium Citrate, Magnesium Oxide and Citrate, Fish Oil

Herb Pharm
Healthy Menopause Tonic (Alcohol Extract)

Chaste Tree (Vitex), Motherwort leaf and flower, **Black Cohosh**, **Licorice**, Pulsatilla

NOW Foods
Herbal Pause™ w/Estro G-100™ (Capsule)

Jerusalem Sage, Swallow-wort, Angelica (Giant)

Christopher's
Hormonal Changease Formula (Capsule and Glycerine Extract)

Black Cohosh, Sarsaparilla, **Ginseng (American)**, **Licorice**, False Unicorn (Helonias, Chamaelirium) root, Blessed Thistle, Squaw Vine (Partridge Berry)

Planetary Herbals
MenoChange™ (Tablet)

Chaste Tree (Vitex), **Dong Quai**, Wild Yam, Anemarrhena (Zhi-Mu) root, Atractylodes (Bai-Zhu) rhizome, Bupleurum, Epimedium (Horny Goat Weed) leaf, Gardenia fruit, Tree Peony, Amur Cork Tree (Phellodendron) bark, Poria Mushroom, Peony (White, Chinese), Ginger, Motherwort leaf, **Licorice**, **Black Cohosh**; Non-Herbal: Calcium Citrate, Magnesium, Sodium, Fiber

Grandma's Herbs
Menopause (Capsule)

Black Cohosh, Lady's Mantle, Squaw Vine (Partridge Berry), Blessed Thistle, Blue Cohosh, False Unicorn (Helonias, Chamaelirium), Eleuthero, Shepherd's Purse leaf, Raspberry (Red), Sarsaparilla, St. John's Wort

Eclectic Institute
Menopause Support (Capsule)

Soybean, **Black Cohosh**, Oat seed (milky)

NOW Foods
Menopause Support (Capsule)

Dong Quai root, Raspberry (Red) leaf, **Chaste Tree (Vitex)**, Red Clover leaf, **Black Cohosh root**, Wild Yam root, **Licorice**, Ginger; Non-Herbal: 5-HTP, Soy Isoflavones (Non-GMO)

Herbs Etc.
Menopautonic™ (Alcohol Extract or Softgel)

Dong Quai root, **Chaste Tree (Vitex) berry**, Hawthorn leaf and flower, Motherwort, False Unicorn (Helonias, Chamaelirium), **Licorice root**, Passionflower, **Black Cohosh root**, Eleuthero root, Pipsissewa, **Ginseng (American) root**

Solaray
Natural Change Blend™ SP-7D™ (Capsule)

Red Clover flower, **Black Cohosh**, Pomegranate seed, Raspberry (Red) leaf, Wild Yam, Fenugreek, Butternut bark, Fennel

Herb Pharm
Phytoestrogen Tonic™ (Alcohol Extract)

Black Cohosh, **Chaste Tree (Vitex)**, Saw Palmetto, Sage, **Licorice**

Herbalist & Alchemist
Replenish Compound™ (Alcohol Extract)

Oat seed (milky), Shatavari root, White Pond Lilly, **Licorice**

Planetary Herbals
Wild Yam-Black Cohosh Complex™ (Tablet)

Black Cohosh, **Dong Quai**, **Dong Quai**, **Ginseng (American)**, Sarsaparilla, **Licorice**, Wild Yam, Wild Yam, Kelp, Ginger, Saw Palmetto, Saw Palmetto, Oregon Grape; Non-Herbal: Calcium, Iodine

Vitanica
Woman's Passage™ (Capsule)

Hops, St. John's Wort, **Black Cohosh**

Vitanica
Women's Phase II™ (Capsule)

Dong Quai, **Licorice**, Burdock root, Motherwort leaf, Wild Yam

Herbalist & Alchemist
Women's Transition Compound™ (Alcohol Extract)

Chaste Tree (Vitex), **Black Cohosh**, Blue Vervain flowering tops, **Dong Quai**, Night Blooming Cereus (Cactus) stem

Menstrual Cramp Formulas

See also *Antispasmodic* and *PMS Relieving Formulas*

This is a subcategory of *Antispasmodic Formulas* aimed at easing cramping associated with a woman's monthly menstrual cycle. These remedies have many of the same key herbs as *Antispasmodic Formulas* and may be used for many of the same problems. See *Dysmenorrhea* and *Cramps (menstrual)* in the *Conditions Section* for additional suggestions. Also consider *PMS Relieving Formulas*.

Key Herbs: Black Cohosh, Blue Cohosh, Cramp Bark, Lobelia and Wild Yam

Planetary Herbals
Cramp Bark Comfort™ (Tablet)

Dong Quai, Squaw Vine (Partridge Berry) aerial parts, **Cramp Bark**, Chaste Tree (Vitex), Poria Mushroom, Cypress rhizome, Ginger; Non-Herbal: Calcium

Vitanica
Cramp Bark Extra™ (Capsule)

Cramp Bark, Valerian, **Black Cohosh**, Ginger; Non-Herbal: Rutin, Vitamin C, Vitamin E, Vitamin B6, Vitamin B3, Calcium , Magnesium

Eclectic Institute
Dong Quai - Wild Yam (Glycerine Extract)

Dong Quai, **Wild Yam**, **Blue Cohosh**, Chaste Tree (Vitex)

Herbalist & Alchemist
Full Moon-Women's Anti-Spasmodic™ (Alcohol Extract)

Black Haw bark, Cypress root, Chamomile flower, **Wild Yam**, Corydalis rhizome, Jamaican Dogwood bark

Nature's Way
PMS with Vitamin B6 & 5-HTP (Capsule)

Black Cohosh, **Wild Yam**, Dandelion leaf, **Lobelia stem, leaf & flower**, **Cramp Bark**; Non-Herbal: L-5-Hydroxytryptophan

Eclectic Institute
Red Raspberry - Squawvine (Glycerine Extract)

Raspberry (Red) leaf, Squaw Vine (Partridge Berry) aerial parts, **Cramp Bark**, **Blue Cohosh**, Raspberry (Red)

Eclectic Institute
Uterine Balance (Capsule)

Cramp Bark, **Cramp Bark**, Kava Kava, Black Haw root & bark, Yarrow flower & leaf

Mineral Formulas

See also *Joint Healing* and *Tissue Healing Formulas*

Our bodies are made from the "dust of the earth" or minerals. Minerals are needed for healthy bones, teeth and connective tissues. Minerals in the form of electrolytes maintain fluid movement throughout the body. Minerals are co-factors for the enzymes that produce hormones, neurotransmitters and other chemicals the body needs to function. Minerals are even involved in detoxification. In short, all body processes require minerals.

The minerals in plants are much more readily absorbed and utilized by the tissues than the typical minerals found in mineral supplements. This is because herbs contain complexes of minerals along with vitamins and co-factors that aid assimilation and utilization.

Herbal *Mineral Formulas* are helpful in supplying minerals for healthy bones, teeth and tissues. They can improve the quality and health of hair, skin and nails. They can speed the healing of broken bones and other injuries. They can also aid recovery from surgery. *Mineral Formulas* can be used much like *Tissue Healing Formulas* and they combine well with *Joint Healing Formulas.*

Key Herbs: Alfalfa, Horsetail, Nettle (Stinging) and Oat

Solaray
Bone & Tissue Blend™ SP-34™ (Capsule)

Horsetail, Plantain, Parsley aerial parts, Marshmallow, Slippery Elm, Burdock root, Myrrh

Nature's Way
Hair & Skin (Capsule)

Capsicum (Cayenne), He Shou Wu (Fo-Ti), **Horsetail**, Kelp, **Nettle (Stinging) leaf**, **Oat straw**, Rosemary, Amla (Indian Gooseberry); Non-Herbal: Methyl Sulfonyl Methane (MSM), Glucosamine, Protease I, Protease II, Peptizyme, Amylase, Lactase, Invertase, Lipase, Celluase, Alpha Galactosidase, Biotin

Solaray
Hair Blend™ SP-38™ (Capsule)

Saw Palmetto, **Horsetail**, Watercress, Juniper berry, Willow (White) bark, Rosemary

Gaia Herbs
Hair, Skin & Nail Support (Liquid Phyto-Caps)

Triphala, **Horsetail**, Burdock root, **Alfalfa aerial parts**, Gotu Kola leaf, **Nettle (Stinging) leaf**; Non-Herbal: Astaxanthin

Herbalist & Alchemist
Herb-Cal™ (Alcohol Tincture)

Horsetail, **Oat seed (milky)**, **Nettle (Stinging) leaf**, **Alfalfa**, Chamomile flower; Non-Herbal: Organic egg shell vinegar

Western Botanicals
Herbal Calcium (Capsule)

Spinach, White Oak bark, Pau d'Arco, Plantain, **Horsetail**, Dandelion leaf, Kelp, Irish Moss, Dulse, **Nettle (Stinging) leaf**

Christopher's
Herbal Calcium Formula (Capsule and Glycerine Extract)

Horsetail, **Nettle (Stinging) leaf**, **Oat straw**, Lobelia

Christopher's
Kid-e-Calc (Vinegar Extract)

Horsetail, **Nettle (Stinging)**, **Oat straw**, Lobelia; Non-Herbal: Apple Cider Vinegar

Grandma's Herbs
Kid-e-Calc (Vinegar Extract)

Horsetail, **Nettle (Stinging) leaf**, **Oat straw**, Valerian; Non-Herbal: Apple Cider Vinegar

Grandma's Herbs
Kid-e-Mins (Glycerine Extract)

Alfalfa, Barley grass, Wheat, Rose, **Oat straw**, Dulse, Ginger, Dandelion, Kelp, Spirulina, Irish Moss root, Beet, Capsicum (Cayenne), Violet, Carrot; Non-Herbal: Nutritional Yeast

Vitanica
Luminous™ (Capsule)

Horsetail, **Nettle (Stinging) leaf**, Gotu Kola, Rosemary, **Oat straw**; Non-Herbal: Vitamin C, Vitamin D2, Vitamin E, Biotin, Calcium, Magnesium, Selenium, Zinc, Silica,

Herbalist & Alchemist
Osteo Herb™ (Capsule)

Nettle (Stinging) leaf, **Alfalfa**, Dandelion leaf, **Horsetail**, **Oat straw**, Black Pepper seed

Herbalist & Alchemist
Osteo Herb™ (Capsule)

Nettle (Stinging) leaf, **Alfalfa**, Dandelion leaf, **Horsetail**, **Oat straw**, Black Pepper

Moistening Lung/Cough Formulas

See also *Cough Remedy, Decongestant* and *Expectorant Formulas*

This is a subcategory of *Cough Remedy Formulas* and is related to *Expectorant* and *Decongestant Formulas.* Key herbs in these formulas are suited to dry, irritated coughs or dehydrated lung tissue where there is very little mucus being produced and/or expelled. They may also be helpful for more chronic, deep-seated respiratory conditions or respiratory irritation brought on by living in dry climates. These contain respiratory herbs with moistening herbs that help hydrate the lungs to promote normal mucus secretions.

Key Herbs: Astragalus, Elecampane, Fritillary, Licorice, Marshmallow, Mullein and Slippery Elm

Nature's Herbs (TwinLab)
CL-7 Formula (Capsule)

Mullein leaf, **Marshmallow root**, **Slippery Elm bark**, Pine (White) bark, Chickweed aerial parts, Hyssop leaf, Black Pepper fruit, Rosemary oil; Non-Herbal: N-Acetyl L-Cysteine, Rice flour, gelatin, medium chain triglycerides, vitamin E

Gaia Herbs
GaiaKids® Cough Syrup for Dry Coughs

Star Anise, Cramp Bark, Ginger, Grindelia (Gumweed), Irish Moss, **Marshmallow**, **Mullein**, Plantain

Western Botanicals
Herbal Cough Syrup (Glycerine Extract)

Cherry (Wild) bark, **Licorice**, **Slippery Elm**, Elder (canadensis) berry, **Marshmallow**, Echinacea root, **Mullein leaf**, Fennel, Horehound, Turkey Rhubarb, Usnea, Lobelia, Lobelia seed, Clove, Ginger, Eucalyptus essential oil, Lemon essential oil, Tea Tree essential oil; Non-Herbal: Pure honey, vegetable glycerine

Herbs for Kids
Horehound Blend™ (Glycerine Extract)

Mullein leaf, **Astragalus**, Horehound, Sage, Orange peel, Oregon Grape, Ginger, Eucalyptus essential oil

Christopher's
Kid-e-Soothe (Glycerine Extract)

Marshmallow, **Astragalus**

Planetary Herbals
Loquat Respiratory Syrup

Loquat leaf, Fritillary bulb, Black Cherry bark, **Slippery Elm**, Platycodon, Trichosanthes seed, Polygala, Poria Mushroom, Schisandra, **Licorice (Chinese)**, Peppermint essential oil; Non-Herbal: Honey, Blackstrap Molasses

Planetary Herbals
Loquat Respiratory Syrup for Kids (Glycerine Extract)

Loquat leaf, Fritillary bulb, Black Cherry bark, **Slippery Elm**, Platycodon, Trichosanthes seed, Polygala, Poria Mushroom, Schisandra, **Licorice**

Christopher's
Lung & Bronchial Formula (Capsule and Glycerine Extract)

Marshmallow leaf, **Mullein**, Chickweed root, Lobelia root, Pleurisy root

Solaray
Lung Caps™ (Capsule)

Pleurisy root, Cherry (Wild) bark, **Slippery Elm**, Clove

Herbalist & Alchemist
Lung Relief Cold/Dry Compound™ (Alcohol Tincture)

Astragalus, Prince Seng root, Asparagus (Chinese) root, **Licorice**, Spikenard

Herbalist & Alchemist
Lung Relief Hot/Dry Compound™ (Alcohol Extract)

Horehound, Platycodon, Red Clover, **Elecampane root**, Ophiopogon

Traditional Medicinals
Throat Coat® Herbal Syrup

Licorice, Cherry (Wild) bark, Fennel fruit, Cinnamon bark, Orange peel, **Slippery Elm**, **Marshmallow**, **Licorice**, Peppermint leaf; Non-Herbal: Honey

Traditional Medicinals
Throat Coat® Lemon Echinacea (Tea)

Echinacea (purpurea) root, **Licorice**, **Licorice**, **Marshmallow leaf**, Lemon Myrtle leaf, **Marshmallow**, Fennel fruit, Orange peel, Cinnamon bark

Gaia Herbs
Throat Shield Tea

Fennel, Grindelia (Gumweed), **Licorice**, **Marshmallow**, Peppermint essential oil, Sage essential oil, Sage

Mushroom Blend Formulas

See also *Immune Balancing* and *Immune Stimulating Formulas*

This is a subcategory of both *Immune Stimulating Formulas* and *Immune Balancing Formulas*. This is because medical mushrooms tend to balance the immune system, strengthening it when it is weak and toning it down if it is overactive.

Mushrooms have long been used in Chinese medicine as tonics to help ward off colds, flu and other contagious diseases. They can be taken during the cold winter months to keep the immune system strong. Key mushrooms found in these formulas include cordyceps, maitake, reishi and shiitake. Other mushrooms in these formulas (but not discussed in this book) are agaricus, turkey tail and snow fungus.

These formulas are also used for both immune deficiency conditions (such as cancer and AIDS) and autoimmune conditions. However, some people with autoimmune conditions may not do well on them. See the caution under *Immune Stimulating Formulas*.

Key Herbs: Cordyceps, Maitake, Reishi (Ganoderma) and Shiitake

New Chapter
LifeShield® Breathe (Capsule)

Cordyceps, **Reishi (Ganoderma)**, Chaga Mushroom, Poria Mushroom

New Chapter
LifeShield® Immunity (Capsule)

Reishi (Ganoderma), **Shiitake Mushroom**, Lion's Mane Mushroom, **Cordyceps**, **Maitake Mushroom**, Poria Mushroom, Mesima Mushroom, Coriolus Mushroom, Chaga Mushroom

New Chapter
LifeShield® Liver Force® (Capsule)

Coriolus Mushroom, **Cordyceps**, Mesima Mushroom, **Reishi (Ganoderma)**, **Shiitake Mushroom**, Poria Mushroom

New Chapter
LifeShield® Mind Force (Capsule)

Lion's Mane Mushroom, **Reishi (Ganoderma)**, **Cordyceps**, Poria Mushroom, Chaga Mushroom

Eclectic Institute
Maitake (Capsule)

Maitake Mushroom, Ginger freeze-dried

Solaray
Mushroom Complete™ (Capsule)

Oyster Mushroom, **Cordyceps**, Turkey Tail Mushroom, Agaricus, Royal, Lion's Mane Mushroom, **Shiitake Mushroom**, **Maitake Mushroom**, Reishi (Ganoderma)

Herbs Etc.
Mushrooms Seven Source™ (Alcohol Extract)

Reishi (Ganoderma), **Shiitake Mushroom**, **Maitake Mushroom**, Oyster Mushroom, Agaricus, Snow fungus, **Cordyceps**

Eclectic Institute
Mycetoblend (Capsule)

Reishi (Ganoderma), **Maitake Mushroom**, Split Gill, Chaga Mushroom, **Shiitake Mushroom**, Turkey Tail Mushroom, Zhu-Ling, Polypore, Ice Man, Polypore, Tinder, Larch (Larix)

Eclectic Institute
Original 7 Mushrooms
(Capsule and Alcohol Extract)

Royal Sun Agaricus, **Cordyceps**, Lion's Mane Mushroom, Turkey Tail Mushroom, **Reishi (Ganoderma)**, **Maitake Mushroom**, Zhu-Ling, **Reishi (Ganoderma)**, **Maitake Mushroom**, Zhu-Ling

Herbalist & Alchemist
Seven Precious Mushrooms™ (Alcohol Extract)

Reishi (Ganoderma), Chaga Mushroom, **Shiitake Mushroom**, **Maitake Mushroom**, **Cordyceps** (militaris)

Nature's Way
Shiitake–Maitake Standardized (Capsule)

Oat seed, **Shiitake Mushroom**, **Shiitake Mushroom**, **Maitake Mushroom**, **Maitake Mushroom**

Nursing Aid Formulas

These formulas are used to enhance the production of breast milk. They may also help to enrich breast milk.

Key Herbs: Blessed Thistle, Fennel, Fenugreek, Marshmallow and Milk Thistle

Gaia Herbs
Lactation Support (Liquid Phyto-Caps)

Fenugreek, **Fennel**, Raspberry (Red) leaf, **Blessed Thistle**, **Marshmallow**

Gaia Herbs
Lactation Support Tea

Fennel, **Fenugreek**, Goat's Rue, Lemon Balm leaf, **Marshmallow**, Nettle (Stinging) leaf

Western Botanicals
Lactation Tea

Raspberry (Red) leaf, Nettle (Stinging) leaf, **Fennel**, Chamomile flower, Oat tops, **Fenugreek**, **Blessed Thistle**, Alfalfa leaf

Vitanica
LactationBlend™ (Capsule)

Goat's Rue aerial parts, **Fennel**, Nettle (Stinging) leaf, **Blessed Thistle**, Vervain, Borage seed, flower & flowering tops, Hops, Oat straw, Raspberry (Red) leaf, Chaste Tree (Vitex), **Fenugreek**, **Milk Thistle seed**

Herb Pharm
Mother's Lactation™ (Alcohol Extract)

Chaste Tree (Vitex), **Fenugreek**, Caraway seed, **Fennel**, Anise seed

Traditional Medicinals
Mother's Milk® (Tea)

Fennel fruit, Anise fruit, Coriander fruit, **Fenugreek**, **Blessed Thistle**, Spearmint, Lemongrass leaf, Lemon Verbena, **Marshmallow**

Yogi Tea
Woman's Nursing Support™ (Tea)

Chamomile flower, **Fennel**, Nettle (Stinging) leaf, Anise seed, **Fenugreek**, Lavender flower

Phytoestrogen Formulas

See also *Female Hormonal Balancing* and *Menopause Balancing Formulas*

Estrogen is not a single hormone. A woman's body makes three different kinds of estrogen. There are also estrogen-like compounds in plants called phytoestrogens. Phytoestrogens bind to estrogen receptor sites and may help protect the body from environmental toxins with estrogenic effects (xenoestrogens). See Avoid *Xenoestrogens* in the *Therapies Section*.

Research suggests that plants containing phytoestrogens may have a protective effect against breast and other estrogen-dependent cancers. They may also be helpful in easing the transition of menopause. *Phytoestrogen Formulas* are related to *Female Hormone Balancing Formulas* and *Menopause Balancing Formulas* and contain some of the same key herbs.

Key Herbs: Black Cohosh, Flax Seed, Hops and Red Clover

Nature's Way
EstroSoy™ (Capsule)

Soybean, **Red Clover flower**; Non-Herbal: Vitamin C

Nature's Way
EstroSoy™ Plus (Capsule)

Soybean, **Red Clover flower**, **Black Cohosh**; Non-Herbal: Vitamin C

Vitanica
HRT Companion™ (Capsule)

Garlic, **Flax seed**, Green Tea, Milk Thistle, Soybean; Non-Herbal: Vitamin C, Vitamin E, Vitamin B6 , Folate, Vitamin B12, DIM (Diindolymethane), Phosphatidylserine,

Grandma's Herbs
Kokoro EstroHerb Cream (Salve)

Black Cohosh, **Red Clover**, Dong Quai, Evening Primrose oil; Non-Herbal: Phytestrogen

Eclectic Institute
Menopause Support (Capsule)

Soybean, **Black Cohosh**, Oat seed (milky)

Vitanica
PhytoEstrogen Herbal™ (Bulk Powder)

Flax seed, Soybean, **Black Cohosh**, Alfalfa leaf, **Red Clover leaf & flower**

PMS Relieving Formulas

See also *Female Hormonal Balancing*, *Menstrual Cramp* and *Uterine Tonic Formulas*

This is a subcategory of *Female Hormonal Balancing Formulas* targeted at PMS. These formulas have some of the benefits of *Menstrual Cramp Formulas*, as well. Since PMS is not a disease but a collection of symptoms that vary widely from one woman to the next, please read about the various types of *PMS* in the *Conditions Section* to help you select appropriate formulas and lifestyle changes for your particular symptoms.

Key Herbs: Black Cohosh, Black Haw, Blessed Thistle, Blue Cohosh, Chastetree (Vitex), Cramp Bark and Wild Yam

Irwin Naturals
Menstrual Relief Hormone Balance (Softgel)

Flax seed, Pumpkin seed, Maca root, Shatavari root, Dandelion root, Raspberry (Red) leaf, **Chaste Tree (Vitex) fruit**, Rose petals, Black Pepper; Non-Herbal: Vitamin B6, Magnesium Citrate, DIM (Diindolymethane)

Herb Pharm
Phytoestrogen Tonic™ (Alcohol Extract)

Black Cohosh, **Chaste Tree (Vitex)**, Saw Palmetto, Sage, Licorice

Herb Pharm
PMS Comfort Tonic™ (Alcohol Extract)

Chaste Tree (Vitex), Dong Quai, Motherwort leaf & flower, Muira Puama stem & bark, Ginger

Eclectic Institute
PMS Support (Capsule)

Chaste Tree (Vitex), Dandelion whole plant, Bladderwrack, Ginger

Nature's Way
PMS with Vitamin B6 & 5-HTP (Capsule)

Black Cohosh, **Wild Yam**, Dandelion leaf, Lobelia stem, leaf & flower, **Cramp Bark**; Non-Herbal: L-5-Hydroxytryptophan

Vitanica
Women's Phase I™ (Capsule)

Kelp, Borage seed, **Wild Yam**, Dandelion leaf, Dong Quai, Passionflower, St. John's Wort, **Chaste Tree (Vitex)**, Ginkgo; Non-Herbal: Chromium, Vitamin E, Vitamin B6, Calcium, Magnesium

Poultice Formulas

See also *Topical Vulnerary Formulas*

A poultice is a paste made of herbs mixed with a little water that is applied topically to promote healing. Poultices can be used where there is swelling and irritation to tissues. They can help draw toxins out of the tissues and speed healing. There are only three commercial formulas listed under this category. One was designed for application to the breast, another for making a vaginal bolus and

Herbal Formulas

the third is an encapsulated product that can be made into a poultice by emptying the contents of the capsule. All of these formulas can be used in applications where a poultice could be helpful.

Poultices can be highly effective in promoting tissue healing. They work like *Topical Vulnerary Formulas* and use similar key herbs. See *Poultice* in the *Therapies Section* to learn how to make a poultice.

Key Herbs: Comfrey, Marshmallow, Plantain and Slippery Elm

Marshmallow, Chamomile, **Plantain**, Yarrow, **Comfrey leaf**

Nature's Sunshine Products
PLS II (Capsule)

Slippery Elm, **Marshmallow**, Goldenseal, Goldenseal, Fenugreek

Christopher's
VB Herbal Bolus (Bulk Powder)

Slippery Elm, Squaw Vine (Partridge Berry), **Comfrey root**, Yellow Dock, **Marshmallow**, Chickweed, Goldenseal, Mullein

Pre-Delivery Formulas

See also *Pregnancy Tonic Formulas*

These formulas are used for the specific purpose of aiding delivery in pregnancy. They are sometimes known as 5-week formulas because they are taken during the last five weeks of pregnancy (starting five weeks from the expected due date). They are used to help prepare the body for labor and delivery and help prevent overdue pregnancies.

Two herbs commonly used in *Pre-Delivery Formulas* are blue cohosh and pennyroyal. Both of these herbs stimulate uterine contractions. Both are contraindicated during the early stages of pregnancy as they may cause miscarriage or damage to the fetus.

Key Herbs: Black Cohosh, Blessed Thistle, Blue Cohosh and Pennyroyal

Nature's Sunshine Products
5-W (Capsule)

Black Cohosh, Dong Quai, Butcher's Broom, Raspberry (Red)

Grandma's Herbs
Deliverease (Capsule)

Raspberry (Red), **Blue Cohosh**, Squaw Vine (Partridge Berry), **Blessed Thistle**, Pennyroyal, Wild Yam, False Unicorn (Helonias, Chamaelirium), Bladder Pod

Christopher's
Prenatal Formula (Capsule)

Squaw Vine (Partridge Berry), **Blessed Thistle**, **Black Cohosh**, Pennyroyal, False Unicorn (Helonias, Chamaelirium) root, Raspberry (Red) leaf, Lobelia

Pregnancy Tonic Formulas

See also *Pre-Delivery* and *Uterine Tonic Formulas*

It is a good idea to be careful when using herbs during pregnancy. However, there are many herbs that are not only safe to use during pregnancy, they are actually beneficial. *Pregnancy Tonic Formulas* contain herbs that can help a woman to have a healthier pregnancy and an easier delivery. Some of the formulas in this group are used to help a woman get pregnant, while others are used as tonics to be used during pregnancy. Read the labels to determine which formulas are used for which purpose.

Key Herbs: Alfalfa, False Unicorn (Helonias), Nettle (Stinging) and Red Raspberry

Vitanica
Maternal Symmetry™ (Capsule)

Kelp, **Raspberry (Red) leaf**, **Nettle (Stinging) leaf**, Squaw Vine (Partridge Berry), Lemon Balm, Oat straw, Dandelion root, Ginger; Non-Herbal: Vitamin A, Vitamin C, Zinc, Vitamin D2 , Folic acid, Vitamin B12,Vitamin B6, Boron, Vitamin B3, Pantothenic Acid, Calcium, Magnesium, Manganese, Vitamin E, Vitamin K, Selenium, Chromium, Thiamin, Copper, Riboflavin, Iron, Iodine Biotin

Western Botanicals
Mother's Tea

Raspberry (Red) leaf, Dandelion leaf, **Nettle (Stinging) leaf**, Peppermint leaf

Vitanica
Pregnancy Prep™ (Capsule)

Tribulus, Rhodiola, Chaste Tree (Vitex), **Raspberry (Red) leaf**, **Alfalfa**, Dong Quai, Motherwort, **False Unicorn (Helonias, Chamaelirium)**; Non-Herbal: Amylase, Protease, Lipase, Cellulose, Lactase

Traditional Medicinals
Pregnancy® Tea

Raspberry (Red) leaf, Strawberry leaf, **Nettle (Stinging) leaf**, Spearmint, Fennel fruit, Rose hips, **Alfalfa leaf**, Lemon Verbena

Yogi Tea
Woman's Mother to Be® (Tea)

Raspberry (Red) leaf, Peppermint leaf, **Nettle (Stinging) leaf**, Spearmint, Dandelion root, Fennel seed, Cardamom seed

Prostate Formulas

See also *Male Glandular Tonic Formulas*

This is a subcategory of *Male Glandular Tonic Formulas* aimed primarily at aiding benign prostate hyperplasia (BPH) and prostatitis (inflammation of the prostate). They help relieve irritation, swelling and enlargement of the prostate gland.

The main key herb used in these formulas is saw palmetto, not because saw palmetto is necessarily the best herb for the prostate, but because scientific studies have been done demonstrating its effectiveness in relieving symptoms of BPH. By combining saw palmetto with other herbs that can help the prostate, formulas are likely to be more effective. For additional information read about *Benign Prostate Hyperplasia* and *Prostatitis* in the *Conditions Section* of this book.

Key Herbs: Buchu, Nettle (Stinging), Pumpkin Seed, Pygeum Bark and Saw Palmetto

Irwin Naturals
Daily Prostate Defense (Tablet)

Saw Palmetto, Tomato, Ginger, Papaya

Planetary Herbals
Damiana Male Potential™ (Tablet)

Saw Palmetto, Sarsaparilla, Damiana (aphrodisiaca) aerial parts, Schisandra, Ophiopogon, Ginseng (Korean, Asian), Cinnamon (cassia) bark, Horny Goat Weed aerial parts, Noni (Morinda) root, Ginkgo

Herb Pharm
Healthy Prostate Tonic™ (Alcohol Extract)

Saw Palmetto, **Nettle (Stinging) root**, Pipsissewa, Cleavers (Bedstraw), Thuja

New Chapter
LycoPom® (Capsule)

Tomato, Pomegranate, Sea Buckthorn seed, Rose hips, Turmeric, Saffron, Rosemary, Calendula (Marigold) flower

Christopher's
Male Urinary Tract Formula (Capsule)

Capsicum (Cayenne), Ginger, Goldenseal, Gravel Root root, Juniper berry, Marshmallow, Parsley root, Uva Ursi, Ginseng (American)

Herbalist & Alchemist
Men's Prostate Tonic™ (Alcohol Extract)

Saw Palmetto, Collinsonia (Stoneroot), **Nettle (Stinging) root**, White Sage

Nature's Answer
Prost-Answer (Glycerine Extract)

Saw Palmetto, Pumpkin seed, Corn Silk, **Buchu leaf**, Bladderwrack, Parsley leaf, Capsicum (Cayenne)

Irwin Naturals
Prosta-Strong (Softgel)

Saw Palmetto, **Nettle (Stinging) leaf**, **Pygeum bark**, Green Tea, Pumpkin seed, Black Pepper, Ginger; Non-Herbal: Zinc Picolinate, Fish Oil, Graminex™ Flower Pollen, Quercetin, 10% Beta-Sitosterol, Lyc-O-Mato Tomato extract

Grandma's Herbs
Prostate (Capsule)

Corn Silk, Parsley leaf, **Saw Palmetto**, **Buchu**, Echinacea, Marshmallow, Dandelion seed, Pumpkin, Uva Ursi

New Chapter
Prostate 5LX® (Softgel)

Saw Palmetto, Green Tea leaf, Pumpkin oil, Ginger, **Nettle (Stinging) root**, Rosemary

Solaray
Prostate Blend™ SP-16™ (Capsule)

Saw Palmetto, Pumpkin seed, Corn Silk, Parsley aerial parts, Ginger, **Nettle (Stinging) root**, Kelp, Burdock root

Solaray
Prostate Caps™ (Capsule)

Parsley leaf, Corn Silk, **Saw Palmetto**, Clove, Capsicum (Cayenne), Pumpkin seed

Gaia Herbs
Prostate Health (Liquid Phyto-Caps)

Nettle (Stinging) root, Green Tea leaf, White Sage aerial parts, Rosemary, Pumpkin oil, Pomegranate arils and seed oil

NOW Foods
Prostate Health Clinical Strength (Capsule)

Saw Palmetto, **Nettle (Stinging) root**, Turmeric, Pumpkin seed oil, Green Tea, Pomegranate fruit, Japanese Knotweed (Hu Zhang), Flax seed; Non-Herbal: Vitamin D-3, Zinc, Selenium, Phytosterols, Quercetin, Lycopene

Christopher's
Prostate Plus Formula (Capsule)

Saw Palmetto, Mullein, Ginkgo

Western Botanicals
Prostate Plus Formula (Capsule and Alcohol Extract)

Saw Palmetto, Ginseng (American), Eleuthero root, Ginkgo, Oat tops, **Pygeum**, Sarsaparilla, Ginseng (Korean, Asian), Mullein leaf & flower, Pumpkin seed, Scullcap (Skullcap), **Buchu leaf**, Capsicum (chinense)

Eclectic Institute
Prostate Support (Capsule)

Saw Palmetto, **Nettle (Stinging) root**, Kava Kava, Corn Silk

NOW Foods
Prostate Support (Softgel)

Saw Palmetto, **Pygeum**, **Nettle (Stinging) root**, Pumpkin seed oil; Non-Herbal: Vitamin B-6, Zinc, Lycopene

New Chapter
Prostate Take Care™ (Softgel)

Saw Palmetto, Green Tea leaf, Pumpkin oil, Ginger, **Nettle (Stinging) root**, Rosemary

Traditional Medicinals
Prostate Tea with Nettle Root

Green Tea leaf, **Nettle (Stinging) root**

Nature's Way
Prostate with Saw Palmetto (Capsule)

Saw Palmetto, Dandelion leaf, Soybean, Oat bran; Non-Herbal: Calcium, Zinc, Beta Glucan Extract

Herbal Formulas

Herbs Etc.

Prostatonic™ (Alcohol Extract)

Saw Palmetto berry, Yarrow flowering tops, Dong Quai root, **Nettle (Stinging) root**, Ginseng (American) root, Damiana (diffusa) leaf, Cleavers (Bedstraw), Pipsissewa, Yerba mansa root, Sarsaparilla root

RidgeCrest Herbals

ProstEase™ (Capsule)

Echinacea root, Eleuthero root, **Nettle (Stinging) leaf**, Parsley, Pumpkin seed, **Pygeum bark**, Sandalwood, **Saw Palmetto berry**, Watermelon seed; Non-Herbal: Agnus Castus 6X, Avena Sativa 6X, Conium Maculatum 12X, Lycopodium Clavatum 12X, Nux Vomica 12X, Phosphoricum Acidum 12X, Selenium Metallicum 12X, Alanine, Glutamic acid, Glycine, Zinc Aspartate

Nature's Way

Prostol™ (Capsule)

Saw Palmetto, **Nettle (Stinging) root**

Nature's Answer

ProstSupport™ w/Ester C (Capsule)

Saw Palmetto, Tomato, Capsicum (Cayenne), **Pygeum**, Pumpkin seed, Maitake Mushroom; Non-Herbal: Vitamin C (as Ester-C), Vitamin E, Zinc, Selenium

NOW Foods

Pygeum & Saw Palmetto (Capsule)

Saw Palmetto, **Pygeum bark**, Pumpkin seed oil

Eclectic Institute

Saw Palmetto - Nettles
(Alcohol Extract and Glycerine Extract)

Saw Palmetto, **Nettle (Stinging) root**, Echinacea (angustifolia) root, Pipsissewa, Ocotillo bark, Red Cedar leaf

Solaray

Saw Palmetto & Nettle Root with Pumpkin (Capsule)

Nettle (Stinging) root, Pumpkin seed, **Saw Palmetto**

Planetary Herbals

Saw Palmetto Classic™ (Tablet)

Saw Palmetto, Pumpkin oil, **Pygeum**, Echinacea (purpurea) root, Echinacea (pallida) root, Gardenia fruit, Asian Water Plantain rhizome, Chinese Salvia root, Gravel Root root, Codonopsis root, Dodder seed, Ligustrum fruit, Asian Water Plantain seed, Dong Quai; Non-Herbal: Sodium, fiber, calcium

New Chapter

Zyflamend® Prostate (Softgel)

Saw Palmetto, Green Tea leaf, Chinese Scullcap (Scute/Huang Qin), Pumpkin oil, Ginger, Rosemary, Turmeric, **Nettle (Stinging) root**, Holy Basil leaf, Japanese Knotweed (Hu Zhang) root, Coptis (Chinese Goldthread,Huang Lian) root, Barberry root, Oregano leaf

Quit Smoking Formulas

See also *Lung* and *Respiratory Tonic Formulas*

Tobacco is a powerful drug and smoking is a very difficult addiction to kick. *Quit Smoking Formulas* are herbal formulas that can aid the process. One of the most important key herbs in these formulas is lobelia. Lobelia contains an alkaloid called lobeline that attaches to the same receptor sites as nicotine. Lobeline, however, relaxes, rather than stimulates, these receptors. This makes lobelia very useful for reducing tobacco cravings.

Other herbs in these formulas can help soothe the nerves and make quitting easier. As part of your stop smoking efforts, it is also important to rebuild the lungs. Use Lung and Respiratory Tonic Formulas to strengthen the lungs and overcome some of the damage caused by smoking. See *Addictions (tobacco smoking or chewing)* in the *Conditions Section*.

Key Herbs: Chamomile (English and Roman), Licorice, Lobelia, Oat, Passionflower and St. John's wort

Grandma's Herbs

Kick-It (Capsule)

Bladder Pod, Mullein leaf, **Passionflower**, Ginseng (Korean, Asian), Valerian, Sarsaparilla, Peppermint, Chaparral (Creosote), Eucalyptus, Kelp, Black Cohosh, Sage, Calamus (Sweet Flag)

Gaia Herbs

Nicotine Relief (Liquid Phyto-Caps)

Lobelia, **Lobelia seed**, **Oat seed (milky)**, **St. John's Wort flowering tops**, **Passionflower vine**, **Licorice**

Herbs Etc.

Smoke Free® (Spray, Softgel)

Lobelia, **Oat seed (milky)**, Osha root, **Licorice root**, **Passionflower**, Pleurisy root, Grindelia (Gumweed) flower, Mullein leaf, Ginger root

Christopher's

Smoke Out (Alcohol Extract)

Oat, **Lobelia**, Rose hips, Capsicum (Cayenne)

Herbalist & Alchemist

Smoker's ResQ™ (Alcohol Extract)

Oat seed (milky), Scullcap (Skullcap) flowering tops, **Licorice**, Plantain, **Lobelia flower**, **Lobelia seed**; Non-Herbal: Apple cider vinegar

Renew Life

Smokers' Cleanse™ (Capsule and Tablet)

Fenugreek, Malabar Nut Tree leaf, Mullein leaf, Wasabi, Pine bark, Orange, Ashwagandha root, Kava Kava, **Chamomile flower**, Hops strobile, Lemon Balm leaf, Meadowsweet, Scullcap (Skullcap); Non-Herbal: Vitamin C, N-Acetyl L-Cysteine, L-Glutamine, GABA, L-Tyrosine, Xylitol, Vitamin B-6, 5-HTP, Cane Juice Extract

Relaxing Nervine Formulas

See also *Antispasmodic* and *Sleep Formulas*

In modern society we face a great deal of mental and emotional stress. As a result we can become chronically "uptight" from excessive activity in our sympathetic nervous system. *Relaxing Nervine Formulas* contain herbs that activate the parasympathetic nervous system and sedate the sympathetic nervous system. This helps a person "unwind" and relax.

The sympathetic nervous system increases heart rate and blood pressure, makes our breathing more rapid and shallow, tenses our muscles and inhibits digestion and elimination. This is part of the reason indigestion, high blood pressure, poor elimination and muscle tension are rampant in our society.

Activating the parasympathetic nervous system helps us digest our food better, lowers our blood pressure and heart rate, improves elimination and eases tension-related problems like tension headaches, neck and shoulder pain and back pain. It can help us sleep more soundly and aid the healing process, as our body heals and repairs in a more parasympathetic mode. Blends of various nervine herbs can provide these benefits.

A subcategory of this therapeutic action is *Sleep Formulas*, which contain many of the same herbs, but are targeted at helping a person relax so they can go to sleep. However, just about any *Relaxing Nervine Formula* will work as an aid to sleep. *Nerve Tonic Formulas* are another subcategory of *Relaxing Nervine Formulas*, but contain ingredients more targeted to rebuilding or tonifying damaged or weakened nerves.

Key Herbs: Blue Vervain, California Poppy, Chamomile (English and Roman), Hops, Kava-kava, Lavender, Lemon Balm, Lobelia, Passionflower, Scullcap (Skullcap) and Valerian

RidgeCrest Herbals
Anxiety Free (Capsule)
Eleuthero root, **Lemon Balm leaf**, **Passionflower**, **Lavender**, Ashwagandha, Holy Basil; Non-Herbal: Vitamins B1, B2, B3/B4, B5, B6 and B12, biotin, folic acid, choline, Inositol, GABA, L-Theanine

Herb Pharm
Anxiety Soother™ (Alcohol Extract)
Kava Kava, **Passionflower**, Bacopa (Water Hyssop), Mimosa (Albizia, Silk Tree) bark, **Lavender (angustifolia) flower and essential oil**

Gaia Herbs
Calm Restore Herbal Drops
Scullcap (Skullcap), **Blue Vervain**, **California Poppy**, **Lavender**, **Lemon Balm**, **Passionflower**

Yogi Tea
Calming™ (Tea)
Chamomile flower, Licorice, Gotu Kola, Hibiscus, Fennel, Lemongrass, Cardamom seed, Orange peel, Barley malt, Rose hips, **Lavender flower**

Herbs for Kids
Chamomile Calm™ (Glycerine Extract)
Chamomile flower, Fennel, **Hops strobile**, Wood Betony (betonica), Catnip

Traditional Medicinals
Chamomile with Lavender (Tea)
Chamomile flower, **Lavender flower**, **Lemon Balm leaf**

Herb Pharm
Children's Herbal (Glycerite)
Chamomile flower, **Lemon Balm leaf & flower**, Catnip leaf & flower, Fennel seed

Traditional Medicinals
Easy Now® (Tea)
Passionflower, **Chamomile flower**, **Lavender flower**, Catnip, Rosemary, Peppermint leaf, Spearmint, Licorice, Stevia

Nature's Way
Ex-Stress® (Capsule)
Lemon Balm leaf, Wood Betony (betonica) stem, leaf & flower, Black Cohosh, **Hops flower**, **Valerian**, Capsicum (Cayenne)

Gaia Herbs
GaiaKids® Sleep & Relax Herbal Syrup
Passionflower leaf, **Lemon Balm leaf**, **Chamomile flower**

Yogi Tea
Honey Lavender Stress Relief™ (Tea)
Rooibos (Redbush), **Chamomile flower**, **Lemon Balm leaf**, Spearmint, Lemongrass, **Lavender flower**, Peppermint leaf, Lemon Myrtle, Sage, **Passionflower**

Urban Moonshine
Joy Tonic (Alcohol Extract)
Motherwort, Linden (Basswood, Tilia), Rose, **Lemon Balm**, Lemongrass, Mugwort

Traditional Medicinals
"Just for Kids" Nighty Night® (Tea)
Passionflower, **Chamomile flower**, Linden (Basswood, Tilia) flower, Catnip, **Hops strobile**, Spearmint, Lemon Verbena, Lemon peel, Lemongrass leaf

Herbs Etc.
Kava Cool Complex™ (Alcohol Extract or Softgel)
Kava Kava root, **Chamomile flower**, St. John's Wort bud, Oat seed (milky), **Passionflower**, **Hops strobile**, **Scullcap (Skullcap)**, Stevia leaf

Eclectic Institute
Kava Kava - Calif. Poppy (Alcohol Extract and Glycerine Extract)
California Poppy, **Passionflower leaf, flower & fruit**, Jamaican Dogwood bark

Yogi Tea
Kava Stress Relief (Tea)

Carob, Sarsaparilla, Cinnamon bark, Ginger, Barley malt, **Kava Kava**, Cardamom seed, Licorice, Cinnamon essential oil

NOW Foods
Kick Back™ Tea

Chamomile flower, Spearmint leaf, Linden (Basswood, Tilia) leaf, Oat straw, **Lavender flower**, Cinnamon (burmannii) bark, Eleuthero root, Stevia leaf; Non-Herbal: Suntheanine® L-Theanine

Christopher's
Kid-e-Trac (Glycerine Extract)

Valerian, **Scullcap (Skullcap)**, Ginkgo, Oregon Grape, St. John's Wort, Mullein leaf, Gotu Kola, Sarsaparilla, Dandelion root, **Lobelia**, Alfalfa, Barley, Wheat grass

Herbalist & Alchemist
Kid's Calmpound Glycerite™ (Glycerine Extract)

Catnip flowering tops, **Chamomile flower**, Oat seed (milky), **Scullcap (Skullcap) flowering tops**

Gaia Herbs
Melissa Supreme, Alcohol-free (Glycerine Extract)

Scullcap (Skullcap), **Chamomile**, Gotu Kola, Kelp, **Lemon Balm**, **Passionflower**, Oat seed

Grandma's Herbs
NaturALL-Calm (Capsule)

St. John's Wort, **Valerian**, **Scullcap (Skullcap)**, Cedar (Juniper) berry, Black Root, **Blue Vervain**, Mistletoe, **Passionflower**, Wild Yam, Peppermint leaf, **Chamomile**, **Hops root**, **Bladder Pod**, Wood Betony (betonica), Feverfew, Blue Cohosh, Cascara Sagrada, Capsicum (Cayenne)

Solaray
Nerve Blend™ SP-14™ (Capsule)

Valerian, **Passionflower flower**, Wood Betony (betonica) aerial parts, Ginger, **Hops flower**, **Scullcap (Skullcap) aerial parts**, **Chamomile flowering tops**

Western Botanicals
Nerve Calm Formula (Capsule and Alcohol Extract)

Black Cohosh, **Valerian**, Blue Cohosh, Wild Yam, **Hops flower**, **Passionflower**, **Scullcap (Skullcap)**, **Lobelia**, **Lobelia seed**, **Chamomile flower**, Wood Betony (betonica)

Christopher's
Nerve Comfort Formula (Glycerine Extract)

Wild (Prickly) Lettuce, **Valerian**

Grandma's Herbs
Nervine (Capsule)

Scullcap (Skullcap), St. John's Wort, **Blue Vervain**, **Valerian**, **Hops flower**, Spearmint, Wood Betony (betonica), Mistletoe, Lady's Slipper, **Bladder Pod**, Capsicum (Cayenne)

Herbs Etc.
Nervine Tonic™ (Alcohol Extract or Softgel)

Passionflower, **Valerian root**, Oat seed (milky), Black Cohosh root, **Scullcap (Skullcap)**, Betony

Grandma's Herbs
Night Nervine (Capsule)

Hops flower, **Valerian**, **Blue Vervain**, **Scullcap (Skullcap)**, St. John's Wort, Black Cohosh, Lady's Slipper, Lily of the Valley, **Bladder Pod**, Mistletoe, Spearmint

Christopher's
Relax-Eze (Capsule and Glycerine Extract)

Black Cohosh, Capsicum (Cayenne), **Hops flower**, **Lobelia**, **Scullcap (Skullcap)**, **Valerian**, Wood Betony (betonica), Mistletoe

Eclectic Institute
Relaxation Support (Capsule)

Kava Kava, **California Poppy flower & leaf**, **Passionflower flower & leaf**

Yogi Tea
Relaxed Mind™ (Tea)

Sage, **Lavender flower**, Nettle (Stinging) leaf, **Scullcap (Skullcap) leaf**, Chrysanthemum flower, Blackberry leaf, Gotu Kola, Helichrysum, Shank Pushpi, Lemon Myrtle

Western Botanicals
Rest Easy Tea

Chamomile flower, **Scullcap (Skullcap)**, Catnip, Peppermint leaf, Stevia, Spearmint, **Passionflower**, **Lemon Balm leaf**, Lemongrass, **Lavender flower**

Herbalist & Alchemist
Serenity Compound™ (Alcohol Extract)

Chamomile flower, Eleuthero root, Linden (Basswood, Tilia) flower, Oat seed (milky), **Scullcap (Skullcap) flowering tops**

Gaia Herbs
Serenity Herbal Elixir (Alcohol Extract)

Passionflower vine, **Scullcap (Skullcap)**, **Kava Kava**, **Chamomile flower**, Oat seed (milky), Mugwort, Peppermint leaf, Hawthorn berry, flower & leaf, Peppermint essential oil; Non-Herbal: Syrup of apricot fruit, Sea Vegetable blend, Vegetable Glycerin, Honey

Gaia Herbs
Serenity with Passionflower (Liquid Phyto-Caps)

Scullcap (Skullcap), **Passionflower vine**, **Kava Kava**, Oat seed (milky), **Chamomile flower**, Mugwort, **Hops strobile**, Peppermint leaf

Gaia Herbs
Sleep & Relax Tea

Chamomile, **Lemon Balm leaf**, Licorice, **Passionflower**

Celestial Seasonings
Sleepytime® Sinus Soother Wellness Tea

Spearmint, Licorice, Peppermint leaf, Tulsi (Holy Basil) leaf, Nettle (Stinging) leaf, Linden (Basswood, Tilia) flower & leaf, Fennel

Planetary Herbals
Stress Free™ (Tablet)

Jujube seed, **Scullcap (Skullcap) aerial parts**, **Hops strobile**, Wood Betony (betonica) aerial parts, Ginseng (American), Hawthorn berry, Ginger, Licorice, **Chamomile flower**, Black Cohosh, Eleuthero root; Non-Herbal: Calcium, Magnesium

Herbs Etc.
Stress ReLeaf® (Alcohol Extract or Softgel)

Holy Basil, **Passionflower**, **Valerian root**, Oat seed (milky), Ashwagandha root, Black Cohosh root, **Scullcap (Skullcap)**, Betony

Irwin Naturals
Stress-Defy™ (Softgel)

Scullcap (Skullcap), Holy Basil, Ginkgo, Rhodiola root, Black Pepper, Ginger, Turmeric; Non-Herbal: Thiamin, Riboflavin, Vitamin B6, Calcium citrate, Magneium citrate, fish oil, L-Theanine, GABA, soy lecithin

Herbalist & Alchemist
Tension Relief™ (Alcohol Extract)

Motherwort flowering tops, Oat seed (milky), Bacopa (Water Hyssop), **Blue Vervain flowering tops**, Polygala

Celestial Seasonings
Tension Tamer® (Tea)

Eleuthero, Peppermint, Cinnamon, Ginger, **Chamomile**, Lemongrass, Licorice, Catnip, Linden (Basswood, Tilia) flower, Soybean, **Hops**; Non-Herbal: Lemon flavor, Vitamins B6, B12

Eclectic Institute
Valerian - Passion Flower (Capsule)

Valerian, **Scullcap (Skullcap) flower and leaf**, **Passionflower flower and leaf**, **Hops**, **Chamomile flower and leaf**

Eclectic Institute
Valerian - Passion Flower (Alcohol Extract and Glycerine Extract)

Valerian, **Passionflower flower and leaf**, **Chamomile flower and leaf**, **Hops strobile**, Anise seed

Gaia Herbs
Valerian Poppy Supreme (Alcohol and Glycerine Extract)

Scullcap (Skullcap), **California Poppy**, **Chamomile**, **Kava Kava**, Mugwort, **Passionflower**, **Valerian**

Herbs for Kids
Valerian Super Calm™ (Glycerine Extract)

Chamomile flower, **Valerian**, Fennel, **Hops strobile**, Wood Betony (betonica), Catnip

Herbalist & Alchemist
Women's Calmpound™ (Alcohol Extract)

Chaste Tree (Vitex), Motherwort flowering tops, **Scullcap (Skullcap) flowering tops**, **Blue Vervain flowering tops**, Pulsatilla root

Sinus Decongestant Formulas

See also *Decongestant* and
Goldenseal & Echinacea Formulas

This is a subcategory of *Decongestant Formulas*. Decongestants break up trapped mucus and help the body expel it. *Sinus Decongestant Remedies* are targeted towards decongesting the sinuses more than the lungs, although they are somewhat interchangeable. See *Congestion (sinus)* in the *Conditions Section* for more information.

Key Herbs: Brigham Tea, Eyebright, Fenugreek, Horehound, Horseradish, Osha and Thyme

Nature's Answer
Allertone (Glycerine Extract)

Echinacea (angustifolia) root, Goldenseal, Red Clover flowering tops, Bayberry bark, Mullein leaf

Herbs Etc.
Congest Free™ (Alcohol Extract)

Xanthium (Shen-chu) fruit, Cinnamon (cassia) twig, Grindelia (Gumweed) flower, Magnolia (acuminata) bud, Cubeb berry, Chinese Mint, **Eyebright**, Chinese Lovage root, **Osha root**, Capsicum (Cayenne) fruit

Herbs for Kids
Echinacea/Eyebright™ (Glycerine Extract)

Peppermint leaf, Echinacea (purpurea) root, **Eyebright**, Oregon Grape, Boneset, Sage

Nature's Way
Fenu-Thyme (Capsule)

Fenugreek, Thyme leaf

NOW Foods
Fenugreek & Thyme (Capsule)

Fenugreek, Thyme leaf

Nature's Herbs (TwinLab)
Fenugreek-Thyme (Capsule)

Fenugreek seed, **Thyme leaf**, Rosemary oil; Non-Herbal: Gelatin, medium chain triglycerides, vitamin E

Gaia Herbs
GaiaKid's® Sniffle Support Herbal Drops

Elder (Black) berry, Elder (canadensis) flower, **Eyebright**, Plantain, **Fenugreek**, **Thyme leaf**, Anise seed

Nature's Way
HAS® Original Blend (Capsule)

Brigham (Mormon) Tea leaf & stem, Marshmallow, Burdock root, Capsicum (Cayenne), Goldenseal, Elecampane root, Parsley leaf, Rosemary, Cleavers (Bedstraw) stem, leaf & & flower

Christopher's
Herbal Eyebright (Capsule and Alcohol Extract)

Bayberry bark, **Eyebright**, Goldenseal, Raspberry (Red) leaf, Capsicum (Cayenne)

Christopher's
Sinus & Lung Extract (Alcohol Extract)

Brigham (Mormon) Tea, **Horseradish**, Capsicum (Cayenne)

New Chapter
Sinus & Respiratory (Softgel)

Garlic, Oregano essential oil, Echinacea (purpurea) leaf & flower, Echinacea (angustifolia) root, Elder (canadensis) berry, Goldenseal, Andrographis leaf, Green Tea leaf, Astragalus, Lemon Balm, Lemon Balm leaf, Myrrh, Wintergreen, Ginger, Eucalyptus essential oil, Peppermint leaf, Meadowsweet, Purple Willow

Herbal Formulas

Western Botanicals
Sinus Allergy Formula (Capsule and Alcohol Extract)

Horseradish, Brigham (Mormon) Tea, Bitter Orange, Goldenseal, Lobelia, Lobelia seed, Nettle (Stinging) leaf, Peppermint leaf, Echinacea (angustifolia) root, Echinacea (pallida) root, **Eyebright**, Yarrow flower, Kola (cola) nut, Capsicum (chinense), Peppermint essential oil

Christopher's
Sinus Plus Formula (Capsule and Glycerine Extract)

Brigham (Mormon) Tea, Marshmallow, Goldenseal, Chaparral (Creosote), Burdock root, Parsley root, Lobelia, Capsicum (Cayenne)

Herbalist & Alchemist
Sinus Support Compound™ (Alcohol Extract)

Echinacea (purpurea) root, **Osha**, **Eyebright**, **Horseradish**, Bayberry root bark

New Chapter
Sinus Take Care™ (Softgel)

Garlic, Oregano leaf, Echinacea (purpurea) leaf & flower, Echinacea (angustifolia) root, Elder (canadensis) berry, Goldenseal, Andrographis leaf, Green Tea leaf, Astragalus, Lemon Balm leaf, Myrrh, Wintergreen, Ginger, Eucalyptus leaf, Peppermint leaf, Meadowsweet, Purple Willow

RidgeCrest Herbals
SinusClear (Capsule)

Chinese Cimicifuga root, Licorice (Chinese) root, Chinese Lovage root, Cnidium root, Angelica root, Green Tea leaf, Magnolia flower, Notopterygium root, Psyllium seed, Siler root, Xanthium (Shenchu) fruit; Non-Herbal: Hepar Sulphuris Calcareum 10X, Silicea 10X, Pulsatilla 10X, Kali Bichromicum 10X

Planetary Herbals
SinusFree™ (Alcohol Extract)

Horseradish, **Thyme leaf**, Yarrow flowering tops, **Eyebright aerial parts**

Planetary Herbals
Three Spices Sinus Complex™ (Tablet)

Ginger, Long Pepper (Pippali) fruit, Black Pepper seed; Non-Herbal: sodium, fiber, Dehydrated Honey

Skin Healing Formulas

See also *Blood Purifier Formulas*

These are typically blood purifier blends that are targeted to work on skin conditions such as acne or eczema. They utilize the same key herbs as *Blood Purifier Formulas* but may contain additional herbs, like horsetail and gotu kola, to support healthy skin.

Key Herbs: Burdock, Gotu kola, Horsetail, Sarsaparilla and Yellow Dock

Nature's Way
AKN® Skin Care (Capsule)

Dandelion root, **Burdock root**, Licorice, Capsicum (Cayenne), **Yellow Dock**, **Sarsaparilla**, Kelp, Echinacea stem, leaf & flower, Plantain

Herb Pharm
Connective Tissue Tonic (Alcohol Extract)

Gotu Kola, Hawthorn berry, Echinacea (purpurea) root, **Horsetail**

Herb Pharm
Dermal Health™ (Alcohol Extract)

Burdock seed, Nettle (Stinging) seed & calyx, **Sarsaparilla**, **Yellow Dock**, Spilanthes, Ginger

Herbalist & Alchemist
Healthy Skin Tonic™ (Alcohol Extract)

Sarsaparilla, **Yellow Dock**, **Burdock seed**, **Horsetail**, Red Alder

Yogi Tea
Skin Detox (Tea)

Green Tea leaf, Rose petals, Honeybush leaf, Hibiscus flower, Red Clover leaf and flower, Cardamom seed, Oregon Grape root, Orange peel, **Burdock root**, Dandelion root, **Yellow Dock root**

Planetary Herbals
Yellow Dock Skin Cleanse™ (Tablet)

Yellow Dock, Echinacea (purpurea) root, Echinacea (pallida) root, Myrrh, Poria Mushroom, Wild Yam, Marshmallow, Gentian, Bupleurum; Non-Herbal: Calcium, Vitamin C

Sleep Formulas

See also *Adaptogen* and *Relaxing Nervine Formulas*

This is a subcategory of *Relaxing Nervine Formulas*. These are strong nervine formulas that relax the nerves to help people fall asleep.

A classic sleep formula is a blend of hops, valerian and skullcap, all key herbs in these blends. Other ingredients tend to be the same key herbs found in *Relaxing Nervine Formulas*. Non-herbal ingredients in *Sleep Formulas* may include l-theanine, GABA, 5-HTP and melatonin.

Adaptogenic Formulas may also promote better sleep when the inability to sleep is brought on by chronic stress. Taking *Relaxing Nervine Formulas* during the day may also improve sleep at night. See *Insomnia* in the *Conditions Section* for more suggestions.

Key Herbs: California Poppy, Corydalis, Hops, Kavakava, Passionflower, Scullcap (Skullcap) and Valerian

Yogi Tea
Bedtime® (Tea)

Licorice, Spearmint, Chamomile flower, **Scullcap (Skullcap) leaf**, Cardamom seed, Cinnamon bark, St. John's Wort leaf & flower, Rose hips, Raspberry (Red) leaf, **Valerian**, Lavender flower, **Passionflower whole plant**

Planetary Herbals
Chamomile Sleep™ (Tablet)

Jujube seed, Chamomile flower, **Hops strobile**, Poria Mushroom, Ginseng (American), Chuan Xiong rhizome, Anemarrhena (Zhi-Mu) rhizome, Licorice; Non-Herbal: Sodium, Calcium

Herbs Etc.
Deep Sleep®
(Alcohol Extract, Glycerine Extract or Softgel)

California Poppy whole plant, **Valerian root**, **Passionflower**, Chamomile flower, Lemon Balm, Oat seed (milky), Orange peel

RidgeCrest Herbals
DreamOn (Capsule)

Pulsatilla, **Passionflower**, **Valerian root**, Black Cohosh root, Chamomile flower, Lemon Balm; Non-Herbal: Chamomilla, Kali Phosphoricum, Coffea Cruda, Causticum, Ferrum Metallicum, Lycopodium Clavatum, Phosphoric acid, Hyoscyaminum, Aconite Napellus, lupulin

Vitanica
GABA Ease™ (Capsule)

Passionflower, **Hops**, **Scullcap (Skullcap) leaf & stem**; Non-Herbal: Vitamin B6, GABA (Gamma-Aminobutyric Acid), L-Theanine,

Traditional Medicinals
"Just for Kids" Nighty Night® (Tea)

Passionflower, Chamomile flower, Linden (Basswood, Tilia) flower, Catnip, **Hops strobile**, Spearmint, Lemon Verbena, Lemon peel, Lemongrass leaf

Grandma's Herbs
Night Nervine (Capsule)

Hops flower, **Valerian**, Blue Vervain, **Scullcap (Skullcap)**, St. John's Wort, Black Cohosh, Lady's Slipper, Lily of the Valley, Bladder Pod, Mistletoe, Spearmint

NOW Foods
Nighttime™ Tea

Spearmint leaf, Chamomile flower, Licorice, Lemon Myrtle leaf, **Scullcap (Skullcap)**, **Passionflower**, Linden (Basswood, Tilia) leaf, Eleuthero root, Stevia leaf

Traditional Medicinals
Nighty Night® Valerian (Tea)

Valerian, **Passionflower**, Lemon Balm leaf, Peppermint leaf, Caraway fruit, Licorice

Herbalist & Alchemist
Phytocalm™ (Alcohol Extract)

Scullcap (Skullcap) flowering tops, **Hops strobile**, Oat seed (milky), **Passionflower**, **California Poppy**, **Valerian**

Irwin Naturals
Power to Sleep PM (Softgel)

Valerian, Ashwagandha root, **Hops**, **Passionflower pericarp**, Lemon Balm; Non-Herbal: Calcium Citrate, Magnesium Citrate, Fish Oil, GABA, L-Theanine, Melatonin

Herb Pharm
Relaxing Sleep (Alcohol Extract)

Valerian, **Passionflower flowering tops**, **Hops strobile**, Chamomile flower, Catnip leaf & flowering tops

Nature's Way
Silent Night with Valerian (Capsule)

Hops flower, **Valerian**, Lemon Balm leaf; Non-Herbal: Dietary Fiber

Grandma's Herbs
Sleep (Capsule)

Chamomile, **Hops flower**, Lemon Balm, **Passionflower**, **Valerian**, Motherwort, Lavender, **Scullcap (Skullcap)**, **Kava Kava**, St. John's Wort, Jujube fruit, Spearmint, Blue Vervain, Bladder Pod

Gaia Herbs
Sleep & Relax (Capsule)

California Poppy, Lavender essential oil, Lemon Balm leaf, Marjoram essential oil, **Passionflower**, **Valerian**

Gaia Herbs
Sleep & Relax Tea

Chamomile, Lemon Balm leaf, Licorice, **Passionflower**

Solaray
Sleep Blend™ SP-17™ (Capsule)

Valerian, **Hops cone**, **Scullcap (Skullcap) aerial parts**, **Passionflower flower**, Dandelion root, Chamomile flowering tops, Marshmallow, Hawthorn berry

Vitanica
SleepBlend™ (Capsule)

Passionflower, **Hops flower**, **Valerian**; Non-Herbal: Riboflavin, Vitamin B6, Vitamin B12, Calcium, Magnesium,,5-Hydroxytryptophan (5-HTP), Melatonin

Gaia Herbs
SleepThru (Liquid Phyto-Caps)

Ashwagandha root, Jujube fruit, Magnolia, **Passionflower**

Celestial Seasonings
Sleepytime® Decaf Lemon Jasmine Green Tea

Chamomile, Green Tea, Spearmint, Lemongrass, Linden (Basswood, Tilia) flower, Hawthorn, Orange flower, Rose bud; Non-Herbal: Ascorbic acid

Celestial Seasonings
Sleepytime® Herbal Tea

Chamomile, Spearmint, Lemongrass, Orange flower, Hawthorn, Rose bud

Celestial Seasonings
Sleepytime® Kids Goodnight Grape Herbal Tea

Chamomile, Lemongrass, Linden (Basswood, Tilia) flower, Spearmint, Blackberry leaf, Orange flower, Hawthorn, Rose bud, Stevia; Non-Herbal: Ascorbic acid

Celestial Seasonings
Sleepytime® Vanilla Herbal Tea

Chamomile, Spearmint, Lemongrass, Hawthorn, Orange flower, Rose bud

Christopher's
Slumber (Capsule)

Valerian, **Passionflower flower**, Mullein leaf, **Hops flower**, Lavender flower, Lobelia, Black Cohosh, Blue Cohosh

Nature's Answer
Slumber (Capsule and Glycerine Extract)
Valerian, **Hops strobile**, **Scullcap (Skullcap) aerial parts**, **Passionflower aerial parts**

Yogi Tea
Soothing Caramel Bedtime® (Tea)
Chamomile flower, Rooibos (Redbush), Chicory root, **Scullcap (Skullcap) leaf**, Nutmeg, Cinnamon bark and essential oil, **California Poppy whole plant**, Cardamom seed and essential oil, Ginger root and essential oil, Clove, Black Pepper seed, Cinnamon essential oil; Non-Herbal: L-Theanine Suntheanine®

Gaia Herbs
Sound Sleep (Liquid Phyto-Caps)
Scullcap (Skullcap), **California Poppy**, **Hops**, **Kava Kava**, **Passionflower**, **Valerian**

Western Botanicals
Sweet Dreams Formula (Capsule and Glycerine Extract)
Scullcap (Skullcap), Chamomile flower, Black Cohosh, Wood Betony (betonica), **Hops flower**, Linden (Basswood, Tilia) flower, **Valerian**, Vanilla, Lobelia, Lobelia seed, Lemon essential oil, Tangerine

New Chapter
Tranquilnite (Softgel)
Valerian, Magnolia bark, Zizyphus seed, **Hops flower**, **Passionflower flower**, Ginger, Chamomile flower, Lavender flower, Peppermint leaf

Eclectic Institute
Valerian - Passion Flower (Capsule)
Valerian, **Scullcap (Skullcap) flower and leaf**, **Passionflower flower and leaf**, **Hops**, Chamomile flower and leaf

Eclectic Institute
Valerian - Passion Flower (Alcohol Extract and Glycerine Extract)
Valerian, **Passionflower flower and leaf**, Chamomile flower and leaf, **Hops strobile**, Anise seed

Nature's Herbs (TwinLab)
Valerian Combination (Capsule)
Valerian root, **Hops flower**, **Scullcap (Skullcap) aerial parts**, Black Cohosh root, **Passionflower aerial parts**, Capsicum (Cayenne) fruit, Black Pepper fruit, Rosemary oil; Non-Herbal: Gelatin, medium chain triglycerides, vitamin E

A. Vogel
Valerian Complex (Alcohol Tincture)
Valerian, **Hops**

Planetary Herbals
Valerian Easy Sleep™ (Tablet)
Valerian, **Valerian**, Jujube seed, **Scullcap (Skullcap) aerial parts**, **Passionflower leaf & flower**, **Hops strobile**, Wood Betony (betonica) aerial parts, Chamomile flower, Dong Quai, Poria Mushroom, Licorice, Amber resin, Ginseng (American), Ginger; Non-Herbal: Calcium, Sodium, Fiber, Magnesium, Taurine

Nature's Way
Valerian Nighttime™ (Tablet)
Valerian, Lemon Balm leaf; Non-Herbal: Calcium

Stimulant Laxative Formulas

See also *Fiber Blend* and *Gentle Laxative Formulas*

Herbal stimulant laxatives rely on plants containing anthraquinone glycosides. These compounds increase peristalsis and inhibit water and electrolyte absorption from the intestines. There is no evidence that they directly irritate or harm the intestinal membranes, but they do contain yellow-brown dyes which, when taken over a long period of time, will stain the bowel. This is something that may show up in a colonoscopy and alarm the doctor.

Stimulant Laxative Formulas are contraindicated in spastic bowel conditions as they can cause griping and discomfort. In herbal formulas these effects are typically moderated by the use of carminatives and antispasmodics. These formulas should not be used long term, as they tend to deplete the energy of the colon and create dependence. They should be used with caution by women who are pregnant or nursing. *Stimulant Laxative Formulas* are best used for occasional irregularity or as an aid to colon or parasite cleansing.

Aloes and senna are the strongest laxative herbs and butternut is the gentlest laxative herb in the key herbs list. For long term constipation problems try *Gentle Laxative Formulas* and *Fiber Blend Formulas*. Also see *Constipation* in the *Conditions Section* for ideas on overcoming chronic constipation.

Key Herbs: Aloe (cape), Buckthorn, Butternut bark, Cascara Sagrada, Senna Leaves and Turkey Rhubarb

Nature's Way
Aloelax® (Capsule)
Aloe vera, Fennel

Nature's Way
AloeMaxLax™ (Capsule)
Aloe vera latex, **Buckthorn bark**, **Cascara Sagrada**, Fennel

Traditional Medicinals
Chocolate Smooth Move® (Tea)
Senna, Breadnut seed, Licorice, Cocoa (Cacao) seed, Carob

Renew Life
CleanseMORE (Capsule)
Aloe (cape) leaf, **Turkey Rhubarb**, Slippery Elm, Marshmallow, Triphala

Zand
Cleansing Laxative (Tablet)
Turkey Rhubarb, **Buckthorn bark**, Gentian, Anise seed, Fennel, Goldenseal, Oregon Grape

Solaray
Colon Blend™ SP-12™ (Capsule)

Butternut bark, **Cascara Sagrada**, **Senna**, Ginger, Burdock root, Irish Moss

Western Botanicals
Colon Cleanse Formula (Capsule)

Aloe (cape) leaf, **Cascara Sagrada**, Barberry root, **Turkey Rhubarb**, **Senna**, Garlic, Ginger, Fennel, Black Walnut hulls, Clove, Wormwood leaf, Capsicum (chinense)

Western Botanicals
Colon Cleanse Syrup (Glycerine Extract)

Fennel, **Senna**, Cherry (Wild) bark, Ginger, Orange peel, **Turkey Rhubarb**, **Cascara Sagrada**; Non-Herbal: Fig syrup, prune syrup, pure maple syrup

Renew Life
Constipation Stop (Capsule)

Aloe (cape) leaf, **Turkey Rhubarb**, **Buckthorn bark**, Okra, Marshmallow, Slippery Elm

Yerba Prima
Fiber Plus® Caps (Capsule)

Psyllium seed, Soybean, Oat bran, Acacia, Apple pectin, Ginger, Red Clover flowering tops, Dandelion root & leaf, **Senna**

Yerba Prima
Fiber Plus® Powder (Bulk Powder)

Psyllium seed, Soybean, Oat bran, Acacia, Apple pectin, Ginger, Red Clover flowering tops, Dandelion root & leaf, **Senna**

Herbalist & Alchemist
Gentlelax™ (Alcohol Extract)

Butternut root bark, **Buckthorn bark**, Culvers root, Dandelion root, Ginger

Western Botanicals
Happy Colon (Capsule)

Aloe (cape) leaf, **Cascara Sagrada**, Slippery Elm, **Senna**, **Turkey Rhubarb**, Psyllium seed, Barberry root bark

Grandma's Herbs
Herbal Colon Cleanser & Tonic (Capsule)

Cascara Sagrada, **Senna**, **Aloe vera**, **Buckthorn root**, Licorice, Psyllium, **Turkey Rhubarb**, Alfalfa, Calamus (Sweet Flag), Barberry, Black Walnut, **Butternut**, Dandelion root, Flax, Gentian, Marshmallow, Plantain, Prune, Red Clover, Sage, Slippery Elm, Blue Flag, Blue Vervain leaf, Calendula (Marigold), Chamomile, Chicory, Clove, Fennel, Ginger, Raspberry (Red), Yucca, Wahoo

Vitanica
LaxaBlend™ (Capsule)

Prune, Ginger, **Aloe vera**, **Cascara Sagrada**, **Turkey Rhubarb**, **Senna**; Non-Herbal: Vitamin C, Magnesium

Celestial Seasonings
LaxaTea Wellness Tea

Senna, Artichoke, Psyllium hulls, Fennel, Licorice, Orange peel, Cinnamon bark, Ginger; Non-Herbal: Rebiana (sweetener from Stevia)

Christopher's
Lower Bowel Formula (Capsule and Glycerine Extract)

Bayberry bark, **Cascara Sagrada**, Capsicum (Cayenne), Ginger, Lobelia, Raspberry (Red) leaf, Fennel, Goldenseal

Gaia Herbs
Natural Laxative (Tablet)

Dandelion root, Chicory root, Fennel, Caraway seed, Boldo leaf, Cumin, Fennel essential oil

Gaia Herbs
Natural Laxative Tea

Senna pod, **Senna**, Caraway seed, Fennel, Lemon Balm leaf, Malva leaf

Christopher's
Quick Colon Cleanse #1 (Capsule)

Aloe vera, **Cascara Sagrada**, Garlic, **Senna**, Ginger, Barberry bark, Capsicum (Cayenne)

Solaray
Rhubarb & Butternut (Capsule)

Turkey Rhubarb, **Butternut bark**

Traditional Medicinals
Smooth Move® Chamomile (Tea)

Senna, Chamomile flower, Fennel fruit, Peppermint leaf

Traditional Medicinals
Smooth Move® Peppermint (Tea)

Senna, Peppermint leaf, Licorice, Fennel fruit

Traditional Medicinals
Smooth Move® Senna (Tea)

Senna, **Senna**, Licorice, Fennel fruit, Orange peel, Cinnamon bark, Coriander fruit, Ginger, Orange oil

Traditional Medicinals
Smooth Move® Senna Capsules

Senna, Ginger, Licorice

Yogi Tea
Soothing Mint Get Regular® (Tea)

Senna, Peppermint leaf, Anise seed, Yellow Dock, Dandelion root, Licorice, Celery seed, Coriander seed, Cinnamon bark, Amla (Indian Gooseberry), Belleric Myrobalan fruit, Chebulic Myrobalan fruit, Cardamom seed, Ginger, Black Pepper

Grandma's Herbs
Super Lax (Capsule)

Cascara Sagrada, Psyllium seed, **Senna**, **Aloe vera**, Barberry root, Slippery Elm

Nature's Way
Thisilyn® Digestive CLEANSE (Capsule)

Cascara Sagrada, Peppermint leaf, Ginger, Fennel, Marshmallow, Triphala, Milk Thistle seed

Western Botanicals
Turkey Rhubarb Formula (Capsule)

Cascara Sagrada, **Senna**, **Turkey Rhubarb**, Psyllium seed, Barberry root bark, Aloe (cape) leaf, Slippery Elm, Capsicum (chinense)

Herbal Formulas

Styptic/Hemostatic Formulas

See also *Uterine Tonic Formulas*

When excessive bleeding needs to be regulated herbalists turn to herbs with styptic, hemostatic and astringent qualities. These herbs help blood clot, tone up tissues and aid wound healing. *Styptic/Hemostatic Formulas* may be helpful when their is excessive bleeding due to menstruation, cuts, lung irritation, and irritation in the intestinal tract or urinary passages. For heavy menstrual bleeding also consider *Uterine Tonic Formulas*, remedies that tone the uterus and can slow menstrual flow.

Of course, internal bleeding and severe arterial bleeding are very serious problems requiring immediate medical attention. However, *Styptic/Homeostatic Formulas* can be used to control non-life threatening bleeding problems or as a first aid remedy en route to medical attention. So, a *Styptic/Hemostatic Formula* is a good thing to keep in your first aid kit.

Key Herbs: Erigeron (Fleabane), Shepherd's Purse, Tienchi Ginseng and Yarrow

Herb Pharm
Erigeron/Cinnamon (Alcohol Extract)

Erigeron (Canadian Fleabane) essential oil, Cinnamon (verum) essential oil

Solaray
Menstrual Blend™ SP-7B™ (Capsule)

Cranesbill (Wild Geranium) root, Witch Hazel leaf, Raspberry (Red) leaf, **Shepherd's Purse aerial parts**, Ginger, Horsetail, Goldenseal, Irish Moss

Herbalist & Alchemist
Reckless Blood Tonic™ (Alcohol Extract)

Shepherd's Purse, Tienchi Ginseng, Yarrow flower, Cinnamon (cassia) bark

Vitanica
Slow Flow™ (Capsule)

Ginger, Cranesbill (Wild Geranium) root, Periwinkle, **Yarrow flower**, Life Root, **Shepherd's Purse**; Non-Herbal: Vitamin A, Vitamin C, Vitamin K1, Bioflavonoids

Sudorific Formulas

See also *Cold* and *Flu Formulas*

Inducing perspiration is a time-tested remedy for colds, flu and fevers. **Sudorific Formulas** contain herbs that move blood to the surface of the skin, opening the sweat glands to expel toxins and cool fever. Sudorific herbs should be taken as hot (or at least warm) teas, or when using extracts, added to warm liquids. They can be used in conjunction with a sweat bath (see *Therapies Section*) to break a fever or rapidly recover from colds. These blends also have antiviral properties.

Key Herbs: Elder, Peppermint and Yarrow

Traditional Medicinals
Echinacea Plus® Elderberry (Tea)

Echinacea (purpurea), **Elder (canadensis) flower**, Echinacea root, **Elder (canadensis) berry**, Ginger, Chamomile flower, **Yarrow flower**, **Peppermint leaf**

Traditional Medicinals
Gypsy Cold Care® (Tea)

Elder (canadensis) flower, Yarrow flower, Peppermint leaf, Hyssop, Rose hips, Cinnamon bark, Ginger, Safflower petals, Clove, Licorice

Traditional Medicinals
"Just for Kids" Cold Care (Tea)

Elder (canadensis) flower, Linden (Basswood, Tilia) flower, Chamomile flower, **Peppermint leaf**

Christopher's
Kid-e-Well (Glycerine Extract)

Yarrow, Elder (canadensis) flower, Peppermint, Echinacea (angustifolia) root

Herbs for Kids
Temp Assure™ (Glycerine Extract)

Echinacea (purpurea) root, **Peppermint leaf, Yarrow flower**, Catnip

Superfood Formulas

In recent years, the idea of superfoods has become a popular concept. The idea of superfoods is based on nutritional density. Many whole foods contain large quantities of natural vitamins, minerals, antioxidants, fiber and other compounds that may be lacking in modern diets of refined and processed foods.

When most people are chronically ill, the first thing they look for is the "magic-bullet" that will make them well. This bullet often takes the shape of a drug that promises to "fix" the problem, but even people who are involved in natural health can end up searching for a "magic" herb or supplement. However, when anyone suffers from chronic health problems, the wisest place to start their healing process is with food.

The body largely heals itself when it has what it needs to do the job. In modern Western culture, however, much of the available food is processed and devoid of essential nutrients. It may also be loaded with preservatives and other non-nutritive chemicals. Just look around the next time you're in the grocery store—the ratio of refined, processed foods to whole, natural foods is about five to one.

Herbal Superfood Formulas contain nutritionally dense plants such as alfalfa, barley grass, wheat grass, spirulina, kelp and fruit and vegetable powders. They are used to supplement nutrition in a whole food form.

Key Herbs: Alfalfa and Spirulina

Western Botanicals
Bountiful Blend (Liquid)

Raspberry (Red), Cherry, Acerola, Cranberry, Blueberry, Camu Camu berry, Elder (canadensis) berry, Strawberry, Schisandra, Pineapple, Lemon, Mango, Orange, Papaya, Kiwifruit, Grape, Grapefruit, Apple, Pomegranate, Prune, Plum, Peach, Pear, Barley, Spinach, Wheat grass, Kale, **Alfalfa**, Parsley, **Spirulina**, Irish Moss, Chlorella, Kelp, Vanilla, Aloe vera vera gel, Stevia, Pine bark, Grape seed, Carrot, Beet, Celery, Asparagus, Tomato, Brussels Sprout, Broccoli, Cauliflower, Peppermint leaf, Spearmint, Cinnamon, Astragalus, Milk Thistle seed, Licorice, Ginger, Nettle (Stinging) leaf, Pau d'Arco, Eleuthero root, He Shou Wu (Fo-Ti), Ashwagandha root, Olive leaf, Turmeric; Non-Herbal: Apple Cider Vinegar, Soy lecithin

Western Botanicals
Earth's Nutrition (Capsule and Powder)

Spirulina, Chlorella, Nettle (Stinging) leaf, Dulse, Wheat grass, Spinach, **Alfalfa**, Barley grass, Astragalus, Rose hips, Orange peel, Lemon peel, Beet; Non-Herbal: Non-Active Nutritional Yeast

NOW Foods
Green PhytoFoods (Bulk Powder)

Alfalfa, Wheat grass, Barley grass and malt, Carrot, Broccoli, Apple pectin, Oat bran, Chlorella, Beet, Ginseng (Korean, Asian), Eleuthero root, Peppermint, Green Tea leaf, Milk Thistle seed, Kelp, Ginkgo leaf, Grape seed, Bilberry fruit, Stevia leaf; Non-Herbal: Brown Rice bran, Royal Jelly powder, Fructooligosaccharides, Trace Mineral concentrate, Plant multi-enzyme blend, Coenzyme Q10, Alpha Lipoic Acid

Christopher's
Jurassic Green (Capsule and Bulk Powder)

Alfalfa, Barley grass, Kamut grass

Grandma's Herbs
Kid-e-Mins (Glycerine Extract)

Alfalfa, Barley grass, Wheat, Rose, Oat straw, Dulse, Ginger, Dandelion, Kelp, **Spirulina**, Irish Moss root, Beet, Capsicum (Cayenne), Violet, Carrot; Non-Herbal: Nutritional Yeast

Irwin Naturals
Super Green Super Food™ (Softgel)

Chlorella, **Spirulina**, Wheat grass, Kelp, Nopal (Prickly Pear) leaf, Sea Buckthorn fruit, Nettle (Stinging) leaf, Broccoli leaf, Brussels Sprout leaf, Carrot, Kale, Onion, Spinach, Tomato, Plum, Blueberry, Cranberry, Strawberry, Blackberry, Bilberry, Apricot, Papaya, Cherry (Sweet), Grape, Orange, Pineapple; Non-Herbal: Red Algae

Planetary Herbals
Vita Greens & Berries™ (Bulk Powder)

Wheat grass, Barley grass, Oat grass, **Spirulina**, Chlorella, Carrot, Broccoli leaf, Spinach, Beet, Tomato, Kale, Cabbage, Parsley leaf, Cauliflower Sprout, Camu Camu fruit, Passion Fruit, Pineapple, Guava, Acerola, Cupuacu fruit, Açaí berry, Blueberry, Cherry, Cranberry, Pomegranate seed, Black Walnut hulls, Schisandra, Artichoke leaf, Milk Thistle seed, Grape seed, Lycium (Wolfberry/ Gogi), Green Tea leaf, Mangosteen, Apple, Turmeric, Bilberry,

Reishi (Ganoderma), Shiitake Mushroom, Turkey Tail Mushroom, Maitake Mushroom, Astragalus, Eleuthero root, Ginseng (Korean, Asian), Stevia; Non-Herbal: Red Wine Powder, Cashew nut, Probiotic Blend

Christopher's
Vitalerbs (Capsule)

Alfalfa, Barley, Kamut, Dandelion, Kelp, Dulse, **Spirulina**, Irish Moss, Rose hips, Beet, Capsicum (Cayenne), Oat straw, Carrot, Ginger; Non-Herbal: Nutritional Yeast

Tissue Healing Formulas

See also *Joint Healing*, *Mineral* and *Topical Vulnerary Formulas*

These formulas contain herbs that promote rapid regeneration of damaged tissues in the body. These blends are taken internally to speed the healing of broken bones, sprains and other injuries. They may help the body heal faster after surgery as well. Many of these blends would also be helpful in healing ulcerations and inflammatory conditions of the gastro-intestinal tract.

Most of the key herbs in *Tissue Healing Formulas* are also used in *Topical Vulnerary Formulas*. Many of them are also found in *Joint Healing Formulas*, which are targeted more at arthritic conditions and *Mineral Formulas*, which also have tissue-healing properties.

Key Herbs: Calendula, Comfrey, Horsetail, Marshmallow, Plantain, Slippery Elm and White Oak

Nature's Way
Bone, Flesh & Cartilage (Capsule)

White Oak bark, Black Walnut hulls, Gravel Root root, **Marshmallow**, Mullein leaf, **Slippery Elm**, **Calendula (Marigold) flower**

Christopher's
Complete Tissue & Bone Formula (Capsule)

White Oak bark, Lungwort root, **Slippery Elm**, **Marshmallow leaf**, Mullein root, Wormwood, Lobelia, Scullcap (Skullcap), **Plantain**, Aloe vera

Western Botanicals
Complete Tissue Repair Syrup (Glycerine Extract)

Plantain, **White Oak bark**, Black Walnut hulls, **Marshmallow**, Gravel Root root, Aloe vera resin, Willow (White) bark, Lobelia, Lobelia seed, Mullein, Mullein flower, **Horsetail**, St. John's Wort flowering tops, Wormwood, Scullcap (Skullcap); Non-Herbal: Pure Honey

Herb Pharm
Connective Tissue Tonic (Alcohol Extract)

Gotu Kola, Hawthorn berry, Echinacea (purpurea) root, **Horsetail**

Grandma's Herbs
Heal (Capsule)

Heal All, Wheat grass, **Horsetail**, **Slippery Elm**, **Marshmallow**, Alfalfa, Nettle (Stinging), Oat straw, **Calendula (Marigold)**, **White Oak bark**, **Plantain**, Yarrow

Vitanica
Opti-Recovery™ (Capsule)

Horse Chestnut, Dandelion leaf, Echinacea (angustifolia) root, Echinacea (purpurea) root, Cleavers (Bedstraw), Blue Flag; Non-Herbal: Vitamin C, Zinc, Bromelain

Herb Pharm
Trauma Drops™ (Alcohol Extract)

Calendula (Marigold) flower, St. John's Wort flowering tops, Arnica flower

Topical Analgesic Formulas

See also *Analgesic Formulas*

These are remedies applied topically to ease pain. They are related to *Analgesic Formulas*, which are taken internally. These lotions, linaments, oils or creams can be massaged into the skin to ease muscle and joint pain. Massaging the neck and shoulders with these blends can help relieve headaches. Many can also be massaged into the chest to ease respiratory congestion or into the neck to ease sore throats.

Key ingredients in *Topical Analgesic Formulas* include camphor and menthol, aromatic compounds that decongest respiratory passages, stimulate blood flow and ease pain. Formulas that contain these ingredients have the best effects for clearing respiratory passages.

Key Herbs: Arnica, Calendula, Camphor, Capsicum (Cayenne), Catnip, Stillingia and Wintergreen

Tiger Balm
Arthritis Rub (Cream)

Camphor, Cajeput essential oil, Cassia essential oil, Clove essential oil, Peppermint essential oil; Non-Herbal: Menthol, Chondroitin Sulfate, Diazolidinyl Urea, Glucosamine Sulfate, Methyl Paraben, MSM, Methyl Glucose Dioleate, Propyl Paraben, Propylene Glycol

Christopher's
Cayenne Heat Massage Oil

Wintergreen essential oil, **Capsicum (Cayenne)**, Olive oil; Non-Herbal: Menthol Crystals

Christopher's
Cayenne Ointment (Salve)

Olive oil, **Capsicum (Cayenne)**, **Wintergreen essential oil**; Non-Herbal: Beeswax, menthol crystals

Herbalist & Alchemist
Compound Arnica Oil

Arnica oil, St. John's Wort essential oil, Lobelia essential oil, Sweet Birch essential oil, White Sage oil; Non-Herbal: Vitamin E

Western Botanicals
Deep Heat Oil

St. John's Wort flowering tops, Lobelia, Lobelia seed, **Arnica flower**, **Calendula (Marigold) flower**, Ginger, Plantain, Capsicum (chinense), **Wintergreen essential oil**, Olive oil, Aloe vera, Birch (White) essential oil; Non-Herbal: Menthol crystals

Western Botanicals
Deep Heat Ointment (Salve/Ointment)

St. John's Wort flowering tops, Lobelia, Lobelia seed, **Arnica flower**, **Calendula (Marigold) flower**, Ginger, White Oak bark, Marshmallow, Plantain, Mullein flower and herb, Black Walnut hulls, Gravel Root root, Wormwood, Scullcap (Skullcap), Willow (White) bark, Horsetail, Capsicum (Cayenne), **Wintergreen essential oil**, Olive oil, Aloe vera, Birch (White) essential oil; Non-Herbal: Menthol crystals, beeswax

Grandma's Herbs
Deep Muscle Massage (Oil)

Eucalyptus essential oil, Cajeput essential oil, Peppermint essential oil, **Wintergreen essential oil**, Hyssop essential oil, Grape oil; Non-Herbal: Grapeseed oil

Herbalist & Alchemist
Dragon's Dream Ointment™ (Salve/Ointment)

Camphor, Eucalyptus essential oil, Peppermint essential oil, Clove essential oil, **Wintergreen essential oil**, Olive oil; Non-Herbal: Menthol, Beeswax

Gaia Herbs
GaiaKids® Warming Chest Rub (Salve/Ointment)

Cocoa (Cacao) butter, Coconut oil, Lavender essential oil, Pine essential oil, Thyme essential oil, Peppermint essential oil, Yarrow essential oil; Non-Herbal: Shea butter

Herbs for Kids
Gum-omile Oil™ (Oil)

Almond oil, Willow bark, Chamomile flower, Clove; Non-Herbal: Vitamin E

Herb Pharm
Joint & Muscle Warming Rub (Alcohol and Glycerine Extract)

St. John's Wort flowering tops, **Arnica flower**, Wormwood leaf & flower, Horse Chestnut seed, Rue fruiting tops, Yarrow flower, **Capsicum (Cayenne)**

Tiger Balm
Liniment (Cream)

Wintergreen essential oil, Eucalyptus essential oil, Lavender essential oil; Non-Herbal: Menthol, Light Mineral oil

Christopher's
Muscle Pain Relief Spray

Capsicum (Cayenne), **Wintergreen essential oil**, Cinnamon essential oil, Eucalyptus essential oil, Orange essential oil, Spearmint essential oil, Coconut oil, Peppermint essential oil, Camphor, Olive oil; Non-Herbal: Menthol crystals

Tiger Balm
Muscle Rub (Cream)

Camphor; Non-Herbal: Menthol, Methyl Salicylate, Cetostearyl Alcohol, Hard Paraffin, Methyl Hydroxybenzoate, Polyoxyethylene Glycol 1000, Propyl Hydroxybenzoate, Purified Water, Sodium Lauryl Sulphate, White Soft Paraffin

Tiger Balm
Neck & Shoulder Rub (Cream)

Camphor, Mint essential oil, Eucalyptus essential oil, Lavender essential oil; Non-Herbal: Menthol, Diazolidinyl Urea, Glycerin, Methyl Glucose Dioleate, Methylparaben, PVM/MA Decadiene

Crosspolymer, Propylene Glycol, Propylparaben, Triethanolamine (TEA)

Olbas
Olbas Analgesic Salve
Peppermint essential oil, Eucalyptus essential oil, Cajeput essential oil, **Wintergreen essential oil**, Juniper essential oil, Clove essential oil; Non-Herbal: Menthol, Hydrogenated peanut oil, White soft paraffin

Olbas
Olbas Herbal Bath (Liquid)
Peppermint essential oil, Eucalyptus essential oil, Cajeput essential oil, **Wintergreen essential oil**, Juniper essential oil, Clove essential oil; Non-Herbal: Sodium Coceth Sulfate and PEG-40 Glycerol Cocoate (Coconut Fatty Esters & Hydrogenated Castor Oil), PEG-6 Caprylic/Capric Glycerides from Coconut and Palm Oils

Olbas
Olbas Oil (Essential Oil)
Peppermint essential oil, Eucalyptus essential oil, Cajeput essential oil, **Wintergreen essential oil**, Juniper essential oil, Clove essential oil

Tiger Balm
Pain Relieving Patch
Camphor, **Capsicum (Cayenne)**, Eucalyptus essential oil, Mint essential oil; Non-Herbal: Menthol, Glycerin, Kaolin, propylene glycol, Sorbitol solution

Tiger Balm
Tiger Balm® Extra (Salve/Ointment)
Camphor, Cajeput essential oil, Cassia essential oil, Clove essential oil, Mint essential oil; Non-Herbal: Menthol, Paraffin Petrolatum

Tiger Balm
Tiger Balm® Regular (Salve/Ointment)
Camphor, Cajeput essential oil, Clove essential oil, Peppermint essential oil; Non-Herbal: Menthol, Peraffin Petrolatum

Tiger Balm
Tiger Balm® Ultra (Salve/Ointment)
Camphor, Cajeput essential oil, Mint essential oil, Clove essential oil, Cassia essential oil; Non-Herbal: Menthol, Paraffin

Herb Pharm
Trauma Oil™
Calendula (Marigold) flower, **Arnica flower**, St. John's Wort flowering tops; Non-Herbal: Olive Oil

White Flower
White Flower Analgesic Balm (Essential Oil)
Camphor, **Wintergreen essential oil**, Eucalyptus essential oil, Lavender essential oil, Peppermint essential oil; Non-Herbal: Menthol

Topical Antiseptic Formulas
See also *Goldenseal & Echinacea Formulas*

These products are applied topically (either to the skin or the gums) to fight infection. A subcategory of this group is *Dental Health Formulas,* which are used to fight gingivitis and gum infections. Liquid *Goldenseal & Echinacea Formulas* can also be used as topical antiseptics.

Key Herbs: Echinacea, Goldenseal, Myrrh, Propolis and Usnea

Herbs Etc.
DermaCillin™ (Spray)
Usnea, Calendula (Marigold) flower, Oregon Grape root, **Propolis gum**, **Myrrh gum resin**, Yerba mansa root, **Echinacea (angustifolia) root**, Lavender (officinalis) essential oil

Eclectic Institute
Ech-Goldenseal Spray
Echinacea (angustifolia) root, **Goldenseal**, Isatis (Woad) root, Cherry (Wild) bark, Slippery Elm, Orange essential oil; Non-Herbal: Kosher vegetable glycerin

Gaia Herbs
Echinacea Goldenseal Propolis Throat Spray
Echinacea (angustifolia) root & aerial parts, **Echinacea (purpurea) root & seed**, **Goldenseal**, Licorice, Oregon Grape, Peppermint, **Propolis**, Thyme

Gaia Herbs
Fresh Breath (Spray)
Clove, Ginger, Ginger, Licorice, Peppermint leaf & essential oil, Prickly Ash (Zanthoxylum americanum), Thyme

Herb Pharm
Friar's Balsam (Alcohol Extract)
Siam Benzoin, Storax balsam, Balsam of Tolu, Balsam of Peru, **Myrrh**, Angelica root

Eclectic Institute
Goldenseal - Propolis Cream (Salve)
Calendula (Marigold) flower, **Myrrh**, **Goldenseal**, **Propolis**, Safflower oil, Almond oil, Avocado oil; Non-Herbal: Kosher Vegetable Glycerin

Western Botanicals
Herbal Antiseptic (Salve/Ointment)
Myrrh, **Goldenseal**, White Oak bark, Olive leaf, Garlic, Plantain, Black Walnut hulls, Capsicum (chinense), Tea Tree essential oil

Western Botanicals
Herbal Mouthwash Concentrate (Alcohol Extract)
White Oak bark, Horsetail, Plantain, Aloe vera, **Echinacea (angustifolia) root**, **Myrrh**, Lobelia, Lobelia seed, Peppermint leaf, **Goldenseal**, Clove essential oil, Peppermint essential oil, Tea Tree essential oil

Herbs Etc.
Mouth Tonic™ (Alcohol Extract)
Echinacea (angustifolia) root, **Myrrh gum resin**, **Goldenseal root**, **Propolis gum**, Yerba mansa root, Bloodroot root

Eclectic Institute
Propolis - Astragalus (Spray)

Propolis, Astragalus, **Echinacea (purpurea) root & seed**, Slippery Elm

Nature's Answer
Sambucus Elder Berry Spray

Elder (Black), Slippery Elm, **Echinacea (purpurea) tops**, Astragalus, Sage, **Propolis**; Non-Herbal: Vegetable glycerin, Purified Water

A. Vogel
Sore Throat Spray

Echinacea (purpurea), Sage leaf

Gaia Herbs
Throat Shield Lozenges

Chicory root, Sage, Aloe vera vera gel, **Myrrh**, Peppermint leaf, Cinnamon bark; Non-Herbal: Freeze dried honey extract, Cane sugar, Mint natural flavor

Gaia Herbs
Throat Shield Spray

Aloe vera, Cinnamon essential oil, **Myrrh**, Peppermint essential oil, Sage; Non-Herbal: Mint natural flavor

Christopher's
X-Ceptic (Alcohol Extract)

White Oak bark, **Goldenseal**, **Myrrh**, Comfrey root, Garlic, Capsicum (Cayenne)

Topical Vulnerary Formulas

See also *Poultice* and *Tissue Healing Formulas*

A vulnerary is an herbal remedy that helps tissues to heal, so *Topical Vulnerary Formulas* are ointments, salves or other products designed to be applied topically to promote rapid healing of tissues. These remedies can be applied to bruises, cuts, scrapes, burns and other injuries to ease pain and speed healing. *Topical Vulnerary Formulas* can be used in combination with *Tissue Healing Formulas* (which are taken internally). Also consider applying a poultice or a compress to injured tissues (see *Therapies Section*).

Key Herbs: Arnica, Calendula, Comfrey, Goldenseal, Lavender, Myrrh, Olive and Plantain

Christopher's
Beauty Facial Cream (Salve)

Olive oil, Aloe vera, Wheat, White Oak bark, Marshmallow, Mullein leaf, Wormwood, Lobelia, Scullcap (Skullcap), **Comfrey root**, Black Walnut leaf, Gravel Root root, Lemon essential oil, Gardenia essential oil; Non-Herbal: Wheat, Vitamin E, Beeswax

Eclectic Institute
C-C-C Cream (Salve)

Calendula (Marigold), **Comfrey root**, Echinacea (angustifolia), Almond oil, Safflower oil; Non-Herbal: Kosher vegetable glycerin, Emulsifying wax

Grandma's Herbs
Chronic Condition Skin Salve

Yarrow, Chaparral (Creosote) leaf, Arrowleaf Balsamroot, Balsam of Peru, St. John's Wort essential oil, Helichrysum; Non-Herbal: Vitamin E

Gaia Herbs
Comfrey Compound (Salve/Ointment)

Scullcap (Skullcap), Black Walnut, **Comfrey**, **Olive**, Gravel Root, Lobelia, Marshmallow, Mullein

Christopher's
Comfrey Ointment (Salve/Ointment)

Comfrey, **Olive oil**; Non-Herbal: Beeswax

Herbalist & Alchemist
Comfrey/Calendula Ointment (Salve/Ointment)

Comfrey root, **Calendula (Marigold) flower**, Propolis, **Olive oil**; Non-Herbal: Vitamin E, Lanolin

Christopher's
Complete Tissue Massage Oil (Oil)

Olive oil, White Oak bark, **Comfrey root**, Mullein leaf, Black Walnut leaf, Marshmallow, Wormwood, Lobelia, Scullcap (Skullcap), Gravel Root root; Non-Herbal: Wheat Germ Oil

Christopher's
Complete Tissue Ointment (Salve/Ointment)

White Oak root, Marshmallow, Mullein root, Wormwood, Lobelia bark, Scullcap (Skullcap), **Comfrey**, Walnut oil, Gravel Root, **Olive**; Non-Herbal: Beeswax

Western Botanicals
Complete Tissue Repair Oil (Salve/Ointment and Oil)

Plantain, White Oak bark, Black Walnut hulls, Marshmallow, Gravel Root root, Aloe vera resin, Willow (White) bark, Lobelia, Lobelia seed, Mullein, Mullein flower, Horsetail, St. John's Wort flowering tops, Wormwood, Scullcap (Skullcap), **Olive oil**; Non-Herbal: Beeswax

Herbalist & Alchemist
Compound Arnica Oil

Arnica oil, St. John's Wort essential oil, Lobelia essential oil, Sweet Birch essential oil, White Sage oil; Non-Herbal: Vitamin E

Western Botanicals
Deep Heat Ointment (Salve/Ointment)

St. John's Wort flowering tops, Lobelia, Lobelia seed, **Arnica flower**, **Calendula (Marigold) flower**, Ginger, White Oak bark, Marshmallow, **Plantain**, Mullein, Mullein flower, Black Walnut hulls, Gravel Root root, Wormwood, Scullcap (Skullcap), Willow (White) bark, Horsetail, Capsicum (chinense), Wintergreen essential oil, **Olive oil**, Aloe vera, Birch (White) essential oil; Non-Herbal: Menthol crystals, Beeswax

Western Botanicals
Essential Skin Care (Lotion)

Plantain, White Oak bark, Black Walnut hulls, Marshmallow, Gravel Root root, Willow (White) bark, Lobelia, Lobelia seed, Mullein leaf, Horsetail, St. John's Wort, Wormwood leaf, Scullcap (Skullcap), Aloe vera vera gel, Grape oil, Jojoba oil, **Olive oil**, Coconut oil, Wheat germ oil, Grapefruit seed; Non-Herbal: Pure Vegetable Glycerine, Emulsifing Plant Wax, Essential Oils

Herb Pharm
Herb Pharm Original Salve™

Comfrey root, St. John's Wort flowers and buds, **Calendula (Marigold) flower**, Chickweed, Mullein leaf, **Plantain**

Western Botanicals
Herbal Throat Spray

Cherry (Wild) bark, Licorice, Slippery Elm, Elder (canadensis) berry, Marshmallow, Echinacea root, Mullein leaf, Fennel, Horehound, Turkey Rhubarb, Usnea, Lobelia, Lobelia seed, Clove, Ginger, Eucalyptus essential oil, Lemon essential oil, Tea Tree essential oil; Non-Herbal: Pure honey, vegetable glycerine

Herbs Etc.
Ivy Itch ReLeaf® (Spray)

Jewelweed, Grindelia (Gumweed) flower, **Plantain leaf**, Licorice root, Echinacea (angustifolia) root

Western Botanicals
Melissa Ointment (Salve/Ointment)

Lemon Balm leaf, White Oak bark, **Plantain**, Aloe vera resin, Black Walnut hulls, Marshmallow, Gravel Root root, Willow (White) bark, Lobelia, Lobelia seed, Wormwood, Horsetail, St. John's Wort flowering tops, Scullcap (Skullcap), Mullein, Mullein flower, **Olive oil**, Aloe vera; Non-Herbal: Beeswax

Christopher's
Nose Ointment (Salve/Ointment)

Spearmint essential oil, Peppermint; Non-Herbal: Vaseline

Christopher's
Rash Formula Ointment (Salve/Ointment)

Comfrey oil, Marshmallow, **Calendula (Marigold)**, Marshmallow; Non-Herbal: Beeswax

Herb Pharm
Soothing Oak & Ivy™ (Alcohol Extract)

Grindelia (Gumweed) flower bud, Sassafras; Non-Herbal: Menthol crystals

Christopher's
Stings & Bites Ointment (Salve/Ointment)

Plantain, **Olive oil**; Non-Herbal: Beeswax

Herbs for Kids
Stingzzz™ Cool Soothing Gel

Citronella essential oil, Aloe vera, **Calendula (Marigold) oil**, Echinacea (purpurea), Lemon Balm, Nettle (Stinging), **Plantain**, Witch Hazel, Yarrow, Grapefruit seed

Herbs for Kids
Super Kids Salve™

Olive oil, Echinacea (purpurea) flower, **Comfrey leaf**, Oregon Grape, Burdock root, Yarrow flower, **Calendula (Marigold) flower**, **Lavender**; Non-Herbal: Vitamin E

Ulcer Healing Formulas

See also *Antibacterial* and *Tissue Healing Formulas*

These formulas are used to soothe irritation and promote healing of stomach and intestinal ulcers. You can also look for *Tissue Healing Formulas* that have similar ingredients. Since ulcers may be related to an overgrowth of *H. pylori* bacteria, *Antibacterial Formulas* may also be helpful. See *Ulcers* in the *Conditions Section* for more information on natural therapy for ulcers.

Key Herbs: Aloe vera and Licorice

Nature's Sunshine Products
Gastro Health Concentrate (Capsule)

Licorice, Pau d'Arco, Clove, Elecampane root, Capsicum (Cayenne)

Solaray
Stomach Blend SP-20B (Capsule)

Mastic gum, Marshmallow, Plantain, Kelp, Capsicum (Cayenne), **Licorice**, Garcinia (Brindleberry)

Urinary Infection Fighting Formulas

See also *Antibacterial, Diuretic, Goldenseal & Echinacea* and *Kidney Tonic Formulas*

This is a subclass of *Diuretic* or *Kidney Tonic Formulas* with herbs that have antimicrobial properties. This makes them more suitable for treating urinary tract infections.

One of the most popular ingredients in *Urinary Infection Fighting Formulas* is cranberry. However, cranberry is more for preventing urinary tract infections than it is for treating them. More important key herbs in these formulas actually do help fight urinary infections, which is why a good formula will often be more effective than just taking cranberry. You can also use *Herbal Antibacterial Formulas* or *Goldenseal & Echinacea Formulas* taken along with a *Diuretic Formula* to fight urinary tract infections.

Key Herbs: Cranberry, Goldenseal, Oregon Grape, Pipsissewa and Uva Ursi

Nature's Answer
Bladdex™ (Glycerine Extract)

Oregon Grape, Couchgrass (Quackgrass) rhizome, **Uva Ursi**, Juniper berry, Marshmallow, Buchu leaf

Traditional Medicinals
Cran-Aid® (Tea)

Cranberry, **Uva Ursi**, Cleavers (Bedstraw), Marshmallow, Hibiscus, Chamomile flower, Rose hips, Peppermint leaf

Herbs Etc.
Cran-Bladder ReLeaf® (Alcohol Extract or Softgel)

Cranberry fruit, **Uva Ursi leaf**, Echinacea (angustifolia) root, Nettle (Stinging), Buchu leaf, Horsetail, **Pipsissewa**, Yarrow flowering tops, Meadowsweet, Licorice root, Stevia leaf

Planetary Herbals
Cranberry Bladder Defense™ (Tablet)

Cranberry, **Uva Ursi**, Poria Mushroom, Echinacea (pallida) root, Coptis (Chinese Goldthread,Huang Lian) root, Zhu-Ling, Marshmallow, Asian Water Plantain rhizome; Non-Herbal: Sugar

Vitanica
CranStat Extra™ (Capsule)

Cranberry, Buchu leaf, **Pipsissewa**, **Uva Ursi**, **Oregon Grape**

Renew Life
Total Kidney Detox™ (Capsule)

Cranberry, Parsley leaf, Horsetail, Nettle (Stinging) leaf, Dandelion leaf, Couchgrass (Quackgrass), White Kidney Bean, Corn Silk, Buchu leaf, **Uva Ursi**; Non-Herbal: Potassium, Arbutin

Gaia Herbs
Urinary Support (Liquid Phyto-Caps)

Coptis (Chinese Goldthread,Huang Lian), Echinacea (angustifolia) root, Echinacea (purpurea) aerial parts, root & seed, Usnea, **Uva Ursi**

Herb Pharm
Urinary System Support (Alcohol Extract)

Goldenrod flowering tops, Corn Silk, Horsetail, **Uva Ursi**, Juniper berry

Eclectic Institute
Urinary Tract Support (Capsule)

Uva Ursi, Marshmallow, **Goldenseal**, Couchgrass (Quackgrass) root, Kava Kava, Corn Silk

Nature's Way
Urinary with Cranberry (Capsule)

Cranberry, Dandelion leaf, Marshmallow, Cleavers (Bedstraw) stem, leaf, fruit & flower, Corn Silk, **Goldenseal**

Gaia Herbs
Usnea Uva Ursi Supreme (Alcohol Extract)

Coptis (Chinese Goldthread,Huang Lian), Echinacea (angustifolia) root, Echinacea (purpurea) aerial parts, root & seed, Usnea, **Uva Ursi**

Herbalist & Alchemist
UT Compound™ (Alcohol Extract)

Cleavers (Bedstraw), Hydrangea, **Uva Ursi**, Agrimony, Corn Silk, **Oregon Grape**

RidgeCrest Herbals
UTIntensive™ (Capsule)

Astragalus root, Gravel Root root, **Uva Ursi fruit**, Burdock root, Juniper berry, Parsley leaf, Alisma (Water Plantain) root, Buchu leaf, Corn Silk, Dandelion root, Birch (White) leaf, Cleavers (Bedstraw), **Cranberry**, Blueberry fruit, Hibiscus; Non-Herbal: Vitamin B6, potassium, magnesium

Eclectic Institute
Uva Ursi - Horsetail (Alcohol Extract)

Uva Ursi, Horsetail, Echinacea root and seed, Goldenrod flowering tops, **Oregon Grape**, Marshmallow

Eclectic Institute
Uva Ursi - Horsetail Cranberry (Glycerine Extract)

Uva Ursi, Horsetail, Echinacea (purpurea) root, Goldenrod flowering tops, **Oregon Grape**, Marshmallow, **Cranberry**

Planetary Herbals
Uva Ursi Diurite™ (Tablet)

Poria Mushroom, Dandelion root, **Uva Ursi**, Ginger, Marshmallow, Parsley root, **Uva Ursi**; Non-Herbal: Calcium

Irwin Naturals
Very Cranberry® (Softgel)

Evening Primrose oil, **Cranberry**, Aloe vera leaf, Rose flower, Black Pepper, Ginger; Non-Herbal: Vitamin C (Ascorbic Acid), Shilajit extract, Citrus Bioflavonoids

Uterine Tonic Formulas

See also *Female Hormonal Balancing, PMS Relieving, Pregnancy Tonic* and *Styptic/Hemostatic Formulas*

This is a subcategory of *Female Hormonal Balancing Formulas*, that are used to strengthen and tone up the uterus. They may also have some of the same properties as *Styptic/Hemostatic Formulas*. This can be helpful in preparing for pregnancy and childbirth or in clearing up heavy menstrual bleeding. These remedies may also be useful for treating a prolapsed uterus.

Key Herbs: Lady's Mantle, Partridge Berry (Squaw Vine) and Red Raspberry

Grandma's Herbs
Fem-Aid (Capsule)

False Unicorn (Helonias, Chamaelirium), Wild Yam, **Lady's Mantle**, Squaw Vine (Partridge Berry), Blessed Thistle, **Raspberry (Red)**, St. John's Wort, Dong Quai, Chamomile, Blue Cohosh, Eleuthero, Cramp Bark, Sarsaparilla, Capsicum (Cayenne)

Gaia Herbs
Fem-Restore (Alcohol Extract)

Fraxinus bark, Red Root, False Unicorn (Helonias, Chamaelirium) root, Cinnamon bark, Mayapple root, Goldenseal root, Ginger rhizome, Lobelia herb and seed

Traditional Medicinals
Female Toner® (Tea)

Raspberry (Red) leaf, Licorice, Strawberry leaf, Nettle (Stinging) leaf, Angelica root, Blessed Thistle, Spearmint, Rose hips, Lemon Verbena, Lemongrass leaf, Ginger, Chamomile flower

Christopher's
Female Tonic Formula (Capsule)

Squaw Vine (Partridge Berry), **Raspberry (Red) leaf**, Nettle (Stinging) leaf, Dandelion leaf, Wild Yam, Cramp Bark, Chickweed, Dulse, Chaste Tree (Vitex), Motherwort, Ginger

Vitanica
Maternal Symmetry™ (Capsule)

Kelp, **Raspberry (Red) leaf**, Nettle (Stinging) leaf, Squaw Vine (Partridge Berry), Lemon Balm, Oat straw, Dandelion root, Ginger; Non-Herbal: Vitamin A, Vitamin C, Zinc, Vitamin D2 , Folic acid, Vitamin B12,Vitamin B6, Boron, Vitamin B3, Pantothenic Acid, Calcium, Magnesium, Manganese, Vitamin E, Vitamin K, Selenium, Chromium, Thiamin, Copper, Riboflavin, Iron, Iodine Biotin

Solaray
Menstrual Blend™ SP-7B™ (Capsule)

Cranesbill (Wild Geranium) root, Witch Hazel leaf, **Raspberry (Red) leaf**, Shepherd's Purse aerial parts, Ginger, Horsetail, Goldenseal, Irish Moss

Traditional Medicinals
Pregnancy® Tea

Raspberry (Red) leaf, Strawberry leaf, Nettle (Stinging) leaf, Spearmint, Fennel fruit, Rose hips, Alfalfa leaf, Lemon Verbena

Eclectic Institute
Red Raspberry - Squawvine (Glycerine Extract)

Raspberry (Red) leaf, Squaw Vine (Partridge Berry) aerial parts, Cramp Bark, Blue Cohosh, **Raspberry (Red)**

Vitanica
Slow Flow™ (Capsule)

Ginger, Cranesbill (Wild Geranium) root, Periwinkle, Yarrow flower, Life Root, Shepherd's Purse; Non-Herbal: Vitamin A, Vitamin C, Vitamin K1, Bioflavonoids

Herbalist & Alchemist
Uterine Tonic™ (Alcohol Extract)

Chaste Tree (Vitex), Dong Quai, Peony (White, Chinese), Cinnamon (cassia) bark, Cypress root, Saw Palmetto, Shepherd's Purse

Herb Pharm
Women's Reproductive Health (Alcohol Extract)

Dong Quai, Shatavari, Chaste Tree (Vitex), Squaw Vine (Partridge Berry), Cramp Bark, Ginger

Vascular Tonic Formulas

These are remedies that tone up flaccid veins. They can help to clear up varicose veins and spider veins. They may also be helpful for hemorrhoids, phlebitis, ulcerations on the skin, venous congestion of the liver, and fatigue and weakness in the legs. These formulas may also reduce the risk of thrombosis (the formation of blood clots in the circulatory system) which can reduce the risk of coronary thrombosis and strokes. See *Varicose Veins* in the *Conditions Section* for more information.

Key Herbs: Butchers Broom, Collinsonia (Stoneroot), Horse Chestnut and Witch Hazel

NOW Foods
Celery Seed Extract (Capsule)

Celery seed, **Horse Chestnut seed**, Hawthorn leaf and flower

Solaray
Cool Cayenne® with Butcher's Broom (Capsule)

Capsicum (Cayenne), **Butcher's Broom root**, Ginger, Guar gum

Herbalist & Alchemist
Ginkgo/Horse Chestnut Compound™ (Alcohol Extract)

Collinsonia (Stoneroot), Ginkgo, Hawthorn berry, Hawthorn flower, Lycium (Wolfberry/Gogi), Cinnamon (cassia) bark, **Horse Chestnut**

Herb Pharm
Healthy Veins Tonic™ (Alcohol Extract)

Horse Chestnut, **Butcher's Broom rhizome**, **Collinsonia (Stoneroot) leaf, flower & root**, Rosemary flowering tops, Prickly Ash

Planetary Herbals
Horse Chestnut Cream (Topical Cream)

Horse Chestnut, **Horse Chestnut**, **Butcher's Broom leaf**, **Witch Hazel bark**, Myrrh, Rosemary essential oil, Aloe vera, Jojoba oil, Grapefruit seed

Planetary Herbals
Horse Chestnut Vein Strength™ (Tablet)

Horse Chestnut, **Witch Hazel bark**, **Butcher's Broom root**, Dong Quai, Ginkgo

Nature's Way
Leg Veins with Tru-OPCs™ (Capsule)

Horse Chestnut, Dandelion leaf, **Butcher's Broom root**, Capsicum (Cayenne), Prickly Ash (Zanthoxylum americanum), Grape seed; Non-Herbal: Vitamin C

Eclectic Institute
Stone Root - Witch Hazel (Alcohol Extract and Glycerine Extract)

Collinsonia (Stoneroot) root, **Witch Hazel bark**, Huckleberry leaf, Prickly Ash, Rosemary

Eclectic Institute
Vein Support (Capsule)

Collinsonia (Stoneroot) root, **Witch Hazel bark**, Bilberry, Gotu Kola leaf

NOW Foods
Vein Supreme™ (Capsule)

Prickly Ash bark, **Horse Chestnut**, **Butcher's Broom root**, Grape seed; Non-Herbal: Rutin, Rice Flour

Herbs Etc.
Vein Tonic™ (Alcohol Extract)

Horse Chestnut nut, **Witch Hazel bark**, **Butcher's Broom root**, Rue, Sweet Clover, Calendula (Marigold) flower, Milk Thistle seed, Ocotillo stem bark, Oregon Grape root, Stevia leaf

Vitanica
VeinoBlend™ (Capsule)

Horse Chestnut, Gotu Kola, Grape seed, **Butcher's Broom**; Non-Herbal: Vitamin C, Bioflavinoids (citrus), Bromelain

Solaray
Venous Blend™ SP-32™ (Capsule)

Witch Hazel leaf, Cranesbill (Wild Geranium) root, Mullein leaf, Slippery Elm, Plantain, Butternut bark, Goldenseal

Vision Supporting Formulas

See also *Antioxidant* and *Eye Wash Formulas*

The eyes are very sensitive to oxidative damage, making it an underlying cause of eye problems like macular degeneration and glaucoma. *Vision Supporting Formulas* help to protect the eyes from oxidative damage. They can also help prevent blindness caused by diabetes when taken regularly.

Besides the key herbs, vision supporting formulas may also contain lutein and zeaxanthin, two carotenoids that have antioxidant properties that have been shown to protect the eyes. Obviously, *Antioxidant Formulas* may also be beneficial for the eyes. Also consider an herbal *Eye Wash Formula*.

Key Herbs: Bilberry (Blueberry, Huckleberry) and Eyebright

NOW Foods
Bilberry Complex (Capsule)

Bilberry fruit, Carrot; Non-Herbal: Riboflavin, citrus bioflavonoids

Yerba Prima
Bilberry Extra Strength (Capsule)

Bilberry, Black Pepper

Planetary Herbals
Bilberry Eye Complex™ (Tablet)

Eyebright aerial parts, **Bilberry**, Rehmannia, Lycium (Wolfberry/Gogi), Chrysanthemum flower, Chinese Yam rhizome, Tree Peony, Tribulus fruit, Poria Mushroom, Asian Water Plantain, Asiatic Dogwood berry; Non-Herbal: Vitamin C, Calcium, Iron

Christopher's
Bilberry Eye Support Formula (Capsule)

Bilberry, **Eyebright**, Ginkgo, Capsicum (Cayenne)

Solaray
Eye Blend™ SP-23™ (Capsule)

Eyebright aerial parts, Goldenseal, Dandelion root, Raspberry (Red) leaf, Fennel, Slippery Elm

Gaia Herbs
Eyebright Bayberry Supreme (Alcohol Extract)

Bayberry, **Eyebright**, Goldenseal, Nettle (Stinging) leaf, Yarrow

Grandma's Herbs
Eyebright-Plus (Capsule)

Eyebright, **Bilberry**, Bayberry, Raspberry (Red), Goldenseal, Blue Vervain, Fennel, Chamomile, Capsicum (Cayenne); Non-Herbal: Lutein

Nature's Way
Ginkgold® Eyes (Capsule)

Bilberry, Ginkgo, Calendula (Marigold) flower; Non-Herbal: Lutein Carotinioid, Zeaxanthin Carotinioid

Western Botanicals
Herbal Eyebright Formula (Capsule)

Bayberry bark, **Eyebright**, Goldenseal, Raspberry (Red) leaf, Capsicum (Cayenne)

Herbalist & Alchemist
Insight Compound™ (Alcohol Extract)

Ginkgo, Lycium (Wolfberry/Gogi), Blueberry, Chrysanthemum flower

Gaia Herbs
Vision Enhancement (Liquid Phyto-Caps)

Bilberry, Grape

Nature's Way
Vision with Lutein & Bilberry (Capsule)

Bilberry, Eleuthero root; Non-Herbal: Vitamin A, Vitamin E, Riboflavin, Biotin, Zinc, Copper, Citrus Bioflavonoids, Taurine, Grape seed extract, Lutein

RidgeCrest Herbals
VisionAid™ (Capsule)

Rehmannia root, Chinese Yam root, Asiatic Dogwood fruit, Poria Mushroom, Tree Peony root bark, Alisma (Water Plantain) root, Cinnamon bark, Aconite (Monkshood) root

Weight Loss Formulas

See also *Adaptogen*, *Fiber Blend*, *General Detoxifying* and *Hypothyroid Formulas*

Weight loss, or what we should really think of as fat loss, can become an ongoing and often frustrating struggle for most people. No pill, herbal or otherwise, is going to make you lose weight if you don't make appropriate modifications in your lifestyle—particularly in the areas of nutrition and physical activity. However, there are a number of herbs that can assist the process.

Weight Loss Formulas are herbal formulas that can assist weight loss by increasing metabolism, enhancing thyroid and digestive function, and reducing hunger.

They may also aid in detoxification, which can help your body let go of fat. The herbal ingredients in Weight Loss Formulas vary considerably. Nevertheless, here are a few key ingredients commonly found in these blends.

Key ingredients in these formulas include caffeine-bearing herbs like guarana and green tea, herbs like kelp and bladderwrack to boost the thyroid, chickweed and Brigham tea. Garcinia is another popular herb in these blends.

Other categories of formulas that may be helpful in weight loss include *Hypothyroid, Fiber Blend, General De-*

toxifying and *Adaptogenic Formulas*. See *Weight Loss (aids for)* in the *Conditions Section* for more suggestions.

Key Herbs: Bladderwrack, Brigham Tea, Chickweed, Guarana, Gymnema, Kelp, Stevia and Tea (Green or Black)

Irwin Naturals
15-Day Weight Loss Cleanse & Flush (Tablet)
Psyllium seed, Uva Ursi leaf, Cascara Sagrada, Fennel seed, Marshmallow root, Capsicum (Cayenne), Black Pepper, Juniper berry, Plum, Beet root, Grapefruit, Oat bran, **Chickweed aerial parts**, Chlorella, Dandelion root, Echinacea (angustifolia), Ginger, Chamomile flower, Fenugreek seed; Non-Herbal: Calcium Carbonate, Fructooligosaccharides (FOS)

NOW Foods
African Mango Diet Support (Capsule)
Mango (African) seed, **Green Tea leaf**

Christopher's
Appetite Formula (Capsule)
Chickweed, Burdock root, Licorice, Saffron, Mandrake root, Fennel leaf, Parsley root, **Kelp**, Black Walnut, Hawthorn, Papaya, Echinacea leaf

Yogi Tea
Caramel Apple Spice Slim Life™ (Tea)
Black Tea, Rooibos (Redbush), Cinnamon bark and essential oil, Schisandra, Apple, Luo han guo (Monk Fruit) fruit, Cardamom seed and essential oil, Ginger root and essential oil, Clove, Black Pepper; Non-Herbal: Salt

Gaia Herbs
Diet Slim Tea
Dandelion, Fennel, Licorice

Gaia Herbs
Diet-Slim (Liquid Phyto-Caps)
Blueberry leaf, Turmeric root, Coleus root, **Green Tea leaf**, Bitter Orange peel, Elder (Black) berry, Ginger root, **Gymnema leaf**, Yohimbe bark, **Bladderwrack fronds**

Yogi Tea
Green Tea Blueberry Slim Life™ (Tea)
Green Tea leaf, Bilberry leaf, Hibiscus, Eleuthero root, Ginseng (Korean, Asian), Garcinia (Brindleberry), Amla (Indian Gooseberry), Belleric Myrobalan fruit, Chebulic Myrobalan fruit

Yogi Tea
Green Tea Slim Life (Tea)
Green Tea leaf, Bilberry leaf, Hibiscus, Orange, Blueberry, **Green Tea**, Eleuthero, Amla (Indian Gooseberry), Belleric Myrobalan fruit, Chebulic Myrobalan fruit, Garcinia (Brindleberry), Licorice

Celestial Seasonings
Metabo Balance Wellness Tea
Green Tea leaf, Garcinia (Brindleberry), Kola (cola) nut, Hibiscus, Orange peel, Rose hips; Non-Herbal: Rebiana (sweetener from Stevia)

Solaray
Metabolic Blend™ SP-18™ (Capsule)
Chickweed aerial parts, Celery seed, Psyllium seed, Horsetail, Fennel, Irish Moss, **Kelp**, Willow (White) bark

Christopher's
Metaburn Herbal Weight Formula (Capsule)
Brigham (Mormon) Tea, Red Clover flower, Capsicum (Cayenne), Oat straw, Damiana leaf, **Chickweed**, Juniper berry, Catnip, Senna, Capsicum (Cayenne)

Grandma's Herbs
Slim (with Caffeine) (Capsule)
Guarana, **Chickweed**, Cascara Sagrada, Cleavers (Bedstraw), Horsetail, Nettle (Stinging), Psyllium, **Bladderwrack**, St. John's Wort, **Kelp**

Grandma's Herbs
Slim Too (Caffeine Free) (Capsule)
Garcinia (Brindleberry), **Bladderwrack**, Cascara Sagrada, Schisandra, Watercress, Fennel, Fennel, Horsetail, **Chickweed**, Chia, Guggul seed, Senna, Psyllium, Grapefruit seed, Celery, Capsicum (Cayenne); Non-Herbal: Vineger Crystals

New Chapter
Supercritical Diet & Energy (Tablet)
Green Tea leaf, **White Tea**, Ginger, Maca, Capsicum (Cayenne), Rhodiola, Cinnamon (verum) bark, Fenugreek, Turmeric, Peppermint leaf, Clove, Rosemary, Sea Buckthorn, Sea Buckthorn seed, Calendula (Marigold) flower; Non-Herbal: Probiotic chromium

Planetary Herbals
Triphala-Garcinia Program™ (Tablet)
Kelp, Guar gum, Atractylodes (Bai-Zhu) root, Cleavers (Bedstraw) leaf & stem, Fennel, **Bladderwrack**, Watercress, Watercress, Licorice, Echinacea root, Astragalus, Ginger, Zizyphus seed, Burdock root, Garcinia (Brindleberry), Spirulina, Harada fruit, Amla (Indian Gooseberry), Bibhitaki (Behada) fruit; Non-Herbal: l-tyroisine, lecithin, apple cider vinegar, Sodium, Dietary Fiber, Protein, Vitamin C, Vitamin B-6, Iron, Iodine

Western Botanicals
Ultra Raspberry Ketone (Capsule)
Raspberry (Red), Mango, Maca, Schisandra, **Green Tea**, Bitter Orange, Brigham (Mormon) Tea

Traditional Medicinals
Weightless® (Tea)
Fennel fruit, Uva Ursi, Cleavers (Bedstraw), Red Clover flower, Parsley leaf, Buchu leaf, Hibiscus, Lemongrass leaf, Flax seed, Spearmint, Stevia

Traditional Medicinals
Weightless® Cranberry (Tea)
Fennel fruit, Red Clover flower, Uva Ursi, Parsley leaf, Cleavers (Bedstraw), Hibiscus, Chicory root, Cranberry, Stevia

Western Botanicals
Weightloss Formula (Capsule and Alcohol Extract)
Burdock root, **Gymnema leaf**, **Chickweed**, Echinacea (angustifolia) root, Black Walnut hulls, Licorice, Fennel, Safflower petals, Parsley leaf, **Bladderwrack**, Hawthorn leaf & flower, Papaya leaf, Shiitake Mushroom, Ginseng (American)

Herbal Formulas

Key Herbs Section

A Guide to Single Herbs Used as Key Herbs in Herbal Formulas and/or Available As Singles From the Companies Listed in this Book

The formulas in this book contain over 700 single herbs, many of which are very obscure and not readily available as singles, so we've focused only on single herbs that are either important herbs of commerce or key herbs in the various product categories in the *Formulas Section*.

For each herb we provide a brief description of what the herb is used for, plus the following information:

Latin Name(s): This is the scientific name or names of the plant being discussed.

Key Herbs: We've also indicated any product categories in which this single herb is a key ingredient. This helps you understand how the herb is used in modern herbalism.

Warnings: Here we list any cautions about the use of this herb. We were overly cautious about these warnings, especially with regard to pregnancy. That is, we've never personally seen these herbs cause some of these problems, but we wanted to make you aware of any potential problems with that herb. Part of these warnings are contraindications (cases in which a remedy shouldn't be used).

Energetics: This refers to how the herb affects biological terrain as previously discussed. It shows if the herb is warming, cooling or neutral; drying, moistening or balancing; and/or constricting, relaxing or nourishing. Here is a review of the basic energetic categories we are using:

Cooling herbs reduce irritation and excess heat.

Warming herbs relieve depression and hypoactivity.

Neutral herbs are neither warming or cooling.

Drying herbs treat stagnation and water retention.

Moistening herbs restore flexiblity and tissue function in atrophy.

Balancing herbs help to bring tissues back to normal from either stagnation or atrophy.

Relaxing herbs ease muscle spasm and improve flow of energy and fluids by easing constriction.

Constricting herbs stop leakage by toning up tissue relaxation.

Nourishing herbs provide nutrients that help the body heal itself and restore normal function.

Properties: These are the major actions of the herb upon the body. The definitions for the properties used in this book can be found in Appendix Three.

Available from: Finally, we've included a list of companies that sell the herb as a single. This will help you locate a source for the herb if you feel you need it. Some herbs are not sold as singles by any of the companies included in the book, but can be found as ingredients in herbal formulas. We included just a couple of remedies we consider very important that are not sold by the companies listed in this book.

These key herbs are all linked with various health conditions in the *Conditions Section*. We recommend that you rely on formulas rather than single herbs to help improve your health. However, you can look in this section for formulas that contain key herbs used for the health conditions you are trying to resolve.

Açaí

Latin name: *Euterpe oleracea*

Like other berries, açaí berries are loaded with antioxidants that help to protect cells from damage that may lead to chronic diseases such as heart disease, diabetes and cancer. Açaí berry contains vitamin A, fiber, calcium, iron, essential fatty acids (omega-9), anthocyanins (antioxidant) and polysterols. The Journal of Agriculture and Food Chemistry published a 2008 study showing that the açaí berry has more antioxidants than blackberries, blueberries, strawberries, raspberries, but fewer antioxidants than red wine and pomegranate juice. A 2006 study by the American Chemical Society showed that açaí mimics the anti-inflammatory effects of prescription medications, such as the COX-1 and COX-2 inhibitors.

Açaí is a key ingredient in *Antioxidant Formulas*

Warnings: No known warnings.

Energetics: Cooling and nourishing

Properties: Anti-inflammatory, antioxidant and nutritive

Available from: Eclectic Institute, Gaia Herbs, Nature's Way, Planetary Herbals and Solaray

Agrimony

Latin name: *Agrimonia eupatoria*

Agrimony has an almost paradoxical action. On one hand, it is an astringent, so it helps stop bleeding in wounds and diarrhea. On the other hand, it relieves tension in the nervous system. Its indication as a flower remedy is a good guide to its herbal use—it helps people who mask their pain behind a facade of cheerfulness. I find it very helpful for people who have a tense pulse and appear friendly and cheerful, but are actually very tense and stressed. It is a great urinary tract remedy and helps urinary tract infections, cystitis and incontinence. It also helps "constricted liver chi," a condition from Chinese medicine that is commonly seen in many Americans. This involves an inner resistance, anger or frustration that constricts blood flow to the liver and creates a tense, wiry pulse. It relaxes blood flow to the liver and helps a person relax and go with the flow of life.

Warnings: No known warnings.

Energetics: Drying and relaxing

Properties: Anti-inflammatory, astringent, hemostatic and vulnerary

Available from: Herbalist & Alchemist

Alfalfa

Latin name: *Medicago sativa*

Alfalfa has been called the king of herbs, and it has been used since ancient times. Roots can grow 30-60 feet deep to pick up minerals and water other plants can't reach. This makes alfalfa a rich source of vitamins, minerals, trace minerals and other nutrients. Its trace mineral content is probably what makes it valuable for the pituitary, since trace mineral deficiencies often affect this gland. It acts as a mild alterative and blood purifier and has been used for arthritis, poor appetite, general weakness and mineral deficiencies. Alfalfa and peppermint make a good tea for digestive troubles.

Alfalfa is a key ingredient in *Iron, Joint Healing, Mineral, Pregnancy Tonic* and *Superfood Formulas*

Warnings: Alfalfa is contraindicated in lupus.

Energetics: Moistening and nourishing

Properties: Anticoagulant (blood thinner), bitter, galactagogue, mineralizer and nutritive

Available from: Eclectic Institute, Grandma's Herbs, Herb Pharm, Herbalist & Alchemist, Nature's Answer, Nature's Way, NOW Foods, Solaray and Western Botanicals

Aloe vera

Latin name: *Aloe vera syn. A. barbadenis*

Aloe vera juice and gel are made from the inner pulp of the aloe vera leaf. Aloe is extremely soothing to irritated skin and mucous membranes, burns and other damaged tissues. Whole leaf aloe vera juice also builds the immune system to help fight arthritis, AIDS, cancer and other degenerative diseases.

Aloe vera gel may be applied full strength topically for burns and skin irritations. Apply liberally and keep the skin moist for best results. Aloe vera works best when fresh. It's easy to keep an aloe plant in the home for treating burns, because they are very easy to grow.

The green part of the leaf is a strong purgative, but is filtered out in the juice and gel. This is why the leaf, which contains anthraquinone glycosides, is a stimulant laxative.

Aloe vera is a key ingredient in *Stimulant Laxative* and *Ulcer Healing Formulas*

Warnings: Some herbalists suggest that children, the elderly and pregnant women should not drink aloe vera juice. However, this may apply only to the green leaf portion (which is strongly cathartic) or to aloe vera concentrates. The diluted juice is a mild, harmless remedy.

Energetics: Cooling and moistening

Properties: Anti-inflammatory, antiseptic, demulcent (mucilant), emollient, laxative (stimulant), purgative (cathartic), soothing and vulnerary

Available from: Nature's Herbs (TwinLab), Nature's Way, New Chapter, Solaray and Western Botanicals

Andrographis

Latin name: *Andrographis paniculata*

Andrographis extracts have been shown to mildly inhibit *Staphylococcus aurea, Psudomonas aeurginosa, Proteus vulgaris, Shigella dysenteriae* and *Escherihia coli*. Extracts have also been shown to inhibit lipid peroxidation and inflammation. It is used in Ayurvedic medicine for diarrhea, dyspepsia, lack of bile flow, hepatitis, malteria, pneumonia, tonsillitis, colds, sinus infections and flu and is used by modern herbalists to treat intestinal parasites, colds, influenza and hepatitis. In a clinical study, patients treated with andrographis for three months were 2.1 times less likely to catch colds than the placebo group.

Warnings: Not for use during pregnancy or lactation.

Energetics: Cooling and drying

Properties: Anti-inflammatory, antibacterial, bitter, cholagogue, febrifuge and immune stimulant

Available from: Herb Pharm, Herbalist & Alchemist, Nature's Way, NOW Foods, Planetary Herbals and Solaray

Angelica

Latin name: *Angelica archangelica*

Angelica is a warming, aromatic tonic useful for many ailments. Angelica helps to warm a cold, stiff, weakened body and is especially warming to the stomach, spleen and intestines. This makes it helpful for poor digestion, colic and intestinal cramps. It promotes perspiration, making it useful for reducing fever. It also helps recovery from colds, flu and congestion in the lungs. Angelica is an important female remedy that helps to regulate menses and balance hormones, as it is related to dong quai and has similar actions. It can also be applied externally for bruises, sprains, muscle and joint pain.

Angelica is a key ingredient in *Digestive Bitter Tonic Formulas*

Warnings: Not for use during pregnancy or while nursing. Also contraindicated in heavy menstrual bleeding.

Energetics: Warming and drying

Properties: Aromatic, decongestant and digestive tonic

Available from: Eclectic Institute, Herb Pharm, Herbalist & Alchemist, Nature's Answer and Western Botanicals

Anise

Latin name: *Pimpinella anisum*

Anise is a soothing aromatic with properties similar to fennel. Tea, tincture or oil can be used to settle the stomach and expel gas. It is useful for colic in infants and helps promote lactation. It is a mucolytic agent and helps to thin and expel mucus from the lungs. It is a common ingredient in formulas for indigestion, but is not a key herb in these formulas.

Warnings: Don't use during pregnancy except under the supervision of a well-trained herbalist (herbiverse.com).

Energetics: Warming and drying

Properties: Aromatic, carminative and galactagogue

Available from: Eclectic Institute and Herb Pharm

Arjuna

Latin name: *Terminalia arjuna (Combretaceae)*

Valued as a remedy for the heart and poor circulation in Ayurvedic medicine, arjuna is used as a treatment for angina, congestive heart failure, heart problems related to smoking, and elevated blood pressure. It is used in a very similar manner to hawthorn and works well when combined with it.

Arjuna is a key ingredient in *Cardiac Tonic Formulas*

Warnings: No known warnings.

Energetics: Cooling and relaxing (slightly)

Properties: Anti-arrhythmic, cardiac, hypotensive and vasodilator

Available from: Planetary Herbals and Solaray

Arnica

Latin name: *Arnica montana*

Arnica is used to reduce swelling, bruising and pain from injury and trauma. It is most often used as a homeopathic preparation both internally and topically to treat swelling, bruises and injuries. It is a good idea to keep homeopathic arnica (both tablets and topical cream) in your first aid kit. Arnica tincture is used topically for these purposes.

Arnica tincture, taken internally, acts as a cardiac tonic and improves the supply of blood through the coronary vessels, but should be taken only under professional supervision as it is highly toxic. It should be highly diluted when used internally—just a few drops diluted in water.

Arnica is a key ingredient in *Topical Analgesic* and *Topical Vulnerary Formulas*

Warnings: Gastric irritation may develop with internal use of the herb. High doses taken internally can cause intoxication, dizziness, tremors, tachycardia, arrhythmia and collapse. Arnica tincture should not be used during pregnancy or nursing. Homeopathic preparations do not cause these problems, but both the herb and the homeopathic preparations should not be applied to broken skin.

Energetics: Warming and drying

Properties: Analgesic (anodyne), anticoagulant (blood thinner), vasodilator and vulnerary

Available from: Eclectic Institute, Herb Pharm, Herbalist & Alchemist and Western Botanicals

Artichoke

Latin name: *Cynara scolymus*

This is the leaf of the globe artichoke that is eaten as a vegetable. It contains cynarin, which has proven liver protection capabilities. Artichoke also contains silymarin, the active constituent of milk thistle. The leaves are used as a digestive bitter for a sluggish liver and poor digestion.

Artichoke is a key ingredient in *Cholagogue* and *Cholesterol Balancing Formulas*

Warnings: No known warnings.

Energetics: Cooling and drying

Properties: Alterative (blood purifier), anticholesteremic, bitter, cholagogue and digestive tonic

Available from: Gaia Herbs, Herb Pharm, Herbalist & Alchemist, Nature's Way, NOW Foods, Planetary Herbals and Solaray

Ashwaganda

Latin name: *Withania somnifera*

An important herb from Ayurvedic medicine, ashwaganda is a nervine and adrenal tonic that helps anxiety, depression, exhaustion and poor muscle tone. It is adaptogenic and reduces the effects of stress, while promoting energy and vitality. It is used as a supporting herb for recovery from debilitating diseases, and is effective for treating sexual dysfunction caused by stress. It is also an effective anti-inflammatory that can relieve symptoms associated with arthritis pain. Ashwaganda is also helpful for boosting the conversion of T4 (the thyroid storage hormone) to T3 (the active thyroid hormone).

Ashwaganda is a key ingredient in *Adaptogen*, *Hypothyroid* and *Immune Balancing Formulas*

Warnings: Use cautiously during pregnancy.

Energetics: Warming (slightly)

Properties: Adaptogen, anti-inflammatory, antidepressant and nervine

Available from: Gaia Herbs, Herb Pharm, Herbalist & Alchemist, Nature's Answer, Nature's Way, NOW Foods, Planetary Herbals, Solaray and Western Botanicals

Astragalus

Latin name: *Astragalus membranaceus (Leguminosae)*

Astragalus is an adaptogenic and tonic herb used in Chinese medicine to boost energy and strengthen immunity. Research suggests that the polysaccharides and saponins in astragalus may be helpful to those with heart disease, improving heart function and providing relief from symptoms. Astragalus appears to restore immune and adrenal function in people whose immune systems have been weakened by chemotherapy or chronic illness. It has antibacterial and antiviral properties, making it useful as a topical treatment for healing wounds. It can be helpful both in preventing and treating common colds and respiratory infections. Astragalus may also have benefits in treating allergic asthma.

Astragalus is a key ingredient in *Adaptogen*, *Antiviral*, *Cold and Flu*, *Digestive Tonic*, *Immune Balancing*, *Immune Stimulating*, *Lung* and *Respiratory Tonic* and *Moistening Lung/Cough Formulas*

Warnings: No known warnings.

Energetics: Warming (slightly) and moistening

Properties: Adaptogen, anti-inflammatory, antiviral, diuretic, hypotensive and immune amphoteric

Available from: Eclectic Institute, Gaia Herbs, Herb Pharm, Herbalist & Alchemist, Herbs Etc., Nature's Answer, Nature's Herbs (TwinLab), Nature's Way, NOW Foods, Planetary Herbals, Solaray and Western Botanicals

Atractylodes

Latin name: *Atractylodes ovata, A. macrocephala*

This Chinese herb is used in digestive and urinary combinations. It may also be helpful for treating fungal and bacterial infections.

Atractylodes is a key ingredient in *Digestive Tonic Formulas*

Warnings: Contraindicated with high fever, excessive sweating, severe inflammation or dehydration.

Energetics: Warming and drying

Properties: Anti-inflammatory, carminative, digestive tonic and diuretic

Available from: Herbalist & Alchemist

Bacopa (Water Hyssop)

Latin name: *Bacopa monnieri*

Used in India to treat nervous disorders such as anxiety, insanity, seizures and poor memory, bacopa has become a popular herb for aiding brain function in Western herbalism. In a recent clinical trial of 98 healthy people over age 55, Bacopa significantly improved memory acquisition and retention.

Bacopa (Water Hyssop) is a key ingredient in *Brain and Memory Tonic Formulas*

Warnings: Not for use with hyperthyroidism.

Energetics: Cooling

Properties: Anti-inflammatory, antioxidant, cerebral tonic and nervine

Available from: Herb Pharm, Herbalist & Alchemist, Planetary Herbals, Solaray

Barberry

Latin name: *Berberis vulgaris or aristata*

One of the best bitter liver tonics, barberry contains the antiseptic berberine for fighting bacterial infection. It also has antifungal properties. It increases bile production. It has been shown to triple bile production for an hour and a half. It is also a common ingredient in blood purifying formulas. This herb can also be helpful for multiple personality disorder either as an herb or a homeopathic.

Barberry is a key ingredient in *Cholagogue* and *General Detoxifying Formulas*

Warnings: Not for use during pregnancy or when emaciated.

Energetics: Cooling and drying

Properties: Alterative (blood purifier), antiseptic, aperient, bitter and cholagogue

Available from: Herbalist & Alchemist, Nature's Answer and Western Botanicals

Bayberry

Latin name: *Myrica cerifera*

A strong astringent with a mild aromatic (stimulant) action, bayberry is a good astringent for the GI tract. It Inhibits or slows bleeding, arrests diarrhea and loosens phlegm to aid the discharge of mucus from the sinuses and gastrointestinal tract.

Bayberry is a key ingredient in *Cough Remedy* and *Eye Wash Formulas*

Warnings: Use with caution during pregnancy.

Energetics: Warming (slightly), drying and constricting

Properties: Astringent, expectorant, hemostatic, styptic and vulnerary

Available from: Eclectic Institute, Herb Pharm, Herbalist & Alchemist, Nature's Answer, Nature's Way, Solaray and Western Botanicals

Bee Pollen

Bee pollen contains every known nutrient in trace amounts. It is highly energizing and therefore used to increase energy, stamina and endurance. It supports the glands and aids the immune system. Bee pollen has been used to overcome allergies to pollen. In overcoming allergies it is best to get bee pollen from local beekeepers and start with a small amount (just a few grains). Gradually increase the dose over a period of several weeks to develop a tolerance to pollen and improve immune function.

Bee Pollen is a key ingredient in *Energy-Boosting Formulas*

Warnings: A few allergic attacks have been reported from use of bee pollen. Symptoms of allergy include itching, dizziness and difficulty swallowing. If you have allergies, be sure to start with a small amount (a few grains).

Energetics: Neutral and nourishing

Properties: Nutritive and stimulant (metabolic)

Available from: Nature's Way, NOW Foods and Solaray

Beet Root

Latin name: *Beta vulgaris*

Due to its high iron content, beet root builds the blood and restores color back to the skin. It also helps produce hydrochloric acid for digestion. Beet root also increases the rate at which free radicals are removed from the body, decreasing one's exposure to their cellular and DNA-damaging effects and reducing the risk of developing cardiovascular disease and cancer. Eating beets is the best way to obtain their benefits.

Beet Root is a key ingredient in *Iron* and *Liver Tonic Formulas*

Warnings: No known warnings.

Energetics: Neutral, moistening and nourishing

Properties: Hepatic and nutritive

Available from: Eclectic Institute, Nature's Way and Solaray

Bilberry (Blueberry, Huckleberry)

Latin name: *Vaccinium myrtillus* and *other species*

Bilberry has been shown to improve night vision and help heal eye irritations. It protects collagen structures in the eyes, thereby preventing and treating macular degeneration and retinopathy. It is also used to tone blood vessels and improve circulation. Scientific studies suggest that this antioxidant-rich berry can protect against diseases of the circulatory system. Blueberries are a cousin of bilberry and can be used interchangeably. Blueberries and Bilberries can improve atherosclerosis and varicose veins. The leaves of huckleberries (and possibly other blueberries) are helpful for reducing blood sugar in diabetes.

Bilberry (Blueberry, Huckleberry) is a key ingredient in *Antioxidant* and *Vision Supporting Formulas*

Warnings: None known for fruit; long-term use of leaves can cause gastric irritation and kidney damage.

Energetics: Cooling, drying (slightly) and nourishing

Properties: Antidiabetic, nutritive, opthalmicum and vascular tonic

Available from: Eclectic Institute, Herbalist & Alchemist, Nature's Way, Planetary Herbals, Solaray and Western Botanicals

Bitter Melon

Latin name: *Momordica charantia*

Bitter melon has long been used in Ayurvedic medicine to treat type 2 diabetes. It is helpful for protecting the pancreas, while improving insulin resistance and lowering blood lipids. Compounds in the plant inhibit H. pylori, which is useful in cases of gastric ulcers. Leaf extracts have demonstrated anticancer and antitumor activity as well as antiviral activity against HIV and herpes simplex. It may be helpful for parasites and intestinal worms and stomach pain or colic accompanied with constipation.

Bitter Melon is a key ingredient in *Blood Sugar Reducing Formulas*

Warnings: May cause diarrhea, stomach ache and bloating. Should not be taken with other diabetes medications without professional supervision.

Energetics: Cooling and drying

Properties: Anthelminthic, antibacterial, anticancer, antidiabetic, antioxidant, antiviral and bitter

Available from: Eclectic Institute, Nature's Herbs (TwinLab), Planetary Herbals, Solaray and Western Botanicals

Black Cohosh

Latin name: *Cimicifuga racemosa (Ranunculaceae)*

Black cohosh is typically used for its estrogenic effects, but it's role as a source of natural estrogens is questionable. It does help to regulate hormones during menopause, however. Black cohosh is also antispasmodic and mildly analgesic. It is a good remedy for venomous bites and stings. Black cohosh can help lower blood pressure and cholesterol, reduce mucus production and enhance circulation. It helps improve dark, gloomy depression and relives dark, twisted emotional congestion.

The many properties of black cohosh make it a useful ingredient in a variety of herbal formulas.

Black Cohosh is a key ingredient in *Analgesic, Antidepressant, Antispasmodic, Female Hormonal Balancing, Menopause Balancing, Menstrual Cramp, Phytoestrogen, PMS Relieving* and *Pre-Delivery Formulas*

Warnings: Black cohosh stimulates uterine contractions. It is contraindicated in early pregnancy but can be used (especially as part of a formula) during the last weeks of pregnancy or during labor. This herb has side-effects in large doses. Can cause headaches, dizziness, irritation of the central nervous system, nausea and vomiting. If headache or dizziness occurs, reduce dose or discontinue use. When black cohosh is used in a formula, it is unlikely to cause any of these effects because the dose is too low.

Energetics: Cooling and relaxing

Properties: Analgesic (anodyne), anti-arrhythmic, antidepressant, antirheumatic, antispasmodic, antivenomous, emmenagogue and hypotensive

Available from: Eclectic Institute, Gaia Herbs, Herb Pharm, Herbalist & Alchemist, Nature's Answer, Nature's Way, NOW Foods, Planetary Herbals, Solaray, Vitanica and Western Botanicals

Key Herbs

Black Haw

Latin name: *Viburnum prunifolium*

Black Haw is used to relieve painful menstruation and low back pain. It is similar in action to cramp bark, though not as strong. Decoctions are useful for menstrual cramps and headaches. It may be added to remedies for high blood pressure.

Black Haw is a key ingredient in *Antispasmodic* and *PMS Relieving Formulas*

Warnings: Contraindicated during pregnancy, except in cases of threatened miscarriage or in the last five weeks. Large doses can be hypotensive.

Energetics: Neutral, drying, relaxing and

Properties: Analgesic (anodyne), anti-abortive and antispasmodic

Available from: Eclectic Institute, Herb Pharm and Herbalist & Alchemist

Black Pepper

Latin name: *Piper nigrum*

Pepper is the world's most traded spice and has been used since ancient times for culinary and medicinal purposes. It stimulates digestion and intestinal mobility to ease gas and bloating.

Black Pepper is a key ingredient in *Carminative Formulas*

Warnings: Large doses can cause gastrointestinal irritation in some people.

Energetics: Warming and drying (slightly)

Properties: Antiseptic, carminative and stimulant (circulatory)

Black Walnut

Latin name: *Juglans nigra*

Black walnut is a remedy for low thyroid, diarrhea, constipation, intestinal flora imbalances, Giardia, parasites, tapeworm, dysentery and Impetigo. It also fights internal and external fungal infections. Externally, it can be applied to athlete's foot, boils, cold sores, fever blisters, poison ivy and ring worm. It also builds tooth enamel when used as a tooth powder.

Black Walnut is a key ingredient in *Antiparasitic Formulas*

Warnings: Not recommended during pregnancy.

Energetics: Warming (slightly), drying and contricting (slightly)

Properties: Anticarious, antifungal, antiparasitic, bitter, immune amphoteric and vermifuge

Available from: Eclectic Institute, Gaia Herbs, Herb Pharm, Herbalist & Alchemist, Nature's Answer, Nature's Way, NOW Foods, Solaray and Western Botanicals

Blackberry

Latin name: *Rubus fruticosus*

This plant's berries are found in jams, jellies and pies. However, the root bark is a very good remedy for diarrhea. It can also be used topically as an astringent for injuries.

Warnings: No known warnings.

Energetics: Drying and constricting

Properties: Antidiarrheal, antifungal, antiseptic and astringent

Available from: Eclectic Institute and Herbalist & Alchemist

Bladderwrack

Latin name: *Fucus vesiculosus*

Bladderwrack contains iodine, which is essential to thyroid health. It also contains alginic acid, which stimulates digestion and metabolism. Bladderwrack is used to help reduce inflammation and pain in joints caused by rheumatoid arthritis. Bladderwrack is filled with fucoidan, a type of fiber that helps lower cholesterol and glucose levels, while removing toxic waste from the body. Fucoidan is known to have a variety of antitumor and antiangiogenic properties.

Bladderwrack is a key ingredient in *Hypothyroid* and *Weight Loss Formulas*

Warnings: Not for use with hyperthyroidism or Grave's disease. Use cautiously with Hashimoto's thyroiditis and during pregnancy.

Energetics: Cooling, moistening and nourishing

Properties: Anti-inflammatory, antirheumatic and nutritive

Available from: Eclectic Institute, Herb Pharm, Herbalist & Alchemist, Nature's Answer, Nature's Way, Solaray and Western Botanicals

Blessed Thistle

Latin name: *Cnicus benedictus*

Blessed thistle is a bitter herb with high mineral content. It is used to strengthen the liver and digestive system with properties similar to milk thistle. It is also taken with marshmallow by nursing mothers to enrich and increase breast milk.

Blessed Thistle is a key ingredient in *Female Hormonal Balancing, Liver Tonic, Nursing Aid, PMS Relieving* and *Pre-Delivery Formulas*

Warnings: Not recommended during pregnancy.

Energetics: Cooling and drying

Properties: Alterative (blood purifier), bitter, cholagogue, galactagogue and hepatic

Available from: Eclectic Institute, Herb Pharm, Herbalist & Alchemist, Nature's Answer, Nature's Herbs (TwinLab), Nature's Way, Solaray and Western Botanicals

Bloodroot

Latin name: *Sanguinaria canadensis*

An expectorant for dry, irritating cough, bloodroot clears mucus from bronchioles and sinuses. It is a very powerful lymph moving herb, but used only in very tiny doses. Externally it is used for fungal infections, eczema, skin disorders, cancer, tumors, ringworm, scabies, warts and venereal sores.

Bloodroot is a key ingredient in *Dental Health Formulas*

Warnings: Used internally in very small doses. Large doses can cause nausea, vomiting, headaches and respiratory failure. Do not use during pregnancy. For use under professional supervision only.

Energetics: Drying and cooling

Properties: Anticancer, antifungal, antiseptic, bitter and lymphatic

Available from: Eclectic Institute, Herb Pharm and Western Botanicals

Blue Cohosh

Latin name: *Caulophyllum thalictroides*

Blue cohosh root is used to help induce labor and support contractions during labor. Today, herbalists use the herb in small doses over a period of time to induce delayed labor. This also works for inducing delayed menstruation. Taken during labor, blue cohosh strengthens contractions and eases the pain of childbirth. Its tonic action actually stimulates and relaxes the uterus at the same time, making it helpful for relieving painful menstrual symptoms such as cramps and breast pain. It can also be used to help ovarian pain.

Blue Cohosh is a key ingredient in *Antispasmodic, Menstrual Cramp, PMS Relieving* and *Pre-Delivery Formulas*

Warnings: Because it stimulates uterine contractions, it should be avoided by pregnant women or women who are trying to become pregnant. It should also be avoided with heavy menstrual bleeding. It can be used by women after their due date to induce labor, but professional supervision is advised. Blue cohosh can be mildly toxic in large doses.

Energetics: Cooling, drying and relaxing

Properties: Antispasmodic, emmenagogue and oxytocic

Available from: Herb Pharm, Herbalist & Alchemist, Nature's Answer, Solaray and Western Botanicals

Blue Flag

Latin name: *Iris versicolor*

This powerful liver cleansing herb is best used in small doses or as part of a combination. It is considered helpful for chronic skin diseases and gallbladder problems involving a lack of bile flow. It helps with hypoglycemia associated with migraines, sugar cravings and red-colored skin.

Blue Flag is a key ingredient in *Cholagogue Formulas*

Warnings: The fresh root is too strong for internal use and can be toxic. Only the dried herb should be used. Large doses of the dried herb can cause nausea, vomiting, intestinal pain and diarrhea. Not for use during pregnancy or lactation.

Energetics: Cooling and drying

Properties: Bitter, cholagogue, emetic and lymphatic

Available from: Herb Pharm and Western Botanicals

Blue Vervain

Latin name: *Verbena hastada (blue vervain) V. officinalis (vervain)*

This herb can be used internally to relax the nerves and combat anxiety. It is very helpful for nervous exhaustion from long term stress or fanatical, hard driving personalities and for people who suffer from neck and shoulder pain, feeling like they're "tied up in knots." It's helpful for rage and women who suffer from anger and tension just before their period. It can alleviate some types of headaches, including migraines associated with PMS. "Detail people" who suffer from surface and peripheral nervous system problems and have neuralgias and skin problems may also benefit from blue vervain. It is beneficial for many spasmodic nervous disorders including tics, Palsy and Tourette's. It can also be helpful for colds, flu, respiratory congestion and mild pain.

Blue Vervain is a key ingredient in *Relaxing Nervine Formulas*

Warnings: Extremely large doses may cause nausea and vomiting. Large doses could potentially stimulate a miscarriage in pregnant women, although in normal doses Blue Vervain was used traditionally to protect against miscarriage.

Energetics: Cooling (slightly), drying and relaxing

Properties: Bitter, diaphoretic/sudorific, diuretic, expectorant, hypotensive, nervine and relaxant

Available from: Eclectic Institute, Herb Pharm, Herbalist & Alchemist, Nature's Answer and Western Botanicals

Boneset

Latin name: *Eupatorium perfoliatum*

An aromatic and bitter herb traditionally used for colds, fevers and flu. Taken as a warm tea it helps to promote perspiration and acts as an emetic. Taken as a cold tea it acts as a tonic. Combined with mint it helps to relieve vomiting and bloating. Combined with ginger and anise it aids coughs. It is very helpful for flu accompanied by aches in the muscles.

Boneset is a key ingredient in *Cold and Flu Formulas*

Warnings: Use cautiously during pregnancy. Long term use is not recommended.

Energetics: Cooling, drying and relaxing (slightly)

Properties: Analgesic (anodyne), bitter, diaphoretic/sudorific and emetic

Available from: Eclectic Institute, Herb Pharm, Herbalist & Alchemist, Nature's Answer and Western Botanicals

Borage

Latin name: *Borago officinalis*

Borage seed oil is high in polyunsaturated fatty acids and is used for inflammation, skin conditions and arthritis. Borage herb is a mood-elevating remedy that boosts adrenal function and lifts sadness and depression. Used as a flower essence it promotes cheerful courage when facing adversity.

Borage is a key ingredient in *Adrenal Tonic Formulas*

Warnings: None for the oil, but the herb itself contains pyrrolizidine alkaloids and should be used with caution. Borage herb is contraindicated in pregnancy.

Energetics: Cooling, moistening and nourishing

Properties: Adrenal tonic, anti-inflammatory, antidepressant, decongestant and expectorant

Available from: Planetary Herbals and Solaray

Boswellia

Latin name: *Boswellia serrata*

Boswellia resin has been used in traditional Ayurvedic medicine as a remedy for arthritis, pulmonary diseases, ringworm and diarrhea. The active constituent in boswellia is boswellic acid, which appears to have anti-inflammatory and anti-arthritic actions. Research studies have shown that Boswellia may be helpful in treating osteoarthritis, rheumatoid arthritis, bursitis, tendonitis, Crohn's disease and ulcerative colitis.

Boswellia is a key ingredient in *Anti-Inflammatory* and *Joint Healing Formulas*

Warnings: No known warnings.

Energetics: Cooling and moistening

Properties: Analgesic (anodyne), anti-inflammatory and expectorant

Available from: Nature's Way, NOW Foods and Solaray

Key Herbs

Brigham Tea

Latin name: *Ephedra sp.*

Brigham tea is a southwestern herb related to Chinese ephedra, which is now illegal to sell. It is a milder stimulant and decongestant than Chinese ephedra.

Brigham Tea is a key ingredient in *Sinus Decongestant* and *Weight Loss Formulas*

Warnings: No known warnings.

Energetics: Warming, drying and contricting (slightly)

Properties: Stimulant (metabolic)

Buchu

Latin name: *Barosma betulina*

A strong diuretic native to Africa, Buchu is used primarily for problems with the urinary tract. It can also be helpful for the prostate.

Buchu is a key ingredient in *Diuretic* and *Prostate Formulas*

Warnings: Contraindicated with dryness. Not recommended for children under two years of age. Not to be used with acute inflammation of the urinary tract.

Energetics: Warming and drying

Properties: Antiseptic, carminative and diuretic

Available from: Eclectic Institute, Herb Pharm, Herbalist & Alchemist and Western Botanicals

Buckthorn

Latin name: *Rhamnus frangula*

A bitter laxative with properties similar to cascara sagrada but not as harsh, buckthorn is most often used to relieve constipation.

Buckthorn is a key ingredient in *General Detoxifying* and *Stimulant Laxative Formulas*

Warnings: Not recommended for use during pregnancy or by persons who are weak. Avoid prolonged use.

Energetics: Cooling and drying

Properties: Anthelminthic, bitter and laxative (stimulant)

Available from: Eclectic Institute, New Chapter, Solaray and Western Botanicals

Bugleweed

Latin name: *Lycopus virginicus*

Bugleweed inhibits iodine metabolism and helps to reduce an overactive thyroid. It is used with lemon balm and motherwort for Grave's disease. It also influences the lungs and heart and can be beneficial for a rapid or irregular heartbeat, especially when it coincides with sleep difficulties.

Bugleweed is a key ingredient in *Hyperthyroid Formulas*

Warnings: Bugleweed should not be used in cases of underactive thyroid (hypothyroidism). It should not be taken during pregnancy or with excessive menstrual bleeding.

Energetics: Cooling and drying

Properties: Antithyrotropic and cardiac

Available from: Herb Pharm and Herbalist & Alchemist

Bupleurum

Latin name: *Bupleurum chinense syn. B. scorzoneraefolium (Umbelliferae)*

A bitter and aromatic Chinese herb, bupleurum is an ingredient in many Chinese formulas for liver, blood and skin conditions. Bupleurum contains saikosides which strengthen liver function while protecting the liver from toxins. It has an anti-inflammatory effect and can reduce the risk of liver cancer in people with cirrhosis.

Bupleurum is a key ingredient in *Antidepressant, Immune Balancing* and *Liver Tonic Formulas*

Warnings: No known warnings.

Energetics: Cooling and drying

Properties: Alterative (blood purifier), antidepressant and carminative

Available from: Herbalist & Alchemist, Nature's Answer and Planetary Herbals

Burdock

Latin name: *Arctium lappa (Compositae)*

A bitter herb used for skin conditions and general liver problems. Stimulates bile function and strengthens the liver. Cleanses the blood of harmful toxins. Also helps with indigestion and clearing up acne and other skin irritations. May be applied as a poultice to infected sores. A strong decoction can be used in baths for itching. Burdock helps to stabilize mast cells which reduces allergic reactions.

Burdock's many properties make it useful in a wide variety of herbal formulas.

Burdock is a key ingredient in *Allergy-Reducing, Anticancer, Blood Purifier, Drawing Salve, Essiac, General Detoxifying, Joint Healing, Lymphatic Drainage* and *Skin Healing Formulas*

Warnings: Use with caution during pregnancy.

Energetics: Cooling, moistening and nourishing

Properties: Alterative (blood purifier), anticancer, bitter, cholagogue, diuretic, hepatic, lymphatic and mast cell stabilizer

Available from: Eclectic Institute, Herb Pharm, Herbalist & Alchemist, Nature's Answer, Nature's Way, NOW Foods, Solaray and Western Botanicals

Butchers Broom

Latin name: *Ruscus aculeatus*

Butcher's broom is a tonic for the vascular system, helping to prevent blood clots and to tone arteries and veins. It is particularly helpful for phlebitis, varicose veins, hemorrhoids and bruises.

Butchers Broom is a key ingredient in *Vascular Tonic Formulas*

Warnings: No known warnings.

Energetics: Cooling, drying and contricting (slightly)

Properties: Vascular tonic

Available from: Herb Pharm, Nature's Way, NOW Foods, Solaray and Western Botanicals

Butterbur Root

Latin name: *Petasites hybridus*

This herb was tested on hay fever (allergic rhinitis) symptoms and found to be as effective as many OTC and prescription drugs. Butterbur has also been shown to reduce the frequency, intensity and duration of migraines. It is also a useful remedy for cramps and asthma.

Butterbur Root is a key ingredient in *Migraine/Headache Formulas*

Warnings: The plant contains pyrrolizidine alkaloids (which can be toxic to the liver), but extracts are available with these alkaloids removed.

Energetics: Cooling and drying

Properties: Analgesic (anodyne), anti-allergenic, antitussive and expectorant

Available from: Planetary Herbals and Solaray

Butternut bark

Latin name: *Juglans cinerea*

Butternut bark is a milder alternative to cascara sagrada and buckthorn. The unripe nut is used to kill intestinal worms.

Butternut bark is a key ingredient in *Stimulant Laxative Formulas*

Warnings: Avoid using during pregnancy and lactation.

Energetics: Cooling and drying

Properties: Bitter, laxative (stimulant) and vermifuge

Available from: Eclectic Institute and Herbalist & Alchemist

Calendula

Latin name: *Calendula officinalis (Compositae)*

Calendula is commonly used topically to speed tissue healing after injuries, burns and bruises, both as an herb and as a homeopathic remedy. It is also a useful remedy for dry skin, eczema and hemorrhoids and can ease pain in minor injuries when applied topically.

Calendula is a key ingredient in *Tissue Healing, Topical Analgesic* and *Topical Vulnerary Formulas*

Warnings: Internal use is contraindicated in pregnancy. Topical use is completely safe.

Energetics: Cooling, drying and constricting

Properties: Astringent, hemostatic, styptic and vulnerary

Available from: Eclectic Institute, Herb Pharm, Herbalist & Alchemist, Nature's Answer, Nature's Way and Western Botanicals

Key Herbs

California Poppy

Latin name: *Eschscholzia californica*

California poppy is in the same family as opium poppy and has mild sedative and analgesic properties, but is not narcotic. It helps to normalize nervous system function to ease nervous tension, anxiety, insomnia and pain (internal and external). It has an affinity for GABA receptors in the brain, calming the mind without depressing the central nervous system.

California Poppy's calming and pain relieving properties.

California Poppy is a key ingredient in *Analgesic, Relaxing Nervine* and *Sleep Formulas*

Warnings: No known warnings.

Energetics: Cooling and relaxing

Properties: Analgesic (anodyne), sedative and soporific (hypnotic)

Available from: Eclectic Institute, Gaia Herbs, Herb Pharm, Herbalist & Alchemist and Western Botanicals

Camphor

Latin name: *Cinnamomum camphora*

Camphor is a local anesthetic, numbing the nerve endings where it is applied. Inhaled, it helps open congested air passages.

Camphor is a key ingredient in *Topical Analgesic Formulas*

Warnings: Use only as part of a *Topical Analgesic Formula*. The herb itself is for professional use only.

Energetics: Warming and relaxing

Properties: Anti-inflammatory, antiseptic, antispasmodic and expectorant

Capsicum (Cayenne)

Latin name: *Capsicum frutescens or C. annuum*

Capsicum is a major stimulant for the circulatory system. It increases circulation to every area of the body it comes in contact with, internally or externally. Capsicum also strengthens the heartbeat. Because adequate blood supply is necessary for all tissues to heal, capsicum has earned a reputation in the West as a kind of "cure-all." Capsicum is also useful for shock, heart attack and trauma. The capsaicin in capsicum blocks pain receptors, giving it an analgesic effect.

Capsicum (Cayenne) is a key ingredient in *Cardiovascular Stimulant, Cold* and *Flu* and *Topical Analgesic Formulas*

Warnings: Due to its irritating nature some people have a hard time taking capsicum. Large doses can be irritating to the stomach and cause painful bowel eliminations. Although capsicum stops bleeding and has been used to heal ulcers, this herb can cause pain when used for these purposes; hence, it should be used with caution. It is best to start with extremely small doses to build up tolerance. Capsicum causes burning sensations in sensitive areas, such as genitals, sinuses, etc. It is not recommended for people with hemorrhoids or anal fissures.

Energetics: Warming and drying

Properties: Analgesic (anodyne), anesthetic, carminative, condiment, counterirritant, diaphoretic/sudorific, hemostatic, hypertensive, hypotensive, stimulant (circulatory), stimulant (metabolic) and styptic

Available from: Eclectic Institute, Grandma's Herbs, Herb Pharm, Herbalist & Alchemist, Nature's Answer, Nature's Herbs (TwinLab), Nature's Way, NOW Foods, Solaray and Western Botanicals

Cardamom

Latin name: *Eletteria cardamomum*

An aromatic spice, cardamon acts as a carminative and digestive aid. It has a reputation as an aphrodisiac and has been used in India for respiratory and kidney ailments.

Cardamom is a key ingredient in *Carminative* and *Digestive Bitter Tonic Formulas*

Warnings: No known warnings.

Energetics: Warming and drying (slightly)

Properties: Aromatic, carminative and condiment

Available from: Herbalist & Alchemist

Cascara Sagrada

Latin name: *Rhamnus purshiana*

A bitter purgative, cascara sagrada increases bile flow and stimulates peristalsis of the colon. The name "cascara sagrada" means holy or sacred bark. It is known for its effectiveness in relieving constipation and colon cleansing.

Cascara Sagrada is a key ingredient in *General Detoxifying* and *Stimulant Laxative Formulas*

Warnings: Not recommended for use during pregnancy or for weak persons. Avoid prolonged use. If a person appears dependent on this or other stimulant laxatives or if cramps or griping become a problem, use nervines or magnesium to counteract bowel spasms. In case of diarrhea caused by excessive use, use charcoal or mucilaginous herbs. Long term use will darken the tissue color of the bowel and create laxative dependency.

Energetics: Cooling and drying

Properties: Bitter, cholagogue, laxative (stimulant) and purgative (cathartic)

Available from: Eclectic Institute, Herb Pharm, Herbalist & Alchemist, Nature's Answer, Nature's Herbs (TwinLab), Nature's Way, NOW Foods, Solaray and Western Botanicals

Catnip

Latin name: *Nepeta cataria*

A mild aromatic herb which is soothing and settling to the stomach and nerves, catnip is helpful for colds, chills, congestion, sore throat and indigestion. It is excellent for colic in infants when combined with fennel. Catnip tea is often used in enemas to bring down fevers or reduce respiratory congestion. It helps produce perspiration without increasing body heat. Catnip can also be used for nervousness or stress and at bedtime as a sleep aid.

Catnip is a key ingredient in *Antacid, Carminative, Catnip & Fennel, Nerve Tonic* and *Topical Analgesic Formulas*

Warnings: Excellent herb for children and babies, mild and extremely safe, but in extremely large doses it can cause vomiting. Avoid during pregnancy.

Energetics: Cooling and drying

Properties: Analgesic (anodyne), antacid, aromatic, carminative, diaphoretic/sudorific, nervine and sedative

Available from: Eclectic Institute, Herb Pharm, Herbalist & Alchemist, Nature's Answer, Nature's Way and Western Botanicals

Cats Claw (Uña de Gato, Gambier)

Latin name: *Uncaria sp.*

Cats claw is one of the very best remedies for normalizing function of the gastrointestinal tract. It is often helpful for ulcers, gastritis, Crohn's disease and irritable bowel syndrome. Aside from inflammation of the bowel and intestines, it can also address inflammation of the joints and muscles. Cats claw seems to have antiviral and anti-mutagenic properties, making it a good complimentary treatment for a variety of degenerative diseases and helping to strengthen the immune system against the effects of chemotherapy.

Cats Claw (Uña de Gato, Gambier) is a key ingredient in *Joint Healing Formulas*

Warnings: No known warnings. Avoid during pregnancy.

Energetics: Cooling and contricting (slightly)

Properties: Anti-inflammatory, anticancer, antimutagenic and antioxidant

Available from: Eclectic Institute, Gaia Herbs, Herb Pharm, Herbalist & Alchemist, Nature's Answer, Nature's Herbs (TwinLab), Nature's Way, NOW Foods, Planetary Herbals, Solaray and Western Botanicals

Celandine

Latin name: *Ranunculus ficaria*

A bitter herb with strong affinity for the liver and gallbladder, celandine is usually used in combination with other herbs. The juice of celandine has traditionally been used for warts, corns and ringworm.

Celandine is a key ingredient in *Cholagogue Formulas*

Warnings: Contraindicated with emaciation or weak digestion. Not for long term use. Not for use during pregnancy.

Energetics: Cooling and drying

Properties: Bitter and cholagogue

Available from: Eclectic Institute, Herb Pharm and Herbalist & Alchemist

Celery

Latin name: *Apium graveolens*

The seeds of celery are used for treating rheumatic conditions and gout. They help the kidneys to dispose of urine and other unwanted waste products. They are useful in arthritis, helping to detoxify the body and improve the circulation of blood to muscles and joints. Celery seeds are effective in treating cystitis, helping to disinfect the bladder and urinary tubules. Celery stalks are good medicine for urinary problems and for alkalizing the body in cases of rheumatism and gout.

Warnings: Use seeds cautiously during pregnancy and while lactating.

Energetics: Warming and drying

Properties: Antirheumatic, condiment and diuretic

Available from: Eclectic Institute, Herb Pharm, Herbalist & Alchemist, Nature's Answer, Nature's Herbs (TwinLab), Solaray and Western Botanicals

Key Herbs

Chamomile (English and Roman)

Latin name: *Chamomilla recutita, Matricaria recutia*

Chamomile has properties similar to catnip and peppermint. It calms the nerves and settles the stomach. It also helps to expel gas. This is an excellent nervine agent, especially for children. Use it homeopathically or make it into a tea and sweeten for colic, hyperactivity, teething, fussiness, fever or irritability in infants and children.

Chamomile is useful for colds and flu in children when combined with elderflower, peppermint and/or yarrow. It contains an anti-inflammatory volatile oil similar to the oil in yarrow. Use it in combination with other nervines and anti-inflammatory agents for pain, swelling and infection. It can be applied topically to help heal injuries and is helpful for quitting smoking when used with lobelia.

Due to its anti-inflammatory properties and its effects on the digestive and nervous systems, chamomile is a common ingredient in herbal formulas.

Chamomile (English and *Roman)* is a key ingredient in *Anti-Inflammatory, Brain Calming, Carminative, Digestive Bitter Tonic, Eye Wash, Intestinal Toning, Nerve Tonic, Quit Smoking* and *Relaxing Nervine Formulas*

Warnings: There have been reports of allergic reactions to chamomile, but these are extremely rare.

Energetics: Cooling and relaxing

Properties: Analgesic (anodyne), antiseptic, antispasmodic, aromatic, carminative, diaphoretic/sudorific, digestive tonic, nervine, opthalmicum and relaxant

Available from: Celestial Seasonings, Eclectic Institute, Herb Pharm, Herbalist & Alchemist, Nature's Answer, Nature's Way, Planetary Herbals, Solaray, Traditional Medicinals, Western Botanicals and Yogi Tea

Chaparral

Latin name: *Larrea tridentada*

A very bitter, acrid herb, chaparral has long been used as a cancer remedy and blood purifier. It contains an antioxidant substance known as NDGA. Chaparral cleanses and tones the liver, blood and lymphatics, making it useful for parasites, bacterial infection, viruses, heavy metal toxicity, drug withdrawal and radiation.

Chaparral is a key ingredient in *Anticancer, Blood Purifier* and *Drawing Salve Formulas*

Warnings: Potentially hepatotoxic, although the evidence is circumstantial. It may be due to taking the plant in capsules instead of its traditional form as a tea. Nevertheless, it is contraindicated in liver disease and when pregnant. It has a strong action on the kidneys and should be taken with ample amounts of water to protect the kidneys.

Energetics: Cooling and drying

Properties: Alterative (blood purifier), anthelminthic, antibacterial, anticancer, antioxidant, antiparasitic, antiseptic and bitter

Available from: Herb Pharm and Western Botanicals

Chastetree (Vitex)

Latin name: *Vitex agnus-castus*

Chastetree helps to regulate female hormones, making it useful for PMS and menopause. It can reduce sex drive in men and was used by Monks under vows of celibacy which is where it gets its name. It is a good remedy to balance reproductive hormones in teenagers and adults. It is generally a better remedy for women than men because it inhibits androgens (male sex hormones). It may take three to six months of use to see optimal results.

Chastetree (Vitex) is a key ingredient in *Female Hormonal Balancing, Menopause Balancing* and *PMS Relieving Formulas*

Warnings: Although a traditional remedy to prevent miscarriages, it has the potential to cause miscarriages in some women. It might reduce the effectiveness of hormonal birth control.

Energetics: Warming and drying

Properties: Anaphrodisiac

Available from: Eclectic Institute, Gaia Herbs, Herb Pharm, Herbalist & Alchemist, Herbs Etc., Planetary Herbals, Solaray, Vitanica and Western Botanicals

Cherry (Wild)

Latin name: *Prunus serotina*

An aromatic and astringent, wild cherry has a long history of use in cough remedies (why so many cough remedies are cherry-flavored). It is a cooling remedy that expels phlegm and soothes and dries out mucus membranes, making it helpful for a variety of respiratory and digestive system problems. It may also help normalize histamine reactions in allergies. In traditional Chinese medicine, it is indicated when there is "heart fire blazing," consisting of palpitations, mental restlessness, agitation, insomnia, rapid pulse, and a yellow-coated tongue with a red tip.

Cherry (Wild) is a key ingredient in *Cough Remedy, Drying Cough/Lung* and *Expectorant Formulas*

Warnings: There is a slight toxicity to wild cherry, so it should not be used in large amounts or for long periods of time. Contains hydrocyanic acid which, in high doses, may cause spasms and difficulty breathing. Medicinal doses have never proven harmful. Not recommended for use by pregnant women.

Energetics: Cooling and drying

Properties: Astringent and expectorant

Available from: Eclectic Institute, Herb Pharm, Herbalist & Alchemist, Nature's Answer and Planetary Herbals

Chickweed

Latin name: *Stellaria media*

Chickweed is a mucilaginous herb thought to break down fats and fatty tumors in the body. It acts as a mild appetite suppressant and weight loss aid when taken one hour before mealtimes. It can be used in poultices for skin irritations and the tea can be used as an eyewash for soothing irritated eyes. Applied topically, it is helpful for reliving itchy skin.

Chickweed is a key ingredient in *Anti-Itch* and *Weight Loss Formulas*

Warnings: No known warnings.

Energetics: Cooling and balancing

Properties: Demulcent (mucilant), emollient and nutritive

Available from: Eclectic Institute, Herb Pharm, Herbalist & Alchemist, Nature's Answer, Nature's Herbs (TwinLab), NOW Foods, Solaray and Western Botanicals

Cilantro/Coriander

Latin name: *Coriandrum sativum*

A widely popular culinary herb, cilantro is used by herbalists to detoxify the body and help remove heavy metals. It has been shown to seek out and bind to toxic metals and fluids in body tissue, such as mercury, lead and aluminum. A Japanese study found that levels of these metals in the body could be significantly reduced when treated with cilantro four times a day for two weeks. Coriander seeds come from the cilantro plant and are used as a carminative and digestive aid.

Cilantro/Coriander is a key ingredient in *Carminative* and *Heavy Metal Cleansing Formulas*

Warnings: No known warnings.

Energetics: Cooling and drying

Properties: Carminative, chelating and condiment

Available from: Herb Pharm, Herbalist & Alchemist, Planetary Herbals and Western Botanicals

Cinnamon

Latin name: *Cinnamomum verum syn. C. zeylanicum (Lauraceae)*

A spicy aromatic herb used in Chinese medicine as a warming stimulant, cinnamon is useful as a digestive and circulatory stimulant. Cinnamon essential oil (*Cassia variety*), has powerful properties for fighting both bacterial and fungal infections. Modern research has shown that cinnamon increases the capability of beta cells in the pancreas to produce insulin, reducing blood glucose levels in diabetics. Daily use of cinnamon was shown in recent studies to triple the efficiency of insulin, which is why it is a key ingredient in many formulas for balancing blood sugar. Cinnamon also has astringent properties and can help control heavy menstrual flows and postpartum bleeding.

Cinnamon is a key ingredient in *Blood Sugar Reducing Formulas*

Warnings: Large amounts of cinnamon oil ingested internally can cause kidney damage or coma. Cinnamon oil and bark is not recommended during pregnancy, except as a seasoning in food. It is also wise to avoid spices like cinnamon while breast feeding. Taking over two grams of cinnamon bark a day can cause gastrointestinal irritation.

Energetics: Warming, drying and constricting

Properties: Analgesic (anodyne), antidiabetic, antiseptic, aromatic, astringent, carminative, condiment and stimulant (metabolic)

Available from: Gaia Herbs, Herb Pharm, Herbalist & Alchemist, Nature's Answer, Nature's Way, New Chapter, NOW Foods, Planetary Herbals, Solaray and Western Botanicals

Cleavers (Bedstraw)

Latin name: *Galium aparine*

Cleavers, also known as bedstraw, are used to promote urination and stimulate the lymphatic system. It has been used externally as a poultice for cancerous growths, tumors, and inflammations and as a decoction for sunburn and freckles.

Cleavers (Bedstraw) is a key ingredient in *Kidney Tonic* and *Lymphatic Drainage Formulas*

Warnings: No known warnings.

Energetics: Cooling and drying

Properties: Diuretic, kidney tonic and lymphatic

Available from: Eclectic Institute, Herb Pharm, Herbalist & Alchemist, Nature's Answer and Western Botanicals

Clove

Latin name: *Eugenia carophyllata syn. Syzgium aromaticum (Myrtaceae)*

A spicy aromatic often used in combination with other herbs, cloves are valuable in liniments, gargles and digestive formulas. Powdered cloves have been used to expel parasites. Clove essential oil applied topically has a numbing effect on the nerves. It has been mixed with olive oil and applied to the gums for teething babies or toothache.

Clove is a key ingredient in *Antiparasitic* and *Dental Health Formulas*

Warnings: Clove can be irritating in large quantities. Clove oil should not be used internally without professional supervision. Use caution in pregnancy.

Energetics: Warming and drying

Properties: Analgesic (anodyne), anesthetic, antiseptic, aromatic, carminative, condiment, counterirritant, stimulant (circulatory) and vermifuge

Available from: Eclectic Institute, Herb Pharm, Herbalist & Alchemist and Western Botanicals

Codonopsis

Latin name: *Codonopsis pilosula*

Used as an expectorant and a tonic, Codonopsis increases vital energy. It can replace ginseng as a milder and safer general tonic for both men and women. It dilates peripheral blood vessels and inhibits adrenal cortex activity (to lower cortisol), thereby lowering blood pressure and improving immune function. Used in Fu Zheng therapies to prevent side effects from chemotherapy or radiation, it also increases hemoglobin levels and red blood cells, stimulates appetite and strengthens the immune system.

Codonopsis is a key ingredient in *Lung and Respiratory Tonic Formulas*

Warnings: No known warnings.

Energetics: Neutral, moistening and nourishing

Properties: Adaptogen, lung tonic and tonic

Available from: Herbalist & Alchemist, Nature's Answer and Planetary Herbals

Coleus

Latin name: *Coleus forskohlii syn. Plectranthus barbatus*

Coleus is used in India for digestive problems, but research showing it increases cAMP levels, which results in an increase in energy production throughout the body, has lead to its use or a variety of cardiac problems. It is used for congestive heart failure, poor coronary blood flow and glaucoma (topical use). When used with hawthorn it can help reduce high blood pressure. Coleus's basic cardiovascular action is to lower blood pressure while simultaneously increasing the contractility of the heart. It is also helpful for asthma and bronchitis.

Coleus is a key ingredient in *Cholesterol Balancing Formulas*

Warnings: Don't take if you have hyperthyroidism or low blood pressure. May interact with cardiac medications.

Energetics: Cooling

Available from: Gaia Herbs and Solaray

Collinsonia (Stoneroot)

Latin name: *Collinsonia canadensis*

Collinsonia is an excellent astringent for rectal problems such as anal fistulae and hemorrhoids. It can be taken orally and applied topically. It is also useful for sore throats and laryngitis, being a specific remedy for speakers and singers who develop throat irritation. It can also be used on skin for poison oak and ivy and as a topical application for injuries.

Collinsonia (Stoneroot) is a key ingredient in *Vascular Tonic Formulas*

Warnings: No known warnings.

Energetics: Cooling and constricting

Properties: Astringent and vascular tonic

Available from: Eclectic Institute, Herb Pharm and Herbalist & Alchemist

Coltsfoot

Latin name: *Tussilago farfara*

Coltsfoot is a great remedy for debilitated individuals with chronic respiratory conditions. It is indicated for asthma and emphysema, as the active constituents can decrease the time for bronchial cilia to recover after damage from smoking. Extracts of the plant have been shown to increase immune resistance. The University of Michigan Health System states that coltsfoot has been found to be just as effective as some allopathic antihistamine medicines in alleviating symptoms, without producing side effects such as drowsiness.

Coltsfoot is a key ingredient in *Cough Remedy Formulas*

Warnings: Not for use during pregnancy and lactation. May be toxic in higher doses. Use only as directed and for no longer than six weeks a year.

Energetics: Cooling and moistening

Properties: Antitussive and expectorant

Available from: Eclectic Institute and Western Botanicals

Comfrey

Latin name: *Symphytum officinale*

Comfrey is a mucilaginous herb with a slight astringent quality. It has been used for generations to aid in the healing of injuries. Not only does it contain important minerals needed in the healing process, it also contains allantoin, a substance with stimulates cell growth. Comfrey is primarily used externally in compresses, poultices and salves,. It has been used internally, but most herbalists no longer use it this way because of a concern about hepatic toxicity.

Comfrey is a key ingredient in *Poultice Formulas* and *Topical Vulnerary Formulas* for external application, but may also be found in some *Tissue Healing Formulas* for internal use.

Comfrey is a key ingredient in *Poultice, Tissue Healing* and *Topical Vulnerary Formulas*

Warnings: Completely safe for topical use. It contains pyrrozolidine alkaloids, which are believed to cause liver problems. Many people have used comfrey internally with no reported ill effects and it is probably safe to use internally for short periods. It should be avoided during pregnancy, where cancer or tumors are present or where there is a history of liver problems.

Energetics: Cooling, moistening and contricting (slightly)

Properties: Cicatrisant, emollient and vulnerary

Available from: Herb Pharm and Solaray

Cordyceps

Latin name: *Cordyceps sinensis, C. miltaris*

Cordyceps entered Western medicine after the Chinese government demonstrated its efficacy at the Olympic games in Beijing, where the Chinese athletes set new world records in nearly every competition they entered. The spectacular performance of the athletes stimulated a burst of pharmacological and clinical research into its health benefits. It is an adaptogen and general health tonic. It benefits the lungs, kidneys, glands and cardiovascular system.

Cordyceps is a key ingredient in *Adaptogen, Energy-Boosting, Exercise, Immune Balancing, Immune Stimulating* and *Mushroom Blend Formulas*

Warnings: No known warnings.

Energetics: Warming (slightly) and balancing

Properties: Adaptogen, anti-inflammatory, anticancer, anticholesteremic, antioxidant, immune amphoteric and tonic

Available from: Eclectic Institute, Herbalist & Alchemist, Planetary Herbals and Solaray

Cornsilk

Latin name: *Zea mays*

A mild, soothing diuretic agent, cornsilk is useful for kidney inflammation and relieving discomfort associated with urinary tract conditions such as inflamed bladder and painful urination.

Cornsilk is a key ingredient in *Kidney Tonic Formulas*

Warnings: No known warnings.

Energetics: Cooling and drying (slightly)

Properties: Demulcent (mucilant), diuretic and soothing

Available from: Eclectic Institute, Herb Pharm, Herbalist & Alchemist, Nature's Answer, Nature's Way and Western Botanicals

Corydalis

Latin name: *Corydalis yanhusuo*

Corydalis is a natural pain reliever that contains an alkaloid called THP, which acts similar to opium poppy but is much milder. It is a good remedy for pain associated with rheumatism, arthritis or menstruation. It can also be used as an aid for sleep.

Corydalis is a key ingredient in *Analgesic* and *Sleep Formulas*

Warnings: Not for use during pregnancy.

Energetics: Warming and relaxing

Properties: Analgesic (anodyne), narcotic, sedative and soporific (hypnotic)

Available from: Herbalist & Alchemist

Cramp Bark

Latin name: *Viburnum opulus*

As it's name implies, cramp bark is used to relax muscle spasms. It is commonly used for women as a uterine tonic since it both relaxes and tones the uterus. It has been used to ease menstrual cramps and prevent miscarriage, but may also be helpful for angina, backache and other problems involving tension.

Cramp Bark is a key ingredient in *Antispasmodic, Menstrual Cramp* and *PMS Relieving Formulas*

Warnings: Don't take with low blood pressure.

Energetics: Relaxing

Properties: Anti-abortive and antispasmodic

Available from: Herb Pharm, Herbalist & Alchemist, Planetary Herbals and Western Botanicals

Cranberry

Latin name: *Vaccinium macrocarpon*

Cranberries contain antioxidants that mitigate the damaging effects of free radicals in the body. They also contain hippuric acid, which is an antibacterial agent. For this reason they are commonly used to prevent urinary tract infections, although they can be used to help prevent other infections. They are high in vitamin C content and were used to prevent scurvy in sailors. Even commercially prepared cranberry juice cocktails have medicinal benefits, although they work better without the added sugar.

Cranberry is a key ingredient in *Urinary Infection Fighting Formulas*

Warnings: No known warnings.

Energetics: Cooling and drying (slightly)

Properties: Antibacterial, antioxidant and nutritive

Available from: Gaia Herbs, Herb Pharm, Nature's Answer, Nature's Herbs (TwinLab), Nature's Way, NOW Foods, Planetary Herbals and Solaray

Culver's root

Latin name: *Leptandra virginica*

A bitter tonic used to cleanse the liver and colon, Culver's root is a strong cholagogue, an agent that stimulates bile flow. It is best used for short periods or in combination with other herbs.

Culver's root is a key ingredient in *Cholagogue Formulas*

Warnings: Contraindicated with emaciation, weak digestion and pregnancy. High doses can cause diarrhea, vomiting, abdominal pain, vertigo and other undesirable effects.

Energetics: Cooling (slightly) and drying

Properties: Bitter and cholagogue

Available from: Herb Pharm and Herbalist & Alchemist

Key Herbs

Damiana

Latin name: *Turnera diffusa syn. T. diffusa var. aphrodisiaca (Turneraceae)*

Damiana is most commonly used to increase libido, but it is really a tonic for stress and low energy. In other words, it works best when low sex drive is due to fatigue and stress. It also has antidepressant effects.

Damiana is a key ingredient in *Antidepressant, Female Aphrodisiac* and *Male Aphrodisiac Formulas*

Warnings: Safe herb, but may want to avoid during pregnancy.

Energetics: Warming

Properties: Antidepressant, aphrodisiac, nervine and stimulant (metabolic)

Available from: Eclectic Institute, Herb Pharm, Herbalist & Alchemist, Nature's Answer, Nature's Way, Planetary Herbals, Solaray and Western Botanicals

Dandelion

Latin name: *Taraxacum officinale (Compositae)*

This common weed in lawns and gardens has a beneficial effect on the digestive system, the urinary system and the pancreas. The root is primarily used to stimulate bile flow and aid the liver, while the leaf is more often employed as a diuretic to aid kidney function. It has a beneficial effect on the microflora of the gut and helps stimulate digestive secretions. Dandelion's many properties cause it to be used in many applications.

Dandelion is a key ingredient in *Blood Purifier, Cholagogue, Digestive Bitter Tonic, Diuretic, General Detoxifying, Hepatoprotective* and *Liver Tonic Formulas*

Warnings: No known warnings.

Energetics: Cooling and drying

Properties: Alterative (blood purifier), bitter, cholagogue, digestive tonic, diuretic, hepatic and hepatoprotective

Available from: Eclectic Institute, Gaia Herbs, Herb Pharm, Herbalist & Alchemist, Nature's Answer, Nature's Herbs (TwinLab), Nature's Way, NOW Foods, Solaray, Traditional Medicinals and Western Botanicals

Devil's Claw

Latin name: *Harpagophytum procumbens (Pedaliaceae)*

Used by indigenous people for thousands of years to treat pain, stomach disorders and fever, Devil's claw is used as an anti-inflammatory in modern herbalism for treating problems like arthritis and low back pain. It Increases mobility in the joints and is a common ingredient in formulas for inflammation and arthritis.

Devil's Claw is a key ingredient in *Anti-Inflammatory* and *Joint Healing Formulas*

Warnings: Contraindicated in gastric and duodenal ulcers.

Energetics: Cooling and drying

Properties: Analgesic (anodyne), anti-inflammatory and bitter

Available from: Eclectic Institute, Herb Pharm, Herbalist & Alchemist, Nature's Answer, Nature's Way, NOW Foods, Solaray and Western Botanicals

Devil's Club

Latin name: *Oplopanax horridus*

Pacific Northwest Indians used devil's club for a myriad of conditions much the same as ginseng is used in Chinese medicine. Although it has numerous potential benefits, it is most often used to help regulate blood sugar. It also helps adrenal burnout, especially people who have dry mucus membranes.

Devil's Club is a key ingredient in *Blood Sugar Reducing Formulas*

Warnings: If collecting devil's club in the wild, be careful to avoid the prickles which may cause painful wounds.

Energetics: Cooling and moistening

Properties: Adaptogen, adrenal tonic, alterative (blood purifier), antidiabetic and tonic

Available from: Eclectic Institute, Herb Pharm, Herbalist & Alchemist and Western Botanicals

Key Herbs

Dong Quai

Latin name: *Angelica sinensis*

Dong quai has been called the female "ginseng" and has been used extensively in the Orient for improving the general health of women. It is a blood tonic and helps to rebuild the blood from the monthly blood loss women experience during their childbearing years. It also eases pain and congestion associated with periods.

Dong Quai is a key ingredient in *Female Hormonal Balancing* and *Menopause Balancing Formulas*

Warnings: Not recommended during pregnancy or with excessive menstrual flow.

Energetics: Warming, moistening and nourishing

Properties: Anticoagulant (blood thinner), aromatic, blood building, emmenagogue and phytoestrogen

Available from: Eclectic Institute, Gaia Herbs, Herb Pharm, Herbalist & Alchemist, Nature's Answer, Nature's Herbs (TwinLab), Nature's Way, NOW Foods, Planetary Herbals, Solaray and Western Botanicals

Dulse

Latin name: *Palmaria palmata*

Dulse is a nourishing food containing numerous trace minerals as well as iodine. It can be used in baths and other topical preparations to promote healthy skin.

Dulse is a key ingredient in *Hypothyroid Formulas*

Warnings: No known warnings.

Energetics: Cooling, moistening and nourishing

Properties: Emollient, mineralizer and nutritive

Available from: Western Botanicals

Echinacea

Latin name: *Echinacea angustifolia & E. purpurea (Compositae)*

Echinacea aids the process of antibody formation and stimulates production of white blood cells. It also helps to strengthen and clear lymph nodes. It inhibits enzymes produced by bacteria to break down compounds that bind cells together, thus inhibiting the spread of infection. Echinacea also helps the body fight viral infections. As an alternative to antibiotics for acute infection or inflammation, take in frequent small doses, and then taper off as condition improves. It is often used to treat colds and flu, but is actually not the best herb for this purpose. Due to its popularity, echinacea is probably overused for many applications where other herbs would be just as effective.

Echinacea is a key ingredient in *Antibacterial, Antiviral, Blood Purifier, Cold* and *Flu, Echinacea Blend, Goldenseal & Echinacea, Immune Stimulating, Lymphatic Drainage* and *Topical Antiseptic Formulas*

Warnings: Echinacea is nontoxic, harmless and has no known contraindications. Many herbalists suggest avoiding it with autoimmune disorders, however. In excessive amounts it can cause excessive salivation and a scratchy, tingling sensation in the throat.

Energetics: Cooling and drying

Properties: Acrid, alterative (blood purifier), analgesic (anodyne), antiseptic, antivenomous, antiviral, immune stimulant and lymphatic

Available from: A. Vogel, Christopher's, Eclectic Institute, Grandma's Herbs, Herb Pharm, Herbalist & Alchemist, Herbs Etc., Nature's Answer, Nature's Herbs (TwinLab), Nature's Way, NOW Foods, Planetary Herbals, Solaray, Western Botanicals and Zand

Elder

Latin name: *Sambucus canadensis, S.nigra*

Elder is a very versatile herb with many useful parts. Elder flowers are an excellent remedy for acute ailments. They help to promote perspiration and reduce inflammation. Research suggests they may have anti-inflammatory, antiviral and anticancer properties, as well as the ability to shorten the duration and severity of flu symptoms. They work especially well in combination with yarrow and mint. They can also be used topically in skin lotions. The fruits (elderberries) have a mild laxative and decongestant action. They are also antiviral and inhibit the spread of viral infections.

Elder is a key ingredient in *Antiviral, Cold* and *Flu* and *Sudorific Formulas*

Warnings: No known warnings for flowers and berries. Stems, bark and root can be toxic.

Energetics: Cooling and drying

Properties: Anti-inflammatory, antiviral, decongestant, diaphoretic/sudorific, febrifuge and nutritive

Available from: Eclectic Institute, Gaia Herbs, Herb Pharm, Herbalist & Alchemist, Nature's Answer, Nature's Way, NOW Foods, Planetary Herbals, Solaray and Western Botanicals

Key Herbs

Elecampane

Latin name: *Inula helenium*

Elecampane is an outstanding remedy for clearing phlegm and mucus from the lungs, urinary system and digestive system. Elecampane is specific for chronic irritation and infection of the respiratory system. It contains inulin which feeds friendly bacteria in the colon.

Elecampane is a key ingredient in *Antiparasitic, Cough Remedy* and *Moistening Lung/Cough Formulas*

Warnings: No known warnings.

Energetics: Warming and drying

Properties: Antiseptic, bitter, diaphoretic/sudorific and expectorant

Available from: Eclectic Institute, Herb Pharm, Herbalist & Alchemist, Nature's Answer and Western Botanicals

Eleuthero (Siberian ginseng)

Latin name: *Eleutherococcus senticosus*

This herb was the first plant identified as an adaptogen by Russian scientists. It not only helps the body cope better with stress, it increases stamina and endurance, stimulates the brain to improve concentration and stimulates male hormone production. Soviet researchers found eleuthero improved athletic performance, aided cosmonauts in preventing space sickness, caused secretaries to make fewer mistakes and helped workers have fewer sick days. In other words, it enhances endurance, immunity, brain function and general good health. Eleuthero aids adrenal function and improves the body's ability to resist disease.

Eleuthero (Siberian ginseng) is a key ingredient in *Adaptogen, Adrenal Tonic, Energy-Boosting, Exercise, Female Aphrodisiac, Immune Balancing* and *Nerve Tonic Formulas*

Warnings: No known warnings.

Energetics: Warming (slightly) and balancing

Properties: Adaptogen, antirheumatic, hypotensive and immune amphoteric

Available from: Eclectic Institute, Gaia Herbs, Herb Pharm, Herbalist & Alchemist, Nature's Answer, Nature's Herbs (TwinLab), Nature's Way, NOW Foods, Solaray and Western Botanicals

Erigeron (Fleabane)

Latin name: *Erigeron canadense*

Erigeron is extremely useful for arresting capillary bleeding from any organ liable to hemorrhage. It also helps to arrest profuse watery secretions from the gastrointestinal tract and excessive urination.

Erigeron (Fleabane) is a key ingredient in *Styptic/ Hemostatic Formulas*

Warnings: No known warnings.

Energetics: Warming and constricting

Properties: Antidiarrheal, antidiuretic, stimulant (circulatory) and styptic

Eucalyptus

Latin name: *Eucaplyptus globulus*

The essential oil of eucalyptus can be inhaled or taken internally in highly diluted, drop doses for respiratory conditions such as coughs, bronchitis, asthma and COPD. The leaves can also be used internally. The oil can also be applied topically as an analgesic in arthritis or to help fight infections in wounds.

Eucalyptus is a key ingredient in *Cough Remedy* and *Decongestant Formulas*

Warnings: Eucalyptus leaf is safe for internal use, but the oil should not be used internally without diluting it and even then it should be used internally only for short periods (7-10 days). Use with caution in young children under the age of four because of possible neurotoxicity.

Energetics: Warming and drying

Properties: Antibacterial, antimicrobial and expectorant

Eyebright

Latin name: *Euphrasia officinalis*

Eyebright is commonly used to treat eye infections and strengthen the eyes. Although it is commonly taken internally for these conditions, it works best when used as an eyewash. The best use of eyebright, however, is as an internal remedy for upper respiratory congestion involving acute irritation of the sinuses and eyes with thin, watery mucus and itching eyes and ears, such as rhinitis or the early stages of a cold. A tincture made from the fresh plant will open the Eustachian tubes in children, allowing the inner ear to drain and thus preventing earaches.

Eyebright is a key ingredient in *Allergy-Reducing, Eye Wash, Sinus Decongestant* and *Vision Supporting Formulas*

Warnings: Eyebright tinctures used as eye drops can cause increased eye pressure, redness, watering and swelling. When using it topically, use the tea.

Energetics: Cooling, drying and contricting (slightly)

Properties: Anti-allergenic, anti-inflammatory, astringent and opthalmicum

Available from: Eclectic Institute, Herb Pharm, Herbalist & Alchemist, Nature's Answer, Nature's Way, NOW Foods, Solaray and Western Botanicals

False Unicorn (Helonias)

Latin name: *Chamaelirium luteum syn. Helonias dioica*

False Unicorn appears to have a progesterone-enhancing effect. It is used as a female tonic to balance excess estrogen and has been used to help prevent miscarriage.

False Unicorn (Helonias) is a key ingredient in *Female Hormonal Balancing* and *Pregnancy Tonic Formulas*

Warnings: Not recommended with emaciation or inflammation.

Energetics: Cooling and moistening

Properties: Anti-abortive, emmenagogue and uterine tonic

Available from: Herb Pharm, Herbalist & Alchemist, Nature's Answer and Western Botanicals

Fennel

Latin name: *Foeniculum vulgare*

Fennel is a wonderful carminative, commonly used in combination with catnip for colic. Catnip and fennel is an excellent remedy for colic, indigestion and diarrhea in infants and young children, as well as adults. Fennel, like most carminatives, stimulates digestion and reduces intestinal gas. It also helps to sweeten and increase breast milk.

Fennel is a key ingredient in *Antacid, Carminative, Catnip & Fennel, Digestive Bitter Tonic* and *Nursing Aid Formulas*

Warnings: Use cautiously during pregnancy.

Energetics: Warming and drying

Properties: Aromatic, carminative, condiment and galactagogue

Available from: Eclectic Institute, Herb Pharm, Herbalist & Alchemist, Nature's Answer, Nature's Way, Solaray and Western Botanicals

Fenugreek

Latin name: *Trigonella foenum-graecum*

Fenugreek encourages weight gain and is helpful for strengthening the body during convalescence. It helps to balance blood sugar and therefore may be helpful for diabetes. Fenugreek also helps to enrich breast milk in nursing mothers. It is a soothing remedy for ulcers, burns, abscesses and other injuries. Used with thyme it helps decongest the sinuses.

Fenugreek is a key ingredient in *Blood Sugar Reducing, Nursing Aid* and *Sinus Decongestant Formulas*

Warnings: Not recommended for use during pregnancy.

Energetics: Warming and drying

Properties: Antidiabetic, condiment, decongestant and galactagogue

Available from: Eclectic Institute, Gaia Herbs, Herb Pharm, Herbalist & Alchemist, Nature's Answer, Nature's Herbs (TwinLab), Nature's Way, NOW Foods, Planetary Herbals, Solaray and Western Botanicals

Feverfew

Latin name: *Tanacetum parthenium (Compositae)*

Feverfew is a very popular natural remedy for migraine headaches. It doesn't work very well once the migraine has started, but taken regularly it helps to prevent migraines and lessen their severity. It has anti-inflammatory properties and its name comes from its traditional use as a remedy for fevers.

Feverfew is a key ingredient in *Analgesic* and *Migraine/Headache Formulas*

Warnings: Because of its emmenagogue properties, some herbalists recommend that it not be used during pregnancy. If mouth soreness or ulcerations develop, reduce dosage or discontinue use. It does not work on migraine headaches caused by weakness or deficiency (i.e., anemia).

Energetics: Cooling and drying

Properties: Analgesic (anodyne), anthelminthic, anti-inflammatory and nervine

Available from: Gaia Herbs, Herb Pharm, Herbalist & Alchemist, Nature's Answer, Nature's Herbs (TwinLab), Nature's Way, NOW Foods, Solaray and Western Botanicals

Key Herbs

Flax Seed

Latin name: *Linum usitatissimum*

Freshly ground flax seed is amazingly healing to an inflamed gut. It is a stool softener and bulk laxative for chronic constipation. Flax lignans are phytoestrogens and may be helpful in preventing estrogen-dependent cancers.

Flax Seed is a key ingredient in *Fiber Blend* and *Phytoestrogen Formulas*

Warnings: Flax sees oxidize very rapidly after being ground. Fresh flax seeds are best.

Energetics: Cooling, moistening and nourishing

Properties: Laxative (bulk) and phytoestrogen

Fringe Tree

Latin name: *Chionathus virginicus*

A bitter tonic with blood purifying, laxative and mild diuretic actions, fringetree is a very effective gallbladder remedy. It stimulates bile flow and helps relieve intestinal gas, bloating and a stuffy feeling under the right rib cage. It is one of the best herbs for gallstones, especially when combined with other liver/gallbladder herbs like wild yam, turmeric, dandelion, barberry and milk thistle.

Fringe Tree is a key ingredient in *Cholagogue Formulas*

Warnings: Should not be used in bile duct obstruction or pregnancy.

Energetics: Cooling and drying

Properties: Anticholesteremic and cholagogue

Available from: Eclectic Institute, Herb Pharm, Herbalist & Alchemist and Western Botanicals

Fritillary

Latin name: *Fritillaria thumbergii* and *other species*

Fritillary bulbs are used in Chinese medicine for dry conditions of the lungs, swollen lymph glands and abscesses. They have a cough suppressing action and are especially helpful for dry cough.

Fritillary is a key ingredient in *Cough Remedy* and *Moistening Lung/Cough Formulas*

Warnings: Raw, unprocessed herb is toxic and should not be taken internally.

Energetics: Cooling, moistening and nourishing

Garlic

Latin name: *Allium sativum*

Garlic has been called Nature's penicillin. It is a strong aromatic herb with powerful antibiotic, antifungal and antiviral action. It acts as an expectorant to expel phlegm from the lungs and as a circulatory tonic to lower high blood pressure and prevent arteriosclerosis. It combines well with other herbs for treating bacterial, viral and fungal infections. It is also helpful for parasites. For hypertension (high blood pressure) and/or high cholesterol, it must be taken daily for at least 3-6 months. The fresh bulb has the best anti-hypertensive (blood pressure lowering) and anti-microbial properties.

Garlic extracted in a vegetable oil can be rubbed on the chest and back to relieve lung congestion. The warm oil can also be dropped into the ears and/or rubbed on the ears and sides of the neck to help relieve earaches. Garlic is useful in enemas for reducing fevers, relieving respiratory congestion, earaches, infection and worms. For a garlic enema, simmer one chopped clove for 10 minutes in 1 pint of water or use 6-8 capsules and steep as tea for 3-5 minutes. Strain before using.

Garlic is a key ingredient in *Antibacterial*, *Antifungal*, *Antiparasitic*, *Cardiovascular Stimulant*, *Cholesterol Balancing*, *Cold* and *Flu*, *Decongestant*, *Ear Drop* and *Hypotensive Formulas*

Warnings: Not for feeble, emaciated or wasting conditions. Gastric irritation is possible; eat or take with food to lessen this effect.

Energetics: Warming and drying

Properties: Anthelminthic, antibacterial, anticholesteremic, anticoagulant (blood thinner), antifungal, antiseptic, antiviral, aphrodisiac, aromatic, condiment, decongestant, diaphoretic/sudorific, expectorant, hypertensive, hypotensive, stimulant (circulatory), stimulant (metabolic) and vermifuge

Available from: Christopher's, Eclectic Institute, Grandma's Herbs, Herb Pharm, Nature's Answer, Nature's Herbs (TwinLab), Nature's Way, New Chapter, NOW Foods, Planetary Herbals, Solaray and Western Botanicals

Key Herbs

Gentian

Latin name: *Gentiana lutea (Gentianaceae)*

This intensely bitter herb is commonly used to stimulate digestive system function. It is often combined with other bitters and carminatives for this purpose. It is best taken in liquid form prior to meals.

Gentian is a key ingredient in *Antacid* and *Digestive Bitter Tonic Formulas*

Warnings: Not for use during pregnancy or acute GI inflammation.

Energetics: Cooling and drying

Properties: Alterative (blood purifier), antacid, anthelminthic, antiseptic, bitter and digestive tonic

Available from: Eclectic Institute, Herb Pharm, Herbalist & Alchemist, Nature's Answer and Western Botanicals

Ginger

Latin name: *Zingiber officinale*

A pungent aromatic, ginger is used to relieve nausea, vomiting and motion sickness. Take capsules or extract before traveling to prevent motion sickness. Taken with or after meals it stimulates digestive secretions. Research indicates that ginger root also enhances immune function, promotes the secretion of bile and gastric fluids and increases blood circulation by inhibiting platelet aggregation. It may also reduce pain and inflammation associated with arthritis and ulcerative colitis. It is very helpful for treating colds and chills.

Ginger is a key ingredient in *Anti-Inflammatory, Cardiovascular Stimulant, Carminative, Cold* and *Flu, Digestive Bitter Tonic* and *Digestive Tonic Formulas*

Warnings: Some authors caution against use during pregnancy, but no adverse effects have been reported by women using ginger for morning sickness.

Energetics: Warming and drying

Properties: Analgesic (anodyne), anti-emetic (antinauseous), aromatic, carminative, condiment, counterirritant, diaphoretic/sudorific, digestive tonic, stimulant (circulatory) and stimulant (metabolic)

Available from: Herb Pharm, Herbalist & Alchemist, Nature's Answer, Nature's Herbs (TwinLab), Nature's Way, New Chapter, NOW Foods, Planetary Herbals, Solaray, Traditional Medicinals and Western Botanicals

Ginkgo

Latin name: *Ginkgo biloba*

Extensive research has been conducted in Europe using concentrated extracts of the flavonoids in this herb. This is one herb that is best used as a standardized extract. Ginkgo is commonly used to enhance memory and brain function. It improves blood flow to the brain and acts as an antioxidant to protect brain cells from damage. It also improves peripheral circulation and may be beneficial in diabetic retinopathy, tinnitus, vertigo and dizziness. Best results are obtained when the herb is used consistently for 2-3 months. Ginkgo is an excellent remedy to take to slow the aging process and protect the nervous and cardiovascular systems.

Ginkgo is a key ingredient in *Antidepressant, Antioxidant, Brain* and *Memory Tonic, Brain Calming* and *Cardiovascular Stimulant Formulas*

Warnings: Use with caution when taking blood thinners. Some authors advise caution during pregnancy, but the herb appears safe. Consult a professional herbalist (findanherbalist.com) for advice.

Energetics: Cooling (slightly)

Properties: Anticoagulant (blood thinner), antioxidant, cerebral tonic, hypotensive and vasodilator

Available from: Eclectic Institute, Gaia Herbs, Herb Pharm, Herbalist & Alchemist, Nature's Answer, Nature's Way, NOW Foods, Planetary Herbals, Solaray, Vitanica and Western Botanicals

Ginseng (American)

Latin name: *Panax quinquefolius*

American ginseng is used as a tonic for strengthening the overall system, improving stamina and resistance to disease. It helps counteract the effects of aging and improves overall health when taken in very small doses. American ginseng is less stimulating than Asian (Korean) ginseng. It helps regulate blood sugar, improves digestion, helps the body cope better with stress, and strengthens adrenal and general glandular function. Ginseng works best in small doses.

Ginseng (American) is a key ingredient in *Adaptogen, Adrenal Tonic, Blood Sugar Reducing, Digestive Tonic, Energy-Boosting* and *Menopause Balancing Formulas*

Warnings: Not toxic, but should not be taken by persons with high blood pressure, fevers, acute inflammation and acute diseases like colds and flu. Regular large doses can cause insomnia and nervous over stimulation.

Energetics: Cooling and moistening

Properties: Adaptogen, adrenal tonic, antidiabetic, aphrodisiac, hypertensive, immune stimulant, stimulant (metabolic) and tonic

Available from: Eclectic Institute, Gaia Herbs, Herb Pharm, Herbalist & Alchemist, Nature's Answer, Nature's Way, NOW Foods, Planetary Herbals, Solaray and Western Botanicals

Ginseng (Asian, Korean)

Latin name: *Panax ginseng*

Ginseng is one of the most highly prized herbs in the world. Asian or Korean ginseng has been shown to increase energy, help fight fatigue and increase physical stamina and agility. It may even enhance the body's ability to recover from physical injuries. Small doses of ginseng are used to slow aging, reduce stress, balance mood and enhance a person's general health. Ginseng may lower the risk of cancer and build up a weakened immune system. Asian ginseng is more warming than American ginseng and is well-suited to older men and women who tend to be cold, pale and easily fatigued. Red ginseng, which is steamed before drying, is more warming in energy, while white ginseng, which is just peeled and dried, is more neutral in energy.

Ginseng (Asian, Korean) is a key ingredient in *Adaptogen, Adrenal Tonic, Energy-Boosting, Female Aphrodisiac, Male Aphrodisiac* and *Male Glandular Tonic Formulas*

Warnings: Has no toxic effects but is contraindicated in acute diseases, high fevers or inflammation.

Energetics: Warming and moistening

Properties: Adaptogen, antioxidant, aphrodisiac, hypertensive, immune stimulant, stimulant (metabolic) and tonic

Available from: Herb Pharm, Herbalist & Alchemist, Nature's Answer, Nature's Herbs (TwinLab), Nature's Way, NOW Foods, Planetary Herbals and Solaray

Goldenrod

Latin name: *Solidago virgaurea, S. canadensis* and *other sp.*

A useful diuretic for urinary tract problems, obstructions, kidney stones and inflammation, goldenrod is very soothing and healing. It is also helpful for hay fever and allergies to cats. It can be helpful for upper respiratory infections and yeast infections like thrush.

Goldenrod is a key ingredient in *Kidney Tonic Formulas*

Warnings: Not for use with edema from kidney failure.

Energetics: Warming and drying

Properties: Anti-inflammatory, antiseptic, diuretic and kidney tonic

Available from: Eclectic Institute, Herb Pharm and Western Botanicals

Goldenseal

Latin name: *Hydrastis canadensis (Ranunculaceae)*

Goldenseal has been considered by many to be a "cure-all" herb. It is a natural antibiotic and immune stimulant with diuretic and antibiotic properties, making it useful in urinary and digestive tract infections. It is particularly helpful for sub acute inflammation of the respiratory, digestive or urinary mucus membranes. Goldenseal lowers blood sugar and stimulates digestion. It is a specific remedy for amoebic dysentery (giardia). Topically, goldenseal heals injuries. It has been used as a wash for sore red eyes and as a topical application for canker sores. Goldenseal has been over harvested and other herbs should be used as substitutes where possible. Coptis root, Oregon grape and barberry all contain berberine alkaloids and have similar antimicrobial properties.

Because of its popularity, goldenseal is a common ingredient in herbal formulas.

Goldenseal is a key ingredient in *Antacid, Antibacterial, Blood Purifier, Blood Sugar Reducing, Digestive Bitter Tonic, Eye Wash, Goldenseal & Echinacea, Immune Stimulating, Topical Antiseptic, Topical Vulnerary* and *Urinary Infection Fighting Formulas*

Warnings: Goldenseal is safe when used at recommended dosages and times, but should not to be used as a single herb for long periods (over 4 weeks). It can cause malabsorption of vitamin B, resulting in fatigue and listlessness, when used for long periods. It is contraindicated for hypoglycemics because it lowers blood sugar levels. Hypoglycemics can use Oregon grape, coptis or myrrh gum instead of goldenseal. It should be used under professional supervision during pregnancy.

Energetics: Cooling, drying and contricting (slightly)

Properties: Alterative (blood purifier), antibacterial, antiparasitic, antiseptic, antiviral, digestive tonic, hemostatic, immune stimulant and opthalmicum

Available from: Eclectic Institute, Gaia Herbs, Herb Pharm, Herbalist & Alchemist, Herbs Etc., Nature's Answer, Nature's Herbs (TwinLab), Nature's Way, Solaray and Western Botanicals

Gotu kola

Latin name: *Centella asiatica syn. Hydrocotyle asiatica (Umbelliferae)*

Gotu kola has a reputation for improving memory and brain function. It also has a positive effect on the adrenals, giving it adaptogenic effects. It is used in India for skin diseases and wasting diseases such as leprosy.

Gotu kola is a key ingredient in *Adrenal Tonic, Brain and Memory Tonic, Energy-Boosting* and *Skin Healing Formulas*

Warnings: Overdose may cause dizziness. Use caution with blood thinning medications. It appears safe during pregnancy and lactation, but some sources suggest caution. Consult with a professional herbalist (herbiverse.com) for advice.

Energetics: Cooling and drying

Properties: Adaptogen and cerebral tonic

Available from: Eclectic Institute, Herb Pharm, Herbalist & Alchemist, Nature's Answer, Nature's Herbs (TwinLab), Nature's Way, NOW Foods, Solaray and Western Botanicals

Gravel root

Latin name: *Eupatorium purpureum*

Gravel root is a diuretic that helps to remove urinary stones and flush the urinary passages. It is also used for kidney infections, prostatitis, pelvic inflammatory disease, gout, and diabetes.

Gravel root is a key ingredient in *Lithotriptic Formulas*

Warnings: Contains pyrrolizidine alkaloids. Not recommended for long term use or for pregnant or nursing women.

Energetics: Cooling and drying

Properties: Diuretic and lithotriptic

Available from: Eclectic Institute and Western Botanicals

Grindelia (Gumweed)

Latin name: *Grindelia spp.*

This resinous expectorant and decongestant is very good at breaking up hardened mucus in the respiratory tract. It eases breathing in bronchitis and asthma. It has antispasmodic action that opens the smaller passages in the lungs and can make breathing easier. Combined with plantain it pulls thick mucus out of the lungs. It has also been applied topically as a salve to heal skin afflictions like poison ivy and rashes. It is also helpful topically for insect bites.

Grindelia (Gumweed) is a key ingredient in *Bronchialdilator, Decongestant* and *Expectorant Formulas*

Warnings: Can be toxic in large doses. Not for long term use or for use by people suffering from kidney or heart disease.

Energetics: Warming, drying and constricting

Properties: Antiseptic, astringent, decongestant and expectorant

Available from: Eclectic Institute and Herb Pharm

Guarana

Latin name: *Paullinia cupana, P. sorbilis*

Guarana has a chemical structure similar to that of caffeine, but it may be more effective than coffee, as it is released more slowly into the body to provide a more sustained energy release.

Guarana is a key ingredient in *Energy-Boosting* and *Weight Loss Formulas*

Warnings: Avoid taking guarana if combined with ephedrine, or if you have high blood pressure, heart disease or sensitivity to caffeine. May cause irregular heartbeat, anxiety, jitteriness and insomnia in susceptible persons.

Energetics: Warming and drying

Properties: Diuretic and stimulant (metabolic)

Available from: Nature's Answer, Solaray and Western Botanicals

Key Herbs

Guggul

Latin name: *Commiphora mukul*

Research has shown that guggul may be able to lower both cholesterol and triglycerides. It also inhibits platelet aggregation and can help prevent and possibly reverse arterial plaque. It mildly stimulates the thyroid and may be helpful for weight loss.

Guggul is a key ingredient in *Cholesterol Balancing Formulas*

Warnings: Because it thins the blood, it should not be used in persons who bleed easily or during pregnancy. Also avoid with hyperthyroid disorders.

Energetics: Warming and drying

Properties: Anti-inflammatory, antibacterial, anticholesteremic and antirheumatic

Available from: Herb Pharm, Herbalist & Alchemist, NOW Foods and Solaray

Gymnema

Latin name: *Gymnema sylvestre*

Ayurvedic practitioners have used gymnema to treat type 2 diabetes for at least 2,000 years. When placed on the tongue, gymnema makes it impossible to taste sugar. It is believed that it not only blocks sweet receptors on the tongue, it also slows absorption of sugar in the digestive tract. Dozens of peer-reviewed studies now support the use of gymnema as a treatment for high blood sugar.

Gymnema is a key ingredient in *Blood Sugar Reducing* and *Weight Loss Formulas*

Warnings: Gymnema is generally regarded as safe and associated with few side effects or drug interactions.

Energetics: Cooling and drying

Properties: Antidiabetic

Available from: Herbalist & Alchemist, Nature's Answer, Nature's Way, NOW Foods, Planetary Herbals, Solaray and Western Botanicals

Hawthorn

Latin name: *Crataegus oxyacantha & C. monogyna (Rosaceae)*

Studies around the world have confirmed that hawthorn berries improve the tone of the cardiac muscle, improve oxygen uptake by the heart, improve circulation in the heart, energize the heart cells and dilate blood vessels in the extremities to reduce strain on the heart. Thus, hawthorn berries are an excellent herbal food for building up the heart muscle. However, it needs to be taken on a regular basis for best results. Generally, it improves cardiac function in heart disorders with or without chest pain. Besides benefiting the heart it helps reduce stress and improves digestion.

Hawthorn is a key ingredient in *Brain Calming*, *Cardiac Tonic* and *Hypotensive Formulas*

Warnings: Completely safe for long-term use.

Energetics: Cooling and moistening

Properties: Anti-arrhythmic, antiseptic, cardiac, hypertensive and hypotensive

Available from: A. Vogel, Christopher's, Eclectic Institute, Gaia Herbs, Herb Pharm, Herbalist & Alchemist, Nature's Answer, Nature's Herbs (TwinLab), Nature's Way, NOW Foods, Planetary Herbals, Solaray and Western Botanicals

He Shou Wu (Ho Shou Wu, Fo-Ti)

Latin name: *Polygonum multiflorum*

This herb is considered an anti-aging tonic and is believed to help prevent (and possibly reverse) the graying of hair when taken regularly. It helps to balance blood sugar levels and increases glycogen reserves in the liver. It helps build up the thyroid and reduces cholesterol.

He Shou Wu (Ho Shou Wu, Fo-Ti) is a key ingredient in *Energy-Boosting* and *Hyperthyroid Formulas*

Warnings: Not for persons with diarrhea, weak digestion and heavy mucus congestion.

Energetics: Neutral and moistening

Properties: Anticholesteremic, blood building, glandular and tonic

Available from: Herb Pharm, Herbalist & Alchemist, Nature's Answer, Nature's Way, NOW Foods and Solaray

Holy Basil

Latin name: *Ocimum sanctum*

Used in Ayurvedic medicine, Holy Basil is considered an adaptogen and general tonic in modern herbalism. It protects the heart from stress, lowers blood pressure and cholesterol levels, and stabilizes blood sugar levels. It reduces feelings of stress and down regulates excessive immune responses in conditions like hay fever (allergic rhinitis) and asthma. At the same time it enhances cerebral circulation, memory, concentration and mental acuity.

Holy Basil is a key ingredient in *Adaptogen* and *Adrenal Tonic Formulas*

Warnings: No known warnings.

Energetics: Cooling and drying

Properties: Adaptogen, antibacterial, antiviral, carminative, hypotensive and immune amphoteric

Available from: Gaia Herbs, Herb Pharm, Herbalist & Alchemist, Nature's Way, New Chapter, Planetary Herbals and Solaray

Hops

Latin name: *Humulus lupulus (Cannabaceae)*

This herb is a powerful nervine and sleep aid, and can be combined with other carminatives for settling a nervous, acidic stomach. It is also estrogenic and has been used to increase sex drive in women and reduce it in men. Hops is indicated for a hot digestive system and/or irritated nervous system. It works best on hot, damp people who are often overweight, red faced with fiery personalities, poor digestion and insomnia.

Hops is a key ingredient in *Phytoestrogen*, *Relaxing Nervine* and *Sleep Formulas*

Warnings: Contraindicated in clinical depression, estrogen dominance or with allergies to hops. Not the best choice in a nervine for young children, but all right as part of a formula. Use during pregnancy with caution because of its estrogenic effects.

Energetics: Cooling and relaxing

Properties: Analgesic (anodyne), anaphrodisiac, antacid, anthelminthic, antispasmodic, nervine, phytoestrogen, sedative and soporific (hypnotic)

Available from: Eclectic Institute, Herb Pharm, Herbalist & Alchemist, Nature's Answer, Nature's Way, Solaray and Western Botanicals

Horehound

Latin name: *Marrubium vulgare*

Horehound has traditionally been used to make cough drops or cough syrup. You can still find horehound drops in some stores. It is an excellent remedy for increasing the secretion of thinner mucus to break up congestion. It is a great remedy for coughing, wheezing and difficult breathing. It stimulates digestion and has a mild cardiac effect.

Horehound is a key ingredient in *Cough Remedy*, *Expectorant* and *Sinus Decongestant Formulas*

Warnings: Use with caution during pregnancy.

Energetics: Cooling and drying

Properties: Anti-arrhythmic, bitter, cardiac, decongestant and expectorant

Available from: Eclectic Institute, Herb Pharm, Herbalist & Alchemist, Nature's Answer and Western Botanicals

Horny Goat Weed (Epimedium)

Latin name: *Epimedium grandiflorum*

Studies have shown that horny goat weed is effective in treating sexual dysfunction, fatigue, arthritis and other conditions. The herb's active constituent, Icariin, acts on the PDE-5 enzyme, which breaks down cyclic guanosine monophosphate (cGMP). cGMP is necessary for an erection in men because it triggers the release of nitric oxide, which dilates genital blood vessels. Many men over 40 have a cGMP deficiency due to excessive PDE-5 activity, resulting in nitric oxide deficiency and erectile dysfunction. Icariin inhibits PDE-5, thereby allowing nitric oxide release sufficient to maintain an erection. It also stimulates the production of osteoblasts, specialized cells involved in building bone mass. The flavonoids in horny goat weed are believed to stimulate the nerves, improving the sensation of touch.

Horny Goat Weed (Epimedium) is a key ingredient in *Male Aphrodisiac* and *Male Glandular Tonic Formulas*

Warnings: High doses of horny goat weed may result in breathing trouble, dizziness, vomiting or thirst and dry mouth.

Energetics: Warming, drying and relaxing (slightly)

Properties: Aphrodisiac and vasodilator

Available from: Nature's Way, Planetary Herbals and Western Botanicals

Horse Chestnut

Latin name: *Aesculus hippocastanum.*

Horse chestnut is a specific a tonic to the vascular system. It improves the tone of veins making it helpful for varicose veins, bruises and hemorrhoids. It can be taken internally or applied topically.

Horse Chestnut is a key ingredient in *Vascular Tonic Formulas*

Warnings: There is some toxicity to the Horse Chestnut plant, but extracts of the seeds are safe when used as directed. Avoid with children, during pregnancy and with nursing mothers. Use cautiously when taking blood thinning medications.

Energetics: Cooling, drying and contricting (slightly)

Properties: Astringent and vascular tonic

Available from: A. Vogel, Eclectic Institute, Herb Pharm, Nature's Way, NOW Foods, Planetary Herbals, Solaray, Vitanica and Western Botanicals

Horseradish

Latin name: *Armoracia rusticana.*

Horseradish is a very good remedy for people who have a hard time digesting and metabolizing protein. Eaten with meat it helps stimulate both the digestion and metabolism of protein. It can be used for colds, flu and other acute ailments and may be helpful for allergies, hay fever and congestion in the lungs.

Horseradish is a key ingredient in *Sinus Decongestant Formulas*

Warnings: Large amounts can cause gastrointestinal upset.

Energetics: Warming and drying

Properties: Carminative, condiment, decongestant, expectorant and stimulant (metabolic)

Available from: Herb Pharm and Western Botanicals

Horsetail

Latin name: *Equisetum arvense*

Horsetail is rich in the mineral silica, which is used with calcium in bones, nails, hair and the skin. Silica adds elasticity to tissues, making them strong but not brittle. It is astringent and is useful for internal bleeding, such as blood in the urine. It has a mild diuretic effect as well.

Horsetail is a key ingredient in *Kidney Tonic, Mineral, Skin Healing* and *Tissue Healing Formulas*

Warnings: Excessive consumption may lead to thiamin deficiencies. Powdered herb not recommended for children, but tea is OK.

Energetics: Cooling, drying and contricting (slightly)

Properties: Diuretic, hemostatic, kidney tonic, mineralizer and vulnerary

Available from: Eclectic Institute, Herb Pharm, Herbalist & Alchemist, Nature's Answer, Nature's Way, Solaray and Western Botanicals

Hydrangea

Latin name: *Hydrangea arborescens*

Used as a diuretic and a calcium solvent, hydrangea is used to help rid the body of kidney stones and calcium deposits. It can also be helpful for bladder pain, back pain and arthritis.

Hydrangea is a key ingredient in *Joint Healing* and *Lithotriptic Formulas*

Warnings: Not recommended for long term use.

Energetics: Cooling and drying

Properties: Analgesic (anodyne), diuretic and lithotriptic

Available from: Eclectic Institute, Herb Pharm, Herbalist & Alchemist, Nature's Answer, Nature's Way and Western Botanicals

Hyssop

Latin name: *Hysopus officinalis*

A traditional remedy that is considered a "cure-all" for respiratory ailments. It helps clear thick and congested phlegm from the lungs to restore free breathing. Having antiseptic properties that are helpful in the treatment of cuts and abrasions, it can also be used to provide immediate relief from insect bites.

Warnings: The essential oil of hyssop is toxic. The herb is GRAS and is safe when used as directed, but should be avoided during pregnancy.

Energetics: Warming and drying

Properties: Antiseptic, antiviral, carminative, decongestant, emmenagogue and expectorant

Available from: Eclectic Institute, Herb Pharm, Herbalist & Alchemist, Nature's Answer, Nature's Way, Solaray and Western Botanicals

Indian Pipe

Latin name: *Monotropa uniflora*

Used primarily to help ease pain, Indian Pipe doesn't actually numb pain. Instead, it has the ability to take your pain and puts it beside you, whether physical or emotional. You remain aware of the pain but you no longer feel it. It can also be helpful for panic attacks from emotional pain and bad "trips" from LSD.

Indian Pipe is a key ingredient in *Analgesic Formulas*

Warnings: Consumption of large doses can bring deep sleep and ultra vivid dreams.

Energetics: Relaxing and cooling

Properties: Antispasmodic, nervine and sedative

Available from: Herbalist & Alchemist

Irish moss

Latin name: *Chondrus crispus*

A seaweed rich in iodine and trace minerals and a source of bromine, protein, amino acids and manganese, Irish moss soothes dry and irritated tissues. It is helpful for chronic, dry lung conditions and sore throat. It soothes dry, irritated membranes and arrests diarrhea, but it may also act as a mild laxative in conditions involving dry, hard stools. Contains a mucilage (carrageenan) which is widely used as a stabilizer in dairy products and cosmetics.

Irish moss is a key ingredient in *Hypothyroid Formulas*

Warnings: No known warnings.

Energetics: Cooling, moistening and nourishing

Properties: Anti-inflammatory, emollient, laxative (bulk), mucliant/mucilaginous and nutritive

Available from: Herbalist & Alchemist and Western Botanicals

Isatis

Latin name: *Isatis tinctoria*

Isatis is a potent antiviral, but is so cooling that if taken for extended periods it can make a person feel like they have an ice cube in their stomach and cause uncontrolled shivering. For this reason it is normally taken only for short periods or combined with ginger. It is used for infections involving fever and inflammation.

Isatis is a key ingredient in *Antiviral Formulas*

Warnings: Isatis is contraindicated for cold, chronic conditions and is not recommended for long term use.

Energetics: Very cooling

Properties: Antiviral and refrigerant

Available from: Herbalist & Alchemist

Jamaican Dogwood

Latin name: *Piscidia erythrina or P. piscipula*

A mild narcotic and anodyne herb, Jamaican dogwood is a relatively potent sedative known as a remedy for migraine headaches, neuralgia, and the treatment of insomnia caused by pain, nervous tension and stress. The bark is anti-inflammatory and antispasmodic and can be used for painful menstrual periods. It is used in combination with other herbs to treat the musculoskeletal pain of arthritis and rheumatism.

Jamaican Dogwood is a key ingredient in *Analgesic* and *Migraine/Headache Formulas*

Warnings: Use with caution with hypotension and with children or pregnant women. May potentiate sedative medications.

Energetics: Cooling and relaxing

Properties: Analgesic (anodyne), antispasmodic, narcotic, sedative and soporific (hypnotic)

Available from: Eclectic Institute, Herb Pharm, Herbalist & Alchemist and Western Botanicals

Jambul

Latin name: *Syzygium cumini*

Most commonly used to treat type II diabetes, Jambul helps to maintain blood sugar levels. The seeds regulate the conversion of starch into sugar, checking the production of glucose. A powder made from the fruit reduces sugar in the urine and abates thirst. It is also helpful for bile insufficiency, gallbladder troubles and hepatitis.

Jambul is a key ingredient in *Blood Sugar Reducing Formulas*

Warnings: No known warnings.

Energetics: Cooling and constricting

Properties: Antidiabetic, antidiarrheal, astringent and bitter

Available from: Herb Pharm

Key Herbs

Jujube

Latin name: *Ziziphus zizyphus*

Jujube dates are a nourishing herb used in Chinese medicine to calm the nervous system, improve stamina and aid recovery from illness.

Jujube is a key ingredient in *Brain Calming Formulas*

Warnings: No known warnings.

Energetics: Cooling, relaxing (slightly) and nourishing

Properties: Sedative

Juniper Berry

Latin name: *Juniperus sp.*

Juniper berry strongly stimulates kidney function and has antiseptic properties. It is commonly used for edema and other urinary problems. It also stimulates digestion. One species of juniper (*J. monosperma*) is sometimes called Cedar Berries and is used in formulas to reduce blood sugar.

Juniper Berry is a key ingredient in *Blood Sugar Reducing* and *Diuretic Formulas*

Warnings: The volatile oils in juniper can be irritating to the kidneys and the nervous system with long-term use. Not recommended when kidneys are inflamed or in cases of nephritis and nephrosis. Not recommended for use in pregnancy.

Energetics: Warming and drying

Properties: Antifungal, antiseptic, aromatic, carminative, diuretic and stimulant (metabolic)

Available from: Eclectic Institute, Herb Pharm, Herbalist & Alchemist, Nature's Answer, Nature's Herbs (TwinLab), Nature's Way, Solaray and Western Botanicals

Kava-kava

Latin name: *Piper methysticum (Piperaceae)*

Kava-kava has long been used to treat stress, anxiety and insomnia. It is used in Polynesian religious ceremonies to reduce anxiety and relax muscles while maintaining a mentally alert state. It also elevates mood. Kava is a diuretic and is also useful for urinary tract infections.

Kava-kava is a key ingredient in *Analgesic, Antidepressant, Relaxing Nervine* and *Sleep Formulas*

Warnings: Large doses over a long period of time may cause liver problems and skin eruptions. Do not drive or operate heavy machinery under the influence of large doses of kava kava as it can impair motor function. If you have liver health problems or drink alcohol regularly you should avoid kava kava.

Energetics: Relaxing, drying and warming

Properties: Acrid, analgesic (anodyne), anesthetic, antidepressant, antiseptic, antispasmodic, diuretic, euphoretic, relaxant, sedative and soporific (hypnotic)

Available from: Eclectic Institute, Gaia Herbs, Herb Pharm, Herbalist & Alchemist, Herbs Etc., NOW Foods and Western Botanicals

Kelp

Latin name: *Laminaria spp.*

A large, fast-growing seaweed or brown algae rich in iodine, minerals, trace minerals, vitamins and chlorophyll, kelp is sometimes considered a super-food because of the many nutrients it contains. Like other seaweeds, it contains sodium alginate, which has proven to be effective at protecting the body from radiation.

Kelp is a key ingredient in *Energy-Boosting, Hypothyroid* and *Weight Loss Formulas*

Warnings: Avoid with hyperthyroid disorders. Use cautiously in Hashimoto's thyroiditis and selenium deficiencies.

Energetics: Cooling, moistening and nourishing

Properties: Emollient and nutritive

Available from: A. Vogel, Herbalist & Alchemist, Nature's Herbs (TwinLab), Nature's Way and Solaray

Khella

Latin name: *Ammi visnaga*

Khella is a vasodilator and calcium channel blocker used to treat cardiovascular problems. Its antispasmodic properties make it helpful for asthma and cramps. It may also be helpful for dissolving stones in the gallbladder and kidneys.

Khella is a key ingredient in *Antispasmodic* and *Bronchialdilator Formulas*

Warnings: Not for use in pregnancy.

Energetics: Warming and relaxing

Properties: Anti-arrhythmic, antispasmodic, bronchial dilator, cardiac, hypotensive and vasodilator

Available from: Herb Pharm

Key Herbs

Kudzu

Latin name: *Pueraria lobata* and *P. thunbergiana*

Kudzu has a history of use in traditional Chinese medicine for counteracting the effects of alcohol. Extracts of the flower are used for treating alcoholism and relieving hangover. The roots are used for neutralizing poisons and viral infections. The roots are also used to treat venous problems and the headache, dizziness and numbness caused by high blood pressure. Kudzu is helpful for leaky gut syndrome, muscle aches, and neck and upper back pain. It is also used for diarrhea, dysentery, and increasing blood flow in patients with arteriosclerosis.

Kudzu is a key ingredient in *Anti-Alcoholic Formulas*

Warnings: No known warnings.

Energetics: Cooling and constricting

Properties: Astringent, demulcent (mucilant) and tonic

Available from: Eclectic Institute, Herbalist & Alchemist, Nature's Way, Planetary Herbals and Solaray

Lady's Mantle

Latin name: *Achemilla vulgaris*

Lady's Mantle is used as a tonic for the uterus and as a remedy for vaginal discharge and heavy menstrual bleeding, internally or externally. It is a styptic and can also be used for other types of bleeding. It has a diuretic effect and eases edema.

Lady's Mantle is a key ingredient in *Uterine Tonic Formulas*

Warnings: Avoid during pregnancy.

Energetics: Drying and constricting

Properties: Antidiarrheal, astringent, styptic, uterine tonic and vulnerary

Available from: Eclectic Institute and Herbalist & Alchemist

Lavender

Latin name: *Lavandula officinalis syn. L. angustifolia (Labiatae)*

Lavender is a relaxing nervine that eases tension and anxiety. It is a specific for high strung, nervous, self-absorbed people who need to relax. It also lifts mood, having a mild antidepressant effect. Lavender has a mild analgesic effect and can ease headaches and migraines (when taken in the early stages). The essential oil of lavender is antifungal and is a great remedy for burns.

Lavender is a key ingredient in *Analgesic, Relaxing Nervine* and *Topical Vulnerary Formulas*

Warnings: No known warnings.

Energetics: Warming (slightly) and relaxing

Properties: Analgesic (anodyne), antifungal, aromatic, cicatrisant, nervine and relaxant

Available from: Herb Pharm, Herbalist & Alchemist, Nature's Answer and Western Botanicals

Lemon

Latin name: *Citrus limon*

Lemon juice has many wonderful medicinal properties. It is used to help fight colds and flu. It has cooling effect on the body and helps with calcium deposits, gallstones and kidney stones. Lemon is used as a flavoring in many herbal teas and remedies.

Warnings: No known warnings.

Energetics: Cooling

Properties: Antiparasitic, antiseptic, condiment, febrifuge, lithotriptic, nutritive and refrigerant

Lemon Balm

Latin name: *Melissa officinalis (Labiatae)*

An aromatic with a mild astringent action and lemony scent, Lemon balm is useful for many acute ailments such as colds, digestive upset and flu. It is used in combination with bugleweed to calm an overactive thyroid. It is helpful for nervousness that affects the heart and digestion. The antiviral properties of lemon balm make it useful for herpes, cold sores, chicken pox and shingles. It also has a positive effect on the brain, helping to ease sadness and depression, calm mania and hysteria, enhance sleep and aid memory and concentration.

Lemon Balm is a key ingredient in *Antidepressant, Antiviral, Brain Calming, Cold* and *Flu, Hyperthyroid* and *Relaxing Nervine Formulas*

Warnings: No known warnings.

Energetics: Cooling and relaxing (slightly)

Properties: Antidepressant, antiseptic, antithyrotropic, antiviral, aromatic, carminative, diaphoretic/sudorific and nervine

Available from: Herb Pharm, Herbalist & Alchemist, Nature's Way, New Chapter, Planetary Herbals, Solaray and Western Botanicals

Licorice

Latin name: *Glycyrrhiza glabra*

Licorice root helps to stabilize blood sugar levels and is useful in treating both hypoglycemia and diabetes. It improves stamina and endurance, increasing energy without being stimulating. Licorice has anti-inflammatory properties and can be used to reduce inflammation and heal ulcerations. The herb also eases dry cough and sore throats when used as a tea or syrup. Licorice has so many valuable properties that it appears as a key herb in numerous herbal formulas.

Licorice is a key ingredient in *Adrenal Tonic, Bronchialdilator, Cough Remedy, Decongestant, Digestive Tonic, Energy-Boosting, Female Hormonal Balancing, Gentle Laxative, Hypoglycemic, Lung* and *Respiratory Tonic, Menopause Balancing, Moistening Lung/Cough, Quit Smoking* and *Ulcer Healing Formulas*

Warnings: Although licorice is a safe herb, some cautions are necessary when taking large doses for long periods of time. Licorice should be avoided in cases of high blood pressure or when taking digitalis. It causes retention of water and sodium and excretion of potassium, which can cause edema (water retention), high blood pressure, heart palpitations or a slowing of the heartbeat. Vertigo (dizziness) and headaches are early symptoms of overuse of licorice. Taking a potassium supplement with licorice can help counteract some of these effects. These effects are much more likely in individuals using licorice extracts or licorice derived drugs than in taking whole licorice root. Deglycyrrhizinated licorice is free of adverse effects. and Use in pregnancy only under the supervision of a qualified herbalist (herbiverse.com) or practitioner. Small quantities as part of a formula are OK during pregnancy.

Energetics: Cooling and moistening

Properties: Adaptogen, adrenal tonic, anti-inflammatory, antitussive, aperient, demulcent (mucilant), expectorant, hypertensive, lung tonic, moistening and phytoestrogen

Available from: Eclectic Institute, Herb Pharm, Herbalist & Alchemist, Nature's Answer, Nature's Way, NOW Foods, Planetary Herbals, Solaray, Traditional Medicinals and Western Botanicals

Lily of the Valley

Latin name: *Convallaria majalis*

Lily of the valley contains cardiac glycosides that affect the heart like digitalis but are less toxic. Lily of the valley normalizes heart action and increases blood pressure in hypotensive people. The crushed leaves of the fresh plant can be applied topically for drawing infection and slivers.

Lily of the Valley is a key ingredient in *Cardiac Tonic* and *Drawing Salve Formulas*

Warnings: This toxic botanical is for professional use only. A toxic dose may cause nausea, vomiting, cardiac arrhythmias, hypertension, restlessness, trembling, confusion, weakness, depression, circulatory collapse and death. Use formulas containing lily of the valley under professional supervision.

Energetics: Warming

Properties: Cardiac, diuretic and drawing

Linden

Latin name: *Tilia sp.*

Linden is a soothing nervine that relaxes tension and reduces blood pressure. It can also be helpful for headaches. It a very pleasant-tasting herbal teas and is a valuable, but underused remedy.

Linden is a key ingredient in *Hypotensive Formulas*

Warnings: No known warnings.

Energetics: Cooling, drying and relaxing

Properties: Antispasmodic, hypotensive, nervine and relaxant

Available from: Herb Pharm, Herbalist & Alchemist, Nature's Answer and Western Botanicals

Lobelia

Latin name: *Lobelia inflata (Campanulaceae)*

Lobelia is a powerful antispasmodic herb. It dilates the bronchial passages to ease asthma attacks and eases pain caused by tension. It helps to clear lymphatic congestion and can be applied topically to insect bites and stings.

Lobelia contains lobeline, which binds to the same receptors in the nervous system as nicotine, but inhibits rather than stimulates them. For this reason, lobelia has been prescribed to help people quit smoking.

Lobelia is a key ingredient in *Analgesic, Antispasmodic, Bronchialdilator, Cough Remedy, Expectorant, Heavy*

Metal Cleansing, Lymphatic Drainage, Menstrual Cramp, Quit Smoking and *Relaxing Nervine Formulas*

Warnings: The FDA considers lobelia to be poisonous; and many sources claim it will cause convulsions, coma and death. These are potential effects of its principle alkaloid lobeline, but there is no record of the whole herb causing these problems in anyone because lobelia is an emetic and makes you throw up if you take too much. Lobelia can produce severe symptoms (nausea, profuse sweating, vomiting and deep relaxation), but these symptoms typically pass quickly and the person feels better afterwards. However, because of these effects, lobelia is not recommended for weak, debilitated persons or persons who are deeply relaxed. Also, lobelia is not recommended for long term use and should be used cautiously during pregnancy. To avoid unpleasant effects such as nausea and vomiting, use small, repeated doses, instead of large infrequent doses, or use it as part of a formula.

Energetics: Warming (slightly), drying (slightly) and relaxing

Properties: Acrid, analgesic (anodyne), anti-arrhythmic, antispasmodic, antitussive, antivenomous, bronchial dilator, decongestant, diaphoretic/sudorific, emetic, expectorant, hypotensive, nervine and vasodilator

Available from: Grandma's Herbs, Herb Pharm, Herbalist & Alchemist, Nature's Answer, Solaray and Western Botanicals

Lomatium

Latin name: *Lomatium dissectum*

An herb with powerful antiviral and antiseptic actions, lomatium is useful for a wide variety of viral conditions. It is also beneficial for respiratory problems. Applied topically it can ease pain and promote healing of wounds, sprains, cuts and other injuries.

Lomatium is a key ingredient in *Antiviral Formulas*

Warnings: Not for use during pregnancy. Discontinue if rash develops.

Energetics: Cooling

Properties: Antiseptic and antiviral

Available from: Herb Pharm, Herbalist & Alchemist, Nature's Answer, Planetary Herbals and Western Botanicals

Lycium (Wolfberry, Gogi)

Latin name: *Lycium chinense (Solanaceae)*

Lycium berries, also known as wolfberries or gogi berries have become very popular due to their antioxidant and anti-inflammatory effects. They are one of the richest sources of vitamin C and contain many other vitamins and nutrients. The berries are used in China as a blood, liver and eye tonic and are also believed to extend human longevity. They are used for cooling hot, irritated tissues.

Lycium (Wolfberry, Gogi) is a key ingredient in *Antioxidant* and *Hepatoprotective Formulas*

Warnings: No known warnings.

Energetics: Cooling and moistening

Properties: Febrifuge, hepatoprotective, nutritive, refrigerant and tonic

Available from: Herbalist & Alchemist, Nature's Way and Planetary Herbals

Maca

Latin name: *Lepidium meyenii*

A rejuvenating tonic for reproductive health in both men and women, scientific studies have shown that maca can be helpful for erectile dysfunction in men and increasing sexual desire in women. Maca has adaptogenic and tonic properties.

Maca is a key ingredient in *Female Aphrodisiac* and *Male Aphrodisiac Formulas*

Warnings: No known warnings.

Energetics: Warming and nourishing

Properties: Testosterone-enhancing and tonic

Available from: Gaia Herbs, Herb Pharm, Herbalist & Alchemist, Nature's Herbs (TwinLab), Nature's Way, NOW Foods, Planetary Herbals, Solaray and Western Botanicals

Maitake

Latin name: *Grifola frondosa*

A powerful immune enhancing mushroom, maitake is used to regulate the immune system. The beta glucans in maitake mushrooms activate and increase production of immune system cells such as macrophages, T-cells, natural killer cells, and neutrophils. These cells help the immune system to fight illness more quickly and efficiently. Maitake may help decrease insulin resistance, thereby increasing insulin sensitivity. It can also help to decrease blood pressure levels, lower total cholesterol levels, and help maintain weight, thereby promoting heart health.

Maitake is a key ingredient in *Immune Balancing, Immune Stimulating* and *Mushroom Blend Formulas*

Warnings: No known warnings.

Energetics: Drying and nourishing

Properties: Anticancer, anticholesteremic, antifungal, antiviral, hepatoprotective, immune amphoteric and tonic

Available from: Eclectic Institute, Herbalist & Alchemist, Nature's Answer, NOW Foods, Planetary Herbals, Solaray and Western Botanicals

Male Fern

Latin name: *Dryopteris filix-mas*

Male fern is employed almost exclusively to expel worms.

Male Fern is a key ingredient in *Antiparasitic Formulas*

Warnings: Male fern can be toxic and is normally used as a small part of a formula. It should be administered by a professional herbalist (herbiverse.com) only.

Energetics: Cooling and drying

Properties: Antiparasitic

Mangosteen

Latin name: *Garcinia mangostana*

Mangosteen fruit is rich in antioxidant polyphenols. In terms of their antioxidant potency, polyphenols are 10 times stronger than vitamin C and 100 times stronger than vitamin E and carotenoids. This gives the body a big boost in fighting free radicals and keeping the immune system strong. Mangosteen rind contains high levels of xanthones. These highly studied constituents promote intestinal, respiratory and immune system health.

Mangosteen is a key ingredient in *Antioxidant Formulas*

Warnings: Very safe remedy.

Energetics: Cooling

Properties: Anti-allergenic, anti-inflammatory, antioxidant and febrifuge

Available from: Solaray

Marshmallow

Latin name: *Althea officinalis*

A mucilaginous herb which aids the bowels, mucous membranes, lungs and kidneys, marshmallow is also a mild, nourishing food. It soothes inflamed and irritated tissues and reduces swelling. Marshmallow is used in combination with other kidney herbs to soothe burning urination, inflamed kidneys and ease the passing of kidney stones. It can also ease respiratory congestion and dry cough. It enriches breast milk in nursing mothers.

Marshmallow is a key ingredient in *Cough Remedy, Intestinal Toning, Moistening Lung/Cough, Nursing Aid, Poultice* and *Tissue Healing Formulas*

Warnings: No known warnings. A very mild and safe remedy for children, infants and elderly persons.

Energetics: Cooling and moistening

Properties: Demulcent (mucilant), diuretic, emollient, expectorant, galactagogue, nutritive and vulnerary

Available from: Eclectic Institute, Herb Pharm, Herbalist & Alchemist, Nature's Answer, Nature's Way, Solaray and Western Botanicals

Meadowsweet

Latin name: *Filipendula ulmaria (Rosaceae)*

Meadowsweet contains salycin, the natural form of aspirin, making it useful for reducing pain and inflammation. It also settles the stomach and acts as a natural antacid. It also contains silica, which aids skin, joints and connective tissues.

Meadowsweet is a key ingredient in *Analgesic, Antacid* and *Anti-Inflammatory Formulas*

Warnings: Because of its natural aspirin content, some herbalists feel it should not be given to small children suffering with fevers from colds, flu or chicken pox. It can cause nausea or vomiting in large doses.

Energetics: Cooling and drying

Properties: Analgesic (anodyne), antacid, anti-inflammatory and stomachic

Available from: Herb Pharm, Herbalist & Alchemist and Western Botanicals

Milk Thistle

Latin name: *Carduus marianus syn. Silybum marianum (Compositae)*

There is good scientific evidence that the silymarin contained in Milk Thistle can protect the liver from various chemicals and toxins and aid in healing liver diseases. Milk thistle can prevent liver cell death from toxins like carbon tetrachloride and even the toxic effects of aminita (death cap) mushrooms. The flavonoids in milk thistle can have an antioxidant effect on the body, which may play a role in reducing one's cancer risk. Milk Thistle enriches breast milk.

Milk Thistle is a key ingredient in *Female Hormonal Balancing, Heavy Metal Cleansing, Hepatoprotective, Liver Tonic* and *Nursing Aid Formulas*

Warnings: No known warnings.

Energetics: Moistening and cooling

Properties: Alterative (blood purifier), cholagogue, galactagogue, hepatic and hepatoprotective

Available from: Eclectic Institute, Gaia Herbs, Herb Pharm, Herbalist & Alchemist, Herbs Etc., Nature's Answer, Nature's Way, NOW Foods, Planetary Herbals, Solaray and Western Botanicals

Mimosa (Albizia, Silk Tree)

Latin name: *Albizia julibrissin*

Also known as Albizia, this herb was traditionally used to calm the spirit, relieve constriction and pain, invigorate the blood, heal bone fractures, and to treat bad temper, depression, insomnia, irritability and poor memory due to suppressed emotions. Modern herbalists use Mimosa to relieve heartache, stress and depression. Animal research shows that the antidepressant action of Mimosa is mediated through 5-HT1A receptors. It is mildly uplifting and yet grounding. The bark slowly stretches one's energy and mood upward and "softens" the heart. The flowers, on the other hand, seem to concentrate energy in the head, causing mild euphoria and giddiness. It is an instant dose of "feel good" that insists you take a walk in nature and enjoy life.

Mimosa (Albizia, Silk Tree) is a key ingredient in *Antidepressant Formulas*

Warnings: Pregnant and breast-feeding women should avoid mimosa, as little is known about its side effects. Additionally, mimosa gum may interact with amoxicillin preventing the body from absorbing this antibiotic.

Energetics: Cooling, moistening and relaxing (slightly)

Properties: Antidepressant, calmative, euphoretic, relaxant and vulnerary

Available from: Herb Pharm

Mistletoe

Latin name: *Viscum album*

Mistletoe is useful for more than getting a kiss at Christmas time. In small doses, it is helpful for hypertension (without fluid retention). In large doses mistletoe induces hypertension. Mistletoe is a powerful nervine and may help relieve vasoconstrictive headaches, Petit mal seizures, and tinnitus. It is oxytocic and has been used during labor to strengthen and normalize uterine contractions.

Mistletoe is a key ingredient in *Hypotensive Formulas*

Warnings: Mistletoe is not a contraceptive, but it may act as an abortifacient, so pregnant women should not take it. There have been some reports of ingestion of mistletoe leading to adverse reaction and even death in animals and small children. Upon further investigation, it was determined in these cases that the substance ingested was probably another species of mistletoe that is not used medicinally. Adults need not fear poisoning unless large amounts are ingested., One other caution; mistletoe contains tyramine. When mixed with a prescription medicine that has a monoamineoxidase inhibitor, a person may experience a sudden drop in blood pressure. So and it should not be taken with prescription blood pressure medications. This is an herb that may require the supervision of a skilled herbalist (herbiverse.com) or a physician.

Energetics: Relaxing

Properties: Cardiac, hypotensive, nervine and sedative

Available from: Herb Pharm, Herbalist & Alchemist and Western Botanicals

Motherwort

Latin name: *Leonurus cardiaca*

As its name implies, motherwort is often used as a remedy for female problems, but is also a calming nervine used to lower blood pressure and aid nervous system related heart problems. It relieves anxiety and nervousness and contains glycosides, which temporarily lower blood pressure and ease the strain on heart muscles. This also makes it useful for tachycardia, heart palpitations, and preventing heart disease. It is valuable for female problems, such as hot flashes, menstrual cramps, scanty menstrual flow and vaginal pain, characterized by weakness, nervous irritability and stress.

Motherwort is a key ingredient in *Hypotensive Formulas*

Warnings: Avoid during pregnancy and menstruation with excessive bleeding.

Energetics: Cooling, drying and relaxing

Properties: Anti-arrhythmic, antispasmodic, antithyrotropic, calmative, cardiac, emmenagogue, hypotensive, nervine, sedative and vasodilator

Available from: Eclectic Institute, Herb Pharm, Herbalist & Alchemist, Nature's Answer, Solaray and Western Botanicals

Muira Puama

Latin name: *Ptychopetalum olacoides*

Muira Puama is a tonic that can help with impotency and performance anxiety in men as well as lack of desire in women. It was used by natives of the Amazon rain forest to promote sexual energy and arousal. It has a relaxing effect and has also been used as a remedy for neuromuscular pain and cramps, rheumatism and poor circulation. It has been used for depression, nervous exhaustion and some mild cases of paralysis.

Muira Puama is a key ingredient in *Female Aphrodisiac, Male Aphrodisiac* and *Male Glandular Tonic Formulas*

Warnings: Not for use during pregnancy.

Energetics: Warming and relaxing

Properties: Antirheumatic, aphrodisiac, nervine, testosterone-enhancing and tonic

Available from: Eclectic Institute, Herb Pharm, Herbalist & Alchemist, Nature's Answer, Solaray and Western Botanicals

Mullein

Latin name: *Verbascum spp.*

Mullein leaves are most commonly used for respiratory complaints. They have a soothing, hydrating effect on the lungs and contain saponins that loosen mucus. It is often used for chronic lung problems such as asthma and COPD, but is also helpful for colds and coughs, particularly dry coughs. Mullein flowers are used to make ear drops to soothe earache.

Mullein is a key ingredient in *Ear Drop, Lung* and *Respiratory Tonic, Lymphatic Drainage* and *Moistening Lung/Cough Formulas*

Warnings: Mullein leaf and flowers are generally regarded as safe. Mullein seeds contain the poisonous substance rotenone.

Energetics: Moistening and cooling

Properties: Anodyne, demulcent (mucilant), expectorant and lung tonic

Available from: Eclectic Institute, Herb Pharm, Herbalist & Alchemist, Nature's Answer, Planetary Herbals, Solaray and Western Botanicals

Myrrh

Latin name: *Commiphora molmol syn. C. myrrha (Burseraceae)*

An aromatic and bitter resin with antiseptic and disinfectant qualities. myrrh combines well with goldenseal, echinacea and other herbs for fighting infection. It is especially helpful when used topically as a gargle, mouthwash or liniment. Myrrh helps heal wounds, and can be blended with aloe vera gel to form a soothing barrier. It is also a bitter tonic for digestion.

Myrrh is a key ingredient in *Antibacterial, Dental Health, Topical Antiseptic* and *Topical Vulnerary Formulas*

Warnings: Avoid taking internally while pregnant.

Energetics: Warming and drying

Properties: Antibacterial, antiseptic, carminative, digestive tonic and disinfectant

Available from: Eclectic Institute, Herb Pharm, Herbalist & Alchemist, Nature's Answer, Nature's Way, Solaray and Western Botanicals

Key Herbs

Nettle (Stinging)

Latin name: *Urtica dioica*

A nourishing herbal food, rich in iron, calcium, magnesium, protein and other nutrients, nettles help to build healthy blood, bones, joints and skin. As a blood-nourishing source of iron, nettles are an excellent remedy for anemia, low blood pressure and general weakness. They expel uric acid and help with rheumatism and gout. They have anti-inflammatory and anti-allergenic properties, making them useful for respiratory allergies, asthma and skin eruptive diseases. A blend of nettles, red raspberry and alfalfa makes a great tea for pregnancy.

Nettle seeds can slow, halt or even partially reverse progressive renal failure. Studies have show the root to improved Benign Prostate Hypertrophy (BPH) symptoms in 81 percent of men taking the herb compared with 16 percent improvement in the placebo group.

Nettle (Stinging) is a key ingredient in *Allergy-Reducing, Iron, Kidney Tonic, Mineral, Pregnancy Tonic* and *Prostate Formulas*

Warnings: Nettle is extremely safe, The live plant can cause contact dermatitis, but the dried plant does not produce this effect. Taken over a period of months, nettle may be moderately hypertensive in some people.

Energetics: Neutral and nourishing

Properties: Anti-allergenic, anti-inflammatory, antihistamine, diuretic, hypertensive, kidney tonic, mast cell stabilizer, mineralizer and tonic

Available from: Eclectic Institute, Gaia Herbs, Herb Pharm, Herbalist & Alchemist, Nature's Answer, Nature's Herbs (TwinLab), Nature's Way, NOW Foods, Planetary Herbals, Solaray, Traditional Medicinals and Western Botanicals

Night Blooming Cereus (Cactus)

Latin name: *Selenicereus grandiflorus*

This species of cactus is used for all types of cardiopulmonary disorders, including angina, tachycardia, palpitations and valvular disease. It has an effect like digitalis, but milder. It stimulates the action of the heart and has been used to aid recovery from heart attacks and combines well with hawthorn and motherwort for this purpose. Cactus and mimosa are favored by some herbalists for people suffering from emotional heartbreak.

Night Blooming Cereus (Cactus) is a key ingredient in *Cardiac Tonic Formulas*

Warnings: Recommended for professional use only.

Energetics: Cooling

Properties: Anti-arrhythmic, cardiac, diuretic, relaxant and sedative

Available from: Herb Pharm and Herbalist & Alchemist

Nopal (Prickly Pear)

Latin name: *Opuntia streptacantha* and *O. ficus-indica*

Nopal is helpful for type II diabetes and has a very low glycemic index. Single doses have reportedly decreased blood sugar by 17 to 46 percent in clinical trials, according to the NMCD. It contains potent antioxidants to reduce inflammation, which is a primary driver of most chronic diseases. It is also helpful for relieving hangover.

Nopal (Prickly Pear) is a key ingredient in *Blood Sugar Reducing Formulas*

Warnings: No known warnings.

Energetics: Cooling and moistening

Properties: Analgesic (anodyne), anti-inflammatory and antidiabetic

Available from: Eclectic Institute, Planetary Herbals and Solaray

Oat

Latin name: *Avena sativa*

The milky (unripe) seeds of the oat grain are used as a remedy for a depleted nervous system. Milky oats is a tonic that combines well with almost every other nervine. However, it works best on people with mental and physical exhaustion, who are irritable and lack focus. They may also experience heart palpitations and loss of libido. They have also been used to aid recovery from drug addiction.

Oat seed and straw is used in remedies for female hormones. Like horsetail, oat straw is rich in silica. It is used as a mineralizer and a mild nervine. Oat bran is used as a bulk laxative and an agent to help lower cholesterol.

Oat is a key ingredient in *Brain Calming, Female Aphrodisiac, Mineral, Nerve Tonic* and *Quit Smoking Formulas*

Warnings: No known warnings.

Energetics: Neutral, moistening and nourishing

Properties: Laxative (bulk), mineralizer, nervine and nutritive

Available from: Eclectic Institute, Herb Pharm, Herbalist & Alchemist, Nature's Answer and Western Botanicals

Ocotillo

Latin name: *Fouquieria splendens*

A plant from the deserts of the Southwest, ocotillo is used for glandular and lymphatic inflammation. It moves fluid through the lymphatic system and may be helpful in chronic pleurisy and water in the lungs.

Ocotillo is a key ingredient in *Lymphatic Drainage Formulas*

Warnings: Not for use during pregnancy.

Energetics: Cooling and drying (slightly)

Properties: Antidiarrheal, astringent and lymphatic

Available from: Eclectic Institute and Herbalist & Alchemist

Olive

Latin name: *Olea europaea folia*

Olive oil is nutritious and helps to lower cholesterol. It is often used in herbal salves and ointments. Olive oil is often used with lemon juice as a natural therapy for gallstones.

The leaf of the olive tree is used, along with other herbs, to treat high blood pressure and angina. Olive leaf is also widely recommended as a broad-spectrum antiviral and antibacterial agent, but it's antimicrobial effects are mild.

Olive is a key ingredient in *Antiviral, Hypotensive* and *Topical Vulnerary Formulas*

Warnings: No known warnings.

Energetics: Cooling, drying and relaxing (slightly)

Properties: Antiviral and hypotensive

Available from: Eclectic Institute, Gaia Herbs, Herb Pharm, Herbalist & Alchemist, Herbs Etc., Nature's Way, NOW Foods, Planetary Herbals, Solaray and Western Botanicals

Orange Peel

Latin name: *Citrus sinensis*

An aromatic and bitter herb which stimulates appetite and digestion, orange peel may also be found in many respiratory formulas.

Orange Peel is a key ingredient in *Digestive Bitter Tonic Formulas*

Warnings: Orange peel is contraindicated with fluid loss and excessive thirst. Some herbalists feel it should be avoided during pregnancy.

Energetics: Warming and drying

Properties: Aromatic, bitter, carminative, decongestant, digestive tonic and stomachic

Available from: Herbalist & Alchemist and Western Botanicals

Oregano

Latin name: *Origanum vulgare*

Oregano is antiseptic and useful for infections of the respiratory and digestive tracts. It is a good remedy for fungal infections, coughs, tonsillitis, bronchitis, asthma and chest congestion. The oil of oregano can be added to bath water or a steamer to clear lungs and bronchials.

Oregano is a key ingredient in *Antifungal Formulas*

Warnings: Oregano should be avoided in large quantities during pregnancy. Oregano oil should not be used internally, except in highly diluted one or two drop doses for short periods of time (one to two weeks) as it is hepatotoxic.

Energetics: Warming and drying

Properties: Antifungal, antimicrobial, aromatic, condiment, expectorant and stimulant (metabolic)

Available from: Gaia Herbs, Herb Pharm, Nature's Answer, Nature's Way, New Chapter, NOW Foods, Planetary Herbals, Solaray and Western Botanicals

Oregon Grape

Latin name: *Berberris repens, B. aquifolium*

Because it has alkaloids similar to goldenseal, Oregon Grape is often used as an alternative to it as goldenseal is becoming endangered. Oregon grape has antimicrobial properties, and is a good lymphatic cleansing herb. It also stimulates bile flow and has been used with other alteratives for liver conditions. It can be used both internally and externally to relieve skin conditions such as acne, boils and eczema and may reduce itching.

Oregon Grape is a key ingredient in *Antibacterial, Blood Purifier, Liver Tonic* and *Urinary Infection Fighting Formulas*

Warnings: Not for use with emaciation or weak digestion. Use with caution during pregnancy.

Energetics: Cooling and drying

Properties: Alterative (blood purifier), antiseptic, cholagogue and lymphatic

Available from: Eclectic Institute, Gaia Herbs, Herb Pharm, Herbalist & Alchemist, Nature's Answer, Solaray and Western Botanicals

Osha

Latin name: *Ligusticum porteri*

Osha is a great remedy for viral infections such as the common cold, flu, sore throat and upper respiratory congestion. It stimulates the digestive and immune systems and expels mucus. It is also used for settling the stomach after vomiting. It can be used with eyebright to prevent and treat earaches in children.

Osha is a key ingredient in *Allergy-Reducing, Drying Cough/Lung, Expectorant* and *Sinus Decongestant Formulas*

Warnings: Not for use during pregnancy.

Energetics: Warming and drying

Properties: Antiviral, decongestant and expectorant

Available from: Eclectic Institute, Gaia Herbs, Herb Pharm, Herbalist & Alchemist, Herbs Etc., Nature's Answer and Western Botanicals

Papaya

Latin name: *Carica papaya*

Papaya fruit contains enzymes that help digest proteins. These enzymes also help expel intestinal worms by digesting their proteins. The seeds of papaya are an even better antiparasitic agent than the fruit.

Papaya is a key ingredient in *Digestive Enzyme Formulas*

Warnings: No known warnings.

Energetics: Cooling and nourishing

Properties: Antiparasitic, condiment and digestant

Available from: Solaray and Western Botanicals

Parsley

Latin name: *Petroselinum crispum*

Parsley is rich in sodium and potassium necessary to regulate fluids in the body. It has a volatile oil that stimulates kidney function and has a mild alkalizing effect on the system. It also helps to lower blood pressure and slow the pulse.

Parsley is a key ingredient in *Kidney Tonic Formulas*

Warnings: Not recommended in cases involving fluid deficiency, wasting or dryness. It is used to dry up breast milk, so it should be avoided while breast feeding.

Energetics: Warming (slightly), drying (slightly) and nourishing

Properties: Antigalactagogue, condiment, diuretic and nutritive

Available from: Eclectic Institute, Nature's Answer, Nature's Way, Solaray and Western Botanicals

Partridge Berry (Squaw Vine)

Latin name: *Mitchella repens*

Partridge Berry was traditionally taken as a tea by Native American women during pregnancy. The natives used the plant to ease the difficulties of pregnancy in the later stages, and make parturition fast and easy. The herb's ability to soothe sore nipples has long been known, and a salve applied after breast feeding worked wonders. It was believed to increase fertility, and it was used to bring about menstruation in irregular cycles. Today, Squaw Vine is used to tone the uterus, which helps in painful, heavy menstruation or periods of irregularity.

Partridge Berry (Squaw Vine) is a key ingredient in *Uterine Tonic Formulas*

Warnings: No known warnings.

Energetics: Warming and drying

Properties: Emmenagogue and uterine tonic

Available from: Herb Pharm and Herbalist & Alchemist

Key Herbs

Passionflower

Latin name: *Passiflora incarnata, P. quadrangularis*

A relaxing nervine, often combined with other nervines for reducing stress and tension and aiding sleep. it helps to quiet mental chatter. Passionflower is also used for restless agitation and exhaustion with or without muscular twitching and spasms.

Passionflower is a key ingredient in *Nerve Tonic, Quit Smoking, Relaxing Nervine* and *Sleep Formulas*

Warnings: No known warnings.

Energetics: Cooling and relaxing

Properties: Analgesic (anodyne), nervine, relaxant, sedative and soporific (hypnotic)

Available from: Eclectic Institute, Gaia Herbs, Herb Pharm, Herbalist & Alchemist, Nature's Answer, NOW Foods, Solaray and Western Botanicals

Pau d' Arco

Latin name: *Tabebuia impetiginosa, T. avellanedae, T. ipe, T. cassanoides, Tecoma ochracea*

Commonly used as an anticancer remedy and an antifungal remedy. It may be helpful for fighting infections in the digestive tract, both bacterial and fungal. Its active constituents include lapachol and beta-lapachone, which have demonstrated potent antifungal properties in laboratory tests.

Pau d' Arco is a key ingredient in *Antifungal, Blood Purifier* and *General Detoxifying Formulas*

Warnings: Contraindicated for blood clotting disorders. Not for pregnant women. Side effects with high doses may include: nausea, vomiting, intestinal discomfort and anticoagulant effects.

Energetics: Cooling (slightly) and drying

Properties: Alterative (blood purifier), anticancer, antifungal, antiseptic and astringent

Available from: Eclectic Institute, Gaia Herbs, Herb Pharm, Herbalist & Alchemist, Nature's Answer, Nature's Herbs (TwinLab), Nature's Way, NOW Foods, Planetary Herbals, Solaray, Traditional Medicinals and Western Botanicals

Paw Paw

Latin name: *Asimina triloba*

The spring twigs, unripe fruit and mature seeds of the American paw paw tree contain compounds called acetogenins, which inhibit energy production in cells. Since cancer cells have a much faster metabolic rate than normal cells, this induces cancer cells to self-destruct. Scientific research demonstrates that paw paw extract is more effective than many chemotherapy drugs at destroying cancer cells, and yet it is completely non-toxic. In a clinical trial involving over 100 people with cancer, a standardized extract of paw paw was shown to reduce tumor markers and tumor sizes, usually within 1-4 weeks, with virtually no side effects. The extract has also been used to kill intestinal parasites and fight fungal and viral infections. Although Native Americans made preparations from the twigs, unripe fruit and seeds, one should rely on the standardized extract for modern applications.

Warnings: The paw paw extract is not toxic to people or animals in normal doses, but it may cause nausea and vomiting when ingested. It is not recommended for healthy people as it will reduce energy levels, causing fatigue. It should only be used by persons with cancer, viral disorders, parasites or other specific health problems. Paw paw may also induce a healing crisis or cleansing reaction if cell die off occurs too rapidly, which may require cleansing herbs to help the body detoxify.

Energetics: Cooling

Properties: Anticancer, antifungal, antiparasitic, antiviral and cytotoxic

Available from: Nature's Sunshine Products

Pennyroyal

Latin name: *Mentha pulegium*

Pennyroyal tea produces sweating and is useful for fevers and flu. The oil is used externally as a mosquito repellent. The herb can be used to regulate menstruation.

Pennyroyal is a key ingredient in *Pre-Delivery Formulas*

Warnings: Avoid during pregnancy, except as part of a formula during the final weeks before the due date, as pennyroyal may cause miscarriage. Pennyroyal oil should not be used internally.

Energetics: Warming, drying and relaxing

Properties: Antispasmodic and diaphoretic/sudorific

Peony

Latin name: *Paeonia lactiflora*

Peony is used as a tonic for women in Chinese medicine. It is also used for abdominal pain, amenorrhea, and to move blood. It is commonly blended with rehmannia, dong quai and ligusticum as a female tonic. It builds the blood and can be helpful for hot flashes or night sweats. It can also relieve abdominal cramps and pain.

Peony is a key ingredient in *Female Hormonal Balancing Formulas*

Warnings: Western peony (*P. officinalis*) should only be used by professionals.

Energetics: Cooling and relaxing

Properties: Alterative (blood purifier), analgesic (anodyne), anti-inflammatory and antispasmodic

Available from: Herbalist & Alchemist

Peppermint

Latin name: *Mentha x piperita (Labiatae)*

A soothing aromatic with primary effects on the nervous system, stomach and colon, peppermint is an excellent ingredient in formulas for acute ailments. It settles the stomach, expels gas and has a mild effect on colds, fevers and headaches.

Peppermint is a key ingredient in *Carminative* and *Sudorific Formulas*

Warnings: Very safe remedy.

Energetics: Cooling and drying

Properties: Analgesic (anodyne), antacid, anti-emetic (antinauseous), antiseptic, aromatic, carminative, condiment, diaphoretic/sudorific, digestive tonic and stimulant (metabolic)

Available from: Celestial Seasonings, Eclectic Institute, Herb Pharm, Herbalist & Alchemist, Nature's Answer, Nature's Way, NOW Foods, Solaray, Traditional Medicinals, Western Botanicals and Yogi Tea

Periwinkle (Lesser)

Latin name: *Vinca minor*

Periwinkle increases blood flow and oxygen to the brain. Clinical studies suggest it may also be helpful in treating dementia, Alzheimer's disease, short-term memory loss caused by some medications, high blood pressure, age-related hearing loss, vertigo, and reducing calcium buildup from dialysis. Used as an astringent against internal bleeding, it can also be helpful for migraines due to vasoconstriction.

Periwinkle (Lesser) is a key ingredient in *Brain* and *Memory Tonic* and *Migraine/Headache Formulas*

Warnings: Do not use during pregnancy. Avoid with low blood pressure and liver and kidney diseases. Periwinkle is best used under professional supervision.

Energetics: Drying and relaxing

Properties: Astringent, hypotensive, sedative and styptic

Available from: Herb Pharm, Herbalist & Alchemist, Nature's Answer and Western Botanicals

Pine (White)

Latin name: *Pinus strobus* and *other species.*

Pine bark is primarily used as an expectorant for coughs. It helps discharge mucus and fight infection. It is particularly helpful for coaxing old, thick, green mucus up and out of the lungs and sinuses and in cases of chronic bronchitis,

The pine gum is a good agent for drawing pus and slivers. It helps wounds to heal. Pine also strengthens muscles and tendons and helps tissue regeneration and repair. The pollen contains testosterone and is used as a male glandular tonic.

Pine (White) is a key ingredient in *Cough Remedy, Drawing Salve, Drying Cough/Lung* and *Expectorant Formulas*

Warnings: No known warnings.

Energetics: Warming and drying

Properties: Antiseptic, aromatic, drawing, expectorant and testosterone-enhancing

Available from: Eclectic Institute and Planetary Herbals

Pipsissewa

Latin name: *Chimaphila umbellata*

Antibacterial and astringent, pipsissewa is used primarily for urinary problems involving inflammation such as cystitis, prostitis and urethritis. It is a great remedy for irritable bladder. It has the same urinary disinfectant compounds as uva ursi, but less tannin, which makes it easier on the kidneys.

Pipsissewa is a key ingredient in *Diuretic*, *Kidney Tonic* and *Urinary Infection Fighting Formulas*

Warnings: No known warnings.

Energetics: Cooling and drying

Properties: Antiseptic and diuretic

Available from: Eclectic Institute, Herb Pharm, Herbalist & Alchemist and Western Botanicals

Plantain

Latin name: *Plantago major*

This common lawn and garden weed is a valuable remedy for bruises, insect bites and injuries when applied topically. It is a common ingredient in poultices. Plantain is used internally for ulcers, inflammatory bowel disorders, and coughs. It is helpful for drawing sticky phlegm out of the lungs, especially when combined with gumweed.

Plantain is a key ingredient in *Anti-Itch*, *Decongestant*, *Drawing Salve*, *Poultice*, *Tissue Healing* and *Topical Vulnerary Formulas*

Warnings: No known warnings.

Energetics: Cooling, moistening and contricting (slightly)

Properties: Antiseptic, antivenomous, astringent, cicatrisant, decongestant, demulcent (mucilant), drawing, emollient and vulnerary

Available from: Eclectic Institute, Herb Pharm, Herbalist & Alchemist, Nature's Answer and Western Botanicals

Platycodon (Balloon Flower)

Latin name: *Platycodon grandiflorus*

This Chinese herb helps decongest the lungs when there is an excess of mucus.

Platycodon (Balloon Flower) is a key ingredient in *Lung and Respiratory Tonic Formulas*

Warnings: No known warnings.

Energetics: Warming (slightly), drying and relaxing (slightly)

Properties: Expectorant

Pleurisy Root

Latin name: *Asclepias tuberosa*

Native American's used pleurisy root for ailments relating to the heart, bronchials and lungs. As its name implies it is one of the best remedies for pleurisy. It eases chest pain and is good for hot, dry conditions of the chest. It also relaxes the peripheral capillaries, increasing perspiration, making it an excellent diaphoretic. It is helpful for respiratory problems where there is dryness in the lungs.

Warnings: Excessive doses may cause vomiting. Not recommended for use during pregnancy.

Energetics: Cooling and moistening

Properties: Anti-inflammatory, diaphoretic/sudorific, diuretic and expectorant

Available from: Eclectic Institute, Herb Pharm, Herbalist & Alchemist, Nature's Answer and Western Botanicals

Poke Root

Latin name: *Phytolacca decandra*

Poke root is a traditional anti-tumor remedy that is also used to clear the lymphatic system. Poke root oil is used topically for swollen lymph nodes, mastitis, or breast cancer. It is similar to applying a castor oil pack, but much stronger. Internally and in SMALL doses a tincture of the berries is used for severe lymphatic congestion and mastitis.

Poke Root is a key ingredient in *Anticancer* and *Drawing Salve Formulas*

Warnings: For professional use only because of its toxicity, especially internally. Not for use during pregnancy.

Key Herbs

Energetics: Cooling

Properties: Alterative (blood purifier), anti-inflammatory, anticancer, immune stimulant and lymphatic

Available from: Herbalist & Alchemist and Western Botanicals

Prickly Ash

Latin name: *Zanthoxylum americanum*

Prickly ash is used internally primarily to aid circulation. It increases peripheral circulation and is indicated for people with cold extremities, Raynaud's disease; peripheral neuropathies or sciatica with damaged, numb, tingling or extremely painful nerves that cause a person to writhe in agony.

Prickly Ash is a key ingredient in *Cardiovascular Stimulant Formulas*

Warnings: Not recommended during pregnancy.

Energetics: Warming and drying

Properties: Alterative (blood purifier), analgesic (anodyne), carminative, diaphoretic/sudorific and stimulant (circulatory)

Available from: Eclectic Institute, Herb Pharm, Herbalist & Alchemist, Nature's Answer and Western Botanicals

Propolis

Propolis is not an herb. It is a substance made by bees that has powerful antibiotic and immune enhancing effects. Warming and stimulating, its antimicrobial activity is due largely to its richness in phenolic aglycones.

Propolis is a key ingredient in *Dental Health* and *Topical Antiseptic Formulas*

Warnings: Avoid propolis if you have bee allergies.

Energetics: Warming and drying

Properties: Antibacterial, antifungal, expectorant and immune amphoteric

Available from: Eclectic Institute, Gaia Herbs, Herb Pharm, Herbalist & Alchemist, Nature's Answer and NOW Foods

Psyllium

Latin name: *Plantago spp. (Plantaginaceae)*

A mucilaginous herb used as a bulk laxative, anti-diarrhea remedy or to soothe intestinal irritation, psyllium is best taken first thing in the morning or right before going to bed. Take before meals to help regulate appetite and blood sugar. It also helps to lower cholesterol. Always take psyllium with plenty of water and liquids.

Psyllium is a key ingredient in *Fiber Blend Formulas*

Warnings: Psyllium is a mild laxative, suitable for use by children, the elderly and during pregnancy, but should be avoided in cases of bowel obstruction or perforations. It can cause constipation when a person is dehydrated.

Energetics: Cooling and moistening

Properties: Absorbent, antidiarrheal, demulcent (mucilant), emollient and laxative (bulk)

Available from: Nature's Herbs (TwinLab), NOW Foods, Solaray, Traditional Medicinals and Yerba Prima

Pygeum Bark

Latin name: *Pygeum africanum, P. gardneri*

Pygeum is a urinary remedy from Africa that has been found to be helpful for prostate swelling. It is most often used in combination with other herbs.

Pygeum Bark is a key ingredient in *Prostate Formulas*

Warnings: No known warnings.

Energetics: Cooling

Properties: Anti-inflammatory and diuretic

Available from: Solaray and Western Botanicals

Quassia

Latin name: *Picrasma excelsa*

Quassia is used in combination with other herbs for parasites. It may also help control infections.

Quassia is a key ingredient in *Antiparasitic Formulas*

Warnings: Excessive doses of the bark may cause irritation of the digestive tract and vomiting. Quassia should not be used during pregnancy.

Energetics: Cooling and drying

Properties: Antibacterial, antispasmodic and antiviral

Available from: Herbalist & Alchemist and Western Botanicals

Red Clover

Latin name: *Trifolium pratense*

A pleasant tasting blood purifier that is used in combination with other blood purifiers for skin conditions, cancer, swollen lymph glands and liver detoxification. Red clover also contains phytoestrogens that block estrogen receptor sites for the stronger xenoestrogens, possibly inhibiting estrogen-dependent cancers.

Red Clover is a key ingredient in *Anticancer, Blood Purifier, Drawing Salve, Lymphatic Drainage* and *Phytoestrogen Formulas*

Warnings: Due to its phytoestrogen content, some herbalists recommend avoiding red clover during pregnancy.

Energetics: Cooling and balancing

Properties: Alterative (blood purifier), antiseptic, lymphatic and phytoestrogen

Available from: Eclectic Institute, Gaia Herbs, Herb Pharm, Herbalist & Alchemist, Nature's Answer, Nature's Herbs (TwinLab), Nature's Way, NOW Foods, Planetary Herbals, Solaray, Vitanica and Western Botanicals

Red Raspberry

Latin name: *Rubus idaeus*

Red raspberry leaves are rich in manganese, an essential element for oxygenation of the cells. It has been used as a tonic to strengthen the uterine muscles for childbirth. It also helps to relieve and prevent morning sickness.

The berries contain anthocyanin, a compound found to contribute to heart health, protect the eyes, guard against cancer, and help protect against diabetes.

Red Raspberry is a key ingredient in *Female Hormonal Balancing, Pregnancy Tonic* and *Uterine Tonic Formulas*

Warnings: No known warnings.

Energetics: Cooling, drying (slightly) and contricting (slightly)

Properties: Antacid, anti-emetic (antinauseous), antidiarrheal and uterine tonic

Available from: Eclectic Institute, Gaia Herbs, Herb Pharm, Herbalist & Alchemist, Nature's Answer, Nature's Way, Solaray, Traditional Medicinals, Western Botanicals and Yogi Tea

Red Root

Latin name: *Ceanothus americanus*

A powerful lymphatic cleanser, red root helps to shrink swollen lymph nodes and reduce an enlarged spleen. It also helps to raise platelet counts. Combined with echinacea it works well for tonsillitis, cysts and infections in the lymph glands. It is very good for AIDS patients with low platelet count, enlarged spleen and/or swollen lymph nodes.

Red Root is a key ingredient in *Lymphatic Drainage Formulas*

Warnings: Not for use during acute inflammation of the spleen.

Energetics: Drying and constricting

Properties: Astringent and lymphatic

Available from: Eclectic Institute, Herb Pharm, Herbalist & Alchemist, Solaray and Western Botanicals

Rehmannia

Latin name: *Rehmannia glutinosa (Scrophulariaceae)*

This Chinese herb is used to cool the blood, reduce fever and rebuild the blood from blood loss. It is also a liver and kidney tonic.

Rehmannia is a key ingredient in *Energy-Boosting* and *Female Hormonal Balancing Formulas*

Warnings: Contraindicated with loss of appetite and diarrhea.

Energetics: Cooling and nourishing

Properties: Antibacterial, blood building and immune amphoteric

Available from: Herb Pharm, Herbalist & Alchemist and Western Botanicals

Reishi (Ganoderma)

Latin name: *Ganoderma lucidum*

This medicinal mushroom has been shown to have immune enhancing effects as well as acting as a general health tonic. Research suggests that reishi relaxes muscles, improves sleep, eases chronic pain, aids heart function, reduces cholesterol and has antioxidant effects.

Reishi (Ganoderma) is a key ingredient in *Immune Balancing, Immune Stimulating* and *Mushroom Blend Formulas*

Warnings: This herb is generally regarded as safe and nontoxic. However, it may be contraindicated with fluid deficiency and dryness.

Energetics: Warming (slightly), balancing and nourishing

Properties: Adaptogen, alterative (blood purifier), anti-allergenic, antibacterial, anticholesteremic, antiviral, immune amphoteric and nutritive

Available from: Eclectic Institute, Herb Pharm, Herbalist & Alchemist, Nature's Answer, Nature's Herbs (TwinLab), NOW Foods, Planetary Herbals, Solaray and Western Botanicals

Rhodiola

Latin name: *Rhodiola rosea*

An adaptogenic tonic, rhodiola aids mental clarity, memory, energy, production and stress reduction.

Rhodiola is a key ingredient in *Adaptogen Formulas*

Warnings: No known warnings.

Energetics: Cooling, drying and constricting

Properties: Adaptogen, antidepressant and astringent

Available from: Gaia Herbs, Herb Pharm, Herbalist & Alchemist, Nature's Answer, Nature's Way, New Chapter, NOW Foods, Planetary Herbals, Solaray and Vitanica

Rose

Latin name: *Rosa sp.*

Rich hips (fruits) are rich in bioflavonoids and vitamin C and strengthen capillaries. They are mildly astringent and can be helpful for acute illnesses like colds.

Rose petals are an uplifting addition to herbal teas. They reduce stress and help heal heartache.

Rose is a key ingredient in *Cold and Flu Formulas*

Warnings: No known warnings.

Energetics: Cooling, drying and contricting (slightly)

Properties: Anti-inflammatory, antibacterial, antidepressant and astringent

Available from: Eclectic Institute

Rosemary

Latin name: *Rosmarinus officinalis (Labiatiae)*

This herb is considered a tonic for elderly people and may help improve circulation to the brain. In Germany, rosemary is approved by the Commission E for use in treating indigestion, joint ailments and stomach problems. Rosemary also has antioxidant properties which protect the brain and blood vessels.

Rosemary is a key ingredient in *Antioxidant* and *Brain and Memory Tonic Formulas*

Warnings: No known warnings.

Energetics: Warming, drying and contricting (slightly)

Properties: Antidepressant, antioxidant, antirheumatic, antiseptic, carminative, cerebral tonic, expectorant and stimulant (metabolic)

Available from: Eclectic Institute, Herb Pharm, Herbalist & Alchemist, Nature's Answer, Nature's Way, Solaray and Western Botanicals

Safflowers

Latin name: *Carthamus tinctorius*

Safflowers aid digestion and neutralize waste acids in the body, particularly lactic acid. A tea of safflowers is a very dependable remedy for relieving muscle soreness from over exertion. It also reduces swelling in breasts, brings on delayed menses, helps move stagnant blood (bruises, blood cots) and heals injuries.

Warnings: No known warnings.

Energetics: Cooling

Properties: Anti-inflammatory, carminative, stomachic and vulnerary

Available from: Solaray and Western Botanicals

Sage

Latin name: *Salvia officinalis (Labiatae)*

Sage can be helpful for colds and fever, especially involving intermittent chills and fever, hoarseness or sweating at night. It is best taken as a cool tea for night sweats and as a hot tea for inducing perspiration. You can also use the tea for sore or horse throat and, laryngitis and as a mouthwash or gargle for irritation of the throat or mouth. Sage's antiseptic properties make it helpful in treating wounds to prevent infection and inflammation. It acts as a nerve tonic, increasing your capacity to handle stress.

Sage is a key ingredient in *Brain and Memory Tonic Formulas*

Warnings: Not recommended as a medicinal herb during pregnancy. Sage will dry up breast milk, so it should be avoided by nursing mothers.

Energetics: Warming, drying and contricting (slightly)

Properties: Antibacterial, antigalactagogue, antiseptic, antisudorific, aromatic, carminative, diaphoretic/sudorific, emmenagogue and nervine

Available from: A. Vogel, Herb Pharm, Herbalist & Alchemist, Nature's Answer, Solaray and Western Botanicals

Sarsaparilla

Latin name: *Smilax sp.*

Sarsaparilla is a member of the ginseng family. It is the major flavoring found in old-fashioned root beer. It is a mild bittersweet herb used for strengthening the liver, purifying the blood and balancing the glands. It helps relieve arthritic pains and clear skin conditions. It also has a reputation as an herb that will enhance testosterone and exercise performance, although there is no evidence that it does either.

Sarsaparilla is a key ingredient in *Blood Purifier, Exercise, Joint Healing, Male Glandular Tonic* and *Skin Healing Formulas*

Warnings: No known warnings.

Energetics: Warming and moistening

Properties: Alterative (blood purifier) and diuretic

Available from: Eclectic Institute, Herb Pharm, Herbalist & Alchemist, Nature's Answer, Nature's Herbs (TwinLab), Nature's Way, Solaray and Western Botanicals

Saw Palmetto

Latin name: *Sabal serrulata syn. Serenoa serrulata (Palmaceae)*

Widely used for prostate enlargement and urinary problems in men, saw palmetto is a general tonic for elderly men and may be helpful with other problems associated with aging. It aids digestion and weight gain in wasting conditions and has a slight effect in stimulating breast tissue in women.

Saw Palmetto is a key ingredient in *Male Glandular Tonic* and *Prostate Formulas*

Warnings: Women who are breast-feeding should avoid this herb, as it inhibits prolactin and may interfere with lactation.

Energetics: Moistening and nourishing

Properties: Antigalactagogue, digestive tonic and expectorant

Available from: A. Vogel, Eclectic Institute, Gaia Herbs, Herb Pharm, Herbalist & Alchemist, Nature's Answer, Nature's Herbs (TwinLab), Nature's Way, NOW Foods, Planetary Herbals, Solaray and Western Botanicals

Schisandra (Schizandra)

Latin name: *Schisandra chinensis*

Used as an adaptogen and general tonic, schizandra Improves circulation, strengthens the heart, aids digestion and increases bile secretion. In traditional Chinese Medicine it is thought to harmonize the body and help one retain energy. It helps to keep the nervous system balanced, increasing both excitatory and inhibitory action. It has hepatoprotective effects like milk thistle.

In one study a concentrated seed extract demonstrated a 76% success rate in treating hepatitis patients.

Schisandra (Schizandra) is a key ingredient in *Adaptogen, Adrenal Tonic, Hepatoprotective, Immune Balancing* and *Lung and Respiratory Tonic Formulas*

Warnings: Contraindicated with acute ailments like colds, flu and fevers.

Energetics: Cooling and moistening

Properties: Adaptogen, antitussive, hepatoprotective, immune amphoteric, lung tonic and moistening

Available from: Eclectic Institute, Gaia Herbs, Herb Pharm, Herbalist & Alchemist, Nature's Answer, Nature's Way, Planetary Herbals, Solaray and Western Botanicals

Scullcap (Skullcap)

Latin name: *Scutellaria lateriflora*

A relaxing nervine, scullcap helps to calm brain function helpful for insomnia and chronic stress. It is also a good remedy for vasoconstrictive (or tension) headaches and migraines. It was used by 19th century herbalists for hysteria, epilepsy, convulsions and schizophrenia. The person who needs scullcap often has an inability to pay attention or a dull headache in the front or base of the skull . Symptoms are worse with noise, odors and light but improve with rest. Scullcap also seems to work well when people feel as if every sound, touch and ray of light is personally attacking them. They are oversensitive to any stimulation, being twitchy even during sleep. A major herb for the nervous system.

Scullcap (Skullcap) is a key ingredient in *Migraine/ Headache, Nerve Tonic, Relaxing Nervine* and *Sleep Formulas*

Warnings: No known warnings.

Energetics: Cooling and relaxing

Properties: Analgesic (anodyne), antispasmodic, nervine, sedative and soporific (hypnotic)

Key Herbs

Available from: Eclectic Institute, Herb Pharm, Herbalist & Alchemist, Nature's Answer, Nature's Herbs (TwinLab), Nature's Way, New Chapter, Solaray and Western Botanicals

Senna Leaves

Latin name: *Cassia senna syn. Senna alexandrina (Leguminosae)*

A very strong stimulant laxative.

Senna Leaves is a key ingredient in *General Detoxifying* and *Stimulant Laxative Formulas*

Warnings: Can be gripping and habit forming but is considered fairly safe.

Energetics: Drying and cooling

Properties: Laxative (stimulant) and purgative (cathartic)

Available from: NOW Foods, Solaray and Western Botanicals

Shatavari

Latin name: *Asparagus racemosa*

A reproductive tonic from Ayurvedic medicine, Shatavari is the root of a species of asparagas. It is has been used as a restorative in people suffering from nervous exhaustion and has been used in a wide range of other ailments.

Shatavari is a key ingredient in *Female Aphrodisiac Formulas*

Warnings: It should be avoided by pregnant women.

Energetics: Cooling and nourishing

Properties: Adaptogen and diuretic

Available from: Herb Pharm, Herbalist & Alchemist, Planetary Herbals and Solaray

Sheep Sorrel

Latin name: *Rumex acetosella*

A salad vegetable, sheep sorrel is an ingredient in the famous anticancer formula Essiac. This makes it a key herb in Herbal *Anticancer Formulas*. It is a detoxifying herb, rich in iron like other members of the dock family. It has a mild laxative and intestinal tonic effect like yellow dock.

Sheep Sorrel is a key ingredient in *Anticancer* and *Essiac Formulas*

Warnings: Contains oxalic acid; don't use if you have a history of kidney stones.

Energetics: Cooling and drying (slightly)

Properties: Anticancer, antiseptic and hepatic

Available from: Herb Pharm and Western Botanicals

Shepherd's Purse

Latin name: *Capsella bursa-pastoris*

One of the best herbs to use for hemorrhaging and heavy bleeding during menstruation. It is an important herb in midwifery because it helps deliver the placenta during childbirth and cuts down on postpartum bleeding. It is one of the few remedies that will increase blood pressure because it helps to constrict blood vessels. It can also be used to soothe the bladder and treat blood in the urine.

Shepherd's Purse is a key ingredient in *Styptic/Hemostatic Formulas*

Warnings: Not for use during pregnancy.

Energetics: Warming, drying and constricting

Properties: Astringent, hypertensive, styptic and vasoconstrictor

Available from: Eclectic Institute, Herb Pharm, Herbalist & Alchemist and Western Botanicals

Shiitake

Latin name: *Lentinula edodes*

This mushroom is finding increasing use as a medicinal treatment for cancer and other health problems. It can be helpful in lowering cholesterol and fighting various types of cancer. It stimulates the immune system to increase the body's ability to fight infections.

Shiitake is a key ingredient in *Immune Stimulating* and *Mushroom Blend Formulas*

Warnings: No known warnings.

Energetics: Balancing and nourishing

Properties: Adaptogen, alterative (blood purifier), anti-allergenic, immune amphoteric and restorative

Available from: Eclectic Institute, Herbalist & Alchemist, Nature's Answer, Planetary Herbals, Solaray and Western Botanicals

Skunk Cabbage

Latin name: *Symplocarpus foetidus*

Skunk cabbage is a powerful antispasmodic, making it useful for cramps and muscle spasms of all kinds. It is a specific for severe bronchial asthmatic spasms associated with emotional distress and coughing to the point of vomiting. It may also be helpful for fluid retention, headache, irritability, nervousness, tightness in the chest and whooping cough.

Skunk Cabbage is a key ingredient in *Antispasmodic* and *Bronchialdilator Formulas*

Warnings: Fresh root can be irritating to mucus membranes. It should be used cautiously by people with a history of kidney stones.

Energetics: Warming (slightly) and relaxing

Properties: Acrid, antispasmodic, emetic and expectorant

Available from: Herb Pharm and Western Botanicals

Slippery Elm

Latin name: *Ulmus rubra (Ulmaceae)*

A soothing and nourishing mucilaginous herb that helps absorb acid and irritants in the stomach, slippery elm is used internally for irritation of the stomach and intestines, diarrhea (especially in children) and as a mild, nourishing food for weak and debilitated persons. In bulk form mix 1-2 teaspoons bulk powder with hot water or

juice (mixes best using a blender). Sweeten to taste and drink (may be slightly "thick" depending on how much powder is used). Externally, slippery elm makes an excellent poultice.

Slippery Elm is a key ingredient in *Fiber Blend, Intestinal Toning, Moistening Lung/Cough, Poultice* and *Tissue Healing Formulas*

Warnings: A mild and very safe remedy.

Energetics: Cooling, moistening and nourishing

Properties: Absorbent, demulcent (mucilant), emollient, mucilant/mucilaginous, nutritive, soothing and vulnerary

Available from: Eclectic Institute, Gaia Herbs, Nature's Answer, Nature's Herbs (TwinLab), Nature's Way, NOW Foods, Solaray and Western Botanicals

Solomon's Seal

Latin name: *Polygonatum multiflorum*

A remedy for the musculo-skeletal system, Solomon's Seal helps tone up loose ligaments and tendons. It helps to heal broken bones and strengthen other bones. It is a kidney tonic and builds reproductive organs.

Warnings: No known warnings.

Energetics: Cooling and balancing

Properties: Demulcent (mucilant) and emollient

Available from: Herbalist & Alchemist

Spilanthes

Latin name: *Spilanthes acmella*

An antibacterial and antifungal herb, spilanthes stimulates mucus membrane secretions and the immune system to fight respiratory infections. It acts as a local anesthetic to ease pain, while reducing inflammation. One of its common names is toothache plant, because it has been applied to the gums around an infected tooth to ease pain and help fight the infection.

Spilanthes is a key ingredient in *Antifungal* and *Dental Health Formulas*

Warnings: No known warnings.

Energetics: Warming and constricting

Properties: Analgesic (anodyne), antibacterial, antifungal and astringent

Available from: Herb Pharm and Herbalist & Alchemist

Spirulina

Latin name: *Spirulina sp.*

Spirulina is rich in essential amino acids, the building blocks of protein. It is considered a "superfood" and helps to stabilize energy and blood sugar levels. It has been used as an appetite suppressant to control food cravings. It's high amino acid content has also given it a reputation as a "brain food."

Spirulina is a key ingredient in *Superfood Formulas*

Warnings: No known warnings.

Energetics: Neutral and nourishing

Properties: Nutritive

Available from: Gaia Herbs, Nature's Way and Solaray

Key Herbs

St. John's wort

Latin name: *Hypericum perforatum (Guttiferae)*

St. John's wort became a popular herb when research suggested it could be helpful for mild to moderate depression. It is helpful for some cases of depression, especially those accompanied by anxiety, but the herb has many other valuable properties. It is a nervine herb that helps to regulate the solar plexus, the nerves which regulate digestion. It can be helpful for insomnia, fear, nerve pain and nerve damage. It stimulates nerve regeneration and repair.

St. John's wort also has antiviral properties and has been used for viral infections such as shingles, herpes, mononucleosis and flu. It also helps to heal wounds.

St. John's wort is a key ingredient in *Antidepressant, Antiviral, Nerve Tonic* and *Quit Smoking Formulas*

Warnings: The fresh plant is photo-toxic. It contains a chemical that changes to a toxin in the body after exposure to sunlight. This does not appear to be a problem when taking St. John's Wort internally. Avoid when taking SSRI antidepressants.

Energetics: Warming (slightly)

Properties: Antidepressant, antiseptic, antiviral, digestive tonic, nervine and vulnerary

Available from: A. Vogel, Gaia Herbs, Herb Pharm, Herbalist & Alchemist, Nature's Answer, Nature's Way, New Chapter, NOW Foods, Planetary Herbals, Solaray, Vitanica and Western Botanicals

Stillingia

Latin name: *Stillingia sp.*

Stillingia, also known as queen's root, is an herb in the Hoxsey anticancer formula. It is used primarily to improve lymphatic drainage.

Stillingia is a key ingredient in *Lymphatic Drainage* and *Topical Analgesic Formulas*

Warnings: No known warnings.

Energetics: Warming and balancing

Properties: Analgesic (anodyne), anesthetic and anti-inflammatory

Available from: Eclectic Institute, Herb Pharm, Herbalist & Alchemist and Western Botanicals

Stone Breaker

Latin name: *Phyllanthus niruri*

Stone Breaker has been shown to inhibit the growth of calcium oxalate crystals, stopping the formation or progress of stones. It also stimulates bile flow and aids in digesting fats. It has hepatoprotective properties and its action on the kidneys may be helpful in hypertension.

Stone Breaker is a key ingredient in *Lithotriptic Formulas*

Warnings: No known warnings.

Energetics: Cooling and drying

Properties: Cholagogue, diuretic and lipotropic

Sweet Annie (Ching-Hao)

Latin name: *Artemesia annua (Compositae)*

A close relative of wormwood, sweet annie is used for malaria and intermittent fevers. It is also a good remedy for parasites.

Sweet Annie (Ching-Hao) is a key ingredient in *Antiparasitic Formulas*

Warnings: Not for use when pregnant or nursing. All artemesia species can be toxic in large doses.

Energetics: Cooling and drying

Properties: Anthelminthic, antibacterial, antiparasitic and antiseptic

Available from: Herbalist & Alchemist and Western Botanicals

Tea (Green or Black)

Latin name: *Camellia sinensis*

Tea is the commonly consumed beverage in the world. t contains compounds that reduce cancer risk and protect the liver. Green tea contains powerful antioxidants and is generally considered healthier to drink. Black tea is made from fermented tea leaves. Tea contains caffeine, but is not as likely to cause jittery feelings.

Tea (Green or Black) is a key ingredient in *Antioxidant, Energy-Boosting* and *Weight Loss Formulas*

Warnings: Excessive caffeine consumption can lead to anxiety and adrenal exhaustion.

Energetics: Warming, drying (slightly) and contricting (slightly)

Properties: Anticarious, antimutagenic, antioxidant and stimulant (metabolic)

Available from: Gaia Herbs, Herb Pharm, Nature's Answer, Nature's Way, Solaray, Vitanica and Yogi Tea

Tea Tree

Latin name: *Melaleuca alternifolia (Myrtaceae)*

This volatile oil has powerful disinfectant and antifungal properties. Externally, apply full strength to aid healing and fight infection in burns, cuts, wounds, abrasions, bites, stings, canker sores and other injuries. It disinfects injuries and speeds healing of tissues without stinging.

Tea Tree is a key ingredient in *Antifungal Formulas*

Warnings: Do not take undiluted oil internally. The oil can irritate the skin of some people, but this is rare.

Energetics: Warming and drying

Properties: Antifungal, antiseptic, antiviral and cicatrisant

Thuja

Latin name: *Thuja occidentalis*

The leaves of thuja are a strong antifungal remedy, useful for candida, athlete's foot and jock itch. They also have antiparasitic effects against ringworm, amoebic dysentery and giardia. The leaves have established antiviral activity. Thuja homeopathic is good for side effects from vaccinations.

Warnings: In the 1930's it was used as an abortifacient in Europe and North America. It is not suggested for use during pregnancy. Not suggested for long term use as the herb may irritate the kidneys.

Energetics: Warming and drying

Properties: Anthelminthic, antifungal, antiparasitic, aromatic, emmenagogue and expectorant

Available from: Herb Pharm, Herbalist & Alchemist and Western Botanicals

Thyme

Latin name: *Thymus vulgaris (Labiatae)*

Thyme is a very powerful remedy for infections of all kinds, especially in the lungs and digestive tract. It is indicated for spasmodic conditions of the respiratory and urinary tract with infectious symptoms. It is a good antifungal remedy and can also be used to treat intestinal parasites in children. The combination of fenugreek and thyme is excellent for clearing sinus congestion. Applied topically it helps with insect bites, stings and minor pain.

Thyme is a key ingredient in *Cough Remedy, Decongestant, Drying Cough/Lung* and *Sinus Decongestant Formulas*

Warnings: Avoid large doses in pregnancy. Culinary use and standard dosages found on products are perfectly safe.

Energetics: Warming and drying

Properties: Antibacterial, antifungal, antiviral, aromatic, carminative, decongestant, emmenagogue and stimulant (circulatory)

Available from: Eclectic Institute, Herb Pharm, Herbalist & Alchemist, Nature's Answer, Solaray and Western Botanicals

Tienchi Ginseng

Latin name: *Panax pseudoginseng notoginseng*

Tienchi ginseng is used to control bleeding and hemorrhaging of all kinds. It is also a mild circulatory stimulant and may be helpful for angina.

Tienchi Ginseng is a key ingredient in *Styptic/Hemostatic Formulas*

Warnings: No known warnings.

Energetics: Warming and constricting

Properties: Stimulant (circulatory) and styptic

Available from: Herbalist & Alchemist

Tribulus

Latin name: *Tribulus terrestris*

Tribulus has long been used as a sexual tonic and as a means of restoring vigor to the body. Modern herbalists use Tribulus as a restorative tonic to assist the male reproductive system and bring about an increase in health and stamina. It is used to support testosterone metabolism and hormone function, especially in aging men. The fruit of Tribulus is used to treat urinary tract infections and kidney stones that make urination painful. It may help to reduce blood fats and cholesterol and has a mild hypotensive effect.

Tribulus is a key ingredient in *Male Glandular Tonic Formulas*

Warnings: No known warnings.

Energetics: Warming (slightly), drying and relaxing (slightly)

Properties: Anticholesteremic, aphrodisiac, hypotensive and testosterone-enhancing

Available from: Solaray and Western Botanicals

Key Herbs

Triphala

Latin name: *Emblica officinalis, Terminalia bellerica, Terminalia chebula*

Triphala is not an herb, but blend of three fruits used in Ayurvedic medicine as a gentle laxative, bowel tonic and blood purifier. The first fruit in this blend is haritaki (*Terminalia chebula*). It has a balanced energy containing five flavors (bitter, sour, astringent, salty and sweet). It is a mild laxative that also tones the intestinal membranes. It lubricates tissues and relaxes muscle spasms.

The second fruit in this blend is Bibhitaki (*Terminalia belerica*), an antispasmodic herb that is pungent and warming. It is an expectorant and decongestant and used to treat asthma, bronchial problems and allergies.

The third and final fruit in triphala is Amalaki or Indian Gooseberry (*Embilica officinalis*) which also has a balanced energy containing five flavors (sour, astringent, sweet, pungent and bitter). It contains a small amount of anthraquinones, but is also astringent, so it has both a laxative action and a bowel toning action. This means it corrects both constipation and diarrhea. It is a cooling remedy and is also used to treat ulcers, intestinal inflammation, burning sensations, skin eruptions and infections.

In various formulas these three fruits may also be referred to as Belleric Myrobalan fruit, Chebulic Myrobalan fruit and Indian Gooseberry fruit, or as Harada fruit, Amla fruit and Behada fruit.

Besides normalizing colon function, triphala improves liver function, protects the liver against environmental toxins and improves digestion. It is antioxidant and anti-inflammatory, so it slows aging and protects the body from degenerative disease. It enhances circulation, lowers blood pressure and protects the heart. It helps expel mucus from the respiratory passages and fights infection. In Ayurvedic medicine, triphala is used for constipation, indigestion, flatulence, poor appetite, digestive headaches, sinus congestion, joint pain and general toxicity.

Triphala is a key ingredient in *Gentle Laxative Formulas*

Warnings: None.

Energetics: Cooling (slightly) and drying (slightly)

Properties: Anti-inflammatory, antioxidant, aperient, decongestant, expectorant and hepatoprotective

Available from: Nature's Way, NOW Foods, Planetary Herbals and Solaray

Turkey Rhubarb

Latin name: *Rheum palmatum*

A common ingredient in stimulant laxatives, this bitter is also used as a digestive tonic.

Turkey Rhubarb is a key ingredient in *Antacid, General Detoxifying* and *Stimulant Laxative Formulas*

Warnings: Some people react with abdominal pain. Ginger or nervine herbs can help to counteract this.

Energetics: Drying and cooling

Properties: Antacid and laxative (stimulant)

Available from: Herb Pharm, Nature's Answer and Western Botanicals

Turmeric

Latin name: *Curcuma longa syn. C. domestica*

Turmeric stimulates digestion and aids assimilation. It is a very good liver and gallbladder remedy. It aids liver function and helps dissolve and prevent gallstones. It's potent ability to reduce inflammation and ease chronic pain make it useful for treating arthritis.

Turmeric is a key ingredient in *Analgesic, Anti-Inflammatory* and *Joint Healing Formulas*

Warnings: No known warnings.

Energetics: Cooling

Properties: Anti-inflammatory, antimutagenic, antioxidant, cholagogue, condiment and hepatoprotective

Available from: Eclectic Institute, Gaia Herbs, Herb Pharm, Herbalist & Alchemist, Nature's Way, New Chapter, Planetary Herbals, Solaray and Western Botanicals

Usnea

Latin name: *Tillandsia usneoides*

Actually a lichen, or a symbiotic combination of algae and fungi, usnea has been used for thousands of years in Chinese, Greek and Egyptian medicine to treat a variety of health conditions. It as antibiotic and antifungal properties that may be helpful for treating lung and upper respiratory infections such as the common cold, sore throat and cough, and as an antibacterial for the mouth to promote oral hygiene. It inhibits the growth of gram-positive bacteria.

Usnea is a key ingredient in *Antifungal* and *Topical Antiseptic Formulas*

Warnings: No known warnings.

Energetics: Cooling and drying

Properties: Antibacterial and antifungal

Available from: Eclectic Institute, Herb Pharm, Herbalist & Alchemist and Western Botanicals

Uva ursi

Latin name: *Arctostaphylos uva-ursi*

A reliable diuretic with strong disinfectant and infection fighting properties, uva ursi is useful for kidney and bladder infections, irritated female organs and other urogenital problems.

Uva ursi is a key ingredient in *Diuretic* and *Urinary Infection Fighting Formulas*

Warnings: Not for use in cases involving fluid deficiency, wasting or dryness. Not recommended for long term use because of strong astringency. Prolonged use may irritate the stomach and cause constipation. Not recommended during pregnancy.

Energetics: Warming, drying and constricting

Properties: Antiseptic and diuretic

Available from: Eclectic Institute, Herb Pharm, Herbalist & Alchemist, Nature's Answer, Nature's Way, Planetary Herbals, Solaray and Western Botanicals

Valerian

Latin name: *Valeriana officinalis*

Valerian is a popular and potent nervine with strong tranquilizing effects on the central nervous system. It has been used to treat a wide variety of nervous system conditions, insomnia and mild pain. Thomas Easley, one of the authors, once had a woman take 20 capsules of Valerian three times a day. This was an excessive dose, but it did help the woman to come off of oxytocin, which she had been taking for 10 years to treat a severed sciatic nerve.

Valerian is a key ingredient in *Analgesic, Antispasmodic, Relaxing Nervine* and *Sleep Formulas*

Warnings: Not recommended for persons with "hot" disorders, i.e., high strung, nervous and excitable. (Skullcap or passion flower are better for such individuals). Not recommended for long term use in large doses, although there is no risk of addiction. Does not generally cause drowsiness that could affect driving. Some people react "backwards" to valerian and find it stimulating rather than sedating. Low thyroid and dosage appears to be a factor. Some persons using

Valerian may experience a "light" feeling, as if floating in air, and they may experience hallucinations at night.

Energetics: Warming (slightly) and relaxing

Properties: Analgesic (anodyne), antispasmodic, nervine, sedative and soporific (hypnotic)

Available from: Eclectic Institute, Gaia Herbs, Herb Pharm, Herbalist & Alchemist, Herbs Etc., Nature's Answer, Nature's Herbs (TwinLab), Nature's Way, NOW Foods, Planetary Herbals, Solaray and Western Botanicals

Venus Fly Trap

Latin name: *Dionaea muscipula*

Venus Fly Trap is used in the cases of malignant conditions such as tumors in advanced stages (mammary, bladder, prostate carcinomas and osteosarcoma) and solid tumors. It is also used for Hodgkin and non-Hodgkin lymphoma and other related conditions.

Warnings: Not for use during pregnancy.

Energetics: Cooling

Properties: Analgesic (anodyne), antimutagenic, antiviral, cytotoxic and immune stimulant

Available from: Eclectic Institute and Herb Pharm

Violet

Latin name: *Viola odorata* and *related sp.*

Violet is good remedy for cooling heat and relieving congestion in the lymphatic and respiratory systems.

Violet is a key ingredient in *Lymphatic Drainage Formulas*

Warnings: No known warnings.

Energetics: Cooling and moistening

Properties: Demulcent (mucilant) and lymphatic

Available from: Herb Pharm and Herbalist & Alchemist

White Oak

Latin name: *Quercus alba* and *other species*

A powerful astringent, white oak bark is used internally for hemorrhoids and varicose veins. A decoction can be used as a rectal injection for hemorrhoids, a douche to stop bleeding or as a fomentation for swelling, varicose veins and other injuries. It can also be used as a gargle for sore throat or use as a mouthwash for bleeding gums. Use white oak bark powder with black walnut powder as a tooth pow-

...der for bleeding gums and loose teeth. The powder may be sprinkled into cuts to stop bleeding.

White Oak is a key ingredient in *Dental Health* and *Tissue Healing Formulas*

Warnings: Can be constipating when taken internally. Can interfere with digestion (take between meals). Contains large amounts of tannin, which may be associated with mouth and stomach cancer with consistent, long term use. Use only for short periods internally. No warnings for external use.

Energetics: Drying and constricting

Properties: Anticarious, antidiarrheal, antiseptic, antivenomous, astringent, hemostatic and styptic

Available from: Eclectic Institute, Herb Pharm, Nature's Answer, Nature's Way, Solaray and Western Botanicals

White Pond Lily

Latin name: *Nymphaea odorata*

A cooling and constricting remedy, white pond lily and white water lily (*N. alba*) have been used to reduce restlessness, inflammation and irritation in tissues. They also have a calming effect on libido (sex drive).

Warnings: No known warnings.

Energetics: Cooling and constricting

Properties: Anaphrodisiac, anti-inflammatory, astringent and uterine tonic

Available from: Eclectic Institute and Herbalist & Alchemist

Wild Indigo (Baptista)

Latin name: *Baptisia tinctoria*

A very valuable remedy for serious infections causing toxicity and blood poisoning, wild indigo is indicated in conditions where there is foul discharge and an odor reminiscent of decaying meat. It works very well for these conditions when combined with echinacea and other anti-infective herbs.

Wild Indigo (Baptista) is a key ingredient in *Antibacterial Formulas*

Warnings: This herb should be used with caution. It is potentially toxic and is a strong purgative and emetic in larger doses.

Energetics: Cooling and drying

Properties: Bitter, cathartic, emetic and lymphatic

Available from: Eclectic Institute, Herb Pharm and Western Botanicals

Wild Yam

Latin name: *Dioscorea villosa (Dioscoreaceae)*

Contrary to popular myth, wild yam is not a source of progesterone and is not a reliable herb for birth control. It contains compounds that are used in the synthetic production of hormones like progesterone, but these compounds are not converted to progesterone in the body, nor do they have a progesterone-like action.

Wild Yam is, however, a valuable antispasmodic and anti-inflammatory remedy. It has bee used to ease menstrual cramps and ovarian pain, and is also helpful for irritable bowel and intestinal cramps (gripping). It has also been used in conditions like arthritis and neuralgia.

Wild Yam is a key ingredient in *Antispasmodic, Menstrual Cramp* and *PMS Relieving Formulas*

Warnings: Overdose may cause nausea, vomiting and diarrhea.

Energetics: Cooling, moistening (slightly) and relaxing

Properties: Analgesic (anodyne), anti-inflammatory and antispasmodic

Available from: Eclectic Institute, Gaia Herbs, Herb Pharm, Herbalist & Alchemist, Nature's Answer, Nature's Herbs (TwinLab), Nature's Way, Solaray and Western Botanicals

Willow

Latin name: *Salix alba, Salix lucida* and *other species*

Willow bark has long been used for pain, fevers and inflammation. Its active compound, salicin, is the original source of the synthetic derivative aspirin. The action of white willow is much weaker than that of the synthetic drug, but is less likely to cause stomach problems. Willow generally works best at easing pain when combined with other analgesic herbs.

Willow is a key ingredient in *Analgesic, Anti-Inflammatory, Joint Healing* and *Migraine/Headache Formulas*

Warnings: Not recommended with ulcers or a weak digestive system. Also not recommended during pregnancy.

Energetics: Cooling and drying (slightly)

Properties: Analgesic (anodyne), anti-inflammatory, antiseptic and febrifuge

Available from: Eclectic Institute, Herb Pharm, Herbalist & Alchemist, Nature's Answer, Nature's Herbs (TwinLab), Nature's Way, Solaray and Western Botanicals

Wintergreen

Latin name: *Gaulteria procumbens*

Wintergreen contains salicylic acid (a natural aspirin) which can help to reduce inflammation and pain. It has been taken internally as a tea to ease pain, but it is seldom used internally today. The oil of wintergreen, however, is frequently used as a topical analgesic.

Wintergreen is a key ingredient in *Lymphatic Drainage* and *Topical Analgesic Formulas*

Warnings: The essential oil of wintergreen can trigger contact dermatitis in some people. The essential oil should never be taken internally. People who are sensitive to aspirin should avoid wintergreen.

Energetics: Cooling

Properties: Analgesic (anodyne), anesthetic and anti-inflammatory

Available from: Eclectic Institute, Herb Pharm, Herbalist & Alchemist and Western Botanicals

Witch Hazel

Latin name: *Hamamelis virginiana (Hamamelidaceae)*

Witch hazel is primarily used topically as an astringent. It can also be used as a suppository for hemorrhoids and anal fistula.

Witch Hazel is a key ingredient in *Anti-Itch* and *Vascular Tonic Formulas*

Warnings: No known warnings.

Energetics: Drying and constricting

Properties: Anti-inflammatory, astringent, styptic and vulnerary

Available from: Eclectic Institute, Herb Pharm, Herbalist & Alchemist, Nature's Answer and Western Botanicals

Wood Betony

Latin name: *Betonica officinalis or Stachys officinalis*

Wood betony is an analgesic nervine that relaxes tension in the muscles. It is frequently used in formulas for headaches an is used to relieve middle back pain and tension, facial pain and muscle tension. It is helpful for people whose minds are overactive and stressed and helps ease tension in one's thoughts and emotions.

Warnings: No known warnings.

Energetics: Cooling and relaxing

Properties: Analgesic (anodyne), nervine and sedative

Available from: Eclectic Institute, Herb Pharm, Herbalist & Alchemist, Nature's Answer, Solaray and Western Botanicals

Wormwood

Latin name: *Artemisia absinthium*

As its name implies, wormwood is a powerful anti-parasitic herb, used for expelling tapeworms and other internal worms and parasites. It is also used to stimulate digestion and appetite.

Wormwood is a key ingredient in *Antiparasitic Formulas*

Warnings: A very strong and potentially toxic herb, wormwood should not be used by pregnant women, nursing mothers or weak persons. It should only be used for short periods of time and preferably as part of a formula.

Energetics: Cooling and drying

Properties: Antiparasitic, bitter, stomachic and vermifuge

Available from: Eclectic Institute, Gaia Herbs, Herb Pharm, Herbalist & Alchemist, Planetary Herbals, Solaray and Western Botanicals

Yarrow

Latin name: *Achillea millefolium (Compositae)*

Yarrow's hemostatic properties (ability to stem bleeding) made it the medication of choice for treating war injuries in ancient times. The leaves may be applied topically to bleeding wounds and the herb can be taken internally to stop internal bleeding. This is why yarrow is a key herb in *Styptic/Hemostatic Formulas* and *Topical Vulnerary Formulas*.

Yarrow flowers are also a strong diaphoretic and are used to cool high fevers and help the body fight infection. A warm tea of yarrow is one of the best remedies for inducing a sweat and breaking a fever. Add a little peppermint to improve the flavor.

Yarrow is a key ingredient in *Cold* and *Flu, Styptic/Hemostatic* and *Sudorific Formulas*

Warnings: Yarrow is a safe remedy, but should be reserved for medicinal use and not taken regularly.

Energetics: Cooling, drying and constricting

Properties: Anti-inflammatory, antiviral, diaphoretic/sudorific, febrifuge, hemostatic, styptic and vulnerary

Available from: Eclectic Institute, Gaia Herbs, Herb Pharm, Herbalist & Alchemist, Nature's Answer, Nature's Way, Solaray and Western Botanicals

Key Herbs

Key Herbs

Yellow Dock

Latin name: *Rumex crispus (Polygonaceae)*

Yellow dock is high in organic iron compounds and liberates iron stored in the liver. This makes it useful for anemia, especially when combined with alfalfa, beets and other iron-rich herbs. It is also used as a blood purifier for skin disorders (acne, boils, etc.) and general liver problems. It stimulates the flow of bile and acts as a mild laxative, while reducing heat and irritation in the digestive tract. It is especially indicated where a person has a geographic tongue (a tongue with heavily coated patches and bare bright red areas) and intestinal inflammation with constipation.

Yellow Dock is a key ingredient in *Blood Purifier*, *General Detoxifying*, *Gentle Laxative*, *Iron* and *Skin Healing Formulas*

Warnings: No known warnings.

Energetics: Cooling and drying (slightly)

Properties: Alterative (blood purifier), aperient, cholagogue and hepatic

Available from: Eclectic Institute, Herb Pharm, Herbalist & Alchemist, Nature's Answer, Nature's Way, Planetary Herbals, Solaray and Western Botanicals

Yerba Santa

Latin name: *Eriodictyon californicum*

A warming and stimulating expectorant, yerba santa clears phlegm from the chest and opens air passages. It is a reliable herb for most respiratory problems, but is especially helpful for asthma, profuse expectoration and respiratory complaints with obscure symptoms. It is also an effective diuretic and urinary antiseptic. It can be applied topically to insect bites and stings, poison oak and ivy, bruises, sprains and cuts.

Yerba Santa is a key ingredient in *Cough Remedy*, *Decongestant*, *Drying Cough/Lung* and *Expectorant Formulas*

Warnings: No known warnings.

Energetics: Warming and drying

Properties: Decongestant and expectorant

Available from: Eclectic Institute, Herb Pharm, Herbalist & Alchemist and Western Botanicals

Yohimbe

Latin name: *Pausinystalia yohimbe*

Yohimbe causes dilation of blood vessels, including those in the genitalia, thus helping men to maintain an erection. This effect also lowers blood pressure.

Yohimbe is a key ingredient in *Male Aphrodisiac* and *Male Glandular Tonic Formulas*

Warnings: Avoid long term use, as it can irritate the urinary tract. Contraindicated in cases of emaciation or inflammation.

Energetics: Warming

Properties: Vasodilator

Available from: Gaia Herbs, Herb Pharm, Nature's Answer, Solaray and Western Botanicals

Yucca

Latin name: *Yucca glauca*

A blood purifier with anti-inflammatory and detergent properties, yucca leaf has antioxidant, anti-inflammatory and antifungal properties. It is helpful as an analgesic and anti-inflammatory in arthritis, neuralgia and other inflammatory conditions.

Yucca is a key ingredient in *Anti-Inflammatory* and *Joint Healing Formulas*

Warnings: Excessive consumption may cause diarrhea, nausea, upset stomach and vomiting. Use only under professional supervision during pregnancy.

Energetics: Cooling and moistening

Properties: Alterative (blood purifier), analgesic (anodyne), anti-inflammatory and antiseptic

Available from: Eclectic Institute, Herb Pharm, Nature's Answer, Nature's Way, NOW Foods and Solaray

Nutrients Section

A Guide to 60 Commonly Used Nutritional Supplements

Although this book is primarily a book about herbs, we felt that it would be more useful to readers if we also included a section on some of the major nutritional supplements available in health food stores. We've included a description of each nutrient and appropriate dosages and linked them to the conditions for which they may be helpful.

5-HTP

5-Hydroxytryptophan is the intermediate metabolite of the amino acid l-tryptophan and a direct precursor to the neurotransmitter serotonin. While a tryptophan deficiency isn't common, stress, insulin resistance, vitamin B6 deficiency, and a magnesium deficiency all inhibit the body's ability to convert tryptophan to 5-HTP and then serotonin. Numerous studies have shown 5-HTP to be as or more effective than many prescription antidepressants. Studies have also shown 5-HTP to be an effective remedy for chronic headaches, insomnia, fibromyalgia and even obesity by cutting down on carbohydrate cravings. While no reports have been published, 5-HTP could cause serotonin syndrome and should not be taken with an SSRI unless under the supervision of a health professional.

Dosage: For depression, headaches, fibromyalgia and obesity start with 50 mg, three times a day with meals and increase to 100-200 mg., three times a day for 2 weeks if necessary. For insomnia take 100-300 mg. before bedtime.

Alpha Lipoic Acid

Alpha Lipoic Acid is a vitamin-like enzyme cofactor or a coenzyme. It is chemically similar to a vitamin, and like vitamin C and E is part of the body's first line of defense against free radicals damage. Alpha-lipoic acid is both water and fat-soluble and is capable of extending the life of other antioxidants in the body like vitamin E, vitamin C and glutathione, while at the same time directly preventing oxidative damage. While ALA is naturally made by the body, we still need to get most of it from our diet or supplements, especially as we age or during disease processes.

Alpha Lipoic Acid is hepatoprotective and is currently being studied in the treatment of liver cirrhosis and fat-

ty liver. It also aids liver detoxification and helps remove toxins like heavy metals, organophosphates, latex and pesticides from the body. In addition ALA is an effective treatment for peripheral neuropathy associated with insulin resistance and while research isn't conclusive might actually help insulin resistance as well. ALA crosses both cell membranes and the blood-brain barrier, protecting the entire body from oxidative damage.

Dosage: 600-1800 mg daily with meals. R-lipoic Acid, the active component of ALA, 200-400 mg daily.

Betaine Hydrochloric Acid (HCl)

Betaine HCL (normally found with pepsin in supplements) is a supplement that adds hydrochloric acid (HCl) to the stomach. HCl assists protein digestion, kills orally ingested pathogens, prevents bacterial and fungal overgrowths in the small intestines and is essential for bile and pancreatic enzyme release. HCl is required for the absorption of folic acid, ascorbic acid, beta-carotene, iron, calcium, magnesium, and zinc. Many studies have shown that HCL production declines with age, and impaired HCl production and secretion is seen in a variety of conditions. It may also be helpful in gallbladder disease, gastric polyps and Sjogren's disease.

Dosage: 200-1200 mg before every meal. Start with small doses and increase until symptoms abate or a burning sensation is felt in the stomach. If you feel stomach burning when you take HCl lower your dose. Do not take HCl if you have ulcers or a history of ulcers.

Bioflavonoids

Bioflavonoids are a class of plant secondary metabolites known for their antioxidant activity. Until the 1950's flavonoids were referred to as Vitamin P, probably due to their beneficial effect on the permeability of vascular capillaries.

Bioflavonoids are found in the rind of green citrus fruits and in rose hips and black currants. They have been used in alternative medicine as an aid to enhance the action of vitamin C, to support blood circulation, treat allergies, viruses, arthritis and other inflammatory conditions, and as an antioxidant.

Dosage: Bioflavonoids are often added to vitamin C and multivitamin formulas. Follow manufacturer's recommendations.

Bromelain

Bromelain is a proteolytic (protein-digesting) enzyme from the pineapple plant. It reduces inflammation by inhibiting the formation of bradykinin and COX2 enzymes. It also inhibits platelet aggregation, preventing blood clot formation. Bromelain has been studied extensively and has been shown to be an effective treatment for musculoskeletal injuries as well as speeding post-operative recovery. It is also useful for people with rheumatoid arthritis, osteoarthritis, prostatitis, sinusitis, cancer, inflammatory bowel disease and helps potentiate some antibiotics, increasing their effectiveness.

Dosage: 300 mg taken four times a day with food or on an empty stomach. Don't take bromelain if you are allergic to pineapples or bees. If you are prone to heart palpitations, limit dosage to 400 mg daily.

Calcium

Calcium is the most abundant mineral in the body and is important for healthy bones and teeth, muscular contractions, nerve function, and many other body processes. Calcium intake in Paleolithic people and among healthy populations in the world today averages between 1500 and 2500 mg daily. Compare that to the average American female's intake of around 500 mg daily.

Calcium cannot be properly utilized unless you have adequate stomach acid. Even if you have good digestion, your body still cannot process more than about 400 mg at a time. Calcium also requires magnesium, boron, vitamin D, vitamin K2 and trace minerals for proper utilization. Women with PMS, leg cramps associated with pregnancy, pre-eclampsia, and people with low bone density should supplement with calcium or increase dietary intake.

Dosage: 400-800 mg daily. Always take calcium with equal amounts of magnesium, and preferably with other trace minerals.

Charcoal (Activated)

Charcoal absorbs a variety of irritants in the digestive tract when taken internally. It is useful for diarrhea, intestinal gas, indigestion and poisoning. It can also be applied topically.

Dosage: For poisoning, hospitals normally administer between 50-100 g, but smaller doses like 1000 mg taken at the first sign of intestinal distress work well. Repeat after two hours if needed, up to a maximum of 10 capsules per day. For severe diarrhea, combine with psyllium seed capsules or bulk slippery elm. For treating poisoning, contact the Poison Control Center and follow their recommendations. First-aid application may require 30 to 200 capsules, depending on quantity and toxicity of the material ingested. and Charcoal can also be applied as a poultice to spider bites. It is even effective with brown recluse bites. Change poultice the every hour for maximum benefit.

Chlorophyll

Chlorophyll is the molecule that makes leaves green and captures the sun's energy during photosynthesis. Chlorophyll has an affinity for human blood, where it prevents the clumping of red blood cells and increases the oxygen-carrying capacity of the blood. It can help to detoxify the blood and accelerate wound healing by increasing oxygen uptake. It is also used for reducing colostomy odor, bad breath, and constipation. Chlorophyll also seems to nutritionally build the blood when taken regularly. Intravenously, chlorophyll is used for treating chronic relapsing pancreatitis.

Natural chlorophyll from green leafy vegetables is a good source of magnesium, a mineral many people are deficient in. Natural chlorophyll is sometimes sold in gel capsules and has a beneficial action on the bowel. Liquid chlorophyll is sodium copper chlorophyllin, which means that the magnesium at the center of the chlorophyll molecule has been displaced by copper and sodium. Copper and zinc are antagonists, so people with high levels of copper and low levels of zinc should not use liquid chlorophyll.

Chlorophyll contains components that are activated by light and can cause mild photosensitization when taken internally. Certain carotenoids such as beta-carotene and canthaxanthin seem to prevent or lessen the photosensitivity that results from taking chlorophyll.

Dosage: Add a small amount of liquid chlorophyll to water and drink, or follow the manufacturer's recommendations.

Chondroitin

Chondroitin is a long chain of repeating sugars found naturally in the joints and connective tissues of healthy people and animals. Chondroitin is available from animal sources such as the gristle near the joints, but is not often consumed. This sulfate is important to healthy joints and when taken as a supplement, studies show that it may treat the inflammation and pain of osteoarthritis. Chondroitin helps produce both new cartilage and enhances synovial fluid viscosity. It interferes with enzymes that destroy cartilage molecules as well as those that prevent nutrients from reaching the cartilage. These actions are especially important to those with osteoarthritis who are often suffering because their cartilage is unable to rebuild or protect itself.

Chondroitin is also beneficial to those with psoriasis and inflammatory bowel disorders. It is found naturally in bone broths, a staple of many cultures and a super food in its own right. The improvements in joint function from chondroitin are not permanent, so continued supplementation is warranted for those who see results.

Dosage: 1200-2000 mg taken once daily.

Chromium

Chromium is a trace mineral that helps to improve sensitivity to insulin. Adequate intake is essential for maintenance of normal blood sugar levels. Not only does it help with type 2 diabetes, it also helps type 1 diabetics improve the action of insulin. It is indicated for people with pre-diabetes and women with Poly Cystic Ovarian Syndrome (PCOS). A couple of small studies have shown that chromium is helpful for people with hypoglycemia. While marketed for weight loss and enhancing lean muscle, studies are conflicting at best for these uses.

Dosage: 500-1000 mcg daily

Co-Q10

Co-Q10 stands for Co-enzyme Q10. Like any other enzyme, it is a catalyst, which in this case, is used by the body primarily for energy production at the cellular level. Co-Q10 assists the mitochondria, our sub-cellular power plants, in producing energy by facilitating the production of ATP, the basic energy molecule in the cell. By helping our cells to produce energy, Co-Q10 also helps them to live longer, be healthier and to reproduce properly.

Most of the research on Co-Q10 has focused on the heart, because of how hard the heart works and its high energy requirements. Co-Q10 has been found to strengthen the heart in people who have suffered heart disease and to

protect it from further damage. Other studies have documented its ability to raise or lower blood pressure.

Co-Q10 also has important antioxidant functions. Unfortunately, although Co-Q10 is found in many foods, the levels in our bodies decline with age. With supplementation we can ensure that our cells, and especially our hearts, stay strong and are protected from free radical damage.

Statin drugs deplete Co-Q10, so this supplement should always be taken by people using statin drugs to lower cholesterol. In addition to statins, the beta blockers propranolol and metoprolol along with phenothiazines and tricyclic antidepressants lower Co-Q10 levels. Anyone taking red yeast rice should also take Co-Q10.

Besides helping the heart and circulation, Co-Q10 can help heal bleeding gums, potentially reduce the side effects of chemotherapy and reduce allergic reactions. Co-Q10 may also be of benefit in Huntington's disease, migraine headaches, HIV/AIDS, and Parkinson's disease. In a well-designed study conducted in 2003, Co-Q10 supplementation reduced the need for dialysis and significantly improved creatine clearance and kidney function in those with renal failure.

Dosage: 60-300 mg daily.

Colloidal Minerals

Cultures around the world, independent of each other, have used minerals for healing since ancient times. In Ayurveda, Shilajit, a fossilized vegetable-based mineral compound is considered a nectar of the gods, given to man to live youthful forever. In TCM a variety of minerals are used, including gypsum, magnetite, and about 45 other mineral compounds.

In the U.S. the entire modern liquid trace minerals industry started many years ago when a rancher in southern Utah, suffering from various health problems, was told by a Native American ranch hand about a spring on his property. This spring was considered sacred by the Native Americans who used the water for healing purposes. The rancher found the spring, started bottling the water and drinking it. His health problems cleared up.

He then started selling the bottled water to friends and family members. They also reported positive benefits from drinking the water.

This naturally made him curious, so he got a geologist to examine the spring. The geologist reported that the water from the spring flowed over the remains of an ancient sea bed. Within the clay from this ancient ocean were the remains of microscopic plants and animals containing a rich supply of minerals. The water was dissolving these minerals. This is not unusual. All over the world, mineral springs and mineral waters have been reported to have wondrous healing properties. Many health retreats have been built around such springs. Furthermore, very healthy and long-lived peoples, like the Hunzas, have consumed water from glacial runoffs rich in trace elements.

Minerals play critical roles in every part of our body, but they are especially needed for healthy bones, teeth and other structural systems of the body. Minerals are also catalysts for all biochemical processes and enzyme systems. Colloidal minerals are used to increase energy, reduce arthritis symptoms, turning gray hair dark again, improve general well-being and reduce aches and pains.

Dosage: 1-2 tablespoons daily in water.

Colloidal Silver

An alternative to antibiotics that has been around for a long time is colloidal silver. It has long been known that silver has an antimicrobial action. Pioneers, for example, learned that they could keep water from going bad by putting a few silver coins in the bottom of the water barrel. Nobility in ancient Europe were less prone to infection than the general population because they ate and drank using silverware. Royalty became known as "blue-blood" due to the fact that ingestion of high amounts of silver causes argyria, a condition characterized by a blue/gray discoloration of the skin and inflammation of the inner eyelids. A solution of just 100 parts per million (ppm) of ionic silver taken daily is enough to cause argyria.

Fortunately there are some new forms of colloidal silver that don't have this toxicity and work at lower potencies. Still, colloidal silver only works as an antimicrobial when it comes in contact with pathogens. Therefore, it is most effective when applied topically or used to treat gastrointestinal infections. In high doses, it can help resolve antibiotic-resistant infections.

Dosage: Colloidal silver can be used as a mouthwash, nasal spray or applied topically to injuries as directed on the bottle by the manufacturer. For internal use, follow the manufacturer's recommendations. Only use colloidal silver to fight an active infection. Do not take daily.

Copper

Copper is an essential mineral required for hemoglobin production, the absorption and use of iron, energy metabolism, the development and repair of bone and connective tissue, the formation of myelin sheath, adrenal hormone production, thyroid hormone production, immunity, and the pigmentation of hair and skin. The lack of accuracy in determining a copper deficiency with a single blood test combined with the potential toxicity of copper supplementation has resulted in many people not being properly treated for this deficiency.

A deficiency of copper causes fatigue, anemia, low level of neutrophils and leukocytes, the impairment of nerve and muscle function, under activity of adrenal and thyroid gland function, reproductive difficulties, premature graying of the hair, brittle bones, premature aging of the skin and varicose veins. Copper is found in liver, oysters, nuts, seeds, whole grain and cocoa. Deficiency can occur with poor diet and malabsorption.

Dosage: Consumption of copper rich foods is best. For supplementation please consult a qualified practitioner. Normal supplementation is with 1-5 mg daily if, and only if, you have signs of a copper deficiency. Toxicity if the form of liver damage, renal failure and death has occurred with doses higher than 10 mg daily.

DHA

DHA is an essential fatty acid, and the most abundant fatty acid in the brain. It is part of the Omega-3 family of fatty acids and is found in cold water fish in combination with EPA. New research indicates that the DHA in cold water fish and Omega-3 supplements is what gives them their potent anti-inflammatory action. The EPA found in fish and supplements can be converted to DHA in the body.

DHA is essential for myelin sheath repair and the development, growth and maintenance of the brain. It may be helpful for brain function, memory, visual function, healthy cholesterol levels, neurological conditions, type 2 diabetes, coronary artery disease (CAD), dementia, attention deficit-hyperactivity disorder (ADHD), preventing and treating depression, and reducing aggressive behavior associated with stress. In combination with EPA, DHA is a systemic anti-inflammatory and is also beneficial for the prevention and reversal of many diseases.

Dosage: The best source is wild caught cold water fish, including tuna, mackerel, salmon, sardines and anchovies. Many fish oil products are of poor quality and don't include guaranteed levels of DHA and EPA. If you choose to supplement with fish oils, take a combined EPA/DHA total of 2,000 mg daily.

DHEA

The adrenal glands produce numerous hormones, but the most abundant hormone they produce is DHEA (dehydroepiandrosterone). Small amounts of DHEA are also made in the testes and ovaries. DHEA is a building block for other hormones, including androgens (male hormones such as testosterone) and estrogens. DHEA levels tend to drop as we age, leading to ideas that enhancing DHEA levels may help counteract aging. While hard evidence is lacking for this claim, DHEA has been shown to be helpful as a supplement in certain conditions.

DHEA has been shown to improve immune function and general well-being in those with low DHEA levels. Low levels are also associated with increased instances of cancer, autoimmune disease, type 2 diabetes, heart disease, osteoporosis, cognitive decline and kidney disease. We should remember though that correlation isn't causation.

Taking a hormone like DHEA as a supplement should be done carefully. When you supplement with a hormone, you tend to lower the body's own production of that hormone. Small doses are best because hormones are very potent substances and getting too much of a particular hormone can be just as bad as getting too little. For this reason, it may be a good idea to have hormone levels tested before taking DHEA supplements.

Excessive levels of DHEA can cause acne and hormonal imbalances like those found in teenagers. It's best to get your hormones tested to determine if you actually need DHEA before taking it for any length of time. DHEA should not be taken by children, teenagers, pregnant women or nursing mothers. It should be avoided by people with reproductive cancers, such as prostate or uterine cancer. High levels of DHEA have been reported to cause symptoms of hypothyroidism, heart palpitations and arrhythmia.

Dosage: 5-15 mg daily for women,
10-30 mg daily for men.

Digestive Enzymes

Digestive enzymes are available as nutritional supplements and by prescription for people whose pancreas cannot make or does not release enough digestive enzymes into the gut to digest their food. Digestive enzymes are useful for indigestion, bloating after meals, gas, malabsorption and for people with pancreatitis, cystic fibrosis and cancer. Digestive enzymes normally contain hydrochloric acid, pancreatic enzymes and bile for aiding in the digestion of fats, proteins and carbohydrates.

Dosage: Take 1-2 capsules during or after meals as an aid to digestion. Continued use may decrease the ability of the body to create digestive secretions on its own. Do not take if you have ulcers. Digestive enzymes may cause gastric irritation in some people.

Fiber

Fiber in your diet is essential for a number of reasons. A diet low in fiber can cause constipation, abnormal blood sugar levels, diverticular disease and excess body weight. Diets high in fiber generally curb one's appetite, prevent overeating, promote regularity and improve cholesterol and blood sugar levels. Fiber is found in many kinds of food and comes in various forms. Obtaining fiber from a variety of food sources is best, and you should get between 25-35 grams every day. Most Americans get only about half the recommended amount of fiber in their diets.

Known for its role in digestion, dietary fiber is associated with a number of other health benefits. It is necessary for gastric motility and regular bowel movements. Fiber helps lower cholesterol and may be helpful in preventing and managing type 2 diabetes by slowing the absorption of sugar. High fiber diets also appear to reduce the risk of colon cancer. Fiber can also be used to absorb diarrhea-causing irritants and to soften the stool to help hemorrhoids and anal fistula to heal.

Choosing whole grains, fruits, vegetables, nuts and legumes while limiting refined, processed foods will help you achieve your fiber goals. If you are making a change from a low-fiber diet to a high-fiber diet, it is recommended that you introduce the high-fiber foods into your diet gradually and drink plenty of water. This will help your body adjust to the change and prevent unpleasant gastric side effects.

Dosage: 1/4-2 teaspoons of a fiber supplement in water or juice or follow the manufacturer's recommendations. Best taken first thing in the morning about 30 minutes before breakfast. Fiber may not be tolerated well if you have Small Intestinal Bacterial Overgrowth (SIBO) or Inflammatory Bowel Disorders. See Gut Healing Diet in the Therapies Section.

Nutrients

Folate (Folic Acid, Vitamin B9)

Folic acid is a water soluble member of the B-Vitamin family, Vitamin B9. Folic acid technically refers to the synthetic compound used in dietary supplements and food fortification. Folate is the correct term for the naturally occurring tetrahydrofolate derivatives found in food. Folic acid must undergo reduction and methylation in the liver utilizing the enzyme dihydrofolate reductase, unlike natural folates that are metabolized in the small intestines. The reduced activity of dihydrofolate reductase in the liver, combined with ingesting high levels of folic acid in fortified foods may result in high levels of synthetic folic acid in the body. Epidemiological studies have linked elevated levels of synthetic folic acid in the body to an increase in all forms of cancer. If you supplement with folic acid, by itself or in a multi, we suggest only taking products that contain 5-MTHF or folate, not folic acid.

Folate prevents and treats folate deficient megaloblastic anemia, helps prevent neural tube defects, reduces miscarriages and reduces the risk of colorectal and cervical cancer. Folate also reduces homocysteine levels, decreasing cardiovascular risk, and improves age related cognitive decline.

Dosage: Folate is readily available in green leafy vegetables and organ meats, particularly liver. Unless folate levels are low (easily checked with blood work), most people don't need to supplement. Women trying to become pregnant, and pregnant women should supplement with 800-1000 mcg of 5-MTHF daily. Dosage to reduce homocysteine levels range from 2-5 mg daily. Women with cervical dysplasia should supplement with 10,000 mcg (10 mg) daily of 5-MTHF. Supplementing with folate might mask an underlying B12 deficiency. It is advisable to supplement with B12 and folate together.

GABA

GABA (Gamma-Amino Butyric Acid) is an amino acid that acts as a major calming neurotransmitter in the brain. It is an inhibitory neurotransmitter, which means it inhibits overactivity of nerve cells in the brain. GABA plays a critical role in normalizing the nervous system. Proper levels of this amino acid in the brain contribute to motor control and vision and calm the mind, reducing anxiety, fear, hyperactivity and stress-related sleep disorders. Many people with anxiety, insomnia, epilepsy, and other brain disorders do not manufacture sufficient levels of GABA.

Research has shown that GABA increases the production of alpha brain waves (a state often achieved by meditation, characterized by being relaxed with greater mental focus and mental alertness) and reduces beta waves (associated with nervousness, scattered thoughts and hyperactivity). GABA also increases mental clarity, while reducing the effects of stress. Valium, Xanax and other benzodiazepene drugs mimic or bind to GABA receptors and have a calming effect, but are addicting, while GABA is not.

Dosage: 50-200 mg, three times a day.

Glucosamine

Glucosamine is an amino acid/sugar substance used by the body to produce connective tissues. It is derived from crab shells. Research done on glucosamine showed that glucosamine sulfate brings relief from joint tenderness, swelling and pain. In tests, people who took at least one gram a day of glucosamine salts, condroitin sulfates, or glucosamine sulfate found a dramatic relief from the pain of osteoarthritis. Not only did they have less pain, but the studies showed that the connective tissues gained the ability of self-healing.

When the patients stopped taking these herbs, the relief lasted for six to twelve weeks. In several clinical trials where glucosamine sulfate was compared to NSAIDs, long-term reductions in pain were greater in patients receiving glucosamine sulfate. Glucosamine is beneficial for osteoarthritis, rheumatoid arthritis, TMJ, joint pain and back pain.

Dosage: 500-1000 mg, three times daily. Don't take glucosamine if you have an allergy to shellfish.

Indole-3 Carbinol (DIM)

Indole-3 carbinol is a constituent of cruciferous vegetables of the Brassica genus including broccoli, cabbage and Brussels sprouts. In fact one head of cabbage contains approximately 1200 mg of Indole-3-carbinol. Researchers think that Indole-3 carbinol is one of several compounds responsible for the reduced risk of cancer in people that have diets high in fruits and vegetables.

Indole-3 carbinol helps with both phase 1 and phase 2 detoxification in the liver. It helps to break down excess estrogen compounds, including xenoestrogens, which may contribute to breast, prostate and uterine cancers. This also makes it useful for PMS symptoms brought on by estrogen dominance. Indole-3 carbinol is also beneficial for BPH, fibromyalgia, cervical dysplasia and lupus.

Dosage: 200-400 mg daily.

Iodine

Iodine is an essential trace mineral in humans and is necessary for the production of thyroid hormones. It is also important for breast, uterus and prostate health as well as adrenal and immune function. Dietary sources of iodine include iodized salt, eggs, seaweed and seafood, cow's milk and navy beans. The U.S. recommended daily intake (RDI) for dietary iodine is 150 mcg for adults, 220 mcg for pregnancy, and 270 mcg during lactation. The safe upper limit has been set at 1,000 mcg (1 mg) daily. People in Japan typically consume 7,000-14,000 mcg daily with some areas consuming as much as 50,000 mcg daily.

Iodine supplementation is greatly promoted in the natural world. However studies clearly show that cultures with high iodine intake have a greater risk of autoimmune thyroid disease. While the research isn't definitive, this could be explained by a concomitant deficiency of selenium. The widespread contamination of food and water supplies with the toxin perchlorate, as well as the ingestion of compounds that displace iodine like chlorine and fluoride may very well warrant supplementation with iodine. Supplementation with iodine should only be undertaken with adequate selenium status and only if autoimmune thyroid disease isn't present.

Iodine supplementation is normally in the form of potassium iodide and iodine combined. Iodine is beneficial for goiters, fibrocystic breast disease, uterine fibroids, cardiovascular disease and preventing and treating breast, uterine, cervical and prostate cancer.

Dosage: 200-5,000 mcg daily in those without autoimmune thyroid disease or selenium deficiency. Iodine should only be used under the guidance of a practitioner in higher supplemental doses and for those with thyroid disease.

Iron

Iron is an essential trace mineral, vital for the production of red blood cells and the synthesis of neurotransmitters including dopamine, norepinephrine and serotonin. The absorption of iron from food depends not only on the source of iron, but also the digestive health of the person. Red meat, poultry, and fish provide iron in heme (40%) and non-heme (60%) forms. Non-heme iron is absorbed at 2%-20% and heme iron is absorbed at a rate of about 23%. Plants only contain non-heme iron.

Iron is used to prevent and treat iron deficiency. Symptoms of an iron deficiency if mild, might go unnoticed. As the deficiency leads to anemia symptoms include extreme fatigue, headache, cold hands and feet, pale skin and gums, brittle nails, fast heartbeat, dizziness, shortness of breath, poor appetite and cravings for non-nutritive things like ice and dirt. Iron deficiency is easily and cheaply diagnosed with blood work. Too much iron can cause organ damage and death. Please get your iron levels tested before supplementation. Iron deficiency is common in ADHD, restless leg syndrome, Crohn's disease, depression, and in women with heavy menstrual cycles.

Dosage: 10-50 mg daily with confirmed iron deficiency. Supplemental heme based iron is now commercially available.

L-Arginine

L-arginine is a semi-essential amino acid. It can be made in the body from the amino acids glutamine, glutamate and proline, however rate of arginine production in the body does not compensate for depletion or inadequate supply. L-arginine is essential in protein production, wound healing, fertility and the production of the chemical messenger nitric oxide, which dilates blood vessels. This enlarging of the blood vessels takes stress off the heart, allows blood to flow more easily through the body and reduces blood pressure. This has several positive benefits for cardiovascular health.

For starters, supplementation with L-arginine has proven beneficial in helping angina. Several studies have shown that oral supplementation with L-arginine decreases angina symptoms and improves tolerance to exercise. It also appears to help in cases of congestive heart failure when used as part of a comprehensive treatment plan. Because of its influence on nitric oxide, L-arginine supplements can be helpful in temporarily reducing high blood pressure, particularly in Type 2 diabetics. It may also improve the effectiveness of angiotensin converting enzyme (ACE) inhibitors used in treating hypertension. It has also been helpful in peripheral arterial disease and improves tolerance to transdermal nitrate medications.

The drug sildenafil citrate (Viagra®) affects nitric oxide by blocking an enzyme that breaks down nitric oxide. It was originally developed as a medication for high blood pressure, but was found to be more helpful in erectile dysfunction. Erections are dependent on good blood flow and the ability of the arteries in the penis to dilate. L-arginine supplements, which help the body make more nitric oxide, have also proven beneficial in erectile dysfunction. A study of 50 men with erectile dysfunction showed that the group taking 5 grams of L-arginine per day had improvement over those on the placebo. L-arginine must be taken daily to have this affect.

By increasing blood flow to the brain, L-arginine can help vasoconstrictive migraines. These are migraines where the head feels like it is being squeezed in a vise or by a belt. Other possible benefits of L-arginine include: improving recovery time after surgery, preventing wasting in AIDS patients, preventing pre-eclampsia, improving senile dementia and helping to recover from recurring interstitial cystitis.

Dosage: 3-15 g daily.

L-Carnitine

Carnitine is primarily derived from animal proteins, especially red meat. Although it is not an essential amino acid, supplementation with l-carnitine can have a number of beneficial actions on health. One of the most important functions of carnitine is that it moves fatty acids into the mitochondria of the cell so they can be converted to energy. Carnitine is helpful for the heart and has been shown to be deficient in the hearts of patients who have died from myocardial infarctions. L-Carnitine is used for cardiovascular problems such as angina, congestive heart failure, peripheral artery disease and recovery from heart attack. L-Carnitine is also beneficial for weight control, lack of energy, chronic fatigue syndrome, ADHD and Reye's Syndrome.

Dosage: Follow the manufacturer's recommendations.

L-Glutamine

Glutamine is not an essential amino acid, but it plays a critical role in many of the body's functions nonetheless. It is converted into glutamic acid and, with the help of Vitamin B6, gamma aminobutryic acid (GABA)—two critical neurotransmitters in the brain. Glutamic acid is involved in mental activity and learning, and GABA is a calming neurotransmitter that helps prevent epilepsy, tics, schizophrenia and "mind chatter." Glutamine improves glucose supply to the brain and has been found to help reduce cravings for sugar and alcohol. L-Glutamine helps repair the intestinal tract in leaky gut syndrome and other inflammatory bowel disorders. L-Glutamine is one of the amino acids needed to make the antioxidant glutathione, which helps the body detoxify heavy metals and recycle other antioxidants. L-Glutamine supplementation may also be helpful for colitis, depression, irritability, Crohn's disease, chemotherapy induced diarrhea, ADHD, and ulcers of the stomach.

Dosage: 1-5 g taken three times daily. L-Glutamine is found naturally in meat and bone broth and contributes greatly to its gut healing properties.

L-Lysine

Lysine is an essential amino acid found in meats and dairy but is deficient in most grains. Insufficient intake causes poor appetite, weight loss and anemia. Lysine helps the immune system manufacture antibodies and has been used for viral infections such as mononucleosis, herpes and shingles. It also helps ensure adequate absorption of calcium and the formation of collagen for bone, cartilage and connective tissue. It is necessary for all amino acid assimilation and assists in the storage of fats.

Dosage: 500-3,000 mg daily.

Lactase Enzymes

Lactase is used for preventing symptoms of lactose intolerance, symptoms of which include cramps, diarrhea and gas. Lactase is a sugar-splitting enzyme that hydrolyzes lactose, a milk sugar, to produce glucose and galactose.

Dosage: No adverse effects of lactase ingestion up to 9,900 IU have been observed. Follow the manufacturer's recommendations.

Lipase Enzymes

Lipase is an enzyme produced by the pancreas to help breakdown fats. Supplementing with lipase, normally in combination with protease and amylase, is useful for anyone who is having problems with poor fat metabolism such as indigestion after eating fats and people with Celiac disease, Crohn's disease, or gall bladder problems. It is very helpful after a person has had their gallbladder surgically removed to help the body break down fats more effectively.

Dosage: The activity of lipase varies product to product. Follow product recommendations.

Lutein

Lutein is a carotenoid that helps protect the macula lutea from oxidative damage. It may also help to improve vision, prevent age-related macular degeneration, cataracts and also has a protective effect against breast cancer. Foods like broccoli, spinach, and kale are the best sources of lutein.

Dosage: 20-40 mg daily.

Nutrients

Lycopene

Lycopene is a bright red carotenoid found in fruits and vegetables like tomatoes, red bell peppers and watermelon. Preliminary research on lycopene has shown an inverse correlation between the consumption of lycopene rich foods and cancer risk. While lycopene is a carotenoid, it isn't converted to Vitamin A, but acts as a strong antioxidant instead. Its strong antioxidant properties are what is theorized to reduce cancer risk as well as to help prevent cardiovascular disease by inhibiting the oxidation of low density lipoproteins.

Lycopene supplements have been shown to increase blood levels of lycopene in the same manner as food lycopene consumption. Cooked tomato products like tomato paste are the best food source of lycopene.

Dosage: 30 mg daily.

Magnesium

A study published in the Journal of the American College of Nutrition and sponsored by the National Institutes of Health found that 68% of Americans are magnesium deficient and many experts consider that number optimistic. Magnesium is used in over 300 enzymatic reactions in the body. It acts as a catalyst in the utilization of carbohydrates, fats, protein, calcium, phosphorus and possibly potassium. This vital mineral helps produce energy inside cells.

Magnesium works hand in hand with calcium in the body. Calcium ions make muscles contract, while magnesium ions help muscles relax. So magnesium helps relieve muscle cramping and spasms, relieves colic and spastic bowel conditions and helps prevent heart attacks. Spastic muscles, nervous twitching, spastic colon, hypersensitivity to noises and calcium deposits are all symptoms of magnesium deficiency, which is far more common than calcium deficiency. In fact, over consumption of calcium as a supplement actually contributes to the development of magnesium deficiency. A magnesium deficiency interferes with Vitamin D utilization as well as contributes to hypertension, cardiac arrhythmias, asthma, insulin resistance, osteoporosis, headaches, chemical sensitivity, PMS and fibromyalgia. Alcohol, diuretics, birth control pills, antibiotics, steroids, acid reflux medication, and fluoride deplete the body's supply of magnesium. We recommend across the board supplementation of magnesium.

Dosage: 100-1000 mg daily in divided doses. Of the commercially available magnesium supplements, magnesium glycinate offers the best absorption. For a gentle and well absorbed magnesium supplement you can take 1 tablespoon of milk of magnesia and dissolve it into 4.5 tablespoons of 5% apple cider or white vinegar. One tablespoon of this mixture added to a quart of water and sipped throughout the day is a great way to increase your magnesium levels. Relatively new to the market is magnesium chloride oil. Applied topically the concentrated magnesium penetrates the skin, relaxing tense muscles. It is not known how well topical magnesium chloride works in restoring intracellular magnesium levels.

Melatonin

Melatonin is a hormone that is primarily produced in the pineal gland, with production also occurring in the gastrointestinal tract, retina, bone marrow and bile. In the body tryptophan and B6 are metabolized into serotonin, which under the influence of darkness is converted to melatonin. In addition to regulating sleep, melatonin is a potent scavenger of free radicals. Melatonin has an up regulating effect on part of the immune system, making supplemental melatonin a beneficial part of cancer treatment programs.

As a supplement, melatonin is primarily used to establish normal circadian rhythms in people who do shift work, or are suffering from jet lag or temporary insomnia. Melatonin also seems to directly interact with GABA receptors, inducing relaxation and combating anxiety in people with low natural production. Because melatonin is a naturally occurring hormone, long-term supplementation may alter the body's ability to produce sufficient amounts of it on its own. Melatonin is not recommended for use by children, adolescents, pregnant or lactating women.

Dosage: 1-9 mg, 1 hour before bed. For cancer treatment, 10-50 mg nightly.

MSM

MethylSulfonylMethane (MSM) is an organic sulfur compound found in vegetables, fruit, meat and dairy products. It is a crystalline derivative of DMSO, the first naturally derived NSAID discovered after Aspirin. MSM is one of hundreds of naturally occurring sulfur compounds in foods.

Sulfur is crucial in the process of maintaining a vital healthy body and mind. It is part of the cellular structure and necessary for effecting repairs in the body. It promotes the health of hair, skin, nails, joints and the immune system. In addition to providing sulfur compounds, MSM is a potent systemic anti-inflammatory. It is helpful in many inflammatory disorders including interstitial cystitis, scleroderma, fibromyalgia, lupus, repetitive stress injuries, and osteoarthritis.

Dosage: 1-3 g two times daily. To promote collagen production, take with vitamin C.

N-Acetyl Cysteine

N-Acetyl-Cysteine (NAC) is a stabilized form of cysteine, a sulfur-containing amino acid found in high protein foods. NAC is produced naturally in the body and is also obtained from the diet. It is a precursor to glutathione, which is the body's most important cellular antioxidant and detoxifier. Supplementing with NAC boosts glutathione levels in the liver, in plasma and in the bronchioles of the lungs.

Glutathione acts as a powerful antioxidant in cells that detoxifies chemicals into less harmful compounds. Glutathione is known to aid in the transport of nutrients to cell membranes and to lymphocytes and phagocytes, two major classes of white blood cells produced by the immune system. Taking Vitamin B6, Folate and B12, along with NAC helps recycle glutathione in the body so that it can continue acting as an antioxidant.

NAC is commonly prescribed for those suffering from bronchitis, emphysema, pneumonia, tuberculosis and smoker's cough. It is a natural expectorant that helps thin mucus and loosen phlegm and bronchial secretions in the lungs. Double blind research has found that dosages of 1,200 mg. per day prevents influenza infection and reduces symptoms and the duration of existing influenza infections. It is being studied in the treatment of cystic fibrosis.

NAC also detoxifies and removes heavy metals like lead, mercury and arsenic from the body. It is recommended to supplement zinc and other trace minerals as NAC increases the excretion of zinc and other essential minerals when taken over an extended period. NAC has been used in hospitals for treating patients with acetaminophen toxicity (found in Tylenol) and for treating other causes of liver failure and septic shock. It is often recommended as a liver support for those taking chemotherapy drugs and those suffering from alcohol poisoning.

Dosage: 600-1200 mg, three times daily.

Omega-3 Essential Fatty Acids

American diets typically contain a 20-30:1 ratio of Omega-6 to Omega-3 essential fatty acid (EFA). This leads to the production of inflammatory prostaglandins, oxidative damage, and significantly raises the risk of heart disease. The consumption of Omega-3 fatty acids helps to reduce inflammation and the risk of cardiovascular disease. It also helps lower triglycerides and reduces insulin resistance in cells.

Both EPA and DHA (the active Omega-3 EFA's) are deemed conditionally essential as the body can synthesize them from ALA, found in plant based Omega-3 containing foods. However, consuming foods like flax, walnut and soy, that are high in ALA (plant omega 3's) does not lead to significant increases in tissue DHA.

Omega-3 EFA's from fish inhibit platelet aggregation lower serum triglyceride levels, suppress cell proliferation, induce apoptosis of cancerous cells, and suppress both breast and colon cancer tumor growth and metastasis. The Omega-3 fatty acids EPA and DHA are used in the treatment of rheumatoid arthritis, acute respiratory distress syndrome, multiple sclerosis, dysmenorrhea, hypertension, lupus, diabetes, ulcerative colitis, Crohn's disease, chronic obstructive pulmonary disease (COPD), migraine headaches, depression, and inflammatory skin conditions such as psoriasis and eczema.

Studies show that it's the ratio of Omega-6 to Omega-3 in the body that matters. Supplementing with EPA/DHA rich fish oils, without reducing the consumption of Omega-6 is like trying to put out a forest fire with a water pistol. To improve your ratio of Omega-6 to Omega-3, eliminate your consumption of industrial nut and seeds oils including: soybean, canola, cottonseed, corn, peanut, safflower, and sunflower oil, while at the same time increasing Omega-3.

Dosage: Your best source of EPA/DHA fatty acids is to eat one pound a week of fatty, cold water fish like sardines, tuna and wild salmon. These can be canned in water, fresh or frozen. If you're not a fish fan, supplement with around 2,000 mg daily of combined EPA/DHA. Many of the cheap fish oil products don't list the potency of EPA and DHA and are ineffective. Cod liver oil is an effective way to get EPA/DHA, while also getting the essential fat soluble nutrients Vitamin A and D.

Pantothenic Acid (Vitamin B5)

Pantothenic acid (Vitamin B5) is essential for the production of Coenzyme A, an enzyme responsible for cellular energy production and liver detoxification. Dietary pantothenic acid is found in a wide variety of foods including meats, vegetables and fruits, making a deficiency rare. However supplemental pantothenic acid has been shown to help with stress, adrenal fatigue, acne, arthritis, chronic fatigue and Parkinson's

Dosage: 50-100 mg daily.

Potassium

Potassium ions are necessary for the function of all living cells. Potassium ion diffusion is a key mechanism in nerve transmission, and potassium deficiency results in various forms of cardiac malfunction.

Potassium is used in treating and preventing hypokalemia, hypertension, Menière's disease, thallium poisoning, hypercalciuria, insulin resistance, myocardial infarction, preventing stroke, relieving symptoms of menopause, and infant colic. Ensuring adequate levels is important in a wide variety of conditions as shown below.

Potassium plays a role in many body functions including acid-base balance, electrodynamic characteristics of the cell, isotonicity, and various enzymatic reactions. It is essential in physiological processes including nerve impulse transmission, cardiac, smooth and skeletal muscle contraction, gastric secretion, renal function, tissue synthesis, and carbohydrate synthesis.

Dosage: Potassium is believed to work with other nutrients to produce beneficial physiological effects. Potassium can be obtained from foods such as parsley, dried apricots, chocolate, nuts (especially almonds and pistachios), potatoes, bamboo shoots, bananas, avocados, soybeans, bran, meat, fish and dried milk. When dietary intake is insufficient, potassium can be obtained from oral supplements. Follow the manufacturer's recommendations.

Proanthocyanidins

Proanthocyanidins refer to a class of polyphenols that include oligomeric proanthocyanidins (OPCs). More complex polyphenols with the same polymeric building block are referred to as tannins. Polyphenols are a family of phytochemicals divided into the subclasses anthocyanidins, flavonols, flavanones and isoflavones. Each subclass contains phytochemicals with potent antioxidants. The flavonol group of antioxidants contain proanthocyanidins. Catechin, resveratrol, epicatechin, epigallocatechin, epicatechin gallate, epigallocatechin gallate, theaflavins and thearubigins are other examples in this group.

Proanthocyanidins appear to correlate positively with oxygen radical absorbence capacity (ORAC). Red wine has received considerable media attention because of its health-promoting flavonoids, yet it has a lower content than other sources.

Proanthocyanidins are also sold as dietary supplements to help protect the body from the damaging effects of free radicals. The health benefits of Proanthocyanidins go beyond their antioxidant properties. They are also anti-inflammatory, antiviral and anti-carcinogenic, while protecting the cardiovascular system. Proanthocyanidins also help wounds heal, reduce the pain from pancreatitis, reduce insulin resistance in diabetics and help protect from drug toxicity.

Proanthocyanidins can help lower your levels of LDL or bad cholesterol. Antioxidants also decrease the oxidation of LDL, which may lead to the build up of plaque on the walls of your arteries. Proanthocyanidins have also been used to improve night vision and slow down the degenerative effects of aging on skin collagen and elastin.

Dosage: Proanthocyanidins can be found in many plants, most notably apples, maritime pine bark, grapes, cinnamon, cocoa beans, acai berries, aronia fruit and red wines. Bilberry, cranberry, black currant, green tea, black tea and other plants also contain these flavonoids, with cocoa beans having the highest concentration. Eating these foods is the best way to get these nutrients. If using a supplement, follow the manufacturer's recommendations as to dose.

Probiotics

Acidophilus, bifidophilus and other species of Lactobacillus are friendly bacteria necessary for colon health. There are two main forms that beneficial probiotic organisms can be ingested, fermented foods and supplements. Fermented foods were consumed in a wide variety of forms in almost every traditional culture in the world. Traditional fermented foods include yogurt, kefir, kimchi, and sauerkraut, but many vegetables can be fermented. Yogurt was traditionally made from *L. delbrueckii* and *S. therrnophilus*, however we now know that these species don't survive the human GI tract so most manufacturers now add *Lactobacillus acidophilus and Bifidobacterium bifidum* to increase their effectiveness.

Probiotics aid in the digestion and assimilation of some nutrients, while protecting the body against yeast and harmful bacteria. They can protect against diarrhea when traveling or after taking antibiotics, and are also beneficial for constipation, lactose intolerance, flatulence, inflammatory bowel disease, irritable bowel syndrome and intestinal hyperpermeability. Your gut's protective bacteria (probiotics) are depleted and destroyed by antibiotics, birth control pills, chlorinated water, sucralose (Splenda) and laxatives.

Probiotics should always be taken after a round of antibiotics and are a good idea for most people to consume, either in supplement form or as a traditionally cultured food. They can be taken orally or used in enemas or douches for yeast infection. They may be sprinkled in the diaper for thrush-related diaper rash.

Dosage: Fermented foods are an ideal way to obtain probiotics. A recent study found that 100 million bacteria taken as yogurt survived the GI tract better than 1 billion bacteria from a probiotic supplement. Studies have also demonstrated the effectiveness of cultured vegetables at replenishing the gut's probiotic species. , For supplements take 10 billion active cultures taken one to three times daily with food or cultured foods eaten daily. Certain strains of probiotics demonstrate better therapeutic action for specific problems. L. rhamnosus GG, is a specific strain of probiotic that has the widest range of use and should be a major component of any probiotic supplement. For infections of the GI tract, products with L. johnsonii, L. plantarurn should be used. While not a probiotic, Saccharomyces boulardii, a strain of beneficial yeast is effective at preventing C-Diff, GI infections and inflammatory bowel disorders. It should not be taken, however and by anyone with a suppressed or compromised immune system.

Protease Enzymes

Protease enzymes are produced in the body and are responsible for a variety of functions, from aiding digestion to inducing programed cell death (*apoptosis*). Commercial preparations of protease are derived from pineapple or bacterial fermentation. The preparations from bacterial fermentation have almost no action in the body because they are destroyed by stomach acid. Protease derived from pineapple (*bromelain*) can withstand the acidic environment of the stomach and exhibits a wide range of beneficial actions in the body. (See *Bromelain* for more information).

Dosage: Follow manufacturer's recommendations.

Quercitin

Quercitin is the most abundant flavonoid found in the plant world. It is found in significant amounts in onions, apples, berries and cruciferous vegetables. Quercitin is a strong antioxidant, reducing inflammation throughout the body. Supplemental quercitin is poorly absorbed, with studies showing only about 2% passing through the gut into the bloodstream. There is a distinct possibility that many of the beneficial effects of quercitin are from a reduction of gut inflammation. Quercitin is most beneficial for people with allergies and allergy-induced asthma. However, studies also found that people with chronic prostatitis and interstitial cystitis saw an improvement in symptoms.

Dosage: 400-500 mg three times daily.

SAM-e

S-adenosylmethionine (abbreviated as SAM-e or SAMe) is a natural substance the body makes to facilitate certain chemical reactions. It is synthesized in the body from the amino acid methionine and adenosine triphosphate (ATP). First discovered in Europe and available there by prescription since 1975, SAM-e has a number of potential therapeutic benefits. It may be helpful for depression, liver problems (such as cirrhosis of the liver, chronic viral hepatitis, jaundice and Gilbert's syndrome), arthritis (especially osteoarthritis) migraine headaches and fibromyalgia.

Studies have suggested that SAM-e can be effective for mild to moderate depression. It helps the body produce more mood-enhancing neurotransmitters such as dopamine and serotonin. It works in conjunction with folic acid, B12 and B6 to produce these neurotransmitters, so it would be wise to use a B-Complex supplement when taking SAM-e. It can also aid energy production. Unfortunately, the dose required to manage depression is quite high. European studies typically use 1200 mg daily. SAM-e can move a person from depression to mania and is therefore contraindicated with bipolar disorder.

SAM-e helps to increase glutathione production. Glutathione is a major antioxidant in the body and helps protect the liver from free radical damage. It also helps in liver detoxification through a process called glutathione conjugation. These properties give SAM-e some benefits in conditions such as cirrhosis of the liver, chronic viral hepatitis and jaundice related to pregnancy.

SAM-e shows particular promise in the treatment of osteoarthritis. In large, well-controlled studies, it has been shown to be as effective as nonsteroidal anti-inflammatories in relieving pain without the side effects. It may also prevent damage to cartilage and may help rebuild cartilage when taken for long periods (more than 3 months).

Several studies have been conducted using SAM-e with fibromyalgia. Patients taking SAM-e reported improvements in pain, fatigue, morning stiffness and mood.

Dosage: The longer SAMe is taken, the better the effects. To prevent nausea start with 200 mg twice daily for the first day, increased to 400 mg twice daily on day 3, then increase to 400 mg three times daily on day 10. Maintain this dose for depression. For all other conditions after 3 weeks at 1200 mg daily, reduce to 200 mg twice daily.

Selenium

Selenium is an essential trace mineral found in soil, water and plants. In plants and soil, selenium is contained in the amino acids selenomethionine, selenocysteine and methylselenocysteine. In these compounds, selenium plays a role similar to that of sulfur.

Certain solids are rich in selenium, and selenium can be concentrated by certain plants.

Although selenium is toxic in large doses, it is an essential micronutrient for humans. Selenium functions as a cofactor in the reduction of antioxidant enzymes such as glutathione peroxidase.

Dietary selenium comes from nuts, cereals, meat, mushrooms, fish and eggs. Brazil nuts contain more selenium than other nuts because the nut doesn't require high levels of the element for its own needs. High levels of selenium are also found in kidney, tuna, crab and lobster.

Oxygen molecules can become overly reactive in the body and damage cells. These free radicals can increase oxidative stress on cellular structures, thereby contributing to degenerative diseases like cancer. Selenium may help prevent oxidative stress by working with other vitamins and nutrients in your body.

Selenium is a free radical scavenger. Research suggests that adequate levels help to protect the body against cancer. It also works well with vitamin E to mitigate the development of rheumatoid arthritis, elevated blood pressure, impaired thyroid function, loss of hair color, whitened fingernail beds, weakened immune system, increased risk of joint inflammation, and increased risk of atherosclerosis.

Dosage: 5-55 mcg per day.

Silicon

Silicon is a trace mineral found in the body as orthosilicic acid. Silicon dioxide, also known as silica, is present in foods such as vegetables, whole gains and seafood. A clear biological function of silicon in humans has not been established. There is some evidence, however, that it may play a role in bone and collagen formation. Most of the silicon in the body can be found in connective tissues such as in the aorta, trachea, bone, tendons and skin. Silicon may also protect against atherogenesis.

Silicon is an essential element in human biology, although only small trace amounts are required. Silicon is currently under consideration for elevation to the status of a "plant beneficial substance" by the Association of American Plant Food Control Officials (AAPFCO). Silicon has been shown in university and field studies to improve plant cell wall strength and structural integrity, improve drought and frost resistance, decrease lodging potential and boost the plant's natural pest and disease fighting systems.

In humans, supplemental silicon is used for osteoporosis, cardiovascular disease, Alzheimer's disease, alopecia, and improving hair and nail quality. It is also used for improving skin healing, treating sprains and strains, and digestive system disorders.

Dosage: Coffee, beer, and unfiltered drinking water are the major sources of dietary silicon, followed by grains, fruits and vegetables - especially bananas, raisins, beans and lentils. The average intake of silicon in adults is 14 to 21 mg per day. Horsetail and dulse are two herbs rich in silicon. Foods from animal sources and silicate food additives (to prevent foaming and caking) are lesser sources.

Sodium Alginate (Algin)

Sodium alginate is the sodium salt of alginic acid, also referred to as algin. Sodium alginate is an anionic polysaccharide distributed widely in the cell walls of brown algae, where it, through binding water, forms a viscous gum. In extracted form it absorbs water quickly, capable of absorbing 200-300 times its own weight in water.

In foods, algin is used in candy, gelatins, puddings, condiments, relishes, processed vegetables, fish products, and imitation dairy products. As a dietary supplement, algin is used to lower serum cholesterol levels and to reduce absorption of strontium, barium, tin, cadmium, manganese, zinc, and mercury. Algin is also used for the prevention and treatment of hypertension.

Algin is believed, but not confirmed, to be indigestible. Its cholesterol lowering effects may be related to viscosity of gel and inhibiting cholesterol absorption. Hypotensive effects may be due to the presence of laminine dioxalate. Due to its ability to absorb water quickly, algin can be changed through a lyophilization process to a new structure that has the ability to expand. This ability has made it popular in the weight loss industry as an appetite suppressant. In March, 2010 researchers at Newcastle University announced that dietary alginates can reduce human fat uptake by more than 75%.

Dosage: 1-2 capsules two or three times daily.

Vitamin A

Vitamin A is not a single compound but a family of fat-soluble compounds including retinol, retinal, retinyl ester and retinoic acid. We also use the term vitamin A to talk about certain plant compounds called carotenoids that are dietary precursors of retinol. Vitamin A is responsible for many actions in the body. It acts as a hormone, controlling the gene expression that governs the growth of epithelial cells. These cells make up not only our skin, but the lining of the intestinal tract, lungs, reproductive and urinary tract and the outer surface of the cornea.

Vitamin A is essential in maintaining the integrity of the mucus membranes and helping in the production of IgA, along with helping our white blood cells function properly. Vitamin A deficiencies are implicated in chronic viral infections, including frequent respiratory infections and HIV. Vitamin A is also essential for eye health. Night blindness, excess sensitivity to light, age related macular degeneration and chronic dry or red eyes are all common signs of a Vitamin A deficiency. Vitamin A deficiencies are common in the developing world and even in America where less than 50% of Americans get the suggested RDA of Vitamin A.

Dietary sources of vitamin A include butter, egg yolks, liver, seafood and fish liver oils. It is commonly thought that beta carotene can be converted to Vitamin A in sufficient quantities to supply your body's requirements. However, in several small studies up to 45% of healthy people could not convert beta carotene to Vitamin A. The conversion is also limited by several other factors including a low-fat diet, low thyroid function, diabetes, zinc deficiency, inflammatory bowel disorders and small bowel surgery. It is particularly impaired in infants and children. This is not to say beta-carotene is bad; carotenoids decrease your risk for many diseases. However, for most people we recommend a diet rich in animal source Vitamin A or supplementing with Vitamin A instead of beta-carotene.

Dosage: 1,000-10,000 IU daily depending on dietary consumption. The balance of Vitamins A and D, along with EPA and DHA make cod liver oil or fermented cod liver oil the preferred form for daily Vitamin A supplementation (try the orange or lemon flavored products). For short term high dose supplementation, emulsified Vitamin A works well. Vitamin A, as with all fat soluble vitamins, should be taken with a fatty meal., To guarantee that your Vitamin A is in the optimal range, especially during pregnancy, ask your doctor for a serum retinol test. This should be done early in pregnancy and several times throughout. You should aim for the medium high to high side of the blood reference range., Toxicity: The toxicity of Vitamin A from foods and supplementation is exaggerated by most sources. In fact, in the 30 years that the National Poison Data System has been keeping records, not a single death has ever been reported from taking vitamins and supplements. There is an average of 30-60 cases of vitamin A overdose reported each year. Most of these cases are in alcoholics who are more prone to the damaging effects of Vitamin A because of liver problems and other nutrient deficiencies. In all of the overdose cases, Vitamin A toxicity is completely reversible. These overdoses are reported frequently with no mention of the one million older Americans who have night vision problems due to a lack of vitamin A. , There are reports of Vitamin A doses higher than 10,000 IU causing birth defects (less than 20 cases in the past 30 years). Other studies conflict with these reports, showing that more than 30,000 IU per day are needed to cause birth defects. The primary side effects associated with chronic vitamin A toxicity are headaches, hair loss, red itchy skin, enlargement of the liver and joint pain. All of these symptoms abate after supplementation is stopped. Adequate intake of Vitamin E and D and K seem to limit the toxicity of high doses of Vitamin A.

Vitamin B-1 (Thiamine)

Thiamine is a water soluble B vitamin that is required for the metabolism of fats, carbohydrates, and amino acids. Thiamine is used in every cell of the body to make ATP and aids in the production of acetylcholine and GABA. It is necessary to maintain and repair myelin sheaths and is essential to the nervous system. A deficiency of Thiamine can manifest as Wernicke-Korsakoff psychosis or Beriberi. Dry Beriberi is characterized by weight loss, intestinal pain and constipation, nerve damage, sleep disturbance and memory loss. Wet Beriberi causes cardiac failure, congestive heart disease, edema, and palpitations.

A thiamine deficiency was thought to only occur in severe malnutrition and alcoholism, however we now know that many drugs deplete thiamine and a diet high in simple carbohydrates and processed food, gastrointestinal surgery, dialysis, longer term diuretic use, and cancer can all lead to a deficiency. Supplementing with thiamine can improve mood, peripheral neuropathy, memory, congestive heart failure and multiple sclerosis.

Dosage: 50-200 mg daily, normally as part of a B-complex.

Vitamin B-12

B-12 is essential for normal formation of red blood cells, metabolism and the nervous system. It acts as a cofactor or essential component in DNA synthesis. This makes B-12 important for the production of all cells in the body, the development of red blood cells, normal myelination or covering of nerve cells and the production of neurotransmitters. The current accepted blood level range for B12 in the U.S. is 200-900 ng/ml. Many experts think this is far too low, and standard ranges in most of Europe and Japan are 550-1800 ng/ml. When using these more appropriate healthy ranges, studies find that almost 40% of Americans, regardless of age or diet are deficient in B12.

B12 is not found in plant foods, so vegetarians and vegans are more prone to B12 deficiency. Other factors like intestinal dysbiosis, gut inflammation, low stomach acid, excessive alcohol consumption, pernicious anemia, and acid suppressing drugs can also cause a B12 deficiency. If you have multiple sclerosis, dementia, Alzheimer's, inflammatory bowel disease, memory loss, fatigue upon waking, tingling or numbness in the fingers or toes, cardiovascular disease, depression, migraines, infertility, cancer or any autoimmune disease you should get your B12 levels checked.

Dosage: The most common form of B12 on the market is cyanocobalamin. This is a cheap synthetic form of B12. Supplementation with methylcobalamin is preferable at a dose of 5,000 mcg sublingually a day. If your serum B12 level is below 350 or your MCV is over 96, shots of methylcobalamin are often necessary.

Vitamin B-2 (Riboflavin)

Riboflavin is a B vitamin used in many pathways of the body and helps the breakdown of fats, carbohydrates and amino acids. Overt deficiency is not common in the U.S. because riboflavin is found in a variety of foods and added to many foods. However around 10% of the population shows signs of a sub-clinical deficiency, most likely due to malabsorption issues. It takes 3-8 months of inadequate dietary intake for clinical signs and symptoms to appear. Symptoms of a riboflavin deficiency include: cracked lips and sides of the mouth, painful inflammation of the tongue and mouth, sore throat, dry skin and iron deficient anemia. Those with anemia, elevated homocysteine levels, migraines, cataracts, and carpal tunnel syndrome should consider supplementing with B2.

Dosage: 30-50 mg daily, normally as part of a B-complex. 400 mg daily to help prevent migraines.

Vitamin B-3 (Niacin)

Also known as B3, niacin is an important nutrient for a variety of functions in the body. A severe niacin deficiency manifest as a disease called Pellagra. Pellagra is characterized by the 4 D's: Diarrhea, Dermatitis, Dementia and Death. While Pellagra is less common now than 100 years ago thanks to the fortification of foods, it still exists and it's early symptoms are often overlooked. In addition to reversing Pellagra, niacin helps improve circulation, as evidenced by the red flushing of the skin from capillaries dilating when a big dose of niacin is taken. It also helps lower cholesterol and is used as a prescription drug for its cholesterol lowering effects.

Niacinamide, the form of B3 that doesn't cause skin flushing, doesn't seem to help with circulation, but it does help prevent pancreas cell damage from Type 1 diabetes, while improving joint function in people with arthritis. Niacinamide also has a long history of use in treating Schizophrenia. Psychiatric journals from the 1940's showed many people with Schizophrenia being cured when food began being fortified with niacin. Since then studies have shown conflicting results using niacinamine for Schizophrenia. It appears that when given in high doses in the initial stages of Schizophrenia, niacinamide can prove an effective cure, but people who have had Schizophrenia for a long time don't see any improvement with supplementation. Niacinamide also helps with skin disorders, the metabolism of nutrients, and the production of hydrochloric acid.

Nutrients

Dosage: For circulatory issues or high cholesterol, start with 50 mg of niacin (nicotinic acid) three times a day. Once a week increase your dose by 50 mg three times daily until you reach 200 mg three times daily. Niacin (in the form of nicotinic acid) should not be taken if you drink alcohol or have liver disease, stomach ulcers or gout. Niacin can cause an elevation of liver enzymes and liver damage in high doses. For Type 1 Diabetes, Schizophrenia, and arthritis, Niacinamide (a flush-free form of niacin) is used in doses ranging from 1.75 g-3.5 g daily. The dosage for children with diabetes is 150-300 mg per year of age, up to 3 grams daily. Taking too much niacinamide can cause nausea, heartburn, vomiting, flatulence, and diarrhea.

Vitamin B-6 (Pyridoxine)

B6 is the primary cofactor for over 100 enzymes that control amino acid metabolism. It is responsible for producing many of the amine based neurotransmitters and hormones, including serotonin, that the body uses to control mood and energy production. B6 is also involved in the formation of antibodies, hemoglobin production and sodium/phosphorus balance in the body. B6 is found in a variety of foods including many vegetables, fruits, meats and nuts. Because of the widespread availability of B6 in foods severe deficiency is uncommon. However your body doesn't store B6, so we need a constant supply from our diet.

Supplemental B6 has been shown to help improve certain types of anemia, carpal tunnel syndrome, morning sickness, elevated homocysteine levels and PMS. Elderly and alcoholics along with people that have liver disease, rheumatoid arthritis, type 1 diabetes, and those infected with HIV are most prone to a B6 deficiency. The metabolically active and most safe form of vitamin B6 is pyridoxal-5-phosphate (P5P).

Dosage: 50-100 mg three times daily of P5P. High doses of Pyridoxine hydrochloride can cause neuropathy. This is not been observed with P5P supplementation. B-6 is commonly taken as part of a B-complex.

Vitamin B-Complex

B-complex vitamins (B1, B2, B3, B5, B6, B7, B9, B12) are essential for the formation of red blood cells, metabolism, nervous system function, promotes normal growth and metabolism of nutrients and proteins. They are needed for the synthesis of RNA and DNA, growth and division of cells, fetal development, especially neural tube development. This group of vitamins also reduces blood levels of homocysteine, which is an amino acid that contributes to cardiovascular disease by damaging the endothelium (thin layer of cells that protect the artery walls).

Deficiencies of B vitamins in pregnant women may cause birth defects. Turkey, tuna, liver, beef and leafy green vegetables are high in most B vitamins. Most of the B vitamins are excreted fairly quickly in the urine, so having a nutrient-dense diet or supplementing with B vitamins is essential for most people. Consider supplementation when dealing with high periods of stress, metabolic disease or any nervous system disorder.

Dosage: 1-3 capsules, three times a day. Refer to manufacturer suggestions.

Vitamin C

Vitamin C is extremely important for tissue integrity (healthy gums, wound healing, etc.), adrenal function (stress, fatigue), the immune system and much more. Vitamin C acts as an antioxidant, protecting the body from the oxidative damage linked to heart disease, diabetes and many chronic inflammatory conditions. Unlike most mammals, humans don't synthesize their own Vitamin C and must obtain it from their diet.

Consuming vitamin C from foods or supplements increases iron absorption and the healing rate of wounds and burns. Vitamin C also stabilizes mast cells and improves immune function, reducing allergic reactions and when taken daily shortens the duration of common viral infections like colds. Vitamin C in very high doses might play a positive role in cancer treatment. Aspirin, most pain medications, alcohol, some antidepressants, steroids, and oral contraceptives may reduce vitamin C levels in the body.

Dosage: 250-10,000 mg. daily. Vitamin C may be taken to bowel tolerance, meaning you can increase the dose until it starts causing diarrhea. If diarrhea occurs with large doses of vitamin C reduce the dose until the diarrhea stops.

Vitamin D

Vitamin D is a fat-soluble vitamin that the body naturally synthesizes during exposure to sunlight. Vitamin D is primarily known for its role in promoting calcium absorption from the intestinal tract. It helps to maintain adequate levels of calcium and phosphorus in the blood to enable the mineralization of bone. Without sufficient vitamin D, bones become thin, brittle or misshapen. A severe deficiency produces the disease known as rickets in children and osteomalacia in adults. Vitamin D is needed to prevent osteoporosis in the elderly as well.

However, the benefits of vitamin D do not end with the role it plays in maintaining proper calcium and phosphorous levels for bone health. Vitamin D also affects the immune system. It promotes phagocytosis (anti-tumor activity) and helps modulate the immune system. Some evidence suggests it may play a role in protecting the body against cancer. Insufficient levels of vitamin D may also be linked to an increased susceptibility to other chronic diseases.

After vitamin D is formed in the skin or taken orally, it is metabolized into two different substances: 25-hydroxyvitamin D, known as calcidiol, and 1,25-dihydroxyvitamin D, known as calcitriol. Calcidiol is the storage form of vitamin D produced in the liver and is what blood tests measure to determine vitamin D status. Calcidiol is converted in the kidneys and other organs of the body to calcitrol, a potent hormone with widespread action. Calcitrol regulates the uptake of calcium from the gut and binds to Vitamin D Receptors (VDR), helping to control the expression of genes that regulate immunity, cell metabolism and many other functions within the body.

Supplemental vitamin D is found in two forms, Vitamin D2 and Vitamin D3. Vitamin D2 is not naturally present in the human body and has actions within the body different than those of vitamin D3. Vitamin D3 is the form of Vitamin D that the body naturally produces and is most effective at treating vitamin D deficiency. Adequate Vitamin D3 blood levels have been shown to help prevent osteoporosis and bone loss, diabetes, cancer, low thyroid and autoimmune disorders. Expert opinions vary on what an adequate blood level of vitamin D3 is. A review of the published literature shows that blood levels of 35-45 ng/ml is the ideal range for most people. However some people with VDR polymorphisms or specific illnesses need to raise their blood levels to 50-70 ng/ml.

Dosage: The dose of supplemental vitamin D3 required to get people to the ideal range varies. Digestion, absorption, weight and genetics are all factors that have an influence on how much you need to take. Some people, with normal sun exposure only need 2000 IU

a day of D3, however some people require 10,000 IU daily to achieve adequate blood levels. It's best to supplement with 5,000 IU daily of Vitamin D3 and after 1 month check your blood level. If your blood level of Vitamin D is too low, increase your dose. If your blood level is too high, decrease your dose. Vitamin D3 and all other fat soluble vitamins absorb better when taken with the largest meal of the day. When supplementing with Vitamin D3 it's best to also consume food or supplement with Vitamins A and K2 found in organ meats and fermented foods. Blood levels of Vitamin D over 70 ng/ml show no concrete benefits and increase your risk of kidney stones.

Vitamin E

Vitamin E is not a single vitamin, but a family of fat soluble vitamins called tocopherols. Alpha-tocopherol is considered the most active form of Vitamin E, but plants also contain beta, gamma and delta tocopherol, all of which have beneficial actions. Vitamin E's primary action is to prevent oxidative damage to cell membranes, but Vitamin E also prevents the oxidation of polyunsaturated fatty acids, helps control gene expression, and inhibits platelets from sticking together.

While studies have found that people who consume more vitamin E from foods have less heart disease, studies have also shown that supplementing with d-alpha tocopherol doesn't seem to increase longevity or decrease heart disease. Small studies indicate that supplementing with mixed tocopherols, instead of just d-alpha tocopherol, might reduce heart disease in addition to improving blood flow in intermittent claudication. Vitamin E is protective against prostate, bladder and colon cancer.

Dosage: 400-800 IU daily of mixed tocopherols. Use caution when taking Vitamin E with prescription blood thinners.

Vitamin K

Vitamin K is not a single vitamin, but actually a family of fat soluble vitamins that include K1 and K2. Vitamin K1 is found in a variety of green vegetables and is essential for normal blood clotting. Healthy gut bacteria can transform K1 into K2, and new research suggest that K1 to K2 conversion can occur in the testes, pancreas and arterial walls as well. K2 helps with blood clotting as well as playing an important role in bone and immune health.

There are several subtype of K2, the most researched being MK4 and MK7. MK4 is the most common type of K2 that the body creates from K1. MK4 strengthens the bones and prevents fractures and bone loss from normal aging as well as bone loss associated with steroid medications, anorexia, post-menopausal bone loss, and cirrhosis of the liver. MK7, the form of K2 derived from fermented soy (natto), seems to have some of the beneficial actions on bone health as MK4. Both MK4 and MK7 in sufficient doses seem to prevent and even reverse the deposition of calcium in the arteries associated with heart disease.

Vitamin K2 (MK4) has a strong action on the immune system. In several studies K2 (MK4) was found both in test tubes and in humans to reduce the growth of several types of cancer. Broad spectrum antibiotics, aspirin and the fat substitute Olestra reduces the synthesis of Vitamin K in the gut.

Dosage: The standard dose for the treatment of osteoporosis in studies is 45 mg of K2 daily. However doses as small as 1.5 mg of K2 a day help prevent osteoporosis in healthy people. The normal dose in studies for cancer ranges from 25 mg-140 mg daily of K2, but the most common dose is 45 mg a day of K2. Vitamin K1 and K2, even at very high doses, have no known toxicity. There is a possibility that a high intake of Vitamin A and/or Vitamin E could interfere with Vitamin K utilization, but more studies are needed to confirm this. Vitamin K1 and to a lesser extent K2 interfere and should not be taken with blood thinning medications that are vitamin K antagonist (such as Warfarin). Vitamin K1 and K2 do not interfere with heparin, antiplatelet agents (asprin, Plavix etc.) and direct thrombin inhibitors (hirudin, argatoban).

Zeaxanthin

Zeaxanthin is one of the most common carotenoids found in nature. It is important in the xanthophyll cycle. Synthesized in plants and some microorganisms, it is the pigment that gives paprika, corn, saffron, wolfberries and many other plants their characteristic color.

Xanthophylls such as zeaxanthin are found in highest quantity in the leaves of most green plants, where they act to modulate light energy and perhaps serve as a non-photochemical quenching agent to deal with triplet chlorophyll (an excited form of chlorophyll), which is overproduced at very high light levels during photosynthesis.

Zeaxanthin is one of the two primary xanthophyll carotenoids contained within the retina of the eye. Within the central macula, zeaxanthin is the dominant component, whereas in the peripheral retina, lutein predominates. Several research studies have connected high dietary intake of foods providing zeaxanthin with lower incidence of age-related macular degeneration (AMD).

Zeaxanthin supplements are used to treat various disorders, primarily those affecting the eyes. There are no reported side effects from taking zeaxanthin supplements.

Dosage: Humans obtain zeaxanthin from dietary foods such as vegetables, fruits and berries. For supplements, follow manufacturer's recommendations.

Zinc

Zinc is important for immune system function, male reproductive function and tissue healing. Zinc is essential for the production of Superoxide Dismutase, a potent antioxidant, and helps protect Vitamin E stores and prevents LDL and VLDL oxidation. Severe deficiencies of zinc are rare, but mild to moderate deficiency occurs regularly in children, elderly, and those with eating disorders, diabetes, renal disease, and gastrointestinal disease. Zinc has been shown to help slow the progression of Alzheimer's, improve sperm count, reduce prostate swelling in BPH, and increase the speed of healing from both gastric ulcers and lower limb ulcers.

Dosage: 10-100 mg. If you supplement above 50 mg take 2 mg of copper to prevent a copper deficiency. Zinc supplementation can reduce the absorption of some antibiotics. Birth control medications and tetracycline can reduce zinc levels in the body. Take zinc supplements separate from acid-reducing medications.

Companies

Contact information and a brief description of the companies whose products are featured in this book.

None of the companies listed below provided any kind of financial support to this book, and the classifications and descriptions we make about the single herbs and formulas are strictly our own.

In choosing the companies to feature in this book, we concentrated primarily on the most popular brands sold in health food stores. We also selected some lesser-known brands because of some of their unique formulas.

All of these companies are required to follow FDA GMP guidelines, but this doesn't mean that all of the companies manufacture to the same standards. We have not toured the manufacturing facilities of these companies, nor have we personally used all of their products. So, we encourage you to visit their websites and learn more about them, so you can decide which brands you want to rely on.

Just because a particular formula may not work for you, doesn't mean that a different formula won't work. You may have to try several formulas to determine which products and brands are best for your needs.

A. Vogel

http://bioforceusa.com

Phone: 518-828-9111
Address: 6 Grandinetti Drive
 Ghent, NY 12075

Alfred Vogel established the company in Roggwil, Thurgau, Switzerland in 1963 to meet the increasing demand for his products. His aim was to provide effective natural remedies, a basic palette of healthy foodstuffs, books, and a monthly magazine containing reliable information on all aspects of health and natural living to a constantly growing number of people.

A. Vogel standardizes their plant remedies. They choose seed varieties of the highest quality, use the best cultivation methods, find the ideal time to harvest and follow a strictly controlled production process. A.Vogel's medicinal plants originate from its own cultivation, managed by contract farmers and from approved wild gathering and sustainable cultivation projects which consider the needs of the resident population. The plants are cultivated according to the strict guidelines of BIO-SUISSE, that is without the use of fertilizers, insecticides, herbicides or fungicides. These procedures help them guarantee consistent effectiveness in their products.

Celestial Seasonings

http://celestialseasonings.com

Phone: 800-351-8175
Address: 4600 Sleepytime Dr.
 Boulder, CO 80301

In 1969, a group of passionate young entrepreneurs founded Celestial Seasonings on the belief that their flavorful, all-natural herbal teas could help people live healthier lives. They harvested fresh herbs from the Rocky Mountains by hand, and then dried, blended and packaged them in hand-sewn muslin bags to be sold at local health food stores. By staying committed to their vision, the founders of Celestial Seasonings turned their cottage industry into an almost overnight success.

Today, Celestial Seasonings is one of the largest specialty tea manufacturers in North America. It serves more than 1.6 billion cups of tea every year, and it sources more than 100 different ingredients from over 35 countries. For more than 40 years, the experts at Celestial Seasonings have traveled to the ends of the earth to find the highest quality, most authentic ingredients for their teas.

Christopher's

http://herbsfirst.com

Phone: 801-228-1901
Address: 501 West 965 North, Suite 3
 Orem, UT 84057

John Christopher was born with rheumatoid arthritis and told by several physicians that he would not live past the age of thirty. He was abandoned by his biological parents and left in an orphanage. Fortunately, he was adopted as a toddler by loving parents. Early on, his life was spared through the use of medicinal herbs, and he was able to overcome the crippling effects of rheumatoid arthritis through the use of herbs, dietary changes, and alternative healing methods. Dr. Christopher went on to became one of the nation's leading authorities on herbal medicine, founding the School of Herbal Medicine. Many of today's top herbalists received some of their early training from Dr. Christopher.

Today, David Christopher carries on his father's tradition. Christopher's carries Doctor Christopher's original formulas. It seeks to continue on the legacy of product excellence and caring service to customers begun by this pioneer in modern herbal medicine.

Eclectic Institute

http://eclecticherb.com

Phone: 800-332-4372
Address: 36350 S.E. Industrial Way
             Sandy, OR 97055

The Eclectic Institute was founded in 1982 by naturopathic physicians, Edward Alstat and Michael Ancharski. At that time, Dr. Alstat was serving as the pharmacist for the Portland Naturopathic clinic at the National College of Naturopathic Medicine. Dr. Ancharski was the Clinic Director. In spite of having access to the latest botanical literature, research and practitioners, they could not find high quality, botanical preparations to use in their clinic. Most herbs on the commercial market simply were not pure, vital or fresh enough to meet their standards. They decided to develop and market their own line of botanical products using only organic herbs carefully grown and harvested and processed while fresh.

Doctors Alstat and Ancharski developed Organol, the only certified organic grape alcohol used in botanical liquid extracts. The company believes that organic grape alcohol offers distinct advantages over distilled grain alcohol. In addition to their line of organic alcohol extracts and alcohol-free glycerites, Eclectic Institute also utilizes freeze-drying to manufacture encapsulated products. They also grow many herbs on their own certified organic farm.

Gaia Herbs

http://gaiaherbs.com

Phone: 800-831-7780
Address: 101 Gaia Herbs Dr.
             Brevard, NC 28712

Gaia Herbs is a certified organic grower and manufacturer of liquid herbal extracts. It is based in Western North Carolina. The Gaia Herb Farm, nestled in a pristine mountain valley, is one of the largest and most productive commercial medicinal herb farms in the United States. On this 250 acre farm, Gaia cultivates over 50 herbs, each of which is certified organic by Oregon Tilth.

A vertically integrated company, Gaia controls every stage of production from organic soil enrichment programs, seed selection, cultivation and harvesting, to research and analysis for correct harvest time. Gaia also tests to validate that their extracts contain the full spectrum of plant compounds, concentrating them to pre-determined levels. The company never purifies or isolates individual properties of its herb, but instead makes medicine that mirrors nature. In 2001, Gaia Herbs introduced its patented Liquid Phyto-Caps™, a technology that delivers a concentrated liquid extract in a vegetarian capsule.

Grandma's Herbs

http://grandmasherbs.com

Phone: 800-724-4689
Address: 221 West 200 South
             Saint George, UT 84770

Since 1979 Grandma's Herbs has been in the business of helping people get well. Their herbal formulas were created by Master Herbalist, Joseph VanSeters. With over 30 years of study he has refined the companies formulas to meet people's health concerns. They seek out the best raw materials and use no fillers.

Herb Pharm

http://herb-pharm.com

Phone: 541-846-6262
Address: P.O. Box 116
             Williams, OR 97544

Herb Pharm was founded in 1974 by Ed Smith and Sara Katz. Both Ed and Sarah are well-known and respected in the professional herbalists community. The Herb Pharm team also includes David Bunting, Herbal Affairs Manager overseeing quality control, and Julie Plunkett, Clinical Herbalist and Health Educator.

Located in a rural valley nestled in the Siskiyou Mountains of southern Oregon, Herb Pharm prides itself in growing its own herbs on an 85-acre organic herb farm certified by Tilth. They are certified Salmon Safe, Bee Friendly and as a Botanical Sanctuary through United Plant Savers. They employ time-honored sustainable agricultural techniques including crop rotation, cover cropping, natural weed control and composting to condition the soil. Herb Pharm is also dedicated to wildcrafting herbs in a responsible and sustainable manner. Throughout the hundreds of steps of their manufacturing processes – from planting the fields to shipping out the finished products – each and every step is controlled through FDA-mandated Good Manufacturing Practices and by strict inspections by their Analytical Laboratory and Quality Assurance Department. All finished batches are tested organoleptically (taste, odor, appearance) and microbiologically to ensure compliance, consistency and safety, as well as ensuring compliance to any label claims.

In recent years, Herb Pharm was awarded the Socially Responsible Business Award by a panel of leading natural products manufacturers, and received the Herbal Industry Leader Award from the American Herbal Products Association (AHPA) for laudable business practices. Ed and Sara believe that the herb and natural products industry should be a model of social and environmental responsibility. Just as the industry has changed the way millions of people view their food and healthcare, Herb Pharm also strives to be an inspiration for how businesses can positively contribute to society and the environment.

Herbalist & Alchemist

http://herbalist-alchemist.com

Phone: 908-689-9020
Address: 51 South Wandling Ave.
Washington, NJ 07882

Located in rural northwestern New Jersey, Herbalist & Alchemist has been crafting high quality, traditional herbal products since 1981. Founded by internationally known ethnobotanist, clinical herbalist, lecturer, and author David Winston, RH (AHG) to manufacture quality herbal products for use with his patients, Herbalist & Alchemist products are based on his 40 years of clinical experience practicing Cherokee, Chinese and Western herbal medicine. Because of his exacting standards and extensive

knowledge, the herbal extracts they manufacture are widely used by clinical herbalists who value their quality and efficacy.

Herbalist and Alchemist's mission is to develop, manufacture and distribute herbal supplements that are of the highest quality, organically grown, ethically wild-crafted or sustainably harvested plant materials. Every employee is committed to achieving the highest standards of excellence possible. The company is dedicated to continually improving its knowledge base, processes and practices in order to maintain its position in the forefront of the herbal products community. Herbalist & Alchemist is likewise committed to providing education and information about the health benefits and uses of herbal medicine.

Herbs Etc.

http://herbsetc.com

Phone: 888-694-3727
Address: 1345 Cerrillos Rd.
Santa Fe, NM 87505

Herbs Etc. was founded by medical herbalist Daniel Gagnon. As a child and a young adult, Daniel suffered from eczema, asthma and allergies. His journey back to health is the driving force that motivates him to share the benefits of natural healing with other individuals. His number one goal is to develop effective herbal medicines that contain only natural and beneficial ingredients that have little or no side effects.

Herbs, Etc. has their own certified organic manufacturing facility. The company uses fresh or dried whole herbs grown on family-owned, certified organic farms. They use a proprietary extraction process known as kinetic maceration, which involves putting the herbs, alcohol and water in a hermetically sealed container and tumbling them non-stop for 12 hours. They also use a cryogenic or ultra-cold grinding process to ensure optimum potency of the active constituents.

Herbs for Kids

http://herbsforkids.com

Phone: 800-648-2704
Address: 1500 Kearns Blvd., Suite 200
Park City, UT 84060

Herbs for Kids was founded in 1990 by herbalist and expectant mother, Sunny Mavor. Sunny has counseled and taught about the joy of herbs at stores, schools and symposiums across the nation. With a background as a practicing herbalist and in retail natural food management, she knew the difficulty of finding herbal products acceptable for children. She wished to create an alternative to alcohol-based products, as most adult formulas often use herbs too strong for children. Also, the typical adult dosage forms (capsules, tablets and teas) are difficult to administer to children.

Sunny created the first company dedicated to Earth-reviving herbal health care for children. Her background as an herbalist has allowed her to create alcohol-free blends that are gentle, safe and effective, and taste good so children will be willing to take them. Even the most bitter of herbs are blended to have a flavor that goes down easily. Herbs for Kids remains the premiere line of traditional herbal extracts for children.

Irwin Naturals

http://irwinnaturals.com

Phone: 800-297-3273
Address: 5310 Beethoven Street
Los Angeles, CA 90066

Irwin Naturals is committed to developing solution-oriented formulas that exceed the highest standards for quality and purity. They invest heavily in research to produce cutting edge formulas. They utilize a Liquid Soft-Gel technology to deliver their formulas.

Nature's Answer

http://naturesanswer.com

Phone: 800-439-2324
Address: 85 Commerce Dr.
Hauppauge, NY 11788

Nature's Answer is a family-owned and operated company dedicated to total health. It was started in 1972, when owner Frank D'amelio created a business from his true passion. From the age of seven Frank Sr. had a powerful interest in the healing and restorative powers of plants. He remembers consulting with his grandmother about the healing powers of herbs until her death. He continued his studies into natural healing and studied botany, herbal healing and chemistry. He dedicated himself to launching a business that would produce high quality herbal extracts and nutritional products to help support, promote and enhance healthier lifestyles.

With one of the most comprehensive herbariums in the world, Nature's Answer has identified Mother Nature's Advanced Botanical Fingerprint Technology™ for over 800 unique plant reference standards. These authenticated samples serve as the standard by which all incoming raw material is judged. They use extraction techniques that capture the holistic balance of each herb.

All the herbs they process are wildcrafted or organically grown with minor exceptions. Whenever possible, they endeavor to use wildcrafted herbs, as both traditional practitioners and current scientific assays confirm the higher activity of herbs grown wild in their natural environment. Having over 40 years experience with wildcrafters and herbal sources; they work to ensure the long term protection of the plant species in the wild.

Nature's Answer holds many certifications, including GMP, NSF (National Safety Foundation), Kosher and Organic (QAI certification). They combine the best of traditional herbal remedies, vitamins and minerals with their knowledge of innovative scientific techniques and phytopharmaceutical manufacturing, to deliver high-quality, naturally-derived products for the entire family.

Nature's Herbs (TwinLab)

http://twinlab.com/brands/natures-herbs

Phone: 212-651-8500
Address: 632 Broadway, Suite 201
New York City, NY 10012

TwinLab was created in 1968 when founder David Blechman leveraged his 20 years of expertise in the pharmaceutical industry to develop and market a liquid protein supplement. Working out of his family's garage, he and his wife named their developing business TwinLab, after the couple's two sets of twins. Sales soared, and in the 1980s, TwinLab branched out to a broader range of vitamins, minerals, herbs and teas.

Since 1968, the TwinLab brand has produced innovative, high performance health and wellness products. In addition to the extensive line of vitamins, minerals and sports nutrition formulas of its namesake brand, TwinLab Corporation manufactures and sells the Nature's Herbs line of herbs and phytonutrients.

TwinLab's plant in American Fork, UT, is a NSF GMP registered facility from which they manufacture, package and distribute over 1,000 products. The NSF program verifies that TwinLab's manufacturing plant has met NSF International's stringent independent registration process guidelines. Facilities registered GMP by NSF conform to the highest verification process including ongoing monitoring via two annual facility inspections, to ensure continued compliance with program requirements. TwinLab also operates its own Research & Development facility in Grand Rapids, MI.

Nature's Sunshine Products

http://naturessunshine.com

Phone: 800-223-8225

Address: 2500 West Executive Parkway, Suite 500
Lehi, UT 84043

Nature's Sunshine Products was a pioneer in encapsulating herbs and has been a leader in quality control for herbal products. Products from this company are sold via network marketing and are not usually found in health food stores. However, we included a few unique products they offer because we have had personal experience with them.

Nature's Way

http://naturesway.com

Phone: 800-962-8873

Address: 3051 West Maple Loop Dr., Suite 125
Lehi, UT 84043

Back in the late 1960s, Tom Murdock, founder of Nature's Way, needed a solution to help his gravely ill wife. After trying conventional medicine without success, they turned to the traditional Native American knowledge of medicinal plants growing in the Arizona desert. As a result, she recovered and lived an additional 25 years. Motivated by a passion to spread natural healing, Tom and his family moved back to the mountain valleys of Utah county, where they started Nature's Way.

Nature's Way is located in what has been called the "silicon valley of the herb industry." They have been a pioneering leader in herbal medicine for over 40 years. It was the first major supplement company to be certified as an organic food processor. The company was also the first to bring clinically proven, European phytomedicines to the U.S. market. It has founded donor groups to protect the world's rain forests and provide nutritional supplements to the poor of developing nations. Nature's Way has a state-of-the-art, pharmaceutically licensed, GMP manufacturing facility and continually updates and reinvests in it.

NatureWorks

http://vitasprings.com/natureworks.html

Phone: 626-579-2668

Address: 2003 N. Tyler Ave.
South El Monte, CA 91733

NatureWorks is a European company that is famous for making a traditional formula created by Paracelsus in the 16th century known as Swedish Bitters.

New Chapter

http://newchapter.com

Phone: 800-543-7279

Address: 90 Technology Drive
Brattleboro, VT 05301

Paul Schulick developed a passion for healing when he accompanied his pediatrician dad on house calls. He recognized that healing wasn't just about medicine, it was also about the loving care his father showed his patients. He started studying alternative healing in the early 1970s and formalized his training by becoming a Master Herbalist through The School of Natural Healing. He and his wife Barbi Schulick founded New Chapter in 1982 in Brattleboro, Vermont.

Recognizing the tremendous healing potential of ginger in the early 1990s, Paul integrated supercritical extraction technology into a full line of ginger products. By 1994, while searching for a reliable source of organic ginger, Paul partnered with Steven Farrell to found Luna Nueva, the first organic and now Biodynamic blue ring ginger farm in Costa Rica. New Chapter believe in using whole food, not synthetic chemical isolates. They use modern science to validate the effectiveness of their products. Most New Chapter products are certified organic and are GMP (Good Manufacturing Practices) certified by NSF International, the world's leading expert in independent GMP audits and product safety.

NOW Foods

http://nowfoods.com

Phone: 888-669-3663

Address: 244 Knollwood Dr., Suite 300
Bloomingdale, IL 60108

NOW Foods manufactures a comprehensive line of natural health products, including dietary supplements, sports nutrition, natural foods, and personal care items.

Companies

Many NOW products are manufactured with organic, raw and non-GMO ingredients, as well as many trademarked ingredients. They have been committed to product excellence since 1968. Its company philosophy is a simple one; high quality nutrition products should not be considered a luxury available only to the wealthiest.

NOW takes great pride in providing value in products and services that empower people to lead healthier lives. NOW is one of the top-selling brands in health food stores. NOW's technical staff and scientific consulting group includes twelve PhD's and one M.D. NOW Foods has developed peer-reviewed, official AOAC and USP methods for the testing of glucosamine, and is currently offering similar methods for SAMe, chondroitin, L-Carnitine and L-Arginine.

NOW was the first for-profit business in Illinois' DuPage County to receive the Earth Flag for Business. It received the Illinois Governor's Award for Pollution Prevention, and was further recognized by Clear Air Counts for its ongoing environmental efforts. NOW conducts seasonal, community-based Forest Preserve cleanup days, provides ongoing safety and environmental education to all employees, and maintains a robust recycling program. NOW believes in the preservation of good health through natural products, education, and sound science. Its personal commitment to a natural lifestyle is the underpinning of its commitment to produce quality natural products.

Olbas

http://pennherb.com/Olbas-Remedies

Phone: 800-523-9971
Address: 10601 Decatur Road
Philadelphia, PA 19154

It was in Switzerland, over 100 years ago, that herbalists and botanists developed a blend of pure essentials oils that came to be known as Olbas Oil. The name Olbas is an acronym for Oleum Basileum, or "Oil from Basle." Basle is enviably nestled on the border of Switzerland, Germany and France in the very heart of Europe, and to this day it is a center of pharmaceutical research in Switzerland. Olbas products are now sold worldwide. The official importer for Olbas products is the Penn Herb Company.

Planetary Herbals

http://planetaryherbals.com

Phone: 800-606-6226
Address: P. O. Box 1760
Soquel, CA 95073

For over 30 years, Planetary Herbals has been integrating the wisdom and principles of the planet's three major herbal traditions—Ayurveda, traditional Chinese medicine (TCM), and Western herbalism—into each of their formulas. Their formulas address body systems, not just symptoms. The majority of their core formulas have been derived from the clinical practice of Michael Tierra, Planetary Herbal's chief formulator and one of the world's foremost and well-respected clinical herbalists. Michael first introduced the Triphala compound to the U.S. natural products market nearly 40 years ago, was primarily responsible for the reintroduction of Echinacea back into modern herbal practice, and was one of the first to bring Ashwagandha seeds into the U.S.

Today, Planetary Herbals has one of the best quality assurance teams in the industry, with expertise in traditional herbal assessment skills, analytical chemistry and biology. Its wildcrafted, organic, non-GMO verified Triphala remains its flagship product and is an example of the quality of their products. For those seeking true and lasting healthcare in their lives, each of Planetary Herbals' 200+ formulas, liquids and single herb products reflects the knowledge of its expert herbalists, decades of human clinical experience, and its extensive knowledge of modern pharmacological science.

Renew Life

http://renewlife.com

Phone: 800-830-1800
Address: 198 Palm Harbor Blvd. (Alt. 19) South
Palm Harbor, FL 34683

ReNew Life was established in 1997 by Brenda Watson and her husband Stan. Brenda has become one of the nation's leading authorities on natural digestive health, detoxification and internal cleansing. She is the author of 5 books on this topic, and she has helped millions of people live longer, healthier lives through improved digestion. For more than a decade RenewLife has been making quality products and functional foods using only the purest ingredients found in nature. Their philosophy is that only through proper digestion and a sensible diet can we obtain the nutrients necessary to improve our overall well being.

The ReNew Life manufacturing process utilizes cutting-edge technology and equipment to produce a quality end product. They adhere to strict cGMP (current Good Manufacturing Practice) standards to ensure the consistency and reliability of each of its natural supplements. They do not use flow agents or lubricants to operate their machinery, opting for a slower manufacturing process that does not require these chemicals.

RidgeCrest Herbals

http://rcherbals.com

Phone: 801-978-9633
Address: 3683 West 2270 South #A
             Salt Lake City, UT 84120-2306

RidgeCrest Herbals is a Utah corporation with deep roots in the natural products industry. Started in 1986, it evolved into a manufacturer and distributor of over-the-counter herbal medicines and other herbal formulations, sold primarily to natural healing professionals (chiropractors, midwives and naturopaths). In 1994, new management and capital came in, and the company was launched in a new direction. To reflect the changes in the company's function, the name was changed to Ridgecrest Herbals in 1996.

As the company's new founders, Clyde St. Clair and Paul Warnock brought unique and valuable assets to their mission of providing eclectic, innovative and effective herbal and homeopathic remedies for professionals and individuals. In 1998, Ridgecrest Herbals established ClearLungs as the best-selling natural lung product in the US market, and a number of other products were also category leaders. But in 2001, health problems forced the two partners to withdraw from the business, and an outside sales management firm was brought in, with Paul's son, Matt, asked to serve as president in 2005.

Since 2005, the company has consistently grown its product line and revenues, moving to a new facility with room for more expansion in 2009. All manufacturing is done in the United States, to company specifications, by highly qualified contract manufacturers. They stand behind their products with an unconditional satisfaction guarantee.

Solaray

http://nutraceutical.com/about/brands/solaray.cfm

Phone: 800-669-8877
Address: 1400 Kearns Blvd.
             Park City, UT 84060

Solaray began in 1973 as a pioneer in formulating and marketing blended herbal products with complementary effects. Since its inception, Solaray has focused on encapsulated products, which offer rapid disintegration and are easy to swallow. By 1984, Solaray became a full line manufacturer, carrying not only high quality herbs, but also a full line of vitamins, minerals and specialty products. Today, Solaray nutraceuticals are sold under many brand names in over 60 countries.

Solaray's passion for helping people become healthier can be seen in its team members and its state-of-the-art manufacturing facility. With the latest technology and committed personnel, Solaray can ensure that quality controls are applied at every level. Solaray knows what goes into their products because every product is subjected to rigorous testing and screening protocols. The process may vary by ingredient, but typically includes organoleptic (taste, touch, smell) testing to compare it to previous batches, and lab assays for microbial, identity, purity and potency validation. Only when an ingredient has passed all of the required assays is it released to manufacturing. Solaray adheres to all current good manufacturing practices (cGMP) and an independent auditing firm audits their facilities, laboratory and manufacturing protocols for compliance with the latest regulations.

Tiger Balm

http://tigerbalm.com/

Phone: 510-887-1899
Address: 3536 Arden Road
             Hayward, CA 94545-3908

Tiger Balm is a Chinese company that makes a popular line of topical analgesic products. It began when Aw Chu Kin, a Chinese herbalist working in the Emperor's court, left China and set up a small medicine shop called Eng Aun Tong in Rangoon in the late 1870s. There he would make and sell his special ointment that was effective in relieving all kinds of aches and pains.

When Aw Chu Kin died in 1908, he left his business to his sons Aw Boon Haw (meaning 'gentle tiger') and Aw Boon Par (meaning 'gentle leopard'). They took the business to Singapore and successfully sold their ointment to surrounding countries like Malaysia, Hong Kong and various cities in China. Aw Boon Haw was the marketing genius who named the product Tiger Balm. Today, Tiger Balm has a 100 year-old track record of success and can be purchased in 100 countries.

Traditional Medicinals

http://traditionalmedicinals.com

Phone: 866-972-6879
Address: 4515 Ross Road
Sebastopol, CA 95472

In early 1974, three young friends started Traditional Medicinals in the back of a small herb shop along the Russian River in Northern California. The company was founded with the intention of providing herbal teas for self care, while preserving the knowledge and herbal formulas of Traditional Herbal Medicine. At the time, traditional herbal tea infusions had all but faded away in the United States. And never before had these reliable formulas been available in convenient tea bags. Over the decades that followed, the company introduced millions of health conscious consumers to traditional herbal tea formulas.

Traditional Medicinals uses pharmacopoeial grade herbs in its products and bases its formulations on the principles and practice of Traditional Herbal Medicine. It uses herbs that are farmed or wild crafted under organic certification. It works with Fair Trade and other certification organizations for the monitoring of equitable trade practices in its supply chain. Traditional Medicinals never uses herbs sterilized by irradiation or ethylene oxide, and it never uses genetically-modified ingredients. The company has incorporated clinical testing and scientific understanding to ensure the reliability of its products, while retaining its reverence for the beauty and mystery of Nature. They are also committed to sustainable harvesting.

Urban Moonshine

http://urbanmoonshine.com

Phone: 802-428-4707
Address: 255 South Champlain St., Suite 3
Burlington, VT 05401

Jovial King is the founder and formulator of Urban Moonshine. She has studied herbal medicine for many years, with an array of terrific teachers including completing apprenticeships with Brigitte Mars, Guido Mase, Rosemary Gladstar, and Hart Brent.

Urban Moonshine is a family business whose mission is to rekindle the relationship between herbal medicine and the modern world. They hope to inspire people to bring herbal medicine "out of the cupboard and onto the counter" in everyday life. That is why they have spent long hours creating a product line that embodies beauty, simplicity and the best quality ingredients. Urban Moonshine is deeply committed to being a socially and environmentally conscious company and makes every effort to support local farmers, cut back on waste and look for green alternatives in their everyday use of resources and packaging.

Urban Moonshine is Certified Organic by the Northeast Farming Association of Vermont (NOFA). They support local farmers by sourcing their ingredients locally whenever possible. They are also a member of United Plant Savers, American Herbal Products Association, NorthEast Herbal Association, and the American Herbalists Guild. Urban Moonshine is GMP compliant and takes great care in quality control and product safety.

Vitanica

http://vitanica.com

Phone: 800-572-4712
Address: P.O. Box 1299
Tualatin, OR 97062

Vitanica takes pride in their service and responsiveness to women's health. All of their products are formulated based on scientific research and/or clinical research and experience as conducted by Dr. Tori Hudson in her women's health practice. Dr. Hudson is a well-respected authority on natural healthcare for women.

Vitanica is committed to using the highest quality, premium grade organic or wildcrafted herbs available. Their herbs and extracts are selected on the basis of purity, bioactivity, and maximal therapeutic benefit. Their product line is run in small batches to ensure the freshest products possible, and the entire line uses vegetarian-friendly, plant-based capsules.

Western Botanicals

http://westernbotanicals.com

Phone: 800-651-4372
Address: 768 East 1950 North
Spanish Fork, UT 84660

Western Botanicals was established in 1996 with the goal of establishing an herbalist in every home. The company is staffed by health-minded individuals and licensed healthcare professionals. They believe that natural herbs are whole foods that build health, in contrast to chemicals designed to simply suppress symptoms. This is why they have built their business with the home herbalist in mind.

Western Botanicals purchases high quality organic and wildcrafted herbs available to ensure pesticide and herbicide free products. They are an organic certified manufacturer through Oregon Tilth and USDA. They are a GMP compliant facility and use HPTLC equipment to identify their raw materials, which are also tested for microbes and foreign materials.

White Flower

http://chineseherbsdirect.com/white-flower-m-45.html

Phone: 877-252-5436
Address: 2675 Skypark Dr., Suite 102
Torrance, CA 90505

This Chinese company makes a famous topical analgesic oil, which is imported into the United States and sold in many health food stores and other outlets.

Yerba Prima

http://yerba.com

Phone: 800-488-4339
Address: 740 Jefferson Avenue
Ashland, OR 97520

Yerba Prima specializes in high quality dietary fiber products, herbal products and internal cleansing/detoxification products. The company was founded in 1980 by a group of health conscious individuals in the San Francisco Bay Area who were learning about the benefits of internal cleansing. Yerba Prima pioneered the first whole body internal cleansing program and first natural dietary fiber line in the U.S. natural products market. After many years in Oakland, California, the company relocated in 1991 to a custom designed corporate office and manufacturing facility in Ashland, Oregon.

From the beginning, Yerba Prima has been dedicated to producing only the highest quality products. Their two primary goals in developing and marketing products are:

1. Products that really work, that provide real benefits for people, and

2. Products that are safe for people to use.

Because they are dedicated to ensuring that their products improve or maintain health, they are continually studying scientific research about herbs and dietary fiber

and they consult with leading researchers. This ensures that their products are based on what has been proven effective.

Manufacturing takes place in accordance with Good Manufacturing Practices (GMPs) that are stricter than normal industry standards to ensure the safety, purity and efficacy of all Yerba Prima products. Extensive testing is done at each step of the manufacturing process, beginning with testing of all incoming ingredients and packaging materials used in Yerba Prima products. Additional microbiological, chemical and physical tests take place during and after each manufacturing cycle to ensure product quality.

Yogi Tea

http://yogiproducts.com

Phone: 800-964-4832
Address: 950 International Way
Springfield, OR 97477

The story of Yogi tea began in 1969 when Yogi Bhajan, a teacher of holistic living, started teaching yoga in the West. He shared the wisdom and knowledge of Ayurveda and healthy living that he had mastered in India with his students while serving a specially spiced tea, which they affectionately named "Yogi Tea." In 1984 this blossomed into the Yogi Tea Company. Packages of the rough, dried spices began to appear in natural foods stores throughout Southern California. As demand increased, the spices were more finely ground, packaged and sealed into individual tea bags. By 1986, Yogi Tea was distributed nationwide.

The holistic teachings of Ayurveda and healthy living are the inspiration behind Yogi. They have continued to expand and evolve their tea blends to address specific health, creating specialized herbal formulas, blended for both flavor and purpose.

Karta Purkh Singh Khalsa, who has studied yoga and Ayurveda for over 40 years, and is currently the president of the American Herbalists Guild (AHG), formulates products for Yogi Tea in conjunction with their research and development team. Yogi Tea strives to support the health and well-being of their consumers by incorporating the highest-quality natural and organic ingredients in their teas.

To ensure consistency and quality, Yogi ingredients are meticulously reviewed and tested for insecticides, pesticides and heavy metals. Yogi Tea follows the USDA's National Organic Program (NOP) for all ingredients, and their facility is Organically Certified by Quality Assurance International (QAI), an independent third party organic certifier.

Yogi tea believes the purpose of business is to serve. It was founded on that belief and still uses it as in guiding principle: "Feel Good, Be Good, Do Good." The holistic teachings of Ayurveda and healthy living are the inspiration behind Yogi and are reflected in how they develop our products.

Zand

http://zand.com

Phone: 800-241-0859

Address: 1441 West Smith Road
Ferndale, WA 98248

Zand combines the best of American and European herbal medicine with the wisdom of traditional Chinese medicine. They embrace the principles of Traditional Chinese Medicine by developing formulas that address the whole body, not just the primary illness. These products are made using today's science and manufacturing technology. The company manufactures its products according to the highest nutraceutical standards, in a facility operating according to FDA pharmaceutical regulations. They are an NSF registered facility.

For over 25 years, Zand has been committed to supporting the herbal industry, herb growers and vendors with a commitment to organic, pesticide-free, sustainable agricultural practices, and long-term purchase and growing agreements. They believe these efforts help to ensure growth of the herbal supply chain, the quality of herbs for their products, and more importantly, help to maintain a healthy and balanced planet.

Company Abbreviations

These are the abbreviations we use to refer to a company's products in the Herbal Formula Index starting on the next page.

AV	A. Vogel
CR	Christopher's
CS	Celestial Seasonings
EI	Eclectic Institute
GH	Gaia Herbs
GH	Grandma's Herbs
H&A	Herbalist & Alchemist
HE	Herbs Etc.
HK	Herbs for Kids
HP	Herb Pharm
IN	Irwin Naturals
NA	Nature's Answer
NC	New Chapter
NF	NOW Foods
NSP	Nature's Sunshine Products
NW	Nature's Way
NWS	NatureWorks
OL	Olbas
PH	Planetary Herbals
RC	RidgeCrest Herbals
RL	Renew Life
SR	Solaray
TB	Tiger Balm
TL	Nature's Herbs (TwinLab)
TM	Traditional Medicinals
UM	Urban Moonshine
VT	Vitanica
WB	Western Botanicals
WF	White Flower
YP	Yerba Prima
YT	Yogi Tea
ZD	Zand

Herbal Formula Index

If you find an herbal formula and want to know what category it fits into, you can look it up here. This index tells you which product category or categories we've classified that formula under. We've also used a two-letter abbreviation for the company that makes it. A key to these abbreviations can be found on the previous page.

Bengal Spice (CS): *Carminative Formulas*

Berry DeTox (YT): *Blood Purifier Formulas*

Berry Enerji Green Tea Energy Shot (CS): *Energy-Boosting Formulas*

Berry Kombucha Energy Shot (CS): *Energy-Boosting Formulas*

Bilberry Complex (NF): *Vision Supporting Formulas*

Bilberry Extra Strength (YP): *Vision Supporting Formulas*

Bilberry Eye Complex (PH): *Vision Supporting Formulas*

Bilberry Eye Support Formula (CR): *Vision Supporting Formulas*

Bitters Compound (H&A): *Digestive Bitter Tonic Formulas*

Bitters Extra (VT): *Digestive Bitter Tonic and Digestive Enzyme Formulas*

Black Cohosh-Kava Kava (EI): *Analgesic and Antispasmodic Formulas*

Black Drawing Ointment (CR): *Drawing Salve Formulas*

Black Ointment (NSP): *Drawing Salve Formulas*

Black Walnut & Wormwood (NA): *Antiparasitic Formulas*

Black Walnut & Wormwood (NA): *Antiparasitic Formulas*

Black Walnut Complex (NA): *Antiparasitic Formulas*

Black Walnut-Wormwood G (EI): *Antiparasitic Formulas*

Black Walnut-Wormwood O (EI): *Antiparasitic Formulas*

Bladder Formula (CR): *Diuretic Formulas*

Bladdex (NA): *Urinary Infection Fighting Formulas*

Bloat-Away (IN): *Diuretic Formulas*

Blood Blend SP-11A (SR): *Blood Purifier Formulas*

Blood Circulation Formula (CR): *Cardiovascular Stimulant Formulas*

Blood Cleanser Phase I (GH): *General Detoxifying Formulas*

Blood Cleanser Phase II (GH): *General Detoxifying, Blood Purifier and Anticancer Formulas*

Blood Cleanser Phase III (GH): *General Detoxifying and Anticancer Formulas*

Blood Cleanser Phase IV (GH): *General Detoxifying and Blood Purifier Formulas*

Blood Cleansing Tea (WB): *Blood Purifier Formulas*

Blood Detox Formula (WB): *Blood Purifier Formulas*

Blood Pressure (GH): *Hypotensive Formulas*

Blood Pressure Formula (RC): *Hypotensive Formulas*

Blood Pressure Health (NF): *Hypotensive Formulas*

Blood Pressure Support (HP): *Hypotensive Formulas*

Blood Pressure Take Care (NC): *Hypotensive Formulas*

Blood Pressurex (NSP): *Hypotensive Formulas*

Blood Stream Formula (CR): *Blood Purifier Formulas*

Blood Sugar Balance (EI): *Blood Sugar Reducing Formulas*

Blood Sugar Balance (RC): *Hypoglycemic Formulas*

Blood Sugar Formula (NSP): *Blood Sugar Reducing Formulas*

Blood Sugar with Gymnema (NW): *Blood Sugar Reducing Formulas*

Blood Support (EI): *Blood Purifier Formulas*

Body Balance (GH): *Female Hormonal Balancing Formulas*

Body-Type Vata (IN): *Adaptogen Formulas*

Bone & Tissue Blend SP-34 (SR): *Mineral Formulas*

Bone, *Flesh & Cartilage (NW): Tissue Healing Formulas*

Bone/Skin Poultice (NSP): *Tissue Healing Formulas*

Bountiful Blend (WB): *Superfood Formulas*

Bowel Cleanse (RL): *Fiber Blend Formulas*

Bowel Detox (NSP): *General Detoxifying Formulas*

BP-X (NSP): *Blood Purifier Formulas*

Brain & Memory (HP): *Brain and Memory Tonic Formulas*

Brain Circulation Formula (WB): *Brain and Memory Tonic Formulas*

Brain Elevate (NF): *Brain and Memory Tonic Formulas*

Brain-Protex w/ Huperzine A (NSP): *Brain and Memory Tonic Formulas*

Brainstorm (NA): *Brain and Memory Tonic Formulas*

Breast Enhance (NSP): *Phytoestrogen Formulas*

Breath Tonic Peppermint (HP): *Carminative Formulas*

Breath Tonic Spearmint (HP): *Carminative Formulas*

Breathe Deep (YT): *Decongestant Formulas*

Breathe Easy (TM): *Decongestant Formulas*

Bronchial Blend SP-22 (SR): *Expectorant Formulas*

Bronchial Formula (NSP): *Lung and Respiratory Tonic Formulas*

Bronchial Wellness Herbal Syrup (GH): *Decongestant Formulas*

Bronchial Wellness Tea (GH): *Decongestant Formulas*

Bronchosan (AV): *Expectorant Formulas*

Broncitone (NA): *Decongestant and Cough Remedy Formulas*

Bubble-B-Gone (NA): *Carminative Formulas*

Buddy Bear Gentle Lax (RL): *Gentle Laxative Formulas*

Bug Itch Releaf (HE): *Anti-Itch Formulas*

Bupleurum Calmative Compound (PH): *Nerve Tonic Formulas*

Bupleurum Liver Cleanse (PH): *Liver Tonic Formulas*

Burdock/Red Root Compound (H&A): *Lymphatic Drainage and Blood Purifier Formulas*

Butterbur Extra (VT): *Migraine/Headache Formulas*

Butterbur with Feverfew (NF): *Migraine/Headache Formulas*

C Food Complex (NC): *Immune Stimulating Formulas*

C-C-C Cream (EI): *Topical Vulnerary Formulas*

C-X (NSP): *Female Hormonal Balancing Formulas*

Calm Breath (HP): *Bronchialdilator Formulas*

Calm Child (PH): *Brain Calming Formulas*

Calm Child Herbal Syrup (PH): *Brain Calming Formulas*

Calm Restore Herbal Drops (GH): *Relaxing Nervine Formulas*

Calm Waters (HP): *Kidney Tonic Formulas*

Calming (YT): *Relaxing Nervine Formulas*

Candida Clear (NF): *Antifungal Formulas*

Candida Digest (PH): *Digestive Tonic Formulas*

Candida Quick Cleanse (ZD): *Antifungal Formulas*

CandidaStat (VT): *Antifungal and Antibacterial Formulas*

CandiGONE (RL): *Antifungal Formulas*

Candistroy (IN): *Antifungal Formulas*

CapsiCool (NW): *Cardiovascular Stimulant Formulas*

Caramel Apple Spice Slim Life (YT): *Weight Loss Formulas*

Cardiaforce Tonic (AV): *Cardiac Tonic Formulas*

Cardio + (WB): *Hypotensive Formulas*

Cardio Assurance (NSP): *Cardiac Tonic Formulas*

Cardio Calmpound (H&A): *Hypotensive Formulas*

CardioBlend (VT): *Cardiovascular Stimulant Formulas*

CardioNutriv (NA): *Hypotensive Formulas*

Carminitive Compound (H&A): *Carminative Formulas*

Catnip & Fennel Extract (2 fl. oz.) (NSP): *Catnip & Fennel Formulas*

Cayenne & Garlic (NW): *Cardiovascular Stimulant Formulas*

Cayenne & Ginger (SR): *Cardiovascular Stimulant Formulas*

Cayenne Heat Massage Oil (CR): *Topical Analgesic Formulas*

Cayenne Ointment (CR): *Topical Analgesic Formulas*

Cayenne With Garlic (SR): *Cardiovascular Stimulant Formulas*

Celery Seed Extract (NF): *Vascular Tonic Formulas*

Cellular Blend SP-29 (SR): *General Detoxifying Formulas*

Chai Black (YT): *Carminative and Energy-Boosting Formulas*

Chai Green (YT): *Carminative Formulas*

Chai Rooibos (YT): *Carminative Formulas*

Chamomile - Catnip kid (EI): *Carminative Formulas*

Chamomile - Catnip O (EI): *Carminative Formulas*

Chamomile Calm (HK): *Relaxing Nervine Formulas*

Chamomile Sleep (PH): *Sleep Formulas*

Chamomile with Lavender (TM): *Relaxing Nervine Formulas*

Change-O-Life (NW): *Menopause Balancing Formulas*

Changes for Women AM/PM Formula (ZD): *Menopause Balancing Formulas*

Chaste Berry-Vitex Extract (NF): *Female Hormonal Balancing Formulas*

Cherry Bark Blend (HK): *Decongestant and Cough Remedy Formulas*

Chest Comfort (CR): *Cold and Flu Formulas*

Chest Rub (GH): *Decongestant Formulas*

Children's Herbal (HP): *Carminative, Relaxing Nervine and Cold and Flu Formulas*

Children's Winter Health (HP): *Cold and Flu Formulas*

Chocolate Smooth Move (TM): *Stimulant Laxative Formulas*

CholestBlend (VT): *Cholesterol Balancing Formulas*

Cholester-Reg II (NSP): *Cholesterol Balancing Formulas*

Cholesterol (GH): *Cholesterol Balancing Formulas*

Cholesterol Blend SP-31 (SR): *Fiber Blend Formulas*

Cholesterol Health (HP): *Cholesterol Balancing and Liver Tonic Formulas*

Cholesterol Maintenance (GH): *Cholesterol Balancing Formulas*

Cholesterol Support (NF): *Cholesterol Balancing Formulas*

CholestGar (PH): *Cholesterol Balancing Formulas*

Chronic Condition Skin Salve (GH): *Topical Vulnerary Formulas*

Cinnamon Apple Spice (CS): *Carminative Formulas*

Cinnamon Glucose Balance (PH): *Blood Sugar Reducing Formulas*

Circulation Blend SP-11B (SR): *Cardiovascular Stimulant Formulas*

Circulatory Support (EI): *Cardiac Tonic Formulas*

Citrus ENERJI Green Tea Energy Shot (CS): *Energy-Boosting Formulas*

Citrus Kombucha Energy Shot (CS): *Energy-Boosting Formulas*

CL-7 Formula (TL): *Moistening Lung/Cough Formulas*

Clarity Compound (H&A): *Brain and Memory Tonic Formulas*

Classic India Spice (YT): *Carminative Formulas*

Cleanse & Detox Tea (GH): *Blood Purifier and Cholagogue Formulas*

Cleanse Today (ZD): *Hepatoprotective and Liver Tonic Formulas*

CleanseMORE (RL): *Stimulant Laxative Formulas*

CleanseSMART (RL): *General Detoxifying Formulas*

Cleansing Fiber (ZD): *Fiber Blend Formulas*

Cleansing Laxative (ZD): *Stimulant Laxative Formulas*

Cleansing Support (EI): *Essiac Formulas*

ClearLungs Chest Rub (RC): *Decongestant Formulas*

ClearLungs Classic (RC): *Decongestant and Lung and Respiratory Tonic Formulas*

ClearLungs Extra Strength (RC): *Lung and Respiratory Tonic Formulas*

ClearLungs Liquid (RC): *Lung and Respiratory Tonic Formulas*

Cold Care P.M. (TM): *Antiviral and Cold and Flu Formulas*

Cold Season (YT): *Cold and Flu Formulas*

Cold Season Immune Formula (CR): *Cold and Flu Formulas*

Colon Blend SP-12 (SR): *Stimulant Laxative Formulas*

Colon Care Caps (YP): *Fiber Blend Formulas*

Colon Care Formula (YP): *Fiber Blend Formulas*

Colon Cleanse Formula (WB): *Stimulant Laxative Formulas*

Colon Cleanse Syrup (WB): *Stimulant Laxative Formulas*

Colon Comfort Formula (WB): *Intestinal Toning Formulas*

Colon Detox Formula (WB): *Fiber Blend Formulas*

Colon Motility Blend (VT): *Digestive Enzyme and Gentle Laxative Formulas*

Comfree Pepsin with Algin (SR): *Intestinal Toning Formulas*

Comfrey Compound (GH): *Topical Vulnerary Formulas*

Comfrey Ointment (CR): *Topical Vulnerary Formulas*

Comfrey/Calendula Ointment (H&A): *Topical Vulnerary Formulas*

Complete Cat's Claw Complex (PH): *Immune Stimulating Formulas*

Complete Tissue & Bone Formula (CR): *Tissue Healing Formulas*

Complete Tissue Massage Oil (CR): *Topical Vulnerary Formulas*

Complete Tissue Ointment (CR): *Topical Vulnerary Formulas*

Complete Tissue Repair Oil (WB): *Topical Vulnerary Formulas*

Complete Tissue Repair Syrup (WB): *Tissue Healing Formulas*

Compound Arnica Oil (H&A): *Topical Vulnerary and Topical Analgesic Formulas*

Compound Biotic (EI): *Antiviral Formulas*

Compound Elixir (EI): *Expectorant Formulas*

Compound Herbal Biotic (EI): *Antiviral Formulas*

Compound Herbal Elixir (EI): *Expectorant* and *Decongestant Formulas*

Compound Mullein Oil (H&A): *Ear Drop Formulas*

Congest Free (HE): *Sinus Decongestant Formulas*

Connective Tissue Tonic (HP): *Tissue Healing* and *Skin Healing Formulas*

Constipation Stop (RL): *Stimulant Laxative Formulas*

Continence with Flowtrol (SR): *Kidney Tonic Formulas*

Cool Cayenne (SR): *Cardiovascular Stimulant Formulas*

Cool Cayenne with Butcher's Broom (SR): *Vascular Tonic* and *Cardiovascular Stimulant Formulas*

Cordyceps Power CS-4 (PH): *Energy-Boosting* and *Exercise Formulas*

Cramp Bark Comfort (PH): *Menstrual Cramp Formulas*

Cramp Bark Extra (VT): *Menstrual Cramp Formulas*

Cramp ReLeaf (HE): *Antispasmodic Formulas*

Cran-Aid (TM): *Urinary Infection Fighting Formulas*

Cran-Bladder ReLeaf (HE): *Urinary Infection Fighting Formulas*

Cranberry Bladder Defense (PH): *Urinary Infection Fighting Formulas*

CranStat Extra (VT): *Urinary Infection Fighting Formulas*

Critical Liver Support (RL): *Liver Tonic Formulas*

D-Flame (NF): *Anti-Inflammatory Formulas*

Daily Fiber Caps (YP): *Fiber Blend Formulas*

Daily Fiber Formula (YP): *Fiber Blend Formulas*

Daily Gentle Cleanse (IN): *Hepatoprotective* and *Gentle Laxative Formulas*

Daily Multi-Detox (RL): *General Detoxifying Formulas*

Daily Prostate Defense (IN): *Prostate Formulas*

Damiana Male Potential (PH): *Male Glandular Tonic* and *Prostate Formulas*

Decaf India Spice Chai Tea (CS): *Carminative Formulas*

Decongest Herbal Formula (ZD): *Decongestant Formulas*

Deep Health (Deep Chi Builder) (HE): *Adaptogen* and *Immune Stimulating Formulas*

Deep Heat Oil (WB): *Topical Analgesic Formulas*

Deep Heat Ointment (WB): *Topical Vulnerary* and *Topical Analgesic Formulas*

Deep Liver Support (GH): *Immune Balancing Formulas*

Deep Muscle Massage (GH): *Topical Analgesic Formulas*

Deep Sleep (HE): *Sleep Formulas*

Defense System (GH): *General Detoxifying* and *Immune Stimulating Formulas*

Deliverease (GH): *Pre-Delivery Formulas*

Depression Formula (WB): *Antidepressant Formulas*

Deprezac (HE): *Antidepressant Formulas*

DermaCillin (HE): *Topical Antiseptic Formulas*

Dermal Health (HP): *Skin Healing Formulas*

DeTox (YT): *Blood Purifier Formulas*

Detox Blend SP-25 (SR): *Fiber Blend Formulas*

Detox Support (NF): *Blood Purifier Formulas*

Devil's Claw - Yucca (EI): *Joint Healing* and *Anti-Inflammatory Formulas*

DiarEASE (RL): *Anti-Diarrhea Formulas*

Diet Slim Tea (GH): *Weight Loss Formulas*

Diet-Slim (GH): *Weight Loss Formulas*

Digestion Aid Formula (WB): *Carminative Formulas*

Digestion Blend SP-27 (SR): *Carminative* and *Digestive Bitter Tonic Formulas*

Digestive Aid (AV): *Digestive Bitter Tonic Formulas*

Digestive Bitters (HP): *Digestive Bitter Tonic Formulas*

Digestive Bitters Tonic (4 fl. oz.) (NSP): *Digestive Bitter Tonic Formulas*

Digestive Comfort (PH): *Digestive Tonic Formulas*

Digestive Grape Bitters (PH): *Digestive Bitter Tonic Formulas*

Digestive Support (EI): *Digestive Bitter Tonic Formulas*

Dong Quai - Wild Yam (EI): *Female Hormonal Balancing* and *Menstrual Cramp Formulas*

Dong Quai Supreme (GH): *Female Hormonal Balancing Formulas*

Dong Quai with Damiana (SR): *Female Hormonal Balancing Formulas*

Dragon's Dream Ointment (H&A): *Topical Analgesic Formulas*

DreamOn (RC): *Sleep Formulas*

E & Selenium Food Complex (NC): *Antioxidant Formulas*

E-KID-nacea (NA): *Echinacea Blend Formulas*

E.P.B. (EI): *Echinacea Blend Formulas*

Ear & Nerve Formula (CR): *Antispasmodic Formulas*

Ear Drops (EI): *Ear Drop Formulas*

Ear Oil with Mullein & St. John's Wort (GH): *Ear Drop Formulas*

Early Alert (HE): *Antibacterial* and *Immune Stimulating Formulas*

Earth's Nutrition (WB): *Superfood Formulas*

Easy Now (TM): *Relaxing Nervine Formulas*

Eater's Digest (TM): *Carminative Formulas*

Eater's Digest Peppermint (TM): *Carminative Formulas*

Ech-Astragalus (EI): *Immune Stimulating Formulas*

Ech-Astragalus kid (EI): *Immune Stimulating Formulas*

Ech-Goldenseal (EI): *Goldenseal & Echinacea Formulas*

Ech-Goldenseal Spray (EI): *Goldenseal & Echinacea Formulas*

Ech-Goldenseal Spray (EI): *Topical Antiseptic Formulas*

Echinace (YP): *Echinacea Blend Formulas*

Echinacea & Goldenseal (NA): *Goldenseal & Echinacea Formulas*

Echinacea & Goldenseal Glycerite (NF): *Goldenseal & Echinacea Formulas*

Echinacea & Goldenseal Plus (NF): *Blood Purifier* and *Goldenseal & Echinacea Formulas*

Echinacea & Goldenseal Root (NA): *Goldenseal & Echinacea Formulas*

Echinacea 50/50 Ang./Purp. (NF): *Echinacea Blend Formulas*

Echinacea and *Elderberry (SR): Antiviral Formulas*

Echinacea Complex (NW): *Echinacea Blend Formulas*

Echinacea Defense Force (PH): *Immune Stimulating Formulas*

Echinacea Elder Herbal Syrup (TM): *Antiviral Formulas*

Echinacea Goldenseal (HP): *Antibacterial* and *Decongestant Formulas*

Echinacea Goldenseal (GH): *Goldenseal & Echinacea Formulas*

Echinacea Goldenseal Propolis Throat Spray (GH): *Topical Antiseptic Formulas*

Echinacea Goldenseal Supreme (GH): *Immune Stimulating* and *Goldenseal & Echinacea Formulas*

Echinacea Goldenseal Supreme, *Alcohol-Free (GH): Antibacterial Formulas*

Echinacea Goldenseal Supreme, *Extra-Stength (GH): Antibacterial Formulas*

Echinacea Immune Support (YT): *Immune Stimulating Formulas*

Echinacea Plus (TM): *Echinacea Blend Formulas*

Echinacea Plus Elderberry (TM): *Antiviral* and *Sudorific Formulas*

Echinacea Premium Blend (EI): *Echinacea Blend Formulas*

Echinacea Purpurea, *Angustifolia (SR): Echinacea Blend Formulas*

Echinacea Red Root Supreme (GH): *Lymphatic Drainage* and *Antibacterial Formulas*

Echinacea Root with Goldenseal Root (SR): *Goldenseal & Echinacea Formulas*

Echinacea Root with Vitamin C & Zinc (SR): *Cold* and *Flu Formulas*

Echinacea Supreme (GH): *Echinacea Blend Formulas*

Echinacea Supreme (GH): *Echinacea Blend Formulas*

Echinacea Supreme, *Extra-Strength (GH): Echinacea Blend Formulas*

Echinacea Triple Source (HE): *Echinacea Blend Formulas*

Echinacea-Astragalus (EI): *Immune Stimulating Formulas*

Echinacea-Elderberry Syrup (PH): *Antiviral* and *Cold* and *Flu Formulas*

Echinacea-Goldenseal (EI): *Goldenseal & Echinacea Formulas*

Echinacea-Goldenseal (EI): *Goldenseal & Echinacea Formulas*

Echinacea-Goldenseal (EI): *Goldenseal & Echinacea Formulas*

Echinacea-Goldenseal Liquid Extract (PH): *Goldenseal & Echinacea Formulas*

Echinacea-Goldenseal O (EI): *Goldenseal & Echinacea Formulas*

Echinacea-Goldenseal with Olive Leaf (PH): *Goldenseal & Echinacea Formulas*

Echinacea-Oregon Grape (EI): *Antibacterial* and *Immune Stimulating Formulas*

Echinacea–Goldenseal (NW): *Goldenseal & Echinacea Formulas*

Echinacea, *Astragalus & Reishi (NW): Immune Stimulating Formulas*

Echinacea/Astragalus (HK): *Antiviral Formulas*

Echinacea/Eyebright (HK): *Sinus Decongestant Formulas*

Echinacea/Golden Seal (NSP): *Goldenseal & Echinacea Formulas*

Echinacea/GoldenRoot Blackberry (HK): *Antibacterial Formulas*

Echinacea/GoldenRoot Orange (HK): *Antibacterial Formulas*

Echinacea/Goldenseal (WB): *Goldenseal & Echinacea Formulas*

Echinacea/Goldenseal Compound (H&A): *Goldenseal & Echinacea Formulas*

Egyptian Licorice Mint (YT): *Carminative Formulas*

Egyptian Licorice (YT): *Carminative Formulas*

Elderberry - Red Root (EI): *Antiviral Formulas*

Elderberry, *Zinc & Echinacea Syrup (NF): Antiviral* and *Cold* and *Flu Formulas*

Eldertussin Elderberry Syrup (HK): *Decongestant Formulas*

Emotional Relief (H&A): *Antidepressant Formulas*

Energizer Green Tea Ginger Tonic (NC): *Carminative* and *Energy-Boosting Formulas*

Energy Tonic (UM): *Adaptogen Formulas*

Energy Vitality (GH): *Energy-Boosting Formulas*

Erigeron/Cinnamon (HP): *Styptic/Hemostatic Formulas*

Essential Skin Care (WB): *Topical Vulnerary Formulas*

Essiac Formula (WB): *Essiac Formulas*

Essiac Tonic (HE): *Essiac Formulas*

EstroPause Menopause Support (IN): *Menopause Balancing Formulas*

EstroSoy (NW): *Phytoestrogen Formulas*

EstroSoy Plus (NW): *Phytoestrogen Formulas*

Estrotone (NC): *Female Hormonal Balancing Formulas*

EveryDay Detox (TM): *Hepatoprotective Formulas*

EveryDay Detox Lemon (TM): *Blood Purifier Formulas*

Ex-Stress (NW): *Relaxing Nervine Formulas*

Eye Blend SP-23 (SR): *Vision Supporting Formulas*

Eyebright Bayberry Supreme (GH): *Vision Supporting Formulas*

Eyebright-Plus (GH): *Vision Supporting Formulas*

False Unicorn & Lobelia (CR): *Female Hormonal Balancing Formulas*

Fast Lane Caffeinated Black Tea (CS): *Energy-Boosting Formulas*

Fat Grabbers (NSP): *Fiber Blend Formulas*

Feelin' Groovy Tea (NF): *Immune Stimulating Formulas*

Fem Rebalance (VT): *Female Hormonal Balancing Formulas*

Fem-Aid (GH): *Female Hormonal Balancing* and *Uterine Tonic Formulas*

Fem-Restore (GH): *Female Hormonal Balancing* and *Uterine Tonic Formulas*

Female Balance Formula (WB): *Female Hormonal Balancing Formulas*

Female Balance (NF): *Female Hormonal Balancing Formulas*

Female Caps (SR): *Female Hormonal Balancing Formulas*

Female Complex (NA): *Female Hormonal Balancing Formulas*

Female Hormone Blend SP-7C (SR): *Female Hormonal Balancing Formulas*

Female Libido Enhancer (GH): *Female Aphrodisiac Formulas*

Female Libido Tonic (HP): *Female Aphrodisiac Formulas*

Female Reproductive Formula (CR): *Female Hormonal Balancing Formulas*

Female Toner (TM): *Female Hormonal Balancing* and *Uterine Tonic Formulas*

Female Tonic Formula (CR): *Female Hormonal Balancing* and *Uterine Tonic Formulas*

Fenu-Thyme (NW): *Sinus Decongestant Formulas*

Fenugreek & Thyme (NF): *Sinus Decongestant Formulas*

Fenugreek-Thyme (TL): *Sinus Decongestant Formulas*

Fertility Blend SP-1 (SR): *Male Glandular Tonic* and *Female Hormonal Balancing Formulas*

Feverfew - Guarana (EI): *Migraine/Headache Formulas*

Feverfew Head Aid (PH): *Migraine/Headache Formulas*

Feverfew Jamaican Dogwood Supreme (GH): *Analgesic Formulas*

Fiber Plus Caps (YP): *Stimulant Laxative Formulas*

Fiber Plus Powder (YP): *Fiber Blend* and *Stimulant Laxative Formulas*

Fiber Smart (RL): *Fiber Blend Formulas*

Fiber-Tastic (RL): *Fiber Blend Formulas*

First Cleanse (RL): *General Detoxifying Formulas*

Fitness Formula (H&A): *Exercise Formulas*

Flex-Ability (PH): *Joint Healing Formulas*

Flex-Ability (PH): *Joint Healing Formulas*

Flexible Joint (HP): *Joint Healing Formulas*

Flu and *Virus Formula (WB): Cold* and *Flu Formulas*

Flush & Be Fit (RL): *General Detoxifying Formulas*

Focus Formula (H&A): *Brain Calming Formulas*

Fresh Breath (GH): *Topical Antiseptic Formulas*

Fresh Green Black Walnut Wormwood Complex (NF): *Antiparasitic Formulas*

Friar's Balsam (HP): *Topical Antiseptic Formulas*

Full Moon-Women's Anti-Spasmodic (H&A): *Menstrual Cramp Formulas*

Full Tilt Tea (NF): *Energy-Boosting Formulas*

Fungus Fighter (HP): *Antifungal Formulas*

GABA Ease (VT): *Sleep Formulas*

GaiaKid's Sniffle Support Herbal Drops (GH): *Antiviral* and *Sinus Decongestant Formulas*

GaiaKids Cough Syrup for Dry Coughs (GH): *Moistening Lung/Cough Formulas*

GaiaKids Cough Syrup for Wet Coughs (GH): *Drying Cough/Lung Formulas*

GaiaKids Cough Syrup with Honey & Lemon (GH): *Decongestant* and *Cough Remedy Formulas*

GaiaKids Ear Drops (GH): *Ear Drop Formulas*

GaiaKids Echinacea Goldenseal (GH): *Goldenseal & Echinacea Formulas*

GaiaKids Kids Defense Herbal Drops (GH): *Immune Stimulating Formulas*

GaiaKids Sleep & Relax Herbal Syrup (GH): *Relaxing Nervine Formulas*

GaiaKids Tummy Tonic Herbal Drops (GH): *Carminative Formulas*

GaiaKids Warming Chest Rub (GH): *Topical Analgesic Formulas*

Gall Bladder Formula (NSP): *Carminative Formulas*

Garlic & Parsley (NW): *Cardiovascular Stimulant Formulas*

Garlic and *Parsley (SR): Cardiovascular Stimulant Formulas*

Garlic Super Complex (NA): *Cardiovascular Stimulant Formulas*

GarliCare with Cool Cayenne (SR): *Cardiovascular Stimulant Formulas*

Garlicin HC (NW): *Cardiac Tonic Formulas*

Garlicin CF (NW): *Antibacterial Formulas*

Gas & Bloating (GH): *Carminative Formulas*

Gas & Bloating Tea (GH): *Carminative Formulas*

Gas Relief (TM): *Carminative Formulas*

Gas-Eze (CR): *Carminative* and *Digestive Enzyme Formulas*

Gastritix (NW): *Carminative Formulas*

Gastro Calm (HP): *Carminative Formulas*

Gastro Health Concentrate (NSP): *Ulcer Healing Formulas*

Gentian-Angelica Bitters (EI): *Digestive Bitter Tonic Formulas*

Gentle-Man (H&A): *Male Glandular Tonic* and *Nerve Tonic Formulas*

Gentlelax (H&A): *Stimulant Laxative Formulas*

GI Blend SP-20 (SR): *Digestive Bitter Tonic Formulas*

Ginger (YT): *Carminative Formulas*

Ginger Aid (TM): *Carminative Formulas*

Ginger Supreme (GH): *Anti-Inflammatory Formulas*

Ginger Warming Compound (PH): *Cardiovascular Stimulant* and *Cold* and *Flu Formulas*

Ginger Yerba Maté (TM): *Energy-Boosting Formulas*

Ginkgo - Gotu Kola (EI): *Brain* and *Memory Tonic Formulas*

Ginkgo - Gotu Kola (EI): *Brain* and *Memory Tonic Formulas*

Ginkgo & Hawthorn Combination (NSP): *Cardiovascular Stimulant Formulas*

Ginkgo Awareness (PH): *Brain* and *Memory Tonic Formulas*

Ginkgo Biloba Extract (NF): *Brain* and *Memory Tonic Formulas*

Ginkgo Clarity (YT): *Brain* and *Memory Tonic Formulas*

Ginkgo Extra Strength (YP): *Brain* and *Memory Tonic Formulas*

Ginkgo Gotu Kola Supreme (GH): *Brain* and *Memory Tonic Formulas*

Ginkgo/Horse Chestnut Compound (H&A): *Vascular Tonic Formulas*

Ginkgold Eyes (NW): *Vision Supporting Formulas*

Ginseng (Siberian) and *Gotu Kola (SR): Brain* and *Memory Tonic Formulas*

Ginseng & Royal Jelly (NF): *Energy-Boosting Formulas*

Ginseng and *Damiana (SR): Male Aphrodisiac* and *Adaptogen Formulas*

Ginseng Classic (PH): *Energy-Boosting Formulas*

Ginseng Elixir (PH): *Digestive Tonic Formulas*

Ginseng Plus Formula (WB): *Adrenal Tonic Formulas*

Ginseng Revitalizer (PH): *Digestive Tonic Formulas*

Ginseng Schisandra Supreme (GH): *Adaptogen Formulas*

Ginseng Supreme (GH): *Adaptogen Formulas*

Ginseng Vitality (YT): *Energy-Boosting* and *Adaptogen Formulas*

Ginseng/Schisandra Compound (H&A): *Adaptogen Formulas*

Ginza-Plus (IN): *Adaptogen Formulas*

Glandular System Formula (CR): *Lymphatic Drainage* and *Bronchialdilator Formulas*

Glandular System Massage Oil (CR): *Lymphatic Drainage* and *Ear Drop Formulas*

GlucoCut Blend Sp-5 (SR): *Blood Sugar Reducing* and *Diuretic Formulas*

Glucosamine-MSM Herbal (PH): *Joint Healing Formulas*

Glycemic Health (GH): *Blood Sugar Reducing Formulas*

Go With The Flow Tea (NF): *Diuretic Formulas*

Golden Ginger (TM): *Carminative Formulas*

Goldenseal - Propolis Cream (EI): *Topical Antiseptic Formulas*

Good Mood (HP): *Antidepressant Formulas*

Green Memory (EI): *Brain* and *Memory Tonic Formulas*

Green PhytoFoods (NF): *Superfood Formulas*

Green Tea Blueberry Slim Life (YT): *Weight Loss Formulas*

Green Tea Energy (YT): *Energy-Boosting* and *Antioxidant Formulas*

Green Tea Goji Berry (YT): *Antioxidant Formulas*

Green Tea Kombucha (YT): *Antioxidant Formulas*

Green Tea Kombucha Decaf (YT): *Antioxidant Formulas*

Green Tea Lemon Ginger (YT): *Carminative Formulas*

Green Tea Muscle Recovery (YT): *Exercise Formulas*

Green Tea Pomegranate (YT): *Antioxidant Formulas*

Green Tea Rejuvenation (YT): *Antioxidant Formulas*

Green Tea Slim Life (YT): *Weight Loss Formulas*

Green Tea Super Antioxidant (YT): *Antioxidant Formulas*

Green Tea Triple Echinacea (YT): *Echinacea Blend Formulas*

Green Tea with Ginger (TM): *Carminative Formulas*

Grief Relief Compound (H&A): *Antidepressant Formulas*

Guggul Cholesterol Compound (PH): *Cholesterol Balancing Formulas*

Gum-omile Oil (HK): *Topical Analgesic Formulas*

Gypsy Cold Care (TM): *Cold* and *Flu* and *Sudorific Formulas*

Hair & Skin (NW): *Mineral Formulas*

Hair Blend SP-38 (SR): *Mineral Formulas*

Hair, *Skin & Nail Support (GH): Mineral Formulas*

Happy Colon (WB): *Stimulant Laxative Formulas*

HAS Original Blend (NW): *Sinus Decongestant* and *Decongestant Formulas*

Hawthorn - Cactus (EI): *Cardiac Tonic Formulas*

Hawthorn Berry Syrup (WB): *Cardiac Tonic Formulas*

Hawthorn Heart (PH): *Cardiac Tonic Formulas*

Hawthorn Plus Extractacap (NA): *Cardiac Tonic Formulas*

HB Pressure Tonic (HE): *Hypotensive Formulas*

Head Soother (HP): *Migraine/Headache Formulas*

Headache Formula (WB): *Migraine/Headache Formulas*

Headache Take Care (NC): *Migraine/Headache Formulas*

Heal (GH): *Tissue Healing Formulas*

Healthy Fasting (YT): *Hypoglycemic Formulas*

Healthy Heart Compound (H&A): *Cardiac Tonic Formulas*

Healthy Kid's Compound (H&A): *Antiviral* and *Antibacterial Formulas*

Healthy Menopause Tonic (HP): *Menopause Balancing Formulas*

Healthy Prostate Tonic (HP): *Prostate Formulas*

Healthy Skin Tonic (H&A): *Skin Healing Formulas*

Healthy Veins Tonic (HP): *Vascular Tonic Formulas*

Heart & Circulatory Health Capsules (AV): *Cardiovascular Stimulant Formulas*

Heart Blend SP-8 (SR): *Cardiac Tonic Formulas*

Heart Caps (SR): *Cardiac Tonic Formulas*

Heart Formula (WB): *Cardiac Tonic Formulas*

Heart Health (HP): *Cardiac Tonic Formulas*

Heart Plus (GH): *Cardiac Tonic Formulas*

Heart Tea (TM): *Cardiac Tonic Formulas*

Heavy Mineral Bugleweed Formula (CR): *Heavy Metal Cleansing Formulas*

HepaFem (VT): *Blood Purifier* and *Cholagogue Formulas*

Herb Cough Elixir (EI): *Expectorant* and *Cough Remedy Formulas*

Herb Pharm Original Salve (HP): *Topical Vulnerary Formulas*

Herb-Cal (H&A): *Mineral Formulas*

Herba Tussin (TM): *Decongestant* and *Cough Remedy Formulas*

Herba Tussin Herbal Syrup (TM): *Decongestant* and *Cough Remedy Formulas*

Herbal Antiseptic (WB): *Topical Antiseptic Formulas*

Herbal Biotic (EI): *Antiviral Formulas*

Herbal Calcium (WB): *Mineral Formulas*

Herbal Calcium Formula (CR): *Mineral Formulas*

Herbal Colon Cleanser & Tonic (GH): *Stimulant Laxative Formulas*

Herbal Cough Syrup (CR): *Expectorant* and *Cough Remedy Formulas*

Herbal Cough Syrup (WB): *Moistening Lung/Cough Formulas*

Herbal Detox (HP): *Antibacterial, Blood Purifier* and *Anticancer Formulas*

Herbal Digest Tea (GH): *Digestive Bitter Tonic Formulas*

Herbal Diuretic (GH): *Diuretic Formulas*

Herbal Ear Drops (WB): *Ear Drop Formulas*

Herbal Eyebright (CR): *Sinus Decongestant* and *Eye Wash Formulas*

Herbal Eyebright Formula (WB): *Vision Supporting Formulas*

Herbal Eyewash Formula with Cayenne Pepper (WB): *Eye Wash Formulas*

Herbal Eyewash Formula without Cayenne Pepper (WB): *Eye Wash Formulas*

Herbal Guard (YP): *Gentle Laxative Formulas*

Herbal Iron Formula (CR): *Iron Formulas*

Herbal Iron Yeast Free (NWS): *Iron Formulas*

Herbal Libido Formula (CR): *Male Aphrodisiac* and *Female Aphrodisiac Formulas*

Herbal Mouthwash Concentrate (WB): *Topical Antiseptic Formulas*

Herbal Parasite Syrup (CR): *Antiparasitic Formulas*

Herbal Pause w/Estro G-100 (NF): *Menopause Balancing Formulas*

Herbal Respiratory Relief (HP): *Decongestant Formulas*

Herbal Snuff Powder (WB): *Decongestant Formulas*

Herbal Super Tonic (WB): *Expectorant* and *Cardiovascular Stimulant Formulas*

Herbal Throat Spray (WB): *Topical Vulnerary Formulas*

Herbal Thyroid Formula (CR): *Energy-Boosting* and *Hypothyroid Formulas*

Herbal Tooth & Gum Powder (CR): *Dental Health Formulas*

Herbal Tooth Powder (WB): *Dental Health Formulas*

HerbalMist (ZD): *Antiviral* and *Antibacterial Formulas*

Herbaprofen (HE): *Analgesic Formulas*

Himalayan Apple Spice (YT): *Carminative Formulas*

Hinga Shtak (PH): *Digestive Tonic Formulas*

Histamine Blend SP-33 (SR): *Expectorant* and *Allergy-Reducing Formulas*

Honey Lavender Stress Relief (YT): *Relaxing Nervine Formulas*

Honey Lemon Ginseng Green Tea (CS): *Energy-Boosting Formulas*

Honey Lemon Throat Comfort (YT): *Expectorant Formulas*

Honey Vanilla White Tea Chai Tea (CS): *Carminative* and *Cardiovascular Stimulant Formulas*

Horehound Blend (HK): *Expectorant* and *Moistening Lung/Cough Formulas*

Hormonal Changease Formula (CR): *Menopause Balancing Formulas*

Horse Chestnut Cream (PH): *Vascular Tonic Formulas*

Horse Chestnut Vein Strength (PH): *Vascular Tonic Formulas*

Hoxsey Red Clover Supreme (GH): *Anticancer Formulas*

HRT Companion (VT): *Female Hormonal Balancing* and *Phytoestrogen Formulas*

HS II (NSP): *Cardiac Tonic Formulas*

Huckleberry - Devil's Club (EI): *Blood Sugar Reducing Formulas*

HY-A (NSP): *Hypoglycemic Formulas*

Immuboost Blend SP-21 (SR): *Antibacterial Formulas*

Immucalm (CR): *Immune Balancing Formulas*

Immune Adapt Caps (H&A): *Immune Balancing Formulas*

Immune Adapt (H&A): *Immune Balancing Formulas*

Immune Balance Compound (H&A): *Immune Balancing Formulas*

Immune Boost (NA): *Antibacterial* and *Immune Stimulating Formulas*

Immune Boost (IN): *Immune Stimulating Formulas*

Immune Boost Formula (WB): *Immune Stimulating Formulas*

Immune Boost Syrup (WB): *Immune Stimulating Formulas*

Immune Defense (HP): *Immune Stimulating Formulas*

Immune Enhancer (GH): *Immune Stimulating Formulas*

Immune Renew (NF): *Immune Balancing Formulas*

Immune Stimulator (NSP): *Mushroom Blend Formulas*

Immune Support (EI): *Antiviral Formulas*

Immune Support Echinacea Ginger Tonic (NC): *Antibacterial Formulas*

Immune Symmetry (VT): *Immune Stimulating Formulas*

Immune System Formula (CR): *Immune Stimulating Formulas*

Immune Tonic (UM): *Immune Balancing Formulas*

Immune Zoom (UM): *Immune Stimulating Formulas*

Immune-Virus Tea (WB): *Blood Purifier* and *Anticancer Formulas*

ImmuneAttack (HP): *Antibacterial Formulas*

Immuno-Shield All Season Wellness (IN): *Immune Stimulating Formulas*

ImmunoBoost (HE): *Immune Stimulating Formulas*

Immunotonic (NA): *Immune Balancing Formulas*

ImmuTain SP-40 (SR): *Immune Balancing Formulas*

IN-X (NSP): *Antibacterial Formulas*

India Spice Chai Tea (CS): *Carminative* and *Cardiovascular Stimulant Formulas*

Indigestion STOP (RL): *Digestive Enzyme Formulas*

Infection Formula (CR): *Antibacterial Formulas*

Infla-Profen (GH): *Joint Healing* and *Anti-Inflammatory Formulas*

Inflama-Care (PH): *Analgesic* and *Anti-Inflammatory Formulas*

Inflama-Dyne (NA): *Anti-Inflammatory Formulas*

Inflamma Response (HP): *Analgesic* and *Anti-Inflammatory Formulas*

Insight Compound (H&A): *Vision Supporting Formulas*

Insure Immune Support (ZD): *Antibacterial Formulas*

Insure Organic Immune Support Unflv (ZD): *Antibacterial Formulas*

Internal Cleanse & Detox (IN): *Intestinal Toning Formulas*

Intestinal Blend SP-24 (SR): *Antiparasitic Formulas*

Intestinal Bowel Soother (RL): *Intestinal Toning Formulas*

Intestinal Bowel Support (RL): *Intestinal Toning Formulas*

Intestinal Calmpound (H&A): *Intestinal Toning Formulas*

Intestinal Soothe & Build (NSP): *Intestinal Toning Formulas*

Intestinal Support (EI): *Antiparasitic Formulas*

Intestinal Tract Defense (HP): *Antiparasitic Formulas*

IntestiNew (RL): *Intestinal Toning Formulas*

Iron Extract (H&A): *Iron Formulas*

Iron Extra (VT): *Iron Formulas*

Itch Ointment (CR): *Anti-Itch Formulas*

Ivy Itch ReLeaf (HE): *Topical Vulnerary* and *Anti-Itch Formulas*

J. Kloss Anti-Spasmodic Compound (H&A): *Antispasmodic Formulas*

Jammin' Lemon Ginger Herbal Tea (CS): *Carminative Formulas*

Joint & Muscle Warming Rub (HP): *Topical Analgesic Formulas*

Joint Blend SP-2 (SR): *Joint Healing Formulas*

Joint Comfort (YT): *Joint Healing Formulas*

Joint Formula (CR): *Joint Healing Formulas*

Joint Health (GH): *Joint Healing* and *Anti-Inflammatory Formulas*

Joint Relief Formula (WB): *Joint Healing Formulas*

Joy Tonic (UM): *Relaxing Nervine Formulas*

Juniper Berry Combination (TL): *Diuretic Formulas*

Jurassic Green (CR): *Superfood Formulas*

"Just for Kids" Cold Care (TM): *Cold* and *Flu* and *Sudorific Formulas*

"Just for Kids" Nighty Night (TM): *Relaxing Nervine* and *Sleep Formulas*

"Just for Kids" Throat Coat (TM): *Expectorant Formulas*

"Just for Kids" Tummy Comfort (TM): *Carminative Formulas*

Kalenite Cleansing Herbs (YP): *General Detoxifying Formulas*

Kava Cool Complex (HE): *Relaxing Nervine Formulas*

Kava Kava - Calif. Poppy (EI): *Relaxing Nervine Formulas*

Kava Stress Relief (YT): *Relaxing Nervine Formulas*

Kick Back Tea (NF): *Relaxing Nervine Formulas*

Kick-It (GH): *Quit Smoking Formulas*

Kid-e-Calc (GH): *Mineral Formulas*

Kid-e-Calc (CR): *Mineral Formulas*

Kid-e-Col (GH): *Catnip & Fennel Formulas*

Kid-e-Col (CR): *Catnip & Fennel Formulas*

Kid-e-Dry (CR): *Kidney Tonic Formulas*

Kid-e-Mins (GH): *Mineral* and *Superfood Formulas*

Kid-e-Reg (GH): *Gentle Laxative Formulas*

Kid-e-Reg (CR): *Gentle Laxative Formulas*

Kid-e-Soothe (GH): *Immune Balancing Formulas*

Kid-e-Soothe (CR): *Moistening Lung/Cough Formulas*

Kid-e-Trac (GH): *Brain Calming Formulas*

Kid-e-Trac (CR): *Relaxing Nervine Formulas*

Kid-e-Well (CR): *Cold* and *Flu* and *Sudorific Formulas*

Kid's Calmpound Glycerite (H&A): *Relaxing Nervine, Brain Calming* and *Nerve Tonic Formulas*

Kid's Tummy Relief (H&A): *Carminative Formulas*

Kidalin (HE): *Brain Calming Formulas*

KidLAX (RL): *Gentle Laxative Formulas*

Kidney (GH): *Diuretic Formulas*

Kidney Bladder Complex (AV): *Kidney Tonic Formulas*

Kidney Blend SP-6 (SR): *Diuretic Formulas*

Kidney Caps (SR): *Kidney Tonic Formulas*

Kidney Formula (CR): *Diuretic Formulas*

Kidney Support Compound (H&A): *Kidney Tonic Formulas*

Kidney Tonic (HE): *Kidney Tonic Formulas*

Kidney-Bladder (NW): *Diuretic Formulas*

Kidney/Bladder Formula (WB): *Diuretic Formulas*

Kidney/Bladder Formula/Tea Combo (WB): *Diuretic* and *Lithotriptic Formulas*

Kidney/Bladder Tea (WB): *Diuretic* and *Lithotriptic Formulas*

KidneyAid (RC): *Kidney Tonic Formulas*

Kids Insure Herbal Formula Orange-Banana (ZD): *Antibacterial Formulas*

Kids Insure Herbal Formula Raspberry (ZD): *Antibacterial Formulas*

Kids' Immune Protect (PH): *Immune Stimulating Formulas*

Kokoro EstroHerb Cream (GH): *Phytoestrogen Formulas*

Kudzu Recovery (PH): *Anti-Alcoholic Formulas*

Kudzu/St.John's Wort (NSP): *Anti-Alcoholic Formulas*

Lactation Support (GH): *Nursing Aid Formulas*

Lactation Support Tea (GH): *Nursing Aid Formulas*

Lactation Tea (WB): *Nursing Aid Formulas*

LactationBlend (VT): *Nursing Aid Formulas*

LaxaBlend (VT): *Stimulant Laxative Formulas*

LaxaTea Wellness Tea (CS): *Stimulant Laxative Formulas*

Leg Veins with Tru-OPCs (NW): *Vascular Tonic Formulas*

Legendary Intestinal Cleanser and *Tonifier (PH): Gentle Laxative Formulas*

Lemon Echinacea Throat Coat (TM): *Lung* and *Respiratory Tonic Formulas*

Lemon Ginger (YT): *Carminative Formulas*

LifeShield Breathe (NC): *Mushroom Blend Formulas*

LifeShield Immunity (NC): *Mushroom Blend Formulas*

LifeShield Liver Force (NC): *Mushroom Blend Formulas*

LifeShield Mind Force (NC): *Mushroom Blend Formulas*

Liniment (TB): *Topical Analgesic Formulas*

Liv-Cleanse Formula (YP): *Hepatoprotective Formulas*

Liver (GH): *Blood Purifier Formulas*

Liver & Gall Bladder Formula (CR): *Cholagogue Formulas*

Liver Blend SP-13 (SR): *Cholagogue Formulas*

Liver Caps (SR): *Hepatoprotective Formulas*

Liver Cleanse (GH): *Blood Purifier* and *Liver Tonic Formulas*

Liver Defense (PH): *Liver Tonic Formulas*

Liver Detox (RL): *Liver Tonic Formulas*

Liver Detox Tea (WB): *Blood Purifier Formulas*

Liver Detoxifier & Regenerator (NF): *Liver Tonic Formulas*

Liver Gallbladder Drops (AV): *Cholagogue Formulas*

Liver Gallbladder Tablets (AV): *Hepatoprotective Formulas*

Liver Health (HP): *Liver Tonic Formulas*

Liver Health (GH): *Hepatoprotective Formulas*

Liver Support (EI): *Liver Tonic Formulas*

Liver Support (NA): *Blood Purifier* and *Liver Tonic Formulas*

Liver Support (NA): *Liver Tonic Formulas*

Liver Take Care (NC): *Hepatoprotective* and *Heavy Metal Cleansing Formulas*

Liver Tone (NA): *Liver Tonic Formulas*

Liver Tonic (HE): *Cholagogue Formulas*

Liver Transition Formula (CR): *Liver Tonic Formulas*

Liver/Gallbladder Formula (WB): *Blood Purifier Formulas*

Liver/Gallbladder Formula/Tea Combo (WB): *Hepatoprotective* and *Cholagogue Formulas*

LiverClean (RC): *Cholagogue Formulas*

Lobelia/Skunk Cabbage (HP): *Antispasmodic* and *Bronchialdilator Formulas*

Lomatium - Osha (EI): *Antiviral Formulas*

Lomatium - Osha Spray (EI): *Antiviral Formulas*

Lomatium & St. John's Wort (NA): *Antiviral Formulas*

Loquat Respiratory Syrup (PH): *Expectorant* and *Moistening Lung/ Cough Formulas*

Loquat Respiratory Syrup for Kids (PH): *Decongestant* and *Moistening Lung/Cough Formulas*

Love Your Heart (RL): *Cardiac Tonic Formulas*

Loviral (HE): *Antiviral Formulas*

Lower Back Support (PH): *Joint Healing Formulas*

Lower Bowel Formula (CR): *Stimulant Laxative Formulas*

Luminous (VT): *Mineral Formulas*

Lung & Bronchial Formula (CR): *Lung* and *Respiratory Tonic* and *Moistening Lung/Cough Formulas*

Lung Caps (SR): *Expectorant* and *Moistening Lung/Cough Formulas*

Lung Relief Antispasmodic Compound (H&A): *Expectorant* and *Bronchialdilator Formulas*

Lung Relief Cold/Damp Compound (H&A): *Decongestant* and *Drying Cough/Lung Formulas*

Lung Relief Cold/Dry Compound (H&A): *Lung* and *Respiratory Tonic* and *Moistening Lung/Cough Formulas*

Lung Relief Hot/Damp Compound (H&A): *Drying Cough/Lung Formulas*

Lung Relief Hot/Dry Compound (H&A): *Moistening Lung/Cough Formulas*

Lung Support (EI): *Decongestant* and *Bronchialdilator Formulas*

Lung Tonic (HE): *Expectorant* and *Lung* and *Respiratory Tonic Formulas*

Lungs Plus Formula (WB): *Decongestant* and *Drying Cough/Lung Formulas*

LycoPom (NC): *Prostate* and *Antioxidant Formulas*

Lymph Gland Cleanse (NSP): *Lymphatic Drainage* and *Antibacterial Formulas*

Lymph Gland Cleanse-HY (NSP): *Lymphatic Drainage* and *Antibacterial Formulas*

Lymphatic Drainage (NSP): *Lymphatic Drainage Formulas*

Lymphatonic (HE): *Lymphatic Drainage* and *Antibacterial Formulas*

Lysine Extra (VT): *Antiviral Formulas*

Maitake (EI): *Mushroom Blend Formulas*

Male Caps (SR): *Male Glandular Tonic Formulas*

Male Complex (NA): *Male Aphrodisiac Formulas*

Male Formula (EI): *Male Aphrodisiac Formulas*

Male Libido (GH): *Male Glandular Tonic* and *Male Aphrodisiac Formulas*

Male Libido Enhancer (GH): *Male Aphrodisiac Formulas*

Male Sexual Vitality (HP): *Male Glandular Tonic Formulas*

Male Stamina Blend Sp-15B (SR): *Male Aphrodisiac Formulas*

Male Tonic Formula (CR): *Male Glandular Tonic Formulas*

Male Urinary Tract Formula (CR): *Diuretic* and *Prostate Formulas*

Master Gland Formula (CR): *Brain* and *Memory Tonic Formulas*

Maternal Symmetry (VT): *Pregnancy Tonic* and *Uterine Tonic Formulas*

Mayan Cocoa Spice (YT): *Carminative Formulas*

Melissa Ointment (WB): *Topical Vulnerary Formulas*

Melissa Supreme, *Alcohol-free* (GH): *Relaxing Nervine Formulas*

Memory (GH): *Brain* and *Memory Tonic Formulas*

Memory Blend SP-30 (SR): *Brain* and *Memory Tonic Formulas*

Memory Plus Formula (CR): *Brain* and *Memory Tonic Formulas*

Men's Formula (H&A): *Male Glandular Tonic Formulas*

Men's Prostate Tonic (H&A): *Prostate Formulas*

Men's Rebuild Internal Cleansing System (YP): *General Detoxifying Formulas*

Men's Rebuild (YP): *Male Glandular Tonic Formulas*

Men's Virility Power (NF): *Male Aphrodisiac Formulas*

MenoChange (PH): *Menopause Balancing Formulas*

Menopause (GH): *Menopause Balancing Formulas*

Menopause Support (EI): *Menopause Balancing* and *Phytoestrogen Formulas*

Menopause Support (NF): *Menopause Balancing Formulas*

Menopautonic (HE): *Menopause Balancing Formulas*

Menstrual Blend SP-7B (SR): *Styptic/Hemostatic* and *Uterine Tonic Formulas*

Menstrual Relief Hormone Balance (IN): *PMS Relieving Formulas*

Mental Alertness (GH): *Brain* and *Memory Tonic Formulas*

MERC-Free Cleanse (RL): *Heavy Metal Cleansing Formulas*

Metabo Balance Wellness Tea (CS): *Weight Loss Formulas*

Metabolic Blend SP-18 (SR): *Weight Loss Formulas*

Metaburn Herbal Weight Formula (CR): *Weight Loss Formulas*

Migra-Free (HE): *Migraine/Headache Formulas*

Migraine Relief (RC): *Migraine/Headache Formulas*

Milk Thistle Extra Strength (YP): *Hepatoprotective Formulas*

Milk Thistle Liver Cleanse (IN): *Hepatoprotective* and *Cholagogue Formulas*

Milk Thistle Yellow Dock Supreme (GH): *Blood Purifier Formulas*

Milk Thistle-Dandelion (EI): *Hepatoprotective Formulas*

MindBlend (VT): *Brain* and *Memory Tonic Formulas*

MindTrac (CR): *Brain* and *Memory Tonic Formulas*

Mint Magic (CS): *Carminative Formulas*

Minty Ginger (HK): *Carminative Formulas*

Mood Aid (NW): *Antidepressant Formulas*

Mood Balance (EI): *Antidepressant Formulas*

Mood Blend SP-39 (SR): *Antidepressant Formulas*

Moroccan Pomegranate Rooibos Tea (CS): *Antioxidant Formulas*

Mother's Lactation (HP): *Nursing Aid Formulas*

Mother's Milk (TM): *Nursing Aid Formulas*

Mother's Tea (WB): *Pregnancy Tonic Formulas*

Motherwort - Black Cohosh G (EI): *Female Hormonal Balancing Formulas*

Motherwort - Black Cohosh O (EI): *Female Hormonal Balancing Formulas*

Mouth Tonic (HE): *Topical Antiseptic* and *Dental Health Formulas*

Mullein Lung Complex (PH): *Decongestant* and *Lung* and *Respiratory Tonic Formulas*

Mullein/Garlic (HP): *Ear Drop* and *Antibacterial Formulas*

Mullein/Garlic Ear Drops (HE): *Ear Drop Formulas*

Multi Gland Caps for Men (SR): *Male Glandular Tonic Formulas*

Multi Gland Caps for Women (SR): *Female Hormonal Balancing Formulas*

Multi-Fiber Cleanse (IN): *General Detoxifying Formulas*

Muscle Pain Relief Spray (CR): *Topical Analgesic Formulas*

Muscle Rub (TB): *Topical Analgesic Formulas*

Muscle/Joint Tonic (H&A): *Anti-Inflammatory Formulas*

Mushroom Complete (SR): *Mushroom Blend Formulas*

Mushrooms Seven Source (HE): *Mushroom Blend Formulas*

Mycetoblend (EI): *Mushroom Blend Formulas*

Myelin Sheath Support (PH): *Nerve Tonic Formulas*

Nasal Support (EI): *Allergy-Reducing Formulas*

Natural Change Blend SP-7D (SR): *Menopause Balancing Formulas*

Natural Detox Wellness Tea (CS): *Blood Purifier Formulas*

Natural Laxative (GH): *Stimulant Laxative Formulas*

Natural Laxative Tea (GH): *Stimulant Laxative Formulas*

NaturALL-Calm (GH): *Relaxing Nervine Formulas*

Nature's Biotic (GH): *Antibacterial Formulas*

Nature's C Complex (WB): *Cold and Flu Formulas*

Nature's Three (NSP): *Fiber Blend Formulas*

NatureWorks Swedish Bitters (NW): *Digestive Bitter Tonic Formulas*

Nausea Ease (VT): *Carminative Formulas*

Neck & Shoulder Rub (TB): *Topical Analgesic Formulas*

Neck and *Shoulders Support (PH): Joint Healing Formulas*

Nerve Blend SP-14 (SR): *Relaxing Nervine Formulas*

Nerve Calm Formula (WB): *Relaxing Nervine and Antispasmodic Formulas*

Nerve Comfort Formula (CR): *Analgesic and Relaxing Nervine Formulas*

Nerve Formula (CR): *Antispasmodic Formulas*

Nerve Repair Formula (WB): *Nerve Tonic Formulas*

Nervine (GH): *Relaxing Nervine Formulas*

Nervine Tonic (HE): *Relaxing Nervine Formulas*

Nervous System Tonic (HP): *Nerve Tonic Formulas*

Nettles - Eyebright (EI): *Allergy-Reducing Formulas*

Nettles & Eyebright (HK): *Allergy-Reducing Formulas*

NeuroZyme (NC): *Brain and Memory Tonic Formulas*

Neutralizing Cordial (EI): *Digestive Bitter Tonic and Antacid Formulas*

Neutralizing Cordial (HP): *Digestive Bitter Tonic and Antacid Formulas*

Nicotine Relief (GH): *Quit Smoking and Bronchialdilator Formulas*

Night Nervine (GH): *Relaxing Nervine and Sleep Formulas*

Nighttime Tea (NF): *Sleep Formulas*

Nighty Night Valerian (TM): *Sleep Formulas*

Nose Ointment (CR): *Topical Vulnerary Formulas*

OctaPower (SR): *Energy-Boosting Formulas*

Oil of Garlic (CR): *Ear Drop Formulas*

Ojibwa Herbal Cleansing Tea (NF): *Anticancer Formulas*

Ojibwa Tea Concentrate (NF): *Essiac Formulas*

Olbas Analgesic Salve (OL): *Topical Analgesic Formulas*

Olbas Cough Syrup (OL): *Cough Remedy Formulas*

Olbas Herbal Bath (OL): *Topical Analgesic Formulas*

Olbas Herbal Tea (OL): *Cold and Flu Formulas*

Olbas Inhaler (OL): *Decongestant Formulas*

Olbas Lozenges (OL): *Decongestant Formulas*

Olbas Oil (OL): *Topical Analgesic Formulas*

Olbas Pastilles (OL): *Cough Remedy Formulas*

Old Indian Syrup for Kids (PH): *Expectorant and Decongestant Formulas*

Old Indian Wild Cherry Bark Syrup (PH): *Expectorant and Drying Cough/Lung Formulas*

Olive Leaf Extract with Echinacea (NF): *Antiviral and Antibacterial Formulas*

Oolong & Matcha Tea (IN): *Energy-Boosting Formulas*

Opti-Recovery (VT): *Tissue Healing and Blood Purifier Formulas*

Oral Health Tonic (HP): *Dental Health Formulas*

Organic Brain Support (IN): *Brain and Memory Tonic Formulas*

Organic Essential Detox (RL): *Blood Purifier Formulas*

Organic Herbalmist Throat Spray (ZD): *Antiviral and Antibacterial Formulas*

Organic Total Body Cleanse (RL): *General Detoxifying Formulas*

Organic Triple Fiber (RL): *Fiber Blend Formulas*

Original 7 Mushrooms (EI): *Mushroom Blend Formulas*

Original Bitters (UM): *Digestive Bitter Tonic Formulas*

Osha Root Cough Syrup (HE): *Expectorant and Drying Cough/Lung Formulas*

Osha Supreme (GH): *Antibacterial and Decongestant Formulas*

Osteo Herb (H&A): *Mineral Formulas*

Osteo Herb (H&A): *Mineral Formulas*

Pain Relief Formula (WB): *Analgesic Formulas*

Pain Relieving Patch (TB): *Topical Analgesic Formulas*

Pain-Aid (GH): *Analgesic Formulas*

Pancreaid (H&A): *Blood Sugar Reducing Formulas*

Pancreas Formula (CR): *Blood Sugar Reducing Formulas*

Pancreas Support Formula (WB): *Blood Sugar Reducing Formulas*

Pancreas-Aid (GH): *Blood Sugar Reducing Formulas*

Para-Shield (GH): *Antiparasitic Formulas*

ParaFree (HE): *Antiparasitic Formulas*

ParaGONE for Kids (RL): *Antiparasitic Formulas*

ParaGONE (RL): *Antiparasitic Formulas*

Parasites & Worms (GH): *Antiparasitic Formulas*

Parastroy (IN): *Antiparasitic Formulas*

Passion Potion (HE): *Female Aphrodisiac Formulas*

Pau d'Arco - Usnea (EI): *Antifungal Formulas*

Pau D'Arco Deep Cleansing (PH): *Blood Purifier Formulas*

Peach DeTox (YT): *Carminative Formulas*

Peak Defense (HE): *Cold and Flu Formulas*

Herbal Formulas

Phytocalm (H&A): *Sleep Formulas*

Phytocillin (HE): *Antifungal* and *Antibacterial Formulas*

Phytodent (H&A): *Dental Health Formulas*

PhytoEstrogen Herbal (VT): *Phytoestrogen Formulas*

Phytoestrogen Tonic (HP): *PMS Relieving* and *Menopause Balancing Formulas*

Pituitary Caps (SR): *Adaptogen Formulas*

Plantain Goldenseal Salve (GH): *Drawing Salve Formulas*

PlantiOxidants (PH): *Antioxidant Formulas*

PMS Comfort Tonic (HP): *PMS Relieving Formulas*

PMS Support (EI): *PMS Relieving Formulas*

PMS Tea (TM): *Diuretic Formulas*

PMS with Vitamin B6 & 5-HTP (NW): *PMS Relieving* and *Menstrual Cramp Formulas*

Pollen Defense (HP): *Allergy-Reducing Formulas*

Pomegranate Green Tea (CS): *Antioxidant Formulas*

Pomegranate Xtreme ENERJI Green Tea Energy Shot (CS): *Energy-Boosting Formulas*

Pomegranate Xtreme Kombucha Energy Shot (CS): *Energy-Boosting Formulas*

Positive Teens & Kids (PH): *Brain Calming Formulas*

Power Cleanse (RL): *General Detoxifying Formulas*

Power to Sleep PM (IN): *Sleep Formulas*

Pregnancy Prep (VT): *Pregnancy Tonic* and *Female Hormonal Balancing Formulas*

Pregnancy Tea (TM): *Pregnancy Tonic* and *Uterine Tonic Formulas*

Prenatal Formula (CR): *Pre-Delivery Formulas*

Propolis - Astragalus (EI): *Topical Antiseptic Formulas*

Propolis Plus Extract (NF): *Antibacterial Formulas*

Prost-Answer (NA): *Prostate Formulas*

Prosta-Strong (IN): *Prostate Formulas*

Prostate (GH): *Prostate Formulas*

Prostate 5LX (NC): *Prostate Formulas*

Prostate Blend SP-16 (SR): *Prostate Formulas*

Prostate Caps (SR): *Prostate Formulas*

Prostate Health (GH): *Prostate Formulas*

Prostate Health Clinical Strength (NF): *Prostate Formulas*

Prostate Plus Formula (CR): *Prostate Formulas*

Prostate Plus Formula (WB): *Prostate Formulas*

Prostate Support (EI): *Prostate Formulas*

Prostate Support (NF): *Prostate Formulas*

Prostate Take Care (NC): *Prostate Formulas*

Prostate Tea with Nettle Root (TM): *Prostate Formulas*

Prostate with Saw Palmetto (NW): *Prostate Formulas*

Prostatonic (HE): *Prostate Formulas*

ProstEase (RC): *Prostate Formulas*

Prostol (NW): *Prostate Formulas*

ProstSupport w/Ester C (NA): *Prostate Formulas*

Pygeum & Saw Palmetto (NF): *Prostate Formulas*

Queeze Ease Tea (NF): *Carminative Formulas*

Quick Colon Cleanse #1 (CR): *Stimulant Laxative Formulas*

Quick Colon Powder #2 (CR): *Fiber Blend Formulas*

Quick Defense (GH): *Antibacterial Formulas*

Quick Digest (ZD): *Digestive Enzyme Formulas*

Quick Digest Citrus (ZD): *Digestive Enzyme Formulas*

Rash Formula Ointment (CR): *Topical Vulnerary Formulas*

Raspberry Passion Perfect Energy (YT): *Energy-Boosting Formulas*

Reckless Blood Tonic (H&A): *Styptic/Hemostatic Formulas*

Red Clover - Burdock (EI): *Blood Purifier Formulas*

Red Clover Cleanser (PH): *Blood Purifier Formulas*

Red Clover Plus Extract (NF): *Blood Purifier Formulas*

Red Clover Supreme (GH): *Blood Purifier Formulas*

Red Clover with Prickly Ash Bark (NW): *Blood Purifier Formulas*

Red Raspberry - Squawvine (EI): *Menstrual Cramp* and *Uterine Tonic Formulas*

Reflux Relief (GH): *Antacid Formulas*

Refreshing Mint Vital Energy (YT): *Energy-Boosting Formulas*

Rehmannia Endurance (PH): *Energy-Boosting Formulas*

Rehmannia Vitalizer (PH): *Energy-Boosting Formulas*

Reishi Mushroom Supreme (PH): *Immune Balancing Formulas*

Rejuve Gentle Daily Fiber (GH): *Fiber Blend Formulas*

Relax-Eze (CR): *Relaxing Nervine Formulas*

Relaxation Support (EI): *Relaxing Nervine Formulas*

Relaxed Mind (YT): *Relaxing Nervine Formulas*

Relaxing Sleep (HP): *Sleep Formulas*

Relief Blend SP-10 (SR): *Analgesic* and *Migraine/Headache Formulas*

Remember Now (HE): *Brain* and *Memory Tonic Formulas*

Replenish Compound (H&A): *Menopause Balancing Formulas*

Respiration Blend SP-3 (SR): *Lung* and *Respiratory Tonic Formulas*

Respiratonic (HE): *Expectorant Formulas*

Respiratory Calmpound (H&A): *Allergy-Reducing* and *Bronchialdilator Formulas*

Respiratory Defense (GH): *Decongestant Formulas*

Respiratory Relief (GH): *Cough Remedy Formulas*

Respiratory Relief Syrup (CR): *Expectorant* and *Antibacterial Formulas*

Respiratory Support & Defense (IN): *Decongestant Formulas*

Rest Easy Tea (WB): *Relaxing Nervine Formulas*

Rhubarb & Butternut (SR): *Stimulant Laxative Formulas*

Sambucus Elder Berry Spray (NA): *Topical Antiseptic Formulas*

Sambucus Immune Syrup (NW): *Antiviral Formulas*

Saw Palmetto - Nettles (EI): *Prostate Formulas*

Saw Palmetto & Nettle Root with Pumpkin (SR): *Prostate Formulas*

Saw Palmetto Classic (PH): *Prostate Formulas*

Schizandra Adrenal Complex (PH): *Adrenal Tonic Formulas*

Scudder's Alterative Compound (GH): *Anticancer Formulas*

Sen Sei Menthol Rub (CR): *Decongestant Formulas*

Sensual Enhancement Formula (WB): *Male Aphrodisiac Formulas*

Serenity Compound (H&A): *Relaxing Nervine Formulas*

Serenity Herbal Elixir (GH): *Relaxing Nervine Formulas*

Serenity with Passionflower (GH): *Relaxing Nervine Formulas*

Seven Precious Mushrooms (H&A): *Mushroom Blend Formulas*

SF (NSP): *Weight Loss Formulas*

Shiitake Mushroom Supreme (PH): *Liver Tonic Formulas*

Shiitake–Maitake Standardized (NW): *Mushroom Blend Formulas*

Silent Night with Valerian (NW): *Sleep Formulas*

Singer's Saving Grace (HE): *Decongestant Formulas*

Sinus & Lung Extract (CR): *Sinus Decongestant Formulas*

Sinus & Respiratory (NC): *Sinus Decongestant* and *Decongestant Formulas*

Sinus Allergy Formula (WB): *Sinus Decongestant Formulas*

Sinus Plus Formula (CR): *Sinus Decongestant Formulas*

Sinus Support Compound (H&A): *Sinus Decongestant Formulas*

Sinus Take Care (NC): *Sinus Decongestant Formulas*

SinusClear (RC): *Sinus Decongestant Formulas*

SinusFree (PH): *Sinus Decongestant Formulas*

Skin Blend SP-4 (SR): *Blood Purifier Formulas*

Skin Detox (YT): *Skin Healing Formulas*

Skullcap - Oats (EI): *Antispasmodic* and *Bronchialdilator Formulas*

Skullcap St. John's Wort Supreme (GH): *Nerve Tonic Formulas*

Sleep (GH): *Sleep Formulas*

Sleep & Relax (GH): *Sleep Formulas*

Sleep & Relax Tea (GH): *Relaxing Nervine* and *Sleep Formulas*

Sleep Blend SP-17 (SR): *Sleep Formulas*

SleepBlend (VT): *Sleep Formulas*

SleepThru (GH): *Sleep Formulas*

Sleepytime Decaf Lemon Jasmine Green Tea (CS): *Sleep Formulas*

Sleepytime Herbal Tea (CS): *Sleep Formulas*

Sleepytime Kids Goodnight Grape Herbal Tea (CS): *Sleep Formulas*

Sleepytime Sinus Soother Wellness Tea (CS): *Relaxing Nervine Formulas*

Sleepytime Vanilla Herbal Tea (CS): *Sleep Formulas*

Slim (with Caffeine) (GH): *Weight Loss Formulas*

Slim Too (Caffeine Free) (GH): *Weight Loss Formulas*

Slow Flow (VT): *Styptic/Hemostatic* and *Uterine Tonic Formulas*

Slumber (CR): *Sleep Formulas*

Slumber (NA): *Sleep Formulas*

Slumber (NA): *Sleep Formulas*

Smoke Free (HE): *Lung* and *Respiratory Tonic* and *Quit Smoking Formulas*

Smoke Out (CR): *Quit Smoking Formulas*

Smoke Take Care (NC): *Antioxidant Formulas*

Smoker's ResQ (H&A): *Quit Smoking Formulas*

Smokers' Cleanse (RL): *Quit Smoking Formulas*

Smooth Move Chamomile (TM): *Stimulant Laxative Formulas*

Smooth Move Peppermint (TM): *Stimulant Laxative Formulas*

Smooth Move Senna (TM): *Stimulant Laxative Formulas*

Smooth Move Senna Capsules (TM): *Stimulant Laxative Formulas*

Soluble Fiber Caps (YP): *Fiber Blend Formulas*

Soluble Fiber Formula (YP): *Fiber Blend Formulas*

Soothing Caramel Bedtime (YT): *Sleep Formulas*

Soothing Coconut & Aloe Natural Laxative (IN): *Gentle Laxative Formulas*

Soothing Mint Get Regular (YT): *Stimulant Laxative Formulas*

Soothing Oak & Ivy (HP): *Topical Vulnerary Formulas*

Soothing Throat Spray (HP): *Antiviral Formulas*

Sore Throat Spray (AV): *Topical Antiseptic Formulas*

Sound Sleep (GH): *Sleep Formulas*

Spleen Activator, *Chinese (NSP): Digestive Tonic Formulas*

St John's Wort (GH): *Topical Vulnerary Formulas*

St. John's Good Mood (TM): *Antidepressant Formulas*

St. John's Wort - Lemon Balm (EI): *Antidepressant Formulas*

St. John's Wort Blues Away (YT): *Antidepressant Formulas*

St. John's Wort Emotional Balance (PH): *Antidepressant Formulas*

Stamina Ginseng Ginger Tonic (NC): *Energy-Boosting* and *Digestive Tonic Formulas*

Steel-Libido (IN): *Male Aphrodisiac Formulas*

Steel-Libido Red (IN): *Male Aphrodisiac Formulas*

Stings & Bites Ointment (CR): *Topical Vulnerary Formulas*

Stingzzz Cool Soothing Gel (HK): *Topical Vulnerary Formulas*

Stomach Blend SP-20B (SR): *Ulcer Healing Formulas*

Stomach Comfort (CR): *Catnip & Fennel Formulas*

Stomach Comfort, *Chewable (NSP): Antacid Formulas*

Stomach Ease (YT): *Antacid Formulas*

Stomach Tonic (HE): *Carminative* and *Antacid Formulas*

Stone Breaker (HP): *Lithotriptic Formulas*

Stone Dissolve Tea (WB): *Lithotriptic Formulas*

Stone Free (PH): *Lithotriptic Formulas*

Stone Root - Witch Hazel (EI): *Vascular Tonic Formulas*

Stop-Ache (CR): *Analgesic Formulas*

Stress Advantage (NC): *Adaptogen Formulas*

Stress Free (PH): *Relaxing Nervine Formulas*

Stress Manager (HP): *Adaptogen Formulas*

Stress ReLeaf (HE): *Adaptogen* and *Relaxing Nervine Formulas*

Stress Response (GH): *Adaptogen Formulas*

Stress Take Care (NC): *Adaptogen Formulas*

Stress-Defy (IN): *Relaxing Nervine Formulas*

Sugar Metabolism (HP): *Blood Sugar Reducing Formulas*

Sugar Plum Spice (CS): *Carminative Formulas*

Sunny Mood (IN): *Antidepressant Formulas*

Super Adrenal Support (WB): *Adrenal Tonic Formulas*

Super Antioxidant (NSP): *Antioxidant Formulas*

Super Antioxidants (NF): *Antioxidant Formulas*

Super Cleanse (IN): *General Detoxifying Formulas*

Super Garlic Immune Formula (CR): *Antibacterial Formulas*

Super Green Super Food (IN): *Superfood Formulas*

Super Kids Salve (HK): *Topical Vulnerary Formulas*

Super Kids Throat Spray (HK): *Antibacterial* and *Immune Stimulating Formulas*

Super Lax (GH): *Stimulant Laxative Formulas*

Super Thisilyn (NW): *Liver Tonic Formulas*

Supercritical Antioxidants (NC): *Antioxidant Formulas*

Supercritical Diet & Energy (NC): *Energy-Boosting* and *Weight Loss Formulas*

Supreme Cleanse (GH): *General Detoxifying Formulas*

Swedish Bitters (NWS): *Digestive Bitter Tonic Formulas*

Sweet Açaí Mango Zinger Ice Herbal Tea (CS): *Antioxidant Formulas*

Sweet Dreams Formula (WB): *Sleep Formulas*

Sweet Tangerine Positive Energy (YT): *Energy-Boosting Formulas*

Sweet Wild Berry Zinger Ice Herbal Tea (CS): *Antioxidant Formulas*

Sweetish Bitters Elixir (GH): *Digestive Bitter Tonic Formulas*

SystemWell Ultimate Immunity (NW): *Immune Stimulating Formulas*

Tei Fu Essential Oil (NSP): *Topical Analgesic Formulas*

Temp Assure (HK): *Cold* and *Flu* and *Sudorific Formulas*

Tension Relief (H&A): *Relaxing Nervine* and *Nerve Tonic Formulas*

Tension Tamer (CS): *Relaxing Nervine Formulas*

TestoJack 200 (NF): *Male Aphrodisiac Formulas*

Think O2 (TM): *Brain* and *Memory Tonic Formulas*

Thisilyn Cleanse (Mineral) (NW): *Blood Purifier Formulas*

Thisilyn Daily Cleanse (NW): *Fiber Blend Formulas*

Thisilyn Digestive CLEANSE (NW): *Stimulant Laxative Formulas*

Thistle Cleanse Formula (ZD): *Blood Purifier Formulas*

Thistles Compound (H&A): *Hepatoprotective Formulas*

Three Spices Sinus Complex (PH): *Carminative* and *Sinus Decongestant Formulas*

Throat Coat (TM): *Intestinal Toning Formulas*

Throat Coat Herbal Syrup (TM): *Expectorant* and *Moistening Lung/Cough Formulas*

Throat Coat Lemon Echinacea (TM): *Decongestant, Cough Remedy* and *Moistening Lung/Cough Formulas*

Throat Comfort (YT): *Expectorant Formulas*

Throat Shield Lozenges (GH): *Topical Antiseptic Formulas*

Throat Shield Spray (GH): *Topical Antiseptic Formulas*

Throat Shield Tea (GH): *Decongestant* and *Moistening Lung/Cough Formulas*

Thymus Plus Caps (SR): *Goldenseal & Echinacea Formulas*

ThyroFem (VT): *Hypothyroid Formulas*

Thyroid (GH): *Hypothyroid Formulas*

Thyroid Blend SP-26 (SR): *Hypothyroid Formulas*

Thyroid Calming (HP): *Hyperthyroid Formulas*

Thyroid Calmpound (H&A): *Hyperthyroid Formulas*

Thyroid Complete (NA): *Hypothyroid Formulas*

Thyroid Formula (WB): *Hypothyroid Formulas*

Thyroid Lifter (HP): *Hypothyroid Formulas*

Thyroid Lift (PH): *Hypothyroid Formulas*

Thyroid Maintenance Formula (CR): *Hypothyroid Formulas*

Thyroid Support (GH): *Hypothyroid Formulas*

Thyroid Thrive (RC): *Hypothyroid Formulas*

Tiger Balm Extra (TB): *Topical Analgesic Formulas*

Tiger Balm Regular (TB): *Topical Analgesic Formulas*

Tiger Balm Ultra (TB): *Topical Analgesic Formulas*

TLC Tea (NF): *Cold* and *Flu Formulas*

Tonic Blend SP-28 (SR): *Adaptogen Formulas*

Total Body Cleanse (RL): *General Detoxifying Formulas*

Total Body Rapid Cleanse (RL): *General Detoxifying Formulas*

Total Kidney Detox (RL): *Urinary Infection Fighting Formulas*

Tranquilnite (NC): *Sleep Formulas*

Trauma Drops (HP): *Tissue Healing Formulas*

Trauma Oil (HP): *Topical Analgesic Formulas*

Tri-Cleanse Complete Internal Cleanser (PH): *Fiber Blend Formulas*

Triphala (PH): *Gentle Laxative Formulas*

Triphala Fruit (GH): *Gentle Laxative Formulas*

Triphala Laxative (PH): *Gentle Laxative Formulas*

Triphala-Garcinia Program (PH): *Weight Loss Formulas*

Tummy Tea (WB): *Carminative Formulas*

Turkey Rhubarb Formula (WB): *Stimulant Laxative Formulas*

Turmeric & Ginger (NA): *Anti-Inflammatory Formulas*

Turmeric Supreme (GH): *Anti-Inflammatory Formulas*

Ultimate Cleanse (IN): *Blood Purifier Formulas*

Ultimate Echinacea (NSP): *Echinacea Blend Formulas*

Ultimate Echinacea (H&A): *Echinacea Blend Formulas*

Ultimate Fiber Cleanse (IN): *Fiber Blend Formulas*

Ultimate Ginseng (HE): *Adaptogen Formulas*

Ultra Raspberry Ketone (WB): *Weight Loss Formulas*

Uplift (VT): *Antidepressant Formulas*

Urinary Support (GH): *Antibacterial* and *Urinary Infection Fighting Formulas*

Urinary Support & Flush (IN): *Diuretic Formulas*

Urinary System Support (HP): *Kidney Tonic* and *Urinary Infection Fighting Formulas*

Urinary Tract Support (EI): *Diuretic* and *Urinary Infection Fighting Formulas*

Urinary with Cranberry (NW): *Diuretic* and *Urinary Infection Fighting Formulas*

Usnea Uva Ursi Supreme (GH): *Antibacterial* and *Urinary Infection Fighting Formulas*

UT Compound (H&A): *Urinary Infection Fighting Formulas*

Uterine Balance (EI): *Menstrual Cramp Formulas*

Uterine Tonic (H&A): *Female Hormonal Balancing* and *Uterine Tonic Formulas*

UTIntensive (RC): *Urinary Infection Fighting Formulas*

Uva Ursi - Horsetail (EI): *Urinary Infection Fighting Formulas*

Uva Ursi - Horsetail Cranberry (EI): *Urinary Infection Fighting Formulas*

Uva Ursi Diurite (PH): *Diuretic* and *Urinary Infection Fighting Formulas*

Valerian - Passion Flower (EI): *Relaxing Nervine* and *Sleep Formulas*

Valerian - Passion Flower (EI): *Relaxing Nervine* and *Sleep Formulas*

Valerian Combination (TL): *Sleep Formulas*

Valerian Complex (AV): *Sleep Formulas*

Valerian Easy Sleep (PH): *Sleep Formulas*

Valerian Nighttime (NW): *Sleep Formulas*

Valerian Poppy Supreme (GH): *Relaxing Nervine Formulas*

Valerian Super Calm (HK): *Relaxing Nervine Formulas*

Vanilla Spice Perfect Energy (YT): *Energy-Boosting Formulas*

Vari-Gone (NSP): *Vascular Tonic Formulas*

Vari-Gone Cream (NSP): *Vascular Tonic Formulas*

Vascular Support (WB): *Hypotensive Formulas*

VB Herbal Bolus (CR): *Poultice Formulas*

Vein Support (EI): *Vascular Tonic Formulas*

Vein Supreme (NF): *Vascular Tonic Formulas*

Vein Tonic (HE): *Vascular Tonic Formulas*

VeinoBlend (VT): *Vascular Tonic Formulas*

Venous Blend SP-32 (SR): *Vascular Tonic Formulas*

Very Berry Antioxidant Blend (SR): *Antioxidant Formulas*

Very Cranberry (IN): *Urinary Infection Fighting Formulas*

Vi Protection Blend (HK): *Antiviral Formulas*

Vibrant Energy (HE): *Energy-Boosting* and *Adrenal Tonic Formulas*

Virattack (HP): *Antiviral Formulas*

Vision Enhancement (GH): *Vision Supporting Formulas*

Vision with Lutein & Bilberry (NW): *Vision Supporting Formulas*

VisionAid (RC): *Vision Supporting Formulas*

Vita Greens & Berries (PH): *Superfood Formulas*

Vitalerbs (CR): *Superfood Formulas*

Vitex Elixir (GH): *Female Hormonal Balancing Formulas*

VX Immune Support (H&A): *Antiviral Formulas*

Warming Circulation Tonic (HP): *Cardiovascular Stimulant Formulas*

Water Out (NF): *Diuretic Formulas*

WaterX (RC): *Diuretic Formulas*

Weightless (TM): *Weight Loss Formulas*

Weightless Cranberry (TM): *Weight Loss Formulas*

Weightloss Formula (WB): *Weight Loss Formulas*

Well Child (PH): *Antiviral* and *Cold* and *Flu Formulas*

Well Child Immune Chewable (PH): *Immune Stimulating Formulas*

White Flower Analgesic Balm (WF): *Topical Analgesic Formulas*

White Willow - Feverfew (EI): *Analgesic* and *Migraine/Headache Formulas*

White Willow with Feverfew Std. (NA): *Analgesic Formulas*

Whole Body Defense (GH): *Immune Stimulating Formulas*

Wild Yam-Black Cohosh Complex (PH): *Menopause Balancing Formulas*

Willow Aid (PH): *Analgesic Formulas*

Willow Pain Response (HP): *Analgesic Formulas*

Willow/Garlic Ear Oil (HK): *Ear Drop Formulas*

Woman's Moon Cycle (YT): *Female Hormonal Balancing Formulas*

Woman's Mother to Be (YT): *Pregnancy Tonic Formulas*

Woman's Nursing Support (YT): *Nursing Aid Formulas*

Woman's Passage (VT): *Menopause Balancing* and *Antidepressant Formulas*

Women's Balance (GH): *Female Hormonal Balancing Formulas*

Women's Calmpound (H&A): *Relaxing Nervine* and *Female Hormonal Balancing Formulas*

Women's Dong Quai Tonifier (PH): *Female Hormonal Balancing Formulas*

Women's Dong Quai Treasure (PH): *Female Hormonal Balancing Formulas*

Women's Formula (H&A): *Female Hormonal Balancing Formulas*

Women's Libido (GH): *Female Aphrodisiac Formulas*

Women's Phase II (VT): *Menopause Balancing Formulas*

Women's Phase I (VT): *PMS Relieving Formulas*

Women's Renew (YP): *Female Hormonal Balancing Formulas*

Women's Renew Internal Cleansing System (YP): *General Detoxifying Formulas*

Women's Reproductive Health (HP): *Uterine Tonic Formulas*

Women's Transition Compound (H&A): *Menopause Balancing Formulas*

Wormwood Black Walnut Supreme (GH): *Antiparasitic Formulas*

X-Ceptic (CR): *Antibacterial* and *Topical Antiseptic Formulas*

Yeast Arrest Suppositories (VT): *Antifungal Formulas*

Yeast Balance (EI): *Antifungal Formulas*

Yeast Blend SP-7A (SR): *Antifungal Formulas*

Yeast ReLeaf (HE): *Antifungal Formulas*

Yellow Dock Skin Cleanse (PH): *Skin Healing Formulas*

Yin Chiao Classic (PH): *Cold* and *Flu Formulas*

Yin Chiao-Echinacea Complex (PH): *Decongestant* and *Immune Stimulating Formulas*

Yohimbe and *Saw Palmetto (SR): Male Aphrodisiac Formulas*

Yohimbe-Plus (IN): *Male Aphrodisiac Formulas*

Zyflamend Breast (NC): *Anti-Inflammatory* and *Antioxidant Formulas*

Zyflamend Nighttime (NC): *Anti-Inflammatory Formulas*

Zyflamend Prostate (NC): *Prostate Formulas*

Zyflamend Tiny Caps (NC): *Anti-Inflammatory Formulas*

Zyflamend Whole Body (NC): *Anti-Inflammatory Formulas*

Herbal Formulas

Property Definitions

Both single herbs and herbal formulas are related to different properties (or actions) of herbs. This is an index that defines what these properties are and how they are used.

Absorbent: A substance used to absorb irritating toxins both internally and externally. May be applied topically as a poultice for bites, stings, or other irritations. Can also be taken internally to absorb toxins. Must be used with a large amounts of water to be effective.

Acrid: A hot, biting, slightly irritating taste. Often found in herbs that are antispasmodic.

Adaptogen: Adaptogens help the body adapt to stressful situations and maintain normal function under mental or physical stress. Strengthen and support adrenal function by adjusting the hypothalamus/pituitary/ adrenal axis to reduce the output of stress hormones. Helps to build the immune system because stress hormones reduce the immune response.

Adrenal Tonic: A substance that builds up and strengthens the function of the adrenal glands.

Alterative (Blood Purifier): Cleanses (or alters) the internal environment of the body without producing noticeable laxative or diuretic effects. Helps remove toxins from the blood, probably by strengthening liver and or lymphatic function. Purifies the blood, helping to combat impurity in the blood and organs. Used to treat torpid or stagnant conditions in the body. Traditionally used to clear up morbid conditions in the body, especially skin diseases, skin eruptions, cancer and wounds with pus.

Analgesic (Anodyne): Helps to relieve pain without causing loss of sensation. An anodyne is a mild analgesic. Useful for minor pains. Don't expect herbal analgesics to have the strength of prescription pain-killing drugs. Often they simply take the "edge" off the pain so it is bearable.

Anaphrodisiac: Decreases sex drive.

Anesthetic: A drug or agent that is used to abolish the sensation of pain by numbing nerve endings.

Anodyne: See *Analgesic*

Antacid: Neutralizes excess stomach acid and/or relaxes the stomach and prevents or treats acid indigestion. Opposite action of digestive tonics. Antacids are used for excess stomach acid that usually occurs in younger people in response to overeating or stress. Indicated by sharp burning pains associated with eating. Dull, burning pains which occur about one to two hours after eating are not symptoms of acid indigestion, but rather a lack of hydrochloric acid and/or enzymes. , Calcium based antacids are generally contraindicated in this latter form of acid indigestion.

However and herbal antacids do not appear to adversely affect acid indigestion caused by lack of hydrochloric acid.

Anthelminthic: A vermifuge, destroying or expelling intestinal worms; an agent that is destructive to parasitic worms. See vermifuge.

Anti-abortive: Helps stop miscarriage or spontaneous abortion. Opposite of abortifacient. Used when bleeding or cramping starts in the early stages of pregnancy to help avoid a miscarriage.

Anti-allergenic: Reduces allergic reactions. Includes herbs listed under antihistamine and mast cell stabilizers. These remedies are used to reduce the allergic responses in mucus membranes of the digestive and respiratory tract. They are useful for hay fever, allergy-induced asthma and earaches.

Anti-arrhythmic: Combating an irregular heart beat; an agent that prevents or alleviates cardiac arrhythmia.

Anti-emetic (Antinauseous): Suppresses vomit reflex, relieves nausea. Used for flu, morning sickness, motion sickness, nausea, etc.

Anti-inflammatory: Reduces inflammation (heat, swelling and pain). Used to reduce inflammatory conditions in the body. Anti-inflammatories vary widely in their mode of action and hence in their specific applications. Almost any herb that heals tissue damage will also act as an anti-inflammatory agent.

Antibacterial: Destroys or inhibits bacteria. Used to fight infection both internally and externally. Many of these remedies do not directly kill bacteria, but act in indirect ways to inhibit their growth or enhance the body's own ability to destroy them.

Anticancer: Remedies that help to fight cancer and shrink tumors.

Anticarious: Preventing or suppressing the development of dental caries (cavities).

Anticholesteremic: Agent that helps to reduce cholesterol.

Anticoagulant (Blood Thinner): Inhibits coagulation of blood and blood clotting. Opposite of blood tonic. Used where there is a risk of thrombosis (blood clots forming in the circulatory system). These remedies also help blood stagnation (thick, heavy blood) which in natural medicine is believed to contribute to a wide variety of conditions including varicose veins, uterine fibroids and liver congestion.

These remedies may be contraindicated in anemia or when the person is already using blood thinners.

Antidepressant: Relieves depression. Helps alleviate depression. Used to help lift the spirits and relieve depression. Caution: do not take people "cold turkey" off antidepressant drugs.

Antidiabetic: An agent that prevents or alleviates diabetes.

Antidiarrheal: Arrests diarrhea.

Antidiuretic: An agent that suppresses the formation of urine.

Antifungal: Kills or inhibits the growth of fungus and yeast. Used for candida and other yeast infections both topically and internally. Synonymous with Fungicide.

Antigalactagogue: Inhibits lactation (flow of breast milk). Opposite of galactagogue. Used for nursing mothers to help dry up breast milk when it is time to stop nursing.

Antihistamine: Helps dry up sinus congestion by counteracting histamine. Similar to anti-allergenic, but more specific. Histamine produces swelling in mucus membranes leading to itchy, watery eyes, runny nose, swollen eustachian tubes, intestinal inflammation and other allergic reactions.

Antimicrobial: An agent that kills microorganisms or suppresses their multiplication or growth.

Antimutagenic: Helps prevent the formation of cancer cells.

Antioxidant: Helps prevent free radical damage by scavenging oxygen radicals, which may help prevent aging and decay.

Antiparasitic: Remedies that destroy parasites. Parasites are difficult to diagnose accurately. However, it is often advisable to take antiparasitic herbs when traveling abroad, or when one has pets or animals, or when one has digestive problems that don't respond to other approaches.

Antirheumatic: An agent that relieves or prevents rheumatism; any substance applied topically or taken internally that reduces pain and inflammation of the joints or other connective tissue.

Antiseptic: Destroys or inhibits micro-organisms (germs). These terms are usually used in reference to herbs that are used on wounds or injuries rather than for internal infections.

Antispasmodic: Relaxes or prevents muscle cramping or spasms. Used for muscle spasms in a variety of applications including: cramps and charley-horses, intestinal cramps (spastic bowel), bronchial spasms in asthma, menstrual cramps, pain during childbirth, pain due to muscle tension, tension headaches.

Antisudorific: Decreases perspiration and elimination through the skin. Used to stop night sweats and/or excessive perspiration. Closes skin pores.

Antithyrotropic: Inhibiting the secretion or actions of thyrotropin.

Antitussive: Suppresses the cough reflex, reducing coughing. Used to arrest coughing when excessive coughing causes chest pain or loss of sleep.

Antivenomous: Counteracts venom from bites and stings by absorbing it or neutralizing it. Used primarily topically for spider bites, bee stings, snake bites, etc. For topical use, moisten powders and apply as a poultice directly to the affected area. It may be necessary to change the poultice several times to obtain the full effect. (Caution: this is a first aid measure and should not replace appropriate medical assistance, especially in the case of allergies to bee stings, or the bite of poisonous snakes and spiders.)

Antiviral: Destroys, inhibits or helps the body to destroy viruses.

Aperient: A very mild laxative. Used to create a gentle laxative action, especially in children or elderly persons.

Aphrodisiac: Increases sex drive. Used for low sex drive, impotency or frigidity. Not recommended for teenagers.

Aromatic: A substance with a strong aroma or smell; odoriferous, stimulant, spicy. This signifies the presence of a significant amount of essential or volatile oils in the plant. Essential oils tend to be stimulating to digestion and circulation, carminative and antiseptic. Aromatic herbs often affect the nerves with relaxing or stimulating effects.

Astringent: Herbs that are astringent contain tannins (and sometimes other compounds) that contract and tone muscle fiber and other tissue. They are used to stop bleeding, arrest discharges (diarrhea, excess mucus, pus, etc.), tone up soft or spongy tissue (varicose veins, hemorrhoids), reduce swelling and/or counteract venom (see anti-venomous). They are contraindicated in tension and dryness.

Bitter: The bitter taste of herbs is due to the presence of alkaloids,diterpenes or glycosides. When taken in liquid form, bitters tend to stimulate digestive secretions. Bitter tasting herbs tend to stimulate elimination, move stagnation and cool and dry tissues. Plants with alkaloids often have a strong effect on the nerves and glands, either stimulating or sedating them. Bitters should generally be avoided by thin, weak, emaciated people.

Blood Building: A concept from Chinese and traditional medicine. Refers to herbs that help overcome anemia and build up the blood. Traditionally used for weak, thin pulse, pale complexion, general weakness.

Bronchial Dilator: Remedies that relax and dilate the bronchials. Used for asthma that is induced by muscular constriction of the air passages due to nervous reactions. These remedies are also good for deep cough, especially whooping cough, where there is constriction of the airways.

Calmative: A mild sedative.

Cardiac: A remedy that tones and strengthens the heart muscle. Used to prevent heart disease or to strengthen the heart when heart disease is already present.

Carminative: Expels gas from the bowel or relieves bloating. Used for people who suffer from severe gas and poor digestive function. These remedies act by stimulating blood flow to the digestive organs and increasing digestive secretions. Most of the gas produced in our colon is absorbed into the blood stream and excreted via the lungs. These remedies increase absorption of gas in the intestines to relieve bloating. They may also help to increase motility (movement) along the digestive tract to push material forward and help to expel trapped gas or food material.

Cathartic: A substance that stimulates the movement of the bowels, which is more powerful that a laxative.

Cerebral Tonic: Improves memory and brain function. Used for loss of memory or concentration due to aging or senility. Also useful for increasing mental alertness and concentration in students or others who need better memory or focus. May be helpful in some cases of ADD.

Chelating: An agent that bonds to metals to facilitate their absorption or removal from the body.

Cholagogue: Increases the flow of bile, helps prevent or dissolve gallstones. Indicated for clay colored stools, some cases of constipation and in gall bladder problems where the gallbladder is congested or has stones. Contraindicated in duodenal ulcers and intestinal inflammation. May also be contraindicated with inflammatory liver diseases.

Cicatrisant: A cicatrisant is a remedy that helps tissues heal without scarring.

Condiment: Condiments are herbs used as seasonings to improve the flavor of food. Condiment herbs are general safe for long term use in low doses.

Counterirritant: A remedy which causes irritation (redness) and thus draws blood away from one area of the body to another. Used topically for temporary relief of pain associated with arthritis, gout, rheumatism, strained muscles, etc. Helps to relieve pain by depleting or blocking substance P neurotransmitters. Pain relief is usually temporary, although increased blood flow may help to stimulate healing. Contraindicated with redness and swelling on the surface of the skin or when the surface of the skin is broken. Not recommended for application after a hot shower or bath. Avoid contact with sensitive areas of the body (eyes, genitals).

Cytotoxic: Kills cancer cells

Decongestant: Relieves (breaks up or loosens) respiratory congestion. Used primarily where mucus has become thick and "stuck" causing difficult breathing, sinus pressure or thick drainage. These remedies tend to thin mucus making it easier to expel.

Demulcent (Mucilant): Demulcents contain complex polysaccharides which are indigestible, but hold water and absorb irritants. Mucilant is a term we coined in to describe this action. It is not found in traditional texts. Applied topically herbs with this property act as a drawing poultice to absorb irritants, reduce inflammation and swelling, and keep tissues moist and pliable. Taken internally they absorb irritants in the digestive tract, help to reduce cholesterol, act as bulk laxatives and moisten dry tissues. They also tend to act as mild nourishing foods to counteract weight loss (wasting). They are indicated in hard, dry, irritated tissue states, including inflammation of the digestive tract, dry, irritating coughs, burning or painful urination, redness and swelling topically. Also indicated in conditions where a person needs mild nourishing foods when recovering from debilitating illnesses. and They are contraindicated with bowel obstruction and should not be applied topically to deep wounds.

Diaphoretic/Sudorific: Increases perspiration and elimination through the skin. Used to bring down fevers. In Chinese medicine these are called "surface-relieving" herbs and are used to relieve "superficial" conditions such as colds, flu, coughs, asthma, edema. Warming sudorifics are used for "wind chill" (mild fever with chills, lack of sweating, white phlegm) and cooling sudorifics are used for "wind-heat" (high fever with chills and sweating, thirst, yellow phlegm). Synonymous with sudorific.

Digestant: Aids digestion of food, generally applied to remedies that contain enzymes or other elements that directly aid in the breakdown of food. Used to supplement digestive secretions and aid in the digestion of food where people are having difficulty manufacturing sufficient hydrochloric acid, enzymes and/or bile salts to breakdown their food. These remedies are especially helpful for older people with poor digestion or people in a wasting condition (where they are losing weight).

Digestive Tonic: Herbs, generally bitter or aromatic, that promote the flow of digestive secretions to aid digestion. They are generally taken about 20-30 minutes prior to meals in a liquid form.

Disinfectant: An agent that disinfects; applied particularly to agents used on inanimate objects; a substance that destroys noxious properties of decaying organic matter. See Antiseptic.

Diuretic: Increases flow of urine to expel excess fluids from the body. Diuretics are used for water retention and various types of kidney problems. They vary widely in their mode of action.

Drawing: Drawing refers to agents that pull morbid material out of the body.

Emetic: Induces vomiting. Used for food or chemical poisoning. Call poison control center for advice before inducing vomiting in cases of chemical poisoning. With caustic agents like lye vomiting should not be induced. Emetics are also used to expel excess phlegm from the system to halt asthma attacks and relieve severe respiratory congestion.

Emmenagogue: Increases (stimulates) and regulates menstrual flow. These herbs have also been called female correctives because they help to regulate the menstrual cycle. They are generally contraindicated during pregnancy.

Emollient: A preparation that soothes and softens external tissue.

Euphoretic: An agent that produces an exaggerated feeling of physical and mental well being, especially when not justified by external reality.

Expectorant: Expels phlegm or mucus from the lungs and sinuses. Increases coughing, sneezing and stimulates drainage.

Febrifuge: Reduces fever and inflammation.

Galactagogue: Enriches and/or increases the flow of breast milk. Opposite of antigalactogogue. Used for nursing mothers to enrich and promote the flow of breast milk. These remedies may also ease colic in nursing babies when taken by the mother to "sweeten" the milk.

Glandular: Influences the glands to produce more of certain hormones. May also mimic hormones. This is a very vague and general term, since specific herbs act on specific glands.

Hemostatic: Stops internal bleeding or hemorrhage. Similar to styptic, but generally used internally. Caution: Seek medical assistance for serious bleeding.

Hepatic: Strengthens liver function.

Hepatoprotective: Protects the liver from toxic chemicals.

Hypertensive: Can help to increase low blood pressure.

Hypotensive: Decreases blood pressure

Immune Amphoteric: Remedies that help to normalize the function of the immune system whether it is underactive (immune weakness) or overactive (autoimmune disorders). These remedies are particularly useful for autoimmune disorders. They appear to enhance communication in the immune system so that it works better without a general stimulating effect that would aggravate autoimmune conditions.

Immune Stimulant: Stimulates the function of the immune system. Used for frequent colds and infection, lowered resistance. May be contraindicated in autoimmune disorders.

Kidney Tonic: Strengthens kidney function and tone. In Chinese medicine the kidneys are thought to be connected to the health of the structural system, so these remedies are helpful for structural weakness, too. They stabilize the structure of the body by acting to balance mineral electrolytes through the kidneys.

Laxative (Bulk): Stimulates elimination through the lower bowel by adding fiber to the intestinal tract. Safer laxatives for long term use. Indicated in high cholesterol, sluggish elimination, elimination problems during pregnancy and general detoxification.

Laxative (Stimulant): A remedy that stimulates bowel movements to relieve constipation. These herbs contain anthraquinone glycosides, which increase peristalsis in the colon and inhibit absorption of water and electrolytes. Long term use of stimulant laxatives can be habit forming.

Lipotropic: Promoting the flow of lipids to and from the liver; acting on fat metabolism by hastening the removal of or decreasing the deposit of fat in the liver.

Lithotriptic: Helps dissolve kidney stones. Used to help people pass kidney stones and/or to prevent their formulation. Will probably help with calcifications elsewhere in the body such as bone spurs.

Lung Tonic: Strengthens lung tissue and function. Used where the lungs are weak and prone to frequent infection, also for conditions where the lungs are dry and leathery and have sustained a loss of elasticity.

Lymphatic: Remedies that act on the lymphatic system. They cleanse, tone or improve the function of the lymph glands and vessels. Indicated with lymphatic swellings, sore throats, mumps, tonsillitis, some cases of breast swelling or tenderness and other problems where there is lymphatic congestion or stagnation.

Mast Cell Stabilizer: Stabilize mast cells to reduce allergic reactions. Used in hay fever, allergenic asthma and other respiratory allergies to reduce allergic reactions.

Mineralizer: Mineralizer is a term we coined at Tree of Light Publishing to describe nutritive herbs which supply trace minerals to aid in tissue healing. Used to build up structural tissues in the body by supplying nutrients to aid tissue regeneration and repair. These herbs are generally rich in calcium and silica.

Moistening: Helps body tissues retain moisture. Used when tissues are dry and don't rehydrate by just drinking water.

Mucliant/Mucilaginous: See Demulcent.

Narcotic: A painkiller that numbs or depresses the central nerves to reduce pain sensations. Do not confuse with hallucinogenic. Narcotics are used for more serious pain than analgesics or anodynes. The herbs below are very mild narcotics.

Nervine: A remedy that strengthens the nervous system. Generally used to refer to remedies that inhibit sympathetic nerves and stimulate parasympathetic nerves to have a calming or relaxing effect. Technically speaking, an agent that does the opposite (stimulates sympathetic nerves and inhibits parasympathetic nerves) could also be called a nervine, but the term is not generally used in this manner. These remedies are used to relax muscles, reduce anxiety and tension, ease stress and aid sleep and relaxation

Nutritive: An herb, food or supplement that supplies essential nutrition.

Opthalmicum: A remedy for diseases of the eye.

Oxytocic: The term oxytocic refers specifically to remedies that have an oxytocin mimicking effect. Oxytocin is the hormone responsible for uterine contractions during labor.

Phytoestrogen: A plant substance that mimics estrogens is called a phytoestrogen. Plants that contain phytoestrogens may or may not enhance estrogenic effects in the body. Some phyoestrogens are very weak, but by binding to estrogen receptor sites they can reduce the risk of estrogen dependent cancers or aid in estrogen-dominant PMS.

Purgative (Cathartic): Purgatives and cathartics are strong laxatives. Useful for occasional purging in high fevers, acute infections or occasional sluggish elimination. Not recommended for long term use (more than 30 days).

Refrigerant: Lowers body temperature and relieves thirst. For fever and "hot" conditions where a person feels hot, thirsty, dry or flushed, but fluids don't seem to hydrate or cool the body.

Relaxant: An agent that reduces tension and helps muscles to relax. Used for muscle tension and stress.

Restorative: An agent that supplies some deficiency in the normal constituents of the body, either directly or by chemical reaction.

Sedative: Sedates the nervous system. Has a calming effect on the body.

Soothing: A remedy that reduces tissue irritation. Used when tissues are inflamed and irritated.

Soporific (Hypnotic): A remedy that helps to induce sleep.

Stimulant (Circulatory): An agent that stimulates circulation. Used for cold hands and feet or other symptoms of poor circulation to the extremities. Also used to aid blood flow to various areas of the body to promote tissue healing.

Stimulant (Metabolic): An agent that stimulates metabolism, increasing heat and energy.

Stomachic: A digestive aid and tonic, which improves stomach function and appetite.

Styptic: A powerful astringent action that closes wounds and stops bleeding. Used to stop internal and external bleeding. Caution: with serious external bleeding one should use these remedies by pouring them into a wound and then applying the standard first aid practice of applying pressure directly to the injury. For serious internal bleeding (hemorrhage) these remedies should be taken internally, preferably in liquid form, while en route to the nearest hospital or medical facility for treatment.

Testosterone-Enhancing: Helps increase testosterone levels in men.

Tonic: Refers to remedies with a general anabolic effect, they build up and strengthen organs and tissues, often causing greater structural density or greater functional strength. Used for weakened conditions of the body or specific organs.

Uterine Tonic: Strengthens and tones the uterine muscle in preparation for childbirth.

Vascular Tonic: Tone up varicose veins. Used for varicose veins, hemorrhoids, pain and swelling in the legs, and other conditions where venous circulation is impaired.

Vasoconstrictor: Constricts blood vessels to reduce circulation. Opposite of vasodilator. Used to raise low blood pressure or help reduce bleeding. Some of these remedies may also aid vasodilative headaches. Contraindicated in high blood pressure.

Vasodilator: Opens and relaxes blood vessels to increase circulation. Opposite of vasoconstrictor. Used for high blood pressure. Contraindicated with low blood pressure and vasodilative headaches.

Vermifuge: Destroys intestinal worms. See also antiparasitics.

Vulnerary: Helps injured tissues to heal, usually without scarring

Suggested Additional Reading

Beiler, Henry G.; *Food is Your Best Medicine*

Chevallier, Andrew; *Encyclopedia of Herbal Medicine*

Crawford, Amanda McQuade; *The Herbal Menopause Book*

Flint, Margi; *The Practicing Herbalist*

Foster, Steven and Hobbs, Christopher; *Western Medicinal Plants and Herbs*

Hall, Dorothy: *Creating Your Herbal Profile*

Haas, Elson M.; *The Detox Diet*

Hoffmann, David; *Medical Herbalism*

Kaminski, Patricia and Katz, Richard; *Flower Essence Repertory*

Kuhn, Merrily A. and Winston, David; *Herbal Therapy and Supplements: A Scientific and Traditional Approach*

McGuffin, Michael; Hobbs, Christopher; Upton, Roy; Goldberg, Alicia; *Botanical Safety Handbook*

McIntyre, Anne; Flower Power: *Flower Remedies for Healing Body and Soul*

Mills, Simon and Bone, Kerry; *Principles and Practices of Phytotherapy*

Mills, Simon and Bone, Kerry; *The Essential Guide to Herbal Safety*

Moore, Micheal; *Medicinal Plants of the Desert and Canyon West*

Moore, Micheal; *Medicinal Plants of the Mountain West*

Moore, Micheal; Southwest School of Botanical Medicine Website (*swsbm.com*)

PDR for Herbal Medicines

Price, Weston A.; *Nutrition and Physical Degeneration*

Smith, Ed; *Therapeutic Herb Manual*

Tierra, Michael; *Plantetary Herbology*

Teirra, Michael; *The Way of Chinese Herbs*

Tillotson, Alan; *The One Earth Herbal Sourcebook*

Willard, Terry; *Edible and Medicinal Plants of the Rocky Mountains and Neighboring Territories*

Winston, David; *Herbal Therapeutics: Specific Indications for Herbs & Herbal Formulas*

Wood, Matthew; *The Book of Herbal Wisdom: Using Plants as Medicine*

Wood, Matthew; *The Earthwise Herbal: A Complete Guide to New World Medicinal Plants*

Wood, Matthew; *The Earthwise Herbal: A Complete Guide to Old World Medicinal Plants*

Wood, Matthew: *The Practice of Traditional Western Herbalism*

Want to Learn More?

Here are three ways to further your knowledge of herbs and natural healing

1. Visit Our Website

Modernherbalmedicine.com is the official website for the *School of Modern Herbal Medicine*, where you'll find additional articles and information about herbs, nutrition and natural healing by Steven Horne and Thomas Easley. Sign up for our mailing list to get updates and learn about classes and other educational opportunities.

2. Explore the Herbiverse

Herbiverse.com is an online resource where you can find herbalists, learn how to become an herbalist, or promote yourself if you have an herbal business or practice. At herbiverse.com you can search for herbalists who can help you with more difficult health issues and for herb courses and training programs.

You can also become a member of herbiverse to learn more about herbs for yourself and/or to help you grow and promote an existing herbal business. Membership to the herbiverse includes all of the following benefits:

Monthly *Herbal Hour* webinar

The *Herbal Hour* is a monthly webinar on a specific health topic. It serves two purposes. First, it allows students of herbalism to expand their knowledge of specific applications related to herbs and natural healing. Second, it offers a tool to help experienced herbalists promote their herbal business or practice, because we allow members to download the PowerPoint presentations and modify them to use in their own classes. The Herbal Hour is taught by Steven Horne and Thomas Easley.

Monthly *Holistic Perspective* webinar

Since 1986, Steven Horne, has been doing emotional healing work as part of his efforts to help others. In the Holistic Perspective webinars, he shares his insights into how to help people heal on an emotional, mental, spiritual and social level. This webinar series can enrich your personal growth and development, and teach you how to resolve past trauma and reduce stress in yourself and others.

Monthly *Business Coaching* webinar

This webinar is for people who are trying to develop a practice or business in herbs and natural healing. Many times people have the herbal knowledge and skills to run a successful herbal shop or practice, but they lack the business expertise required to achieve their dreams. This unique and valuable webinar series can help people who are just getting started in their herbal careers as well as provide established herbalists with ideas on how they can better grow and manage their existing business.

Access to the Member Archives

Membership includes access to a library of over 90 past webinars. All past webinars are available in the member area in both windows media video (wmv) and audio (mp3) formats. You'll also be able to download handouts of the PowerPoint presentations in pdf form (both 3 and 6 slide per page formats).

Discounts on Books and Courses

Members get discounts on all our other courses, books and educational materials.

Optional: Searchable Herbalist Profile

If you have an herbal business or practice you can also get an online listing to promote yourself.

One Month Free Trial

You can try out the Herbiverse for one month free! During your one-month free trial, you'll have access to all of the member benefits, including access to the webinar archives, participation in live webinars, online listing and discounts on our other materials.

To get started, visit us online at herbiverse.com or call us at 800-416-2887. Remember that you can cancel at any time, so try us out today and discover the benefits of being a member at *herbiverse.com*.

3. Study with Us

The *School of Modern Herbal Medicine* offers correspondence courses, webinars and live training programs. Here is a sample of the courses we offer.

Fundamentals of Natural Healing

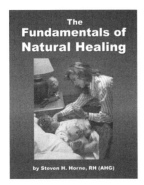

A Practical Guide to Natural Health Care

Wouldn't it be great to be able to quickly and effectively treat common injuries and illnesses in the home? In this course you will learn how to overcome many health problems in less time than it takes to get an appointment to see the doctor. You'll also learn:

- How to relieve pain and reverse damage from common injuries such as bumps, bruises, sprains, cuts, insect bites and stings, and other minor injuries—typically in only 5-20 minutes.

- How the basic categories of herbs help the body heal.

- How to help the body recover quickly from acute illnesses such as colds, flu, sore throats, earaches, headaches, coughs, congestion, rashes, and such—usually in less than 24 hours and often in as little as an hour or two.

- How to build better overall health, reduce the incidence of disease in your home, and reverse many chronic ailments by using the basic ABC principles of health care (Activate, Build and Cleanse).

All of this can be accomplished without drugs or medications— just safe, natural methods. This course is great for anyone who would like to learn how to improve the quality of their own health and the health of family and friends by natural means.

The ABC+D Approach to Natural Health Consulting

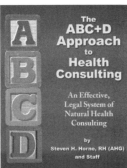

The key to helping people with herbs, nutrition and other natural healing modalities is results. People want to see improvement in their health conditions. Learning how to select the products that will help each person feel better has traditionally been a lengthy process of trial and error. We've made the process much easier by creating the *ABC+D Approach to Natural Health Consulting*.

Instead of trying to memorize various natural treatments for disease conditions, a very difficult and complicated process, the ABC+D system helps you understand the root causes of disease and how to identify and correct them. This by-passes the need to diagnose and treat specific diseases (something that is only legal for licensed doctors to do anyway). Based on The Disease Tree™, the ABC+D system helps you understand that there are four root causes of disease, six imbalances in biological terrain, and 11 body systems. By helping people modify their lifestyle to remove the root causes and by providing Direct Aids to balance biological terrain and support the function of the various body systems, one is able to get dependable results without the need to diagnose diseases. This enables the consultant to get consistent results without risking themselves legally.

Certified Herbal Consultant Program

The Fundamentals of Natural Healing and *ABC+D Approach* are just two of the eight courses in our Certified Herbal Consultant program. This series of correspondence courses is designed to help people knowledgeably sell commercial herbs, herbal formulas and supplements.

The CHC program uses the Body Systems Approach, the Disease Tree™ and other models to make it easy to learn how to use herbs, supplements and other natural healing modalities in a systematic manner. This systematic approach helps you obtain consistent and dependable results.

To learn more visit modernherbalmedicine.com/store/category/certified-herbal-consultant/ or call 800-416-2887.

Advanced Herbal Training Program

Steven Horne and Thomas Easley put the *Advanced Herbal Training Program* together to help people move beyond the limitations of commercial herbalism and help people understand herbal remedies in depth. The program consists of nine modules that take an in-depth look at herbs for various systems of the body and a tenth module that discusses field botany and plant identification. The program comes with a manual and recordings of the internet classes taught by Steven and Thomas.

To learn more visit schoolofmodernherbalmedicine.com/store/category/advanced-herbal-training/ or call 800-416-2887.

Satisfaction Guaranteed

All of our courses, books and educational materials come with a 30-day money-back guarantee. If you're dissatisfied with a product after receiving it, simply return it within 30 days and we'll refund your money.

About the Authors

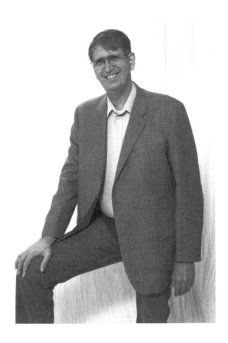 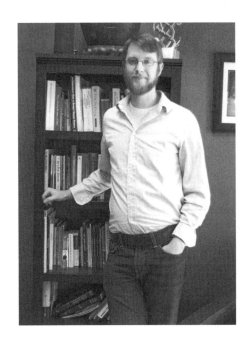

Steven Horne is a professional member and past president of the American Herbalists Guild. He became interested in herbs 45 years ago while learning about edible and medicinal plants as a boy scout. In his early 20s, after many years of failing to find answers to his chronic sinus and respiratory problems in modern medicine, he was able to recover his health through nutrition, herbs and chiropractic care.

Steven obtained a bachelor's degree in communications which he combined with his love of herbs to teach people how to improve their health naturally. He founded Tree of Light and later the School of Modern Herbal Medicine to further share his knowledge with others. He has produced numerous courses, books and videos on natural healing, including the *Certified Herbal Consultant* courses. Steven has also served a consultant and product formulator for several herb companies.

Thomas Easley is a Clinical Herbalist and professional member of the American Herbalists Guild. He has been in full time clinical practice for 12 years. He is the co-developer of the School of Modern Herbal Medicine's *Advanced Herbal Training Program*. Thomas believes in using foods as primary medicine and uses intensive diets as well as stress reduction techniques, nutritional supplements and exercise to help people achieve their health goals.

Thomas is the founder and primary instructor for the Eclectic School of Herbal Medicine. His philosophy integrates modern science and traditional herbalism into a unified and systematic approach to health and healing. He is trained in and uses functional medicine theory, as well as modern naturopathic therapies along with traditional western herbalism. His approach is influenced strongly by both the Eclectic and Physiomedical Physicians of the 19th century.